Modeling Inhibitors of Matrix Metalloproteinases

Matrix metalloproteinases (MMPs) have been established as promising biomolecular targets for novel drug design and discovery against numerous major disease conditions, including various cancers, cardiovascular diseases, neurodegenerative diseases, inflammatory diseases, and more. This book covers various modern molecular modeling methodologies, particularly those related to MMP inhibitors. The text includes descriptions of ligand- and structure-based drug design modeling strategies for designing potential and target-specific or selective MMPIs. This book will benefit those looking for an in-depth text on the design and discovery processes of novel and selective MMPIs.

Features

- Describes modeling strategies applied to MMPs
- Elaborates on the designing strategies of MMPs specifically
- Includes in-depth analyses of related case studies
- Acts as a guide for medicinal chemists, not only from pharmaceutical industries but also from academia
- Covers various modern molecular modeling methodologies, particularly related to MMPIs

QSAR in Environmental and Health Sciences

James Devillers

CTIS, Rillieux La Pape, France

About the Series:

The aim of the book series is to publish cutting-edge research and the latest developments in QSAR modeling applied to environmental and health issues. Its aim is also to publish routinely used QSAR methodologies to provide newcomers to the field with a basic grounding in the correct use of these computer tools. The series is of primary interest to those whose research or professional activity is directly concerned with the development and application of SAR and QSAR models in toxicology and ecotoxicology. It is also intended to provide graduate and postgraduate students with clear and accessible books covering the different aspects of QSARs.

Modeling Inhibitors of Matrix Metalloproteinases

Edited By

Tarun Jha

Natural Science Laboratory, Division of Medicinal and Pharmaceutical Chemistry, Department of Pharmaceutical Technology, Jadavpur University, Kolkata

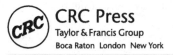

CRC Press
Taylor & Francis Group
Boca Raton London New York

CRC Press is an imprint of the
Taylor & Francis Group, an **informa** business

First edition published 2024
by CRC Press
2385 Executive Center Drive, Suite 320, Boca Raton, FL 33431

and by CRC Press
4 Park Square, Milton Park, Abingdon, Oxon, OX14 4RN

Library of Congress Cataloging-in-Publication Data
Names: Jha, Tarun, editor.
Title: Modeling inhibitors of matrix metalloproteinases / edited by Tarun
Jha, Natural Science Laboratory, Division of Medicinal and
Pharmaceutical Chemistry, Department of Pharmaceutical Technology,
Jadavpur University, Kolkata.
Description: First edition. | Boca Raton : CRC Press, 2024. | Series: QSAR
in environmental and health sciences | Includes bibliographical
references and index. | Summary: "Matrix metalloproteinases (MMPs) have
been established as promising biomolecular targets for novel drug design and discovery
against numerous major disease conditions including
various cancers, cardiovascular, neurodegenerative, inflammatory
diseases, and more. This book covers various modern molecular modeling
methodologies particularly related to MMP inhibitors. Included in the
text are descriptions of ligand-based drug designing and structure-based
drug designing modeling strategies for designing potential and target
specific or selective MMPIs. This book will benefit those who are looking for an in-depth text on
the design and discovery processes of novel and selective MMPIs"-- Provided by publisher.
Identifiers: LCCN 2023031094 (print) | LCCN 2023031095 (ebook) | ISBN
9781032289267 (hardback) | ISBN 9781032300610 (paperback) | ISBN
9781032300610 (ebook)
Subjects: LCSH: Metalloproteinases--Inhibitors. | Extracellular matrix
proteins. | Metalloproteinases--Inhibitors--Structure-activity
relationships. | Metalloproteinases--Inhibitors--Design. |
Molecules--Models.
Classification: LCC RM666.M512 M63 2024 (print) | LCC RM666.M512 (ebook)
| DDC 615.7--dc23/eng/20231020
LC record available at https://lccn.loc.gov/2023031094
LC ebook record available at https://lccn.loc.gov/2023031095

ISBN: 978-1-032-28926-7 (hbk)
ISBN: 978-1-032-30061-0 (pbk)
ISBN: 978-1-003-30328-2 (ebk)

DOI: 10.1201/9781003303282

Typeset in Times

by Deanta Global Publishing Services, Chennai, India

Dedicated to the fond memory of Prof. Arun Uday De,
one of the pioneers of Drug Design in India and
who introduced Drug Design in M. Pharm. class way back in 1972

Contents

PART A   Fundamentals of Molecular Modeling

PART B   Matrix Metalloproteinases and Their Inhibitors

PART C   *Modeling of MMP Inhibitors*

PART D   Conclusion and Future Perspective

Acknowledgment

I thankfully acknowledge Dr. Nilanjan Adhikari, who conducted his MPharm dissertation, PhD thesis, and post-doctoral work under my supervision. He is now an Assistant Professor in the Department of Pharmaceutical Technology at Jadavpur University. Besides his heavy class load, he contributed greatly to this book. I also thankfully acknowledge the services of Dr. Shovanlal Gayen and Dr. Balaram Ghosh. They did their MPharm dissertation under my guidance. Dr. Shovanlal Gayen is an Assistant Professor in the Department of Pharmaceutical Technology of Jadavpur University, and Dr. Balaram Ghosh is an Associate Professor in the Department of Pharmacy, BITS-Pilani, Hyderabad campus. Dr. Gayen and Dr. Ghosh contributed to chapters of this book. I also gratefully acknowledge the services of Mr. Sandip Kr. Baidya and Mr. Suvankar Banerjee, Research Scholars, who are doing their PhD work under my supervision. With effective research work, they also contributed greatly to this book. I also gratefully acknowledge the contribution of Dr. Sk. Abdul Amin, who did his PhD under my guidance and is now an Assistant Professor at JIS University, Kolkata. I thankfully acknowledge the contribution of Mr. Sanjib Das, who conducted his MPharm dissertation and is doing his PhD under my supervision. Finally, I acknowledge the service of Ms. Shamima Khatun, a Research Scholar. Ms. Khatun is doing her PhD under Dr. Shovanlal Gayen, one of my students, and contributed to a chapter.

Last, but not least, I thankfully acknowledge Prof. James Devillers, editor of the journal "SAR and QSAR in Environmental Research" and of the book series "QSAR in Environmental and Health Sciences," who encouraged me to author the book with my students. He also sent timely reminders to complete the work. I also thankfully acknowledge Ms. Hilary Lafoe and Ms. Sukirti Singh, who helped me by sending reminders to finish the work.

Tarun Jha

Series Introduction

The correlation between the toxicity of molecules and their physicochemical properties can be traced to the 19th century. Indeed, in a French thesis entitled *Action de l'alcool amylique sur l'organisme* (Action of amyl alcohol on the body), which was presented in 1863 by A. Cros before the Faculty of Medicine at the University of Strasbourg, an empirical relationship was made between the toxicity of alcohols, their number of carbon atoms, and their solubility. In 1875, Dujardin-Beaumetz and Audigé were the first to stress the mathematical character of the relationship between the toxicity of alcohols and their chain length and molecular weight. In 1899, Hans Horst Meyer and Fritz Baum, at the University of Marburg, showed that narcosis or hypnotic activity was, in fact, linked to the affinity of substances to water and lipid sites within the organism. At the same time, at the University of Zurich, Ernest Overton came to the same conclusion, providing the foundation of the lipoid theory of narcosis. The next important step was made in the 1930s by Lazarev in St. Petersburg, who first demonstrated that different physiological and toxicological effects of molecules were correlated with their oil-water partition coefficient through formal mathematical equations in the form: $\log C = a \log_{Poil/water} + b$. Thus, the Quantitative Structure-Activity Relationship (QSAR) discipline was born. Its foundations were definitively fixed in the early 1960s by the seminal works contributed by C. Hansch and T. Fujita. Since that period, the discipline has gained tremendous interest and now the 2D and 3D QSAR models represent key tools in the development of drugs as well as in the hazard assessment of chemicals.

In 1993, the journal *SAR and QSAR in Environmental Research* was launched by Gordon and Breach to focus on all the important works published in the field and to provide an international forum for the rapid publication of SAR (Structure-Activity Relationship) and QSAR models in (eco)toxicology, agrochemistry, and pharmacology. Today, the journal, which is now owned by Taylor and Francis and publishes three times more issues per year, continues to promote research in the QSAR field by favoring the publication of new molecular descriptors, statistical techniques, and original SAR and QSAR models. This field continues to grow rapidly and many subject areas that require larger developments are unsuitable for publication in a journal due to space limitations.

This prompted us to develop a series of books entitled *QSAR in Environmental and Health Sciences* to act in synergy with the journal. I am extremely grateful to Colin Bulpitt and Fiona Macdonald for their enthusiasm and invaluable help in making the project become a reality.

This book is the seventh in the series and the first dedicated to matrix metalloproteinases (MMPs). MMPs are a family of zinc-dependent endopeptidases with proteolytic properties, and they play key roles in numerous physiological and pathological processes. This timely book focusing on MMP inhibitors and their modeling is therefore of utmost importance.

I gratefully acknowledge Hilary Lafoe for her willingness to assist me in the development of this series.

James Devillers

Preface

The first matrix metalloproteinase was isolated more than 60 years ago. Numerous inhibitors of matrix metalloproteinases have been discovered to date. Except for repurposed doxycycline, no inhibitors of matrix metalloproteinases have come out as drugs. This encourages us to view the whole scenario of inhibitors of matrix metalloproteinases and their designs. Thus, we have been encouraged to write this book.

This book, "Modeling Inhibitors of Matrix Metalloproteinases," has four parts and consists of 16 chapters. The first part (Part A) is named "Fundamentals of Molecular Modeling" and has three chapters. The first chapter (Chapter 1) is "2D-QSAR Studies: Regression and Classification-Based QSAR Studies." Chapter 2 is "3D-QSAR Studies: CoMFA, CoMSIA, and Topomer CoMFA Methods." Chapter 3 consists of "Other Modeling Approaches: Pharmacophore Mapping, Molecular Docking, and Molecular Dynamic Simulation Studies." Going through these three chapters, I think any reader can get an idea of various molecular modeling studies.

Part B is "Matrix Metalloproteinases and Their Inhibitors" and has six chapters. Chapter 4 is named "Collagenases and Their Inhibitors"; Chapter 5 consists of "Gelatinases and Their Inhibitors"; Chapter 6 deals with "Stromelysins and Their Inhibitors"; Chapter 7 introduces "Matrilysins and Their Inhibitors"; Chapter 8 is "Membrane-Type MMPs and Their Inhibitors"; and Chapter 9 corresponds to "Other MMPs and Their Inhibitors." In my opinion, the reader can find all matrix metalloproteinases and most of their inhibitors to date.

Part C of this book consists of "Modeling of MMP Inhibitors," with six chapters. Chapter 10 is called "Modeling Inhibitors of Collagenases"; Chapter 11 deals with gelatinases, Chapter 12 with stromelysins, and Chapter 13 with "Modeling Inhibitors of Matrilysins." Chapters 14 and 15 are modeling inhibitors of membrane-type MMPs and other MMPs, respectively. In these six chapters, a reader can find modeling of inhibitors of all MMPs.

Part D (Chapter 16) deals with the conclusion and future perspectives. In this chapter, the reader may get an idea of the message of the book and the future direction of research.

While writing the preface, I have seen more than 50 articles dealing with various matrix metalloproteinases in the literature. In this period, three publications [1–3] came out on modeling inhibitors of matrix metalloproteinases that show the significance of the subject.

1. Tabti K, Ahmad I, Zafar I, et al. Profiling the structural determinants of pyrrolidine derivative as gelatinases (MMP-2 and MMP-9) inhibitors using in silico approaches. *Comput Biol Chem.* 2023;104:107855.
2. Banerjee S, Baidya SK, Ghosh B, et al. Exploration of structural alerts and fingerprints for novel anticancer therapeutics: A robust classification-QSAR dependent structural analysis of drug-like MMP-9 inhibitors. *SAR QSAR Environ Res.* 2023;34(4):299-319.

3. Malekipour MH, Shirani F, Moradi S, et al. Cinnamic acid derivatives as potential matrix metalloproteinase-9 inhibitors: Molecular docking and dynamics simulations. *Genomics Inform.* 2023;21(1):e9.

Finally, if any reader finds this book useful, that will be satisfactory for us. However, any mistake, if pointed out, can be rectified in the future.

Tarun Jha
Jadavpur University
Kolkata, India
15th June 2023

Editor Biography

Tarun Jha is the senior Professor of the Department of Pharmaceutical Technology, Jadavpur University, Kolkata, India. He has already supervised 20 PhD students and is guiding four more. He also guided six post-doctoral fellows and completed nine research projects. He has published 200 research articles and ten book chapters and has jointly edited a book. Prof. Jha is one of the Editorial Board Members of the journal "SAR and QSAR in Environmental Research," published by Taylor & Francis. He is also serving as a reviewer of 26 internationally reputed journals. His research area includes the design, synthesis, and biological evaluation of anticancer small molecules, especially inhibitors of zinc-dependent metalloenzymes.

List of Contributors

Nilanjan Adhikari
Natural Science Laboratory
Department of Pharmaceutical
    Technology
Jadavpur University, Kolkata,
    West Bengal, India

Sk Abdul Amin
Natural Science Laboratory
Department of Pharmaceutical
    Technology
Jadavpur University
Kolkata, West Bengal, India

Sandip Kumar Baidya
Natural Science Laboratory
Department of Pharmaceutical
    Technology,
Jadavpur University
Kolkata, West Bengal, India

Suvankar Banerjee
Natural Science Laboratory
Department of Pharmaceutical
    Technology,
Jadavpur University
Kolkata, West Bengal, India

Sanjib Das
Natural Science Laboratory
Department of Pharmaceutical
    Technology
Jadavpur University
Kolkata, West Bengal, India

Dr. Shovanlal Gayen
Department of Pharmaceutical
    Technology
Jadavpur University
Kolkata, West Bengal, India

Balaram Ghosh
Department of Pharmacy
BITS-Pilani Hyderabad Campus
Hyderabad, India

Tarun Jha
Department of Pharmaceutical
    Technology
Jadavpur University
Kolkata, West Bengal, India

Samima Khatun
Department of Pharmaceutical
    Technology
Jadavpur University
Kolkata, West Bengal, India

Part A

Fundamentals of
Molecular Modeling

1 2D-QSAR Studies

Regression and Classification-Based QSAR Studies

Sanjib Das, Sk. Abdul Amin, Shovanlal Gayen, and Tarun Jha

CONTENTS

ABSTRACT

In this chapter, the implication of 2D-QSAR in drug design and discovery is explained in detail. Various types of QSAR methodologies, such as linear regression-dependent QSARs (namely 2D-QSAR, linear discriminant analysis), as well as non-linear QSARs (namely artificial neural network, support vector machine, Bayesian classification, and recursive partitioning), are described. The implication of descriptors and statistical validation metrics is explained in detail. In addition, various types of

DOI: 10.1201/9781003303282-2

software useful in performing such QSAR analysis are also mentioned. This chapter clearly illustrates the 2D-QSAR methodologies aiding in drug discovery processes.

Keywords: Regression-based 2D-QSAR; Classification-based 2D-QSAR; Bayesian classification modeling; Linear discriminant analysis (LDA); Support vector machine (SVM); Artificial neural network (ANN)

1.1 INTRODUCTION

Drug discovery is a time-consuming, overpriced, risky, and multistep endeavor that begins with target identification and subsequent validation, followed by hit-to-lead production, lead optimization, preclinical studies, and several phases of clinical trials. A journey of 10–15 years and an expenditure of around US$2.5 billion is required to bring a new drug candidate from a basic research laboratory to the shelf of a chemist's shop [1–3]. To reduce the time and costs related to drug discovery, high-throughput screening and combinatorial methodologies were developed in the 1990s to speed up the synthesis and screening of large libraries. Unfortunately, no remarkable success was achieved, and little progress was made regarding the development of new chemical entities [4]. Later, a combination of biological science, chemical synthesis, and advanced computational techniques was introduced to facilitate the discovery process [4]. In 1981, the cover article of *Fortune* magazine entitled "The next industrial revolution: designing drugs by computer at Merck" was published. Since 1981, computer-aided drug discovery (CADD) has begun to fulfill its promise [5]. There has been persistent hopeful anticipation that CADD could step-up drug discovery. Although there were attempts by many research groups and companies up to 2010, little development was made toward speeding up drug discovery by computational modeling [6]. Advanced computational techniques have emerged over the last decade, and several remarkable initiatives have progressed. Computational methods can now be utilized to progress all stages of preclinical drug discovery, such as target selection and validation, lead discovery and optimization, as well as preclinical tests (Figure 1.1) [7].

Breakthrough initiative regarding the application of CADD into drug discovery programs emerged in 2009 with the foundation of Nimbus Discovery [8]. With a unique drug discovery partnership with Schrödinger Inc., USA, an ultra-lean "virtually integrated, globally distributed" R and D operating model, and a novel asset-centric corporate structure, Nimbus Discovery succeeded in advancing an acetyl-CoA carboxylase (ACC) inhibitor (NDI-010976) into clinical studies within 16 months or treating non-alcoholic steatohepatitis (NASH) [9]. Nimbus initiated a phase I clinical trial of NDI-010976 (GS-0976), which was sponsored by Gilead Sciences [9]. Later, Gilead acquired the asset and further advanced GS-0976 or Firsocostat into a phase II clinical trial [10]. Nimbus has continued its discovery programs with the help of advanced computational modeling and in collaboration with Innovaderm Research Inc., has succeeded in developing NDI-034858, a highly selective tyrosine kinase 2 (TYK2) inhibitor intended for psoriasis pathogenesis that is currently in phase IIb

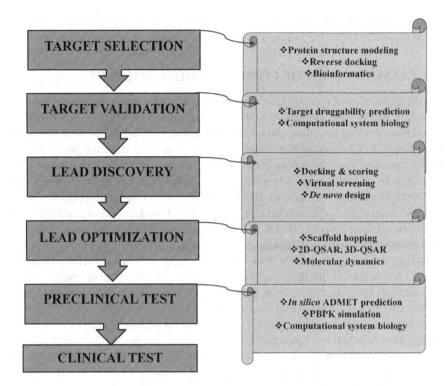

FIGURE 1.1 Application of computer-aided drug design (CADD) in different stages of drug discovery.

clinical trial [11]. Following in the strides of Nimbus, Morphic Therapeutics also advanced MORF-057, an α4β7 integrin inhibitor, into clinical trials for the management of inflammatory bowel disease [12]. MORF-057 is currently in a phase IIa clinical trial [13]. Using computational modeling, Relay Therapeutics developed RLY-1971, an orally active, promising, and selective inhibitor of the protein tyrosine phosphatase (SHP2) for patients bearing advanced or metastatic solid tumors [14]. RLY-1971 is now in a phase I clinical trial [15]. Other clinical candidates of Relay Therapeutics originating from computational modeling are RLY-4008 and RLY-2608 [14]. RLY-4008 is an orally active small molecule, selective fibroblast growth factor receptor 2 (FGFR2) inhibitor intended for metastatic solid tumors and presently has been advanced into a phase I clinical trial [14, 16]. RLY-2608 is the first allosteric pan-mutant (H1047X, E542X, and E545X) and isoform-selective phosphoinositide 3-kinase α (PI3Kα) inhibitor [14]. Presently, RLY-2608 has advanced into a phase I clinical trial for patients suffering from unresectable or metastatic solid tumors, and RLY-2608 in combination with fulvestrant produced fruitful outcomes for patients bearing HR-positive/HER2-negative locally advanced or metastatic breast cancer [17]. The initial success of the above-mentioned startup biotech companies for the rapid development of small molecules under clinical studies has influenced large pharma giants, namely Bayer and AstraZeneca, to provide sophisticated computational modeling techniques in their in-house drug discovery programs [18–20].

1.2 CLASSIFICATION OF COMPUTER-AIDED DRUG DESIGN

For the application of computers in drug development, the term computer-aided drug design (CADD) was adopted. CADD provides several algorithms and computational tools that can save time and costs for drug discovery [4]. In the drug discovery workflow, CADD encompasses many applications ranging from the predictions of interactions and binding affinity between drugs and receptors to the design of compounds with expected physiochemical properties and activity profiles, along with the management and screening of digital repositories of compounds [21, 22]. CADD may be broadly grouped into two classes: structure-based drug design (SBDD) and ligand-based drug design (LBDD). The prerequisite for SBDD is structural information about drug targets. SBDD engages with several computational techniques like homology modeling, molecular docking, and molecular dynamic (MD) simulation. These computational SBDD techniques are used to identify a target molecule that may be an enzyme associated with the disease of interest and to design new biologically active molecules [4]. LBDD is used when 3D structural information of a target molecule or protein is unavailable [3]. LBDD aims at a general approach for determining the contribution of physicochemical and structural features of compounds or ligands with their biological responses [4]. In the case of LBDD, available data on ligands and their biological activities are utilized for the generation of new effective drug candidates [4]. LBDD is generally based on supposition that compounds with similar structural features share similar biological properties and interact with or inhibit similar target molecules [4]. Some of the important techniques used in LBDD are quantitative structure-activity relationships (QSARs), pharmacophore modeling, and artificial intelligence (AI) [3].

1.3 APPLICATION OF QSAR IN THE EARLY STAGES OF DRUG DISCOVERY

The contemporary pipeline to discover hit molecules is a data-driven technique which depends on the biological activity data generated from high throughput screening (HTS) campaigns [23]. However, the cost of procuring new hit molecules in HTS campaigns is quite high. A prodigious amount of chemical and biological information is being stored in different databases. In Chemical Abstract Services, more than 74 million molecules are recorded. There are approximately 1060 molecules that are recognized as new drug-like compounds [24]. The QSAR study is a ligand-based chemometric drug discovery method that quantitatively provides a mathematical correlation between structural alterations of chemical compounds and respective changes in biological activities [25]. The QSAR methods play major roles in the drug discovery pipeline by improving the potency, efficacy, and selectivity of the lead molecules intended for clinical studies [25]. The QSAR analysis is a cost-effective and powerful *in-silico* drug discovery process due to its high and fast throughput as well as good hit rate obtained from ligand-based virtual screening (LBVS) studies of large database compounds [26]. QSAR modeling plays a pivotal role in reducing the number of molecules to be synthesized and biologically evaluated [26]. Nevertheless, QSAR models are useful for hit discovery, hit-to-lead, and lead optimization [26]. In recent decades, the strong dominance of the QSAR approaches has been observed to guide lead optimization. QSAR modeling is not only practiced in research institutes and/or industries, but it is also globally accepted by government agencies such as the US Food and Drug Administration (FDA), Health Canada, and European Union (EU) authorities [27]. The regulatory authority of Canada utilizes QSAR models in order to assess and prioritize the Canadian inventory of existing substances (i.e., domestic substances list, DSL) under the New Substances Provisions of the Canadian Environmental Protection Act (1999). Also, in the EU, the Danish Environmental Protection Agency (EPA) uses QSAR models to predict the endpoint of ecological and health hazard substances whose experimental results are unavailable [27].

QSARs deal with the construction and development of predictive models correlating to the bioactivity of chemicals with attributes or descriptors that are representative of molecular structures [28]. Similar analogs with slight variations in their molecular structures may show either various magnitudes of a particular biological activity or may produce quite different types of biological potential. The objective of the QSAR model is to understand the relationship between molecular structures and the respective alterations in biological activities quantitatively [29, 30]. QSAR analysis utilizes statistical methods as preliminary tools to study the correlation of biological activity with the structural and physicochemical properties of compounds [28]. In order to generate QSAR equations, several regressions and classification-based approaches are available. To establish the reliability and predictability of developed QSAR models, various diagnostic statistics are utilized. From constructed QSAR equations, one may be able to predict the biological activities of novel molecules [30].

1.4 VARIOUS TYPES OF QSAR STUDIES

QSAR methodologies may be categorized in three ways: based on the dimension of descriptors, chemometric methods, and the number of targets (Figure 1.2).

In QSAR analysis, molecular descriptors encode the chemical information that represents the behavior of the compound. By using a suitable algorithm, descriptors are calculated in numerical form, and they are used as the independent variables for QSAR model development [31]. On the other hand, the dimension of an object may be ascribed as the minimum number of coordinates required for explaining a point in it. Dimension is an intrinsic property that does not depend on the space of the object [32]. In QSAR analysis, a higher level of structural information is obtained with the addition of dimension in descriptors. The dimension in QSAR methodology acts as a constraint that regulates the nature of the analysis. The dimensional increment of descriptors in developing the QSAR model is related to the complexity of the modeling method. A descriptor's dimension belongs to the compound's dimension, which particularly represents that molecular feature. Therefore, the dimension of the QSAR analysis belongs to the dimension of the computed descriptors, which is utilized to

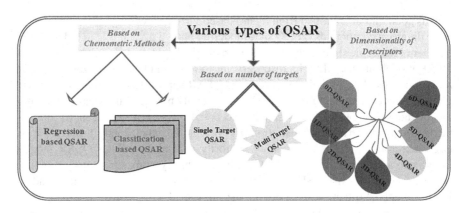

FIGURE 1.2   Various types of QSAR studies.

construct the QSAR model [31]. Based on the dimensionality of descriptors, QSAR methodologies may be classified as zero-dimensional (0D)-QSAR, one-dimensional (1D)-QSAR, two-dimensional (2D)-QSAR, three-dimensional (3D)-QSAR, four-dimensional (4D)-QSAR, five-dimensional (5D)-QSAR, and six-dimensional (6D)-QSAR. The 0D-QSAR model is constructed based on descriptors obtained from information on molecules, namely molecular weight, atom numbers, and atom types, as well as the sum of atomic properties. The 1D-QSAR model matches up the activity or property with global molecular properties, namely pKa, solubility, hydrophobic parameter, and functional groups [33]. Similarly, the 2D-QSAR model is found to correlate the activity with structural decorations. The descriptors derived from the topological portrayal of a compound are the core of predictor variables used for 2D-QSAR model development. For the development of successful QSAR models, various topological indices that contemplate the internal atomic orchestration of molecules are used as 2D descriptors [31]. Topological parameters encode information associated with molecular shape and size, branching, and the existence of multiple bonds, as well as the number of heteroatoms present. These 2D descriptors have a notable function in the modeling of diverse biological endpoints and the physicochemical characters of molecules. For example, a molecular graph represents the topology of a chemical compound, and mathematically it is symbolized as G = (V, E), where V is a set of vertices representing the atoms of the compound and E is a set of elements corresponding to the binary association between pairs of vertices. These molecular graphs depict a non-numeric formation of the chemical structure. The numerical transformation of chemical graphs is crucial. Specific algorithms are used for the determination of topological indices [34]. Among the various numbers of topological descriptors, the most commonly used topological indices are the connectivity indices, the Wiener index, Kier shape, Zagreb indices, and the Balaban J index, where the Wiener index is the most frequently used descriptors and connectivity indices are the most successful descriptors in QSAR studies [34]. The computation of topological indices is very fast and structured because only hydrogen-suppressed two-dimensional information related to the structure of compounds is required [34].

Apart from topological descriptors, various other physicochemical properties of molecules are also considered to be indispensable segments of 2D-QSAR analysis. Again, in 2D-QSAR modeling, three principal classes of physicochemical descriptors are commonly used: hydrophobic, electronic, and steric features. These physicochemical descriptors can be obtained from some experiments or even computable from the structure of the compound without considering the operation of energy minimization or conformational analysis. Various physicochemical features of the compound, like acid dissociation constant (*pKa*), partition coefficient (logP), molar refractivity (MR), spectroscopic signals, rate constants, and so on, may be designated as the whole molecular descriptors or these may demonstrate particular molecular parts. The 2D-QSAR analysis also incorporates other structural features that are directly computable either from molecular structure or molecular formula. These are molecular weight (*MW*), number of hydrogen bond acceptors (*nHBA*), number of hydrogen bond donors (*nHBD*), and counts of several other atoms, fragments, and bonds [31]. On the other hand, 3D-QSAR methodology represents the molecular organization in 3D space [35–37] and correlates the activity or property with non-covalent interaction fields (steric and electrostatic) related to the molecules [38]. Similarly, 4D-QSAR includes an additional combination of ligand configurations in 3D-QSAR by designating each compound in different conformations, stereoisomers, orientations, tautomers, or protonation states. On the other hand, 5D-QSAR perfectly designates various induced-fit models in 4D-QSAR. Again, 6D-QSAR encompasses various solvation models in 5D-QSAR [39].

QSAR analyses can be categorized as linear and non-linear depending on the type of chemometric approaches. In the case of linear methods, these incorporate linear regression (LR), multiple linear regression (MLR), stepwise multiple linear regression (S-MLR) [40], partial least square (PLS), principal component analysis (PCA), and genetic function approximation (GFA). Again, newer evolutions in chemometrics have produced various newer techniques of constructing predictive models encompassing non-linear and algorithmic methodologies such as support vector machine (SVM) [41, 42], artificial neural networks (ANN) [42, 43], k-nearest neighbors (kNN) [44], and Bayesian neural nets [45]. Based on the number of dependent variables, like the number of biological targets, QSAR may also be categorized as single-target or multi-target QSAR (Figure 1.2). Recent reports point out that multi-target drug compounds are highly effective in combating diseases such as Alzheimer's disease, cancer, diabetes, malaria, and tuberculosis. Therefore, these studies point out that a multi-target drug development strategy is an up-to-date research area in the drug discovery field [46–48].

1.5 TWO-DIMENSIONAL-QSAR MODEL DEVELOPMENT

As per the Organization for Economic Co-operation and Development (OECD) guidelines, a QSAR model must be constructed having a specified endpoint, an unambiguous algorithm to undertake model transparency, a specified applicability domain, genuine procedures of validation together with internal execution (decided by goodness-of-fit and robustness) and predictability (determined by external validation), and a probable mechanistic explanation [49]. General steps for 2D-QSAR model development include dataset selection and the pre-processing of data, dataset division (the training set and the test set), calculation of molecular descriptors, feature selection, 2D-QSAR modeling, appropriate validation measures of the 2D-QSAR model, and applicability domain analysis [50]. A short description of the general methods associated with the 2D-QSAR model development will be discussed in the subsequent subsections.

1.5.1 DATASET SELECTION AND PRE-PROCESSING OF DATA

The first step of QSAR analysis is to prepare a dataset free from error, noise, and redundancy [50, 51]. Biological or other response data should be collected from an original source. If the standard error of any experiment is more than the specific response value, it should be eliminated [51]. The dataset of a group of compounds should obey a normal distribution pattern compared with the biological endpoint [51]. If data are collected from the laboratory of different research groups, extra care should be taken. It is necessary to check whether the experimental protocols of different research groups are the same or different. All the dataset compounds and their response values considered for QSAR model generation must originate from the same experimental protocol [51]. The total number of compounds considered for QSAR model development should not be too small because there may be a chance of overfitting [52]. In the case of a continuous response parameter, a minimum number of compounds should not be less than 40, with 20 compounds in the training set and ten compounds in each of the test and external evaluation sets [52]. However, in the case of a category or classification response variable, a minimum number of molecules should not be less than 20, with ten molecules in the training set and five compounds in each of the test and external evaluation sets [52]. It was also suggested that a dataset size with 150–300 molecules in total is ideal for the construction of the QSAR model, and in the case of classification-dependent QSAR, an approximately equal number of molecules in the category or class may provide a better result [52]. For better interpolation, the range of the biological response/activity should be about a three-fold order of magnitude on the logarithmic scale [53–55]. When the dataset is taken from any databases available online, all these compounds and their biological endpoint values should be checked manually to reduce the chance of errors [51]. If the number of descriptors is very high, a descriptor thinning procedure should be utilized [51]. Descriptors or parameters having constant values for all observations and descriptors or parameters having very low variance must be discarded [51]. In the case of descriptors exhibiting excessive mutual inter-correlation, only one should be considered [51]. If some descriptors show a very low correlation with the biological endpoint values, these should also be omitted to reduce the size of the descriptor matrix [51].

1.5.2 DATASET DIVISION (TRAINING SET AND TEST SET)

The dataset is divided into two subsets: one is called the training set and the other is the test set [50]. The training set is taken into consideration for QSAR model development, and the test set is subsequently utilized to judge the predictability and accuracy of the model [50]. An appropriate dataset-splitting technique is necessary to improve the model's quality and predictability. Various methods used for QSAR dataset division are random selection, k-means clustering, Kennard–Stone selection, statistical molecular design, Kohonen's self-organizing map (SOM) selection, sphere exclusion, and extrapolation-oriented test set selection [50, 56]. A detailed discussion of the dataset division method is available in the literature [57, 58].

1.5.3 CALCULATING MOLECULAR DESCRIPTORS

According to Tropsha [59], descriptors are the crucial component for any success-ful QSAR model development [60]. The molecular features considered for QSAR modeling require to be converted into numbers, and this translated structural infor-mation is called descriptors. Molecular descriptors are the numerical presentation of information installed in any chemical structure [56, 60]. In a QSAR study, molecu-lar descriptors are predictors (X) of the dependent parameter (Y) [56]. Molecular descriptors can be divided into two types: structure-based descriptors that can be theoretically computed from molecular representation and non-structure-based descriptors like Log P, pKa, dipole moment, molar refractivity, and polarizability [60]. We have already mentioned in an earlier section that molecular descriptors can also be classified according to their dimension (D) such as 0D, 1D, 2D, 3D, 4D, and so forth [60–62]. Zero-dimensional descriptors are the type of parameters that are independent of molecular connectivity, conformation, and structure. Constitutional descriptors, counts of atoms, and bond type are examples of 0D descriptors. One-dimensional molecular descriptors represent counts of molecular groups as frag-ments and fingerprints, and they also represent the physicochemical properties of compounds. Sybyl line notation (SLN) and the simplified molecular input line entry system (SMILES) are examples of 1D descriptors; 2D descriptors are acquired from molecular graph theory where topological properties of molecules like molecular connectivity indices, shape, size, and branching are contained, and they are also independent of molecular conformation. Graph theory maps the molecules into a graph where the atoms and bonds are represented as vertices and edges, respec-tively. Kier–Hall connectivity indices, the Weiner index, and the Randić connectiv-ity index are examples of 2D descriptors [60]. For the 2D-QSAR model building, 2D descriptors are computed to build the QSAR table. Three-dimensional descriptors are descriptors that correspond to the 3D representation of compounds and relate to the geometrical properties of the molecules. Weighted holistic invariant molecular (WHIM) descriptors, geometry, topology, and atom-weights assembly (GETAWAY) descriptors, molecular representation of structures based on electronic diffraction (3D-MoRSE) descriptors, potential energy descriptors, surface area, shape, and volume descriptors, and quantum chemical parameters are some examples of 3D descriptors [60, 63–65]. Four-dimensional descriptors are related to reference grids and MD simulations [50]. Molecular descriptors have been well discussed in the literature [38, 60, 66]. Various software used for calculating molecular descriptors is listed in Table 1.1 [34].

TABLE 1.1

List of Various Software and Web Servers Available for the Calculation of Molecular Descriptors

Software	Type of descriptors	No. of descriptors	Web address	Paid/Free
PaDEL descriptor	1D, 2D, 3D descriptors, molecular fingerprints	1,875	www.padel.nus.edu.sg	Free
CDK	Topological, electronic, geometrical, constitutional	–	http://cdk.github.io	Free
E-DRAGON	Molecular descriptors		www.vcclab.org/lab/edragon/	Free
ALOGPS2.1	log P, log S	–	www.vcclab.org/lab/alogps/	Free
ACD/labs	log P, log S, log D, pKa	–	www.acdlabs.com	Free
ChemDes	Molecular descriptors	3,679	www.scbdd.com/chemdes	Free (web)
PreADMET	Constitutional, physicochemical, geometrical, topological	>2,000	https://preadmet.webservice.bmdrc.org/preadmet-pc-version-2-0/	Paid
PowerMV	Constitutional, atom pairs, BCUT, fingerprints	1,000	www.niss.org/PowerMV	Free
ADAPT	Topological, physicochemical, geometrical, electronic	260	www.research.chem.psu.edu	Free
MOLD2	1D, 2D	779	www.fda.gov	Free
JOELib	Counting, topological, geometrical properties, etc.	40	www.ra.cs.uni-tuebingen.de	Free
MODEL	Molecular descriptors	3,778	http://jing.cz3.nus.edu.sg/cgi-bin/model/model.cgi	Free (web)
DRAGON	2D-autocorrelations, constitutional, topological, geometrical, GETAWAY, WHIM, RDF, functional groups, etc.	4,885	www.talete.mi.it	Paid

(Continued)

TABLE 1.1 (CONTINUED)

List of Various Software and Web Servers Available for the Calculation of Molecular Descriptors

Software	Type of descriptors	No. of descriptors	Web address	Paid/Free
ADMET predictor	Constitutional, topological, functional group counts, E-state, acid-base ionization, molecular patterns, empirical estimates of quantum, 3D descriptors	297	www.simulations-plus.com	Paid
ADRIANA. Code	Constitutional, topological, functional group counts, E-state, Meylan flags, Moriguchi, 3D descriptors, etc.	1,244	www.molecularnetworks.com	Paid
CODESSA	Constitutional, geometrical, topological, semi-empirical, charge-related, thermodynamical	1,500	www.codessa-pro.com	Paid
MOE	Topological, structural keys, physical properties, etc.	300	www.chemcomp.com	Paid
MOLCONN-Z	Topological	40	www.edusoft-lc.com/molconn	Paid
MOLGEN-QSPR	Constitutional, geometrical, topological, etc.	707	www.molgen.molgenqspr.html	Paid
Sarchitect	Constitutional, 2D, 3D	1,084	www.strandls.com/sarchitect/index .html	Paid

1.5.4 FEATURE SELECTION TECHNIQUE

Due to the availability of a huge number of molecular descriptors for a single molecule, the selection of a proper subset of descriptors from a large pool of initial descriptors is called the feature selection technique, which is a salient step for the development of the QSAR model [67]. The objective of the feature selection process is to identify salient predictor variables to build interrelationships with the response variable [67]. The feature selection process decreases the chance of model complexity and the risk of overtraining and overfitting [67]. Appropriate subset selection of molecular descriptors is directly associated with the predictive quality, stability, reliability, and robustness of developed QSAR models [68, 69]. In QSAR model development techniques, Khan and Roy [69] broadly classified feature selection methods into three major groups: a) classical feature selection methods, namely forward selection, backward elimination, stepwise regression, variable selection, and the modeling method based on the prediction and Leaps-and-Bounds regression method; b) feature selection applying artificial intelligence algorithms such as genetic algorithm (GA), ANN, the particle swarm optimization (PSO) method, the ant colony optimization (ACO) method, the simulated annealing (SA) method, the automatic relevance determination (ARD) method, and so on; and c) miscellaneous methods such as the replacement method (RM), the k-nearest neighbors (k-NN) method, the successive projections algorithm (SPA), and so on. Feature selection techniques are also classified as filter, wrapper, and hybrid methods concerning their dependency on a learning algorithm [68]. Filter methods are unsupervised feature or variable selection techniques that do not recruit any learning algorithm in the variable selection process [68]. In the case of the filter method, feature selection depends only on the descriptors without any dependency on the learning algorithm [68]. In the case of the wrapper method, feature selection depends on both the descriptors and a learning algorithm. In the wrapper method, a classifier or regressor uses an objective function for the selection of descriptors [68]. In the wrapper method, descriptor selection depends on both dependent and independent variables [68]. Filter methods utilize approaches like the GSS coefficient, Shannon entropy, odds ratio, correlation-based feature selection, chi-square analysis, Kolmogorov–Smirnov statistics, Fisher score, the distance-based method, and principal component analysis [50]. Bayesian regularized neural network, recursive feature elimination, genetic algorithm, k-nearest neighbor, backward elimination, forward selection, and variable selection, as well as modeling based on the prediction, factor analysis, and combinatorial protocol, are generally used wrapper methods [50]. Hybrid feature selection methods are a combination of filter and wrapper methods. A detailed account of feature selection techniques is available in the literature [68, 69].

1.5.5 TWO-DIMENSIONAL-QSAR MODEL BUILDING

Two-dimensional-QSAR model-building approaches are considered to build the mathematical relationship between descriptors and the biological endpoint or response values where a set of descriptors, predictor variables, or independent variables are a function of biological endpoint values, response variables, or dependent variables [52]. Statistical techniques used for 2D-QSAR modeling are broadly classified into two classes: linear QSAR models and non-linear QSAR models [70].

1.5.5.1 Linear 2D-QSAR Models

Linear methods are used most extensively in the 2D-QSAR model building because linear 2D-QSAR models are simple, easily interpretable, and reproducible. To develop linear-based 2D-QSAR models, different regression- and classification-based methods are utilized [71]. When the biological response of chemical compounds is completely numerical or quantitative, regression-based statistical approaches are employed. Classification-based statistical techniques are generally used for qualitative or semi-quantitative biological responses to chemical compounds [71]. In both regression-based and classification-based statistical approaches, the descriptor values will be quantitative [71]. In the case of regression-based statistical techniques, the quantitative prediction of biological endpoints is employed, whereas classification-based statistical techniques enable the classification or categorization of chemical compounds into various classes or groups with respect to their biological endpoints, such as active and inactive [71].

1.5.5.1.1 Regression-Based 2D-QSAR Model

MLR and PLS methods are examples of regression-based linear statistical techniques for QSAR model development [68].

1.5.5.1.1.1 Multiple Linear Regression Analysis

MLR analysis is the most frequently used statistical method in 2D-QSAR analysis because it is simple, transparent, reproducible, and easily interpretable. The MLR analysis is an extension of simple linear regression (SLR) where multiple numbers of independent variables are involved. SLR is based on the following mathematical equation:

$$Y = mX + c \qquad (1.1)$$

Equation **1.1** is a two-dimensional linear equation where Y is the dependent or response parameter, X is the independent parameter or input value, m is the slope, and c is the constant. On the other hand, the mathematical model for MLR is as follows:

$$Y = a_0 + a_1X_1 + a_2X_2 + a_3X_3 + a_4X_4 + \ldots + a_nX_n \qquad (1.2)$$

Equation **2.2** is a multi-dimensional linear equation where Y is the dependent or response variable or biological endpoint value; a_0 is the slope of the line; X_1, X_2, X_3, ... X_n is the independent variables or input values or molecular descriptors with their respective coefficients a_1, a_2, a_3, a_4, ...a_n [51, 71, 72].

1.5.5.1.1.2 PLS Method
In the case of the partial least square method, the dependent variables or descriptors (X) and the independent variables or biological response values (Y) are often transformed into new variables named latent variables (LVs). LVs (t_1, ..., t_n) are linear combinations of the descriptors (X_1, ..., X_m) [72]. Before applying the PLS technique, the response or dependent variables (Y) are usually transformed into a logarithmic scale, and the independent variables (X) should be scaled appropriately [71]. If the number of LVs is equal to the number of original variables, the PLS model becomes an MLR model [71]. The mathematical equations for the PLS method are given below in equations **1.3–1.6**:

$$Y = a_1t_1 + a_2t_2 + ... + a_nt_n \tag{1.3}$$

$$t_1 = b_{11}X_1 + b_{12}X_2 + ... + b_{1m}X_m \tag{1.4}$$

$$t_2 = b_{21}X_1 + b_{22}X_2 + ... + b_{2m}X_m \tag{1.5}$$

$$....$$

$$....$$

$$t_n = b_{n1}X_1 + b_{n2}X_2 + ... + b_{nm}X_m \tag{1.6}$$

Here, t_1, ..., t_n are latent variables that are orthogonal to each other and originated from independent variables (X_1, ..., X_m) [72]. The LVs express the variations of both descriptors (X) and biological activities (Y) [72]. The PLS method is especially applicable for data with a large number of X variables that are strongly collinear, noisy, and correlated. If the number of molecular parameters is too large and close to the number of response variables, there is a chance of overfitting. In such cases, the PLS method is preferred over MLR analysis [51].

1.5.5.1.1.3 Principal Component Analysis
Principal component analysis (PCA) is a multivariate analysis and data reduction tool. PCA helps to reduce the dimensionality of large datasets by converting a large set of variables into a smaller one without losing the information of a large dataset to a major extent. Before performing PCA, the initial dataset needs to be standardized because if there are high differences between the ranges of initial parameters, those parameters with larger ranges will govern over those comprising small ranges. After standardization, the next step is the computation of the covariance matrix of variables to understand how variables are correlated among themselves. Highly correlated variables sometimes result in redundant information, which can be identified from the covariance matrix. Then, eigenvectors and eigenvalues are calculated from the covariance matrix for determining the principal components (PCs) related to the data. Here, the PCs are the new parameters that are built as linear combinations of the initial parameters in such a way that the new parameters or PCs are not

correlated, and most of the information among the initial parameters is compressed into the first PC. If the initial dataset has an "*n*" number of variables or dimensions, the number of PCs will be "*n*." The eigenvector with the highest eigenvalue will be considered the first PC, the eigenvector with the second-highest eigenvalue will be considered the second PC, and so on. Among all PCAs, the first component will contain the highest possible information, then the maximum remaining information in the second, and so on. Now, computing the eigenvectors and sequencing these as per their eigenvalues in descending order results in the order of importance of the PCs. After discarding lesser significant PCs, a matrix of vectors containing the remaining ones, which are named feature vectors, is computed. Finally, with the help of the feature vector produced using the eigenvectors of the covariance matrix, the data from the actual axes are transformed or reoriented to the ones designated by the PCs. From the above discussion, it is clear how PCA works as a data reduction tool [73, 74]. PCA is used extensively in the 2D-QSAR study for the analysis of complex datasets and the identification of outliers [75]. Although PCA is used extensively in the 2D-QSAR study, PCA has some limitations. If the relationship between descriptors is non-linear, PCA is not applicable. PCA cannot operate with missing values and mixed descriptors. Interpretation of PCs, as well as their correspondence to the descriptors, is preferably subjective and irrational [75].

1.5.5.1.1.4 Statistical Metrics for Regression-Based 2D-QSAR Models

The different statistical metrics that are employed for the justification of regression-based 2D-QSAR models are correlation coefficient (R), squared correlation coefficient (R^2), adjusted R^2 (R^2_a), and variance ratio (F) at specified degrees of freedom (df), as well as the standard error of the estimate (SEE) [28]. These statistical metrics are not the validation parameters of the constructed 2D-QSAR models. To validate the predictive ability of a regression-based 2D-QSAR model on a new set of data, several internal and external validation features are employed [76]. Generally, leave one out (LOO) cross-validated R^2 (Q^2) [70], the sum of squared deviations between the actual and predicted properties of the test set compounds (PRESS), and the sum of squared deviations error of prediction (SDEP) values are considered as internal validation parameters, whereas R^2_{pred} is usually considered as the model external validation parameter [28, 77].

1.5.5.1.1.5 Model Quality Parameters of Regression-Based 2D-QSAR Study

Among model qualities, the correlation coefficient (R) justifies how intimately the observed data follows the fitted regression line. The R^2 was calculated as per equation **1.7**.

$$R^2 = 1 - \frac{\sum \left(y_{obs} - y_{calc} \right)^2}{\sum \left(y_{obs} - y_{mean} \right)^2} \tag{1.7}$$

Where y_{obs} and y_{calc} are the respective actual and predicted activity of molecules belonging to the training set and y_{mean} is the mean biological response values of the training set molecules. In equation **1.7** of the squared correlation coefficient, the number of descriptors is not considered, which may decrease the degree of freedom and lead to poor statistical reliability [58]. In order to overcome the drawbacks associated with the value of R^2, R^2_a was also calculated from equation **1.8** where n is the number of scores and p is the number of descriptors.

$$R^2_a = \frac{(n-1) \times R^2 - p}{n - p - 1}$$
(1.8)

The SEE was also calculated for the residuals as per equation **1.9**.

$$SEE = \sqrt{\frac{\Sigma(y_{obs} - y_{calc})^2}{n - p - 1}}$$
(1.9)

Where y_{obs} and y_{calc} are the actual and predicted responses of the training set, n is the total number of data points, and p is the total number of molecular descriptors. The lower value of SEE recommends a better model quality.

1.5.5.1.1.6 Model Validation Parameters of Regression-Based 2D-QSAR Study
The predictive ability of any regression-based 2D-QSAR model may be judged by LOO cross-validation Q^2 and SDEP. Each molecule was eliminated from the training set at each time and the activity of the deleted molecule was predicted simultaneously by using the model constructed from the remaining compounds of the training set. The LOO Q^2 value was calculated as per equation **1.10**.

$$Q^2 = 1 - \frac{\Sigma(y_{obs} - y_i)^2}{\Sigma(y_{obs} - y_{mean})^2}$$
(1.10)

Where y_{obs} and y_i are the respective actual and predicted biological responses of the ith compound belonging to the training set and y_{mean} denotes the mean biological response of the training set molecules. Further, PRESS and SDEP values are determined for judging the internal predictability of the model.

The external predictability of the developed 2D-QSAR models is also justified by external validation of the test set molecules. The R^2_{pred} is the external validation criteria, which is calculated as per equation **1.11**.

$$R^2_{pred} = 1 - \frac{\Sigma(y_{obs} - y_i)^2}{\Sigma(y_{obs} - y_{mean})^2}$$
(1.11)

Where y_{obs} and y_i are the respective actual and predicted biological response of the ith molecule of the training dataset, and y_{mean} is the mean biological response of the test dataset.

The R^2_{pred} value is not sufficient to confirm the external predictability of a model. The value of R^2_{pred} is generally governed by the sum of squared differences between observed biological activities of the test set compounds and the mean of biological activities of the training set molecules. Therefore, it may not truly reflect the predictability of the model [62]. For this reason, R^2_m metrics ($R^2_{m(LOO)}$, $R^2_{m(test)}$, and $R^2_{m(Overall)}$) are used to estimate the closeness between the values of the predicted and the observed biological activities of the training set, the test set, and the total dataset, respectively. The R^2_m value should be greater than 0.50 and is calculated as per equation **1.12** [58].

$$R^2_{m(test)} = R^2 \times \left(1 - \sqrt{R^2 - R^2_0} \right) \tag{1.12}$$

Where R^2 and R^2_0 are the squared correlation coefficients between the actual and predicted biological responses of the test set molecules.

1.5.5.1.1.7 Y-Randomization Test
The Y-randomization test is a universally applied technique for ensuring the robustness and validation of a 2D-QSAR model [78]. Here, the dependent or response variable (Y) is randomly and repeatedly shuffled, and new QSAR models are generated with the help of the independent-variable matrix. The expectation of the Y-randomization test is that the 2D-QSAR models should normally have low R^2 and low LOO-Q^2 values. Sometimes, a high Q^2 value may be produced because of a chance correlation of the compounds belonging to the training set. If all QSAR models generated during this Y-randomization test possess comparatively high R^2 and LOO-Q^2 values, an acceptable QSAR model may not be constructed by the current modeling method for the given dataset of compounds [79].

1.5.5.1.2 Classification-Based 2D-QSAR Model
Popular approaches to classification-dependent QSAR studies are linear discriminant analysis (LDA), Bayesian classification modeling, and recursive partitioning.

1.5.5.1.2.1 Linear Discriminant Analysis-QSAR Model
Linear discriminant analysis is a pattern-recognition technique with a classification-based model and is specially used for dimensionality reduction [80]. Like MLR, LDA also performs a similar kind of task by predicting an output when the response variable is a categorical variable and molecular properties are continuous variables [51].

1.5.5.1.2.1.1 Validation Parameters for LDAThe statistical validation parameters for LDA include accuracy, sensitivity, specificity, precision, Matthews's correlation coefficient (MCC), F1 measure, and so on. The quality of the training set is rationalized with the Wilks' parameter (λ). The relative importance of the selected parameters of the LDA-QSAR model is substantiated based on the Fisher–Snedecor parameter (F) [81–84].

These statistical validation parameters of LDA, like sensitivity, specificity, precision, accuracy, and F1 measure, as well as MCC, are calculated as per equations **1.13–1.18**.

$$Sensetivity = \frac{TP}{(TP + FN)} \tag{1.13}$$

$$Specificity = \frac{TN}{(TN + FP)} \tag{1.14}$$

$$Precision = \frac{TP}{(TP + FP)} \tag{1.15}$$

$$Accuracy = \frac{(TP + TN)}{(TP + FP + TN + FN)} \tag{1.16}$$

$$F1 = \frac{2TP}{(2TP + FP + FN)} \tag{1.17}$$

$$MCC = \frac{(TP*TN) - (FP*FN)}{\sqrt{(TP + FP)(TP + FN)(TN + FP)(TN + FN)}} \tag{1.18}$$

Where TP is the true positive or "active" compound that is predicted as "active" in the model. The FN is the false negative where the "active" compound is predicted as "inactive." The TN denotes the true negative where the "inactive" molecules are predicted as "inactive." The FP is false positive where the "inactive" molecules are predicted as "active" compounds.

Some other validation parameters for the constructed LDA model are the receiver operating characteristics curve Euclidean distance (ROCED) and the receiver operating characteristics curve Euclidean distance corrected with fitness function (ROCFIT) [76]. ROCED and ROCFIT are calculated by the following formulae [78, 81] in equations **1.19–1.21**:

$$d_i = \sqrt{(1 - Sensitivity)^2 + (1 - Specificity)^2} \tag{1.19}$$

$$ROCED = (|d_1 - d_2| + 1)(d_1 + d_2)(d_2 + 1) \tag{1.20}$$

$$ROCFIT = \frac{ROCED}{\lambda} \tag{1.21}$$

Where d_i = Euclidean distance between the perfect and a real classifier, i = 1 designates the training set, i = 2 designates the test set, and λ = Wilk's parameter.

The performance of the LDA-QSAR model is decided by evaluating of the area under the receiver operating characteristic curve (AUROC) [85].

1.5.5.1.2.2 Bayesian Classification Model

The Bayesian classification study is formulated depending on the Bayes theorem [86, 87] provided below in equation **1.22**.

$$P(M/N) = \frac{P(N/M)P(M)}{P(N)} \tag{1.22}$$

Where M denotes the model and N represents the observed data. The P(M/N) designates posterior probability, while P (N/M) indicates the likelihood. The P(M) and P(N) signify the prior belief and evidence data, respectively.

The Bayesian classification modeling study helps to classify or discriminate the important good and bad sub-structural features in molecules [88, 89]. A variety of structural and physiochemical descriptors such as lipophilicity, number of rotatable bonds, molecular weight, the total number of rings and the total number of aromatic rings, number of hydrogen bond donors and number of hydrogen bond acceptors, and molecular polar surface area and molecular extended connectivity fingerprints of maximum diameter 6 (ECFP_6) are usually considered for developing the Bayesian model [89–93].

1.5.5.1.2.2.1 Validation Parameters for Bayesian Classification Model The validation parameters for the Bayesian model are LOO cross-validation and five-fold cross-validation [89–93]. Like the LDA method, the internal and external predictability of the Bayesian classification model is also justified by evaluating the AUROC and the parameters, namely accuracy, specificity, sensitivity, precision, F1 measure, MCC, and so on of both the training and the test set compounds [86–90].

1.5.5.1.2.3 Recursive Partitioning Method

The recursive partitioning (RP) method is another classification-based QSAR approach that builds one or more decision trees to explain the relationship between a dependent or biological response variable (Y) and a set of independent variables or molecular descriptors (X). The RP method categorizes data by utilizing a set of hierarchical regulations to scrap a dataset into smaller subsets. The output of the RP method is a decision tree that is built by a recursive partitioning process. The splitting of study samples has occurred in such a way that a specific selected predictor is more a selected cutoff value or not. At each step of splitting, all the molecular parameters are consecutively examined to identify the best benchmark for subdividing compounds. Once the best feature is set, a similar course of action is repeated for each of the obtained classes of molecules [94, 95].

1.5.5.2 Non-Linear QSAR Models

For investigating the probable non-linear relationship between the descriptors and biological endpoints or response values, several machine learning approaches are used. SVMs and ANNs frequently use machine learning techniques for non-linear QSAR model development [41, 42, 93, 96, 97]. SVM parameters such as exponent value (ε), complexity parameter (C), and the kernel type and related parameters (γ) and ANN parameters such as the number of hidden nodes, learning momentum, learning rate, and training time are optimized with Autoweka software [23]. The regression-dependent non-linear models are generated with optimized parameters by using Weka software [98].

1.5.5.2.1 Support Vector Machine Technique

SVM [98] is developed by non-linear mapping of the input parameter into the higher dimensional feature space through kernel function [99–101]. It signifies the evalua-tion of model parameters with the help of the convex optimization approach [99–101]. The SVM is useful to resolve problems related to classification studies. This learning method is also compliant with regression-related problems [42]. Several kernel func-tions are assimilated into the SVM method, such as linear, polynomial, and sigmoid kernels along with the radial basis function (RBF) kernel [42]. In the SVM-based non-linear QSAR study, the descriptor matrix is projected into a high-dimensional feature space from the input feature space with the help of kernel functions [K (x, y)]. Mathematically, kernel function [K (x, y)] is described by equation **1.23**.

$$K (x, y) = \{\emptyset (x) * \emptyset (y)\} \tag{1.23}$$

Where K is a kernel function and $\emptyset$ is a mapping from input space X $\in$ x, y to the feature space F.

1.5.5.2.2 Artificial Neural Network Method

ANN [102–104] is also a very popular tool to build QSAR models [97]. The ANN resembles the human brain framework where ANN nodes are analogous to the biological neurons and ANN layers (input, hidden, and output layers) are compa-rable with the neuronal synaptic weights. In the ANN-based QSAR method, the molecular information from the descriptors initially comes to the input layer and then is transferred to the hidden layer nodes and finally goes to the output layer for processing [102]. The frequently used ANNs in QSAR are Bayesian regularized neural networks, back propagation neural networks, probabilistic neural networks, and Kohonen self-organizing maps. The ANN models are highly adaptable and suc-cessfully employed in the case of a non-linear system having high variability in the dataset. Superior models can be built by the algorithms of ANNs in comparison with traditional linear models like MLR or PLS [50]. However, ANNs also have some drawbacks. ANN does not give explicit knowledge in the form of rules or some way of easy interpretation and possesses a greater computational burden. The model is indirect and hidden in the network structure. The nature of ANN model development is empirical and has a tendency of overfitting [105].

1.5.5.3 Validation Parameters for Non-Linear QSAR Study

Pearson's correlation coefficient for the training set (r_{train}), cross-validated correla-tion coefficient (r_{cv}), the test set correlation coefficient (r_{test}), and the corresponding root mean squared error (RMSE) are statistical parameters that are used for the validation and robustness of SVM and ANN models [96].

1.5.6 INTERPRETATION AND APPLICABILITY DOMAIN ANALYSIS

The descriptors for building the QSAR model should be interpretable. The influence of descriptors on the predicted activity should be understood in a mechanistic way. Applicability domain (AD) analysis is helpful to understand the applicability or predictive ability of the QSAR model on a new set of compounds [50, 58]. The AD is designated as the theoretical region in the chemical space of molecular properties associated to construct the QSAR model with response variables [106]. The prediction of response values by a QSAR model is relevant only if the molecule being predicted lives in the AD of the QSAR model [58]. Different methods are employed for the identification or estimation of the theoretical region in the chemical space. The most common methods or approaches for applicability domain estimation are distance-based methods, geometrical methods, probability density distribution, range in descriptor space, and the range of response variables [107]. The method utilized for interpolation space characterization in cases of distance-based methods, geometrical methods, probability density distribution, and ranges in descriptor space is dependent on the model descriptor space, whereas the methodology used for the range of response variable depends solely on the response space of the training set compounds. In the case of the ranges approach, a compound is considered out of the domain of applicability if at least one parameter is out of the span of the ranges approach. In the case of the distance-based method, if the distance between the chemical and the center of the training dataset surpasses the threshold for distance approaches, the compound is called as out of the applicability domain [58].

1.6 SOFTWARE, DATABASE, AND WEB SERVICES AVAILABLE FOR QSAR STUDY

Various commercial, non-commercial, and open-source QSAR modeling software and tools have been published in the last two decades. Some of these important software and tools [108–123] are summarized in Table 1.2.

1.7 SUMMARY

The phrase "2D-QSAR" proclaims the build-out of QSAR models using 2D descriptors. These 2D descriptors are the most practiced predictor variables reported in QSAR model building. Because they are simple and easy to calculate, a direct mathematical algorithm is involved for computation and reproducible operability. Two-dimensional descriptors contribute extensively to extracting chemical attributes from molecules, and they are also competent to represent 3D molecular features to some extent. A summary of the 2D-QSAR model building is given in Figure 1.3.

TABLE 1.2

List of Different Commercial and Open-Source Software and Web Services for QSAR Studies [108–123]

Entry	Software	Description	Paid/Free
1	cQSAR	A database of regression-based QSAR models having more than 21,000 QSAR equations relating biochemical and physical-chemical activities to molecular descriptors.	Paid
2	QSARPro	QSAR software for calculating molecular descriptor QSAR model building (linear or non-linear regression) and also for predicting the activities of the test or a new set of molecules. It offers another patent pending QSAR technique named group-based QSAR (GQSAR). Works on Linux and Windows.	Paid
3	MedChem Studio (formerly ClassPharmer)	Used for QSAR model building and ADMET property prediction.	Paid
4	Codessa	Procures molecular descriptors using quantum mechanical results from AMPAC, which are then used to develop QSAR/QSPR models.	Paid
5	OpenMolGRID	Grid-enabled QSAR approach for modeling large and complex datasets.	Paid
6	CODESSA Pro	Program for calculating descriptors, developing multi-linear and non-linear QSAR/QSPR models, and interpreting the developed model.	Paid
7	MCASE	Machine learning-based QSAR software for modeling and predicting toxicities of chemicals.	Paid
8	smirep	SAR/QSAR tool for predicting the structural activity of chemical compounds. It works on the Linux platform.	Free
9	AutoWeka	Automated data mining software for QSAR.	Free
10	DTC Lab tools	2D QSAR tools.	Free
11	MOLE db	Online molecular descriptors database comprised of 1,124 molecular descriptors, which are calculated for 234,773 molecules.	Free
12	Datasets of Milano Chemometrics and QSAR Research Group	Reference datasets.	Free
13	OCHEM Database	Online database of experimental measurements of chemical and biological data integrated with a modeling environment. Users can submit experimental data or use the data uploaded by other users to build predictive QSAR models.	Free

(*Continued*)

TABLE 1.2   (CONTINUED)
List of Different Commercial and Open-Source Software and Web Services for QSAR Studies [108–123]

Entry	Software	Description	Paid/Free
14	ChemSAR	Web-based pipeline platform for classification-based models of small molecules. It includes standardization and validation of molecules, calculation of descriptors (1D, 2D, and FP), feature selection, model building, and interpretation.	Free
15	Chembench	Chembench provides robust model building, property and activity predictions, and virtual libraries of available compounds with predicted biological activities and drug-like properties. It also provides special tools for designing chemical libraries.	Free
16	Partial Least Squares Regression (PLSR)	Construct QSAR/QSPR models and predict activity/property using the PLSR technique.	Free

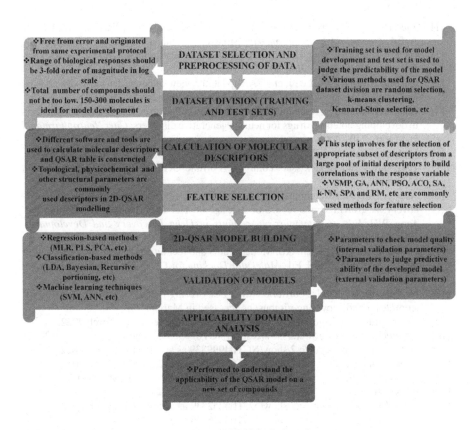

FIGURE 1.3   Schematic representation of 2D-QSAR model development.

For the development of 2D-QSAR, model 2D descriptors provide enormous information to expose the chemistry of a compound, such as size, shape, bonding information, branching, lipophilicity, and so on. For the better predictive ability of the 2D-QSAR model, along with 2D descriptors, higher-dimensional descriptors can also be used for model building [31]. A particular class of descriptors cannot be the final solution for good QSAR practices. Therefore, researchers should practice a mixed approach comprising the topology, electronic configuration, and geometric features of molecules for 2D-QSAR model building. The utility of 2D descriptors may be expanded to a greater extent by incorporating an appropriate and specific extraction algorithm [31]; 2D-QSAR models often suffer from inter-correlation among descriptors, insufficient chemical information, and lack of interpretation. However, on the other hand, by following rational approaches, like using reliable and high-quality data and reasonable and honest uses of statistics, using novel 2D descriptors, considering the appropriate set of compounds that reside in the domain of applicability, and discarding the outliers, using appropriate algorithms may be helpful to eliminate various problems to solve the uncountable chemical mysteries still unknown by 2D-QSAR analysis [53].

REFERENCES

[1].   Tautermann CS. Current and future challenges in modern drug discovery. In: Heifetz A, Ed., *Quantum Mechanics in Drug Discovery*. Humana, New York, 2020, pp. 1–17.

[2].   Hu ZZ, Huang H, Wu CH, et al. Omics-based molecular target and biomarker identification. *Methods Mol Biol* 2011;719:547–571.

[3].   Gurung AB, Ali MA, Lee J, et al. An updated review of computer-aided drug design and its application to COVID-19. *BioMed Res Int* 2021;2021:1–19.

[4].   Baig MH, Ahmad K, Rabbani G, et al. Computer-aided drug design and its application to developing potential drugs for neurodegenerative disorders. *Curr Neuropharmacol* 2018;16(6):740–748.

[5].   Fortune. The next Industrial Revolution: Designing drugs by computer at Merck, 1981. https://www.backissues.com/issue/Fortune-October-05-1981 as accessed in March 2022.

[6].   Abel R. Advanced computational modeling accelerating small-molecule drug discovery: A growing track record of success. In: Huang X, Robert G, Aslanian RG, Tang WH, Eds., *Contemporary Accounts in Drug Discovery and Development*. Wiley, Hoboken, 2022, pp. 9–25.

[7].   Anwar T, Kumar P, Khan AU. Modern tools and techniques in computer-aided drug design. In: Coumar MS, Ed., *Molecular Docking for Computer-Aided Drug Design*. Academic Press, London, UK, 2021, Ch. 1, pp. 1–30.

[8].   New Business Models, Portfolio News. *Discovering Nimbus*, 2011. https://lifescivc.com/2011/03/discovering-nimbus/ as accessed in March 2022.

[9].   https://clinicaltrials.gov/ct2/show/NCT02876796 as accessed in March 2022.

[10]. https://clinicaltrials.gov/ct2/show/results/NCT02856555 as accessed in March 2022.

[11]. https://clinicaltrials.gov/ct2/show/NCT04999839 as accessed in March 2022.

[12]. https://clinicaltrials.gov/ct2/show/NCT04580745 as accessed in March 2022.

[13]. https://clinicaltrials.gov/ct2/show/NCT05291689 as accessed in March 2022.

[14]. https://relaytx.com/pipeline/ as accessed in March 2022.

[15]. https://clinicaltrials.gov/ct2/show/NCT04252339 as accessed in March 2022.

[16]. https://clinicaltrials.gov/ct2/show/NCT04526106 as accessed in March 2022.

[17]. https://clinicaltrials.gov/ct2/show/NCT05216432?term=relay+therapeutics&draw=2 &rank=1 as accessed in March 2022.

[18]. Business Wire. Schrödinger and Bayer collaborate to co-develop de novo design technology to accelerate drug discovery, 2020. https://www.businesswire.com/news /home/20200108005059/en/Schr%C3%B6dinger-and-Bayer-Collaborate-to-Co -Develop-de-novo-Design-Technology-to-Accelerate-Drug-Discovery as accessed in March 2022.

[19]. Business Wire. Schrödinger announces collaboration with AstraZeneca to deploy advanced computing technology for drug discovery, 2019. https://www.busi-nesswire.com/news/home/20190904005166/en/Schr%C3%B6dinger-Announces -Collaboration-with-AstraZeneca-to-Deploy-Advanced-Computing-Technology-for -Drug-Discovery as accessed in March 2022.

[20]. Business Wire. Schrödinger announces expanded collaboration with AstraZeneca to extend computational modeling solutions to biologics, 2020. https://www.busi-nesswire.com/news/home/20200323005050/en/Schr%C3%B6dinger-Announces -Expanded-Collaboration-AstraZeneca-Extend-Computational (as accessed in March 2022.

[21]. Veselovsky AV, Zharkova MS, Poroikov VV, et al. Computer-aided design and discovery of protein-protein interaction inhibitors as agents for anti-HIV therapy. *SAR QSAR Environ Res* 2014;25(6):457–471.

[22]. Suay-García B, Bueso-Bordils JI, Falcó A, et al. Virtual combinatorial chemistry and pharmacological screening: A short guide to drug design. *Int J Mol Sci* 2022;23(3):1620.

[23]. Nantasenamat C, Prachayasittikul V. Maximizing computational tools for successful drug discovery. *Expert Opin Drug Discov* 2015;10(4):321–329.

[24]. Achary PGR. Applications of quantitative structure-activity relationships (QSAR) based virtual screening in drug design: A review. *Mini Rev Med Chem* 2020;20(14):1375–1388.

[25]. Sharma S, Bhatia V. Recent trends in QSAR in modeling of drug-protein and protein-protein interactions. *Comb Chem High Throughput Screen* 2021;24(7):1031–1041.

[26]. Neves BJ, Braga RC, Melo-Filho CC, et al. QSAR-based virtual screening: Advances and applications in drug discovery. *Front Pharmacol* 2018;9:1275.

[27]. Kar S, Sanderson H, Roy K, et al. Ecotoxicological assessment of pharmaceuticals and personal care products using predictive toxicology approaches. *Green Chem* 2020;22(5):1458–1516.

[28]. Amin SA, Gayen S. Modeling the cytotoxic activity of pyrazolo-triazole hybrids using descriptors calculated from the open source tool "PaDEL-descriptor." *J Taibah Univ Sci* 2016;10(6):896–905.

[29]. Roy PP, Paul S, Mitra I, et al. On two novel parameters for validation of predictive QSAR models. *Molecules* 2009;14(5):1660–1701.

[30]. Cherkasov A, Muratov EN, Fourches D, et al. QSAR modeling: Where have you been? Where are you going to? *J Med Chem* 2014;57(12):4977–5010.

[31]. Roy K, Das RN. A review on principles, theory and practices of 2D-QSAR. *Curr Drug Metab* 2014;15(4):346–379.

[32]. Crilly T, Johnson D. The emergence of topological dimension theory. In: James IM, Ed., *History of Topology*. Elsevier, Amsterdam, 1999.

[33]. Todeschini R, Consonni V. Molecular descriptors for chemoinformatics. In: Mannhold R, Kubinyi H, Folkers G, Eds., Methods and Principles in Medicinal Chemistry, *Book Series*. Wiley-VCH, Weinheim, 2009.

[34]. Danishuddin KAU. Descriptors and their selection methods in QSAR analysis: Paradigm for drug design. *Drug Discov.* 2016;21(8):1291–1302.

[35]. Tosco P, Balle T. Open 3DQSAR: A new open-source software aimed at high-throughput chemometric analysis of molecular interaction fields. *J Mol Model* 2011;17(1):201–208.

[36]. Cramer RD. Rethinking 3D-QSAR. *J Comput Aid Mol Des* 2011;25(3):197–201.

[37]. Cramer RD. The inevitable QSAR renaissance. *J Comput Aid Mol Des* 2012;26(1):35–38.

[38]. Doweyko AM. 3D-QSAR illusions. *J Comput Aid Mol Des* 2004;18(7–9):587–596.

[39]. Scior T, Bender A, Tresadern G, et al. Recognizing pitfalls in virtual screening: A critical review. *J Chem Inf Model* 2012;52(4):867–881.

[40]. Sendecor GW, Cochran WG. *Multiple Regression in Statistical Methods*, 6th ed., Oxford & IBH, New Delhi, 1967.

[41]. Nantasenamat C, Isarankura-Na-Ayudhya C, Naenna T, et al. Prediction of bond dissociation enthalpy of antioxidant phenols by support vector machine. *J Mol Graph Modell* 2008;27(2):188–196.

[42]. Nantasenamat C, Worachartcheewan A, Prachayasittikul S, et al. QSAR modeling of aromatase inhibitory activity of 1-substituted 1,2,3-triazole analogs of letrozole. *Eur J Med Chem* 2013;69:99–114.

[43]. Worachartcheewan A, Nantasenamat C, Naenna T, et al. Modeling the activity of furin inhibitors using artificial neural network. *Eur J Med Chem* 2009;44(4):1664–1673.

[44]. Ajmani S, Jadhav K, Kulkarni SA. Three-dimensional QSAR using the k-nearest neighbor method and its interpretation. *J Chem Inf Model* 2006;46(1):24–31.

[45]. Klon AE, Lowrie JF, Diller DJ. Improved naïve Bayesian modeling of numerical data for absorption, distribution, metabolism and excretion (ADME) property prediction. *J Chem Inf Model* 2006;46(5):1945–1956.

[46]. Ling Y, Liu J, Qian J, et al. Recent advances in multi-target drugs targeting protein kinases and histone deacetylases in cancer therapy. *Curr Med Chem* 2020;27(42):7264–7288.

[47]. Benek O, Korabecny J, Soukup O. A perspective on multi-target drugs for Alzheimer's disease. *Trends Pharmacol Sci* 2020;41(7):434–445.

[48]. Makhoba XH, Viegas C Jr, Mosa RA, et al. Potential impact of the multi-target drug approach in the treatment of some complex diseases. *Drug Des Devel Ther* 2020;14:3235–3249.

[49]. Organisation for economic co-operation and development (OECD). The report from the expert group on (quantitative) structure-activity relationships [(Q)SARs] on the principles for the validation of (Q) SARs. *Series on Testing and Assessment*, 2004, p. 206.

[50]. Peter SC, Dhanjal JK, Malik V, et al. Quantitative structure-activity relationship (QSAR): Modeling approaches to biological applications. In: Ranganathan S, Gribskov M, Nakai K, Schönbach C, Eds., *Encyclopedia of Bioinformatics and Computational Biology*. Academic Press, London, UK, 2019, pp. 661–676.

[51]. Roy K, Kar S, Das RN. Selected statistical methods in QSAR. In: Roy K, Kar S, Das RN, Eds., *Understanding the Basics of QSAR for Applications in Pharmaceutical Sciences and Risk Assessment*. Academic Press, 2015, Ch. 6, pp. 191–229.

[52]. Tropsha A. Best practices for QSAR model development, validation, and exploitation. *Mol Inform* 2010;29(6–7):476–488.

[53]. Scior T, Medina-Franco JL, Do QT, et al. How to recognize and workaround pitfalls in QSAR studies: A critical review. *Curr Med Chem* 2009;16(32):4297–4313.

[54]. Gedeck P, Rohde B, Bartels C. QSAR–how good is it in practice? Comparison of descriptor sets on an unbiased cross section of corporate data sets. *J Chem Inf Model* 2006;46(5):1924–1936.

[55]. Hamzeh-Mivehroud M, Sokouti B, Dastmalchi S. An introduction to the basic concepts in QSAR-aided drug design. In: Roy K, Ed., *Quantitative Structure-Activity Relationships in Drug Design, Predictive Toxicology, and Risk Assessment*. IGI Global, Hershey, 2015, pp. 1–47.

[56]. De P, Kar S, Ambure P, et al. Prediction reliability of QSAR models: An overview of various validation tools. *Arch Toxicol* 2022.

[57].   Golbraikh A, Tropsha A. Predictive QSAR modeling based on diversity sampling of experimental datasets for the training and test set selection. *J Comput Aid Mol Des* 2002;16(5–6):357–369.

[58].   Roy K, Kar S, Das RN. Validation of QSAR models. In: Roy K, Kar S, Das RN, Eds., *Understanding the Basics of QSAR for Applications in Pharmaceutical Sciences and Risk Assessment*. Academic Press, London, UK, 2015, Ch. 7, pp. 231–289.

[59].   Tropsha A. Recent trends in quantitative structure-activity relationships. In: Abraham DJ, Ed., *Burger's Medicinal Chemistry and Drug Discovery*. John Wiley & Sons, Hoboken, 2003, pp. 49–76.

[60].   Dastmalchi S, Hamzeh-Mivehroud M, Sokouti B. Molecular descriptors. In: *Quantitative Structure–Activity Relationship: A Practical Approach*. CRC Press, Boca Raton, 2018, Ch. 3, pp. 11–24.

[61].   Engel T. Cheminformatics in diverse dimensions. In: Clark T, Banting L, Eds., *Drug Design Strategies Computational Techniques and Applications*. The Royal Society of Chemistry, Cambridge, 2012, pp. 164–183.

[62].   Roy K, Mitra I. Electrotopological state atom (E-state) index in drug design, QSAR, property prediction and toxicity assessment. *Curr Comput Aid Drug Des* 2012;8(2):135–158.

[63].   Consonni V, Todeschini R, Pavan M. Structure/response correlations and similarity/diversity analysis by GETAWAY descriptors. 1. Theory of the novel 3D molecular descriptors. *J Chem Inf Comput Sci* 2002;42(3):682–692.

[64].   Todeschini R, Gramatica P. New 3D molecular descriptors: The WHIM theory and QSAR applications. In: Kubinyi H, Folkers G, Martin YC, Eds., *3D QSAR in Drug Design*. Springer, Dordrecht, 2002, pp. 355–380.

[65].   Devinyak O, Havrylyuk D, Lesyk R. 3D-MoRSE descriptors explained. *J Mol Graph Modell* 2014;54:194–203.

[66].   Mauri A, Consonni V, Todeschini R. Molecular descriptors. In: Leszczynski J, Ed., *Handbook of Computational Chemistry*. Springer, Dordrecht, 2016, pp. 1–29.

[67].   Goodarzi M, Dejaegher B, Vander Heyden Y. Feature selection methods in QSAR studies. *J AOAC Int* 2012;95(3):636–651.

[68].   Shahlaei M. Descriptor selection methods in quantitative structure-activity relationship studies: A review study. *Chem Rev* 2013;113(10):8093–8103.

[69].   Khan PM, Roy K. Current approaches for choosing feature selection and learning algorithms in quantitative structure-activity relationships (QSAR). *Expert Opin Drug Discov* 2018;13(12):1075–1089.

[70].   Golbraikh A, Tropsha A. Beware of q2! *J Mol Graph Modell* 2002;20(4):269–276.

[71].   Roy K, Kar S, Das RN. Statistical methods in QSAR/QSPR. In: *A Primer on QSAR/QSPR Modeling Fundamental Concepts*. Springer, Cham, 2015.

[72].   Dastmalchi S, Hamzeh-Mivehroud M, Sokouti B. Model building. In: *Quantitative Structure–Activity Relationship: A Practical Approach*. CRC Press, Boca Raton, 2018, Ch. 5, pp. 35–51.

[73].   Jolliffe IT. *Principal Component Analysis*, 2nd ed., Springer, New York, 2002, pp. 1–457.

[74].   Johnson RA, Wichern DW. Principal components. In: *Applied Multivariate Statistical Analysis*, 6th ed., Pearson Prentice Hall, 2007, Ch. 8, pp. 430–480.

[75].   Yoo C, Shahlaei M. The applications of PCA in QSAR studies: A case study on CCR5 antagonists. *Chem Biol Drug Des* 2018;91(1):137–152.

[76].   Golbraikh A, Shen M, Xiao Z, et al. Rational selection of training and test sets for the development of validated QSAR models. *J Comput Aid Mol Des* 2003;17(2–4):241–253.

[77].   Todeschini R, Ballabio D, Grisoni F. Beware of unreliable Q2! A comparative study of regression metrics for predictivity assessment of QSAR models. *J Chem Inf Model* 2016;56(10):1905–1913.

[78]. Rücker C, Rücker G, Meringer M. Y-randomization and its variants in QSPR/QSAR. *J Chem Inf Model* 2007;47(6):2345–2357.

[79]. Tropsha A, Gramatica P, Gombar VK. The importance of being earnest: Validation is the absolute essential for successful application and interpretation of QSPR models. *QSAR Comb Sci* 2003;22(1):69–77.

[80]. Ren YY, Zhou LC, Yang L, et al. Predicting the aquatic toxicity mode of action using logistic regression and linear discriminant analysis. *SAR QSAR Environ Res* 2016;27(9):721–746.

[81]. Pérez-Garrido A, Helguera AM, Borges F, et al. Two new parameters based on distances in a receiver operating characteristic chart for the selection of classification models. *J Chem Inf Model* 2011;51(10):2746–2759.

[82]. Gálvez-Llompart M, Recio MC, García-Domenech R. Topological virtual screening: A way to find new compounds active in ulcerative colitis by inhibiting NF-κB. *Mol Divers* 2011;15(4):917–926.

[83]. Roy K, Mitra I. On various metrics used for validation of predictive QSAR models with applications in virtual screening and focused library design. *Comb Chem High Throughput Screen* 2011;14(6):450–474.

[84]. Roy K, Kar S, Das RN. Validation of QSAR model. In: Roy K, Kar S, Das RN, Eds., *Understanding the Basics of QSAR for Applications in Pharmaceutical Sciences and Risk Assessment*. Academic Press, London, UK, 2015, Ch. 7, pp. 231–286.

[85]. Fawcett T. An introduction to ROC analysis. *Pattern Recognit Lett* 2006;27(8):861–874.

[86]. Zhang H, Ding L, Zou Y, et al. Predicting drug-induced liver injury in human with Naïve Bayes classifier approach. *J Comput Aid Mol Des* 2016;30(10):889–898.

[87]. Liu LL, Lu J, Lu Y, et al. Novel Bayesian classification models for predicting compounds blocking hERG potassium channels. *Acta Pharmacol Sin* 2014;35(8):1093–1102.

[88]. Klon AE, Lowrie JF, Diller DJ. Improved naïve Bayesian modeling of numerical data for absorption, distribution, metabolism and excretion (ADME) property prediction. *J Chem Inf Model* 2006;46(5):1945–1956.

[89]. Das S, Amin SA, Jha T. Insight into the structural requirement of arylsulphonamide based gelatinases (MMP-2 and MMP-9) inhibitors - Part I: 2D-QSAR, 3D-QSAR topomer CoMFA and Naïve Bayes studies - First report of 3D-QSAR topomer CoMFA analysis for MMP-9 inhibitors and jointly inhibitors of gelatinases together. *SAR QSAR Environ Res* 2021;32(8):655–687.

[90]. Adhikari N, Amin SA, Saha A, et al. Structural exploration for the refinement of anticancer matrix metalloproteinase-2 inhibitor designing approaches through robust validated multi-QSARs. *J Mol Struct* 2018;1156:501–515.

[91]. Adhikari N, Amin SA, Saha A. et al. Exploring in house glutamate inhibitors of matrix metalloproteinase-2 through validated robust chemico-biological quantitative approaches. *Struct Chem* 2018;29(1):285–297.

[92]. Jha T, Adhikari N, Saha A, et al. Multiple molecular modeling studies on some derivatives and analogues of glutamic acid as matrix metalloproteinase-2 inhibitors. *SAR QSAR Environ Res* 2018;29(1):43–68.

[93]. Das S, Amin SA, Gayen S, et al. Insight into the structural requirements of gelatinases (MMP-2 and MMP-9) inhibitors by multiple validated molecular modeling approaches: Part II. *SAR QSAR Environ Res* 2022;33(3):167–192.

[94]. Amin SA, Adhikari N, Jha T. Development of decision trees to discriminate HDAC8 inhibitors and non-inhibitors using recursive partitioning. *J Biomol Struct Dyn* 2021;39(1):1–8.

[95]. Chen L, Li Y, Zhao Q, et al. ADME evaluation in drug discovery. 10. Predictions of P-glycoprotein inhibitors using recursive partitioning and naive Bayesian classification techniques. *Mol Pharm* 2011;8(3):889–900.

[96]. Amin SA, Adhikari N, Jha T, et al. First molecular modeling report on novel arylpyrimidine kynurenine monooxygenase inhibitors through multi-QSAR analysis against Huntington's disease: A proposal to chemists! *Bioorg Med Chem Lett* 2016;26(23):5712–5718.

[97]. Amin SA, Adhikari N, Jha T, et al. An integrated multi-QSAR modeling approach for designing knoevenagel-type indoles with enhancing cytotoxic profiles. *Curr Comput Aid Drug Des* 2017;13(4):336–345.

[98]. Hall M, Frank E, Holmes G, et al. The WEKA data mining software: An update. *ACM SIGKDD Explor Newslett* 2009;11(1):10–18.

[99]. Vapnik VN. The support vector method for estimating indicator functions. In: *Statistical Learning Theory.* John Wiley & Sons, New York, 1998, pp. 401–440.

[100]. Yao XJ, Panaye A, Doucet JP, et al. Comparative study of QSAR/QSPR correlations using support vector machines, radial basis function neural networks, and multiple linear regression. *J Chem Inf Comput Sci* 2004;44(4):1257–1266.

[101]. Evgeniou T, Pontil M. Support vector machines: Theory and applications. In: Paliouras G, Karkaletsis V, Spyropoulos CD, Eds., *Machine Learning and Its Applications. ACAI 1999. Lecture Notes in Computer Science.* Springer, Berlin, Heidelberg, 2001, pp. 249–257.

[102]. Livingstone DJ, Manallack DT. Statistics using neural networks: Chance effects. *J Med Chem* 1993;36(9):1295–1297.

[103]. Tetko. IV, Livingstone DJ, Luik AI. Neural network studies. 1. Comparison of overfitting and overtraining. *J Chem Inf Model* 1995;35(5):826–833.

[104]. Livingstone DJ, Manallack DT, Tetko IV. Data modeling with neural networks: Advantages and limitations. *J Comput Aid Mol Des* 1997;11(2):135–142.

[105]. Shi W, Zhang X, Shen Q. Quantitative structure-activity relationships studies of CCR5 inhibitors and toxicity of aromatic compounds using gene expression programming. *Eur J Med Chem* 2010;45(1):49–54.

[106]. Gramatica P. Principles of QSAR models validation: Internal and external. *QSAR Comb Sci* 2007;26(5):694–701.

[107]. Jaworska J, Nikolova-Jeliazkova N, Aldenberg T. QSAR applicabilty domain estimation by projection of the training set descriptor space: A review. *Altern Lab Anim* 2005;33(5):445–459.

[108]. http://www.biobyte.com/bb/prod/cqsar.html as accessed in April 2022.

[109]. https://www.vlifesciences.com/products/QSARPro/Product_QSARpro.php as accessed in April 2022.

[110]. https://www.simulations-plus.com/software/admetpredictor/medchem-studio/ as accessed in April 2022.

[111]. http://www.semichem.com/codessa/default.php as accessed in April 2022.

[112]. http://www.openmolgrid.org/?m=1&s=11 as accessed in April 2022.

[113]. https://www.compudrug.com/codessa_pro as accessed in April 2022.

[114]. http://www.multicase.com/case-ultra as accessed in April 2022.

[115]. https://www.karwath.org/smirep/ as accessed in April 2022.

[116]. https://mt.mahidol.ac.th/autoweka/ as accessed in April 2022.

[117]. https://dtclab.webs.com/software-tools as accessed in April 2022.

[118]. http://michem.disat.unimib.it/mole_db/ as accessed in April 2022.

[119]. https://michem.unimib.it/download/data/ as accessed in April 2022.

[120]. https://www.ochem.eu/home/show.do as accessed in April 2022.

[121]. http://chemsar.scbdd.com/ as accessed in April 2022.

[122]. https://chembench.mml.unc.edu/ as accessed in April 2022.

[123]. http://www.vcclab.org/lab/pls/ as accessed in April 2022.

2 3D-QSAR Studies
CoMFA, CoMSIA, and Topomer CoMFA Methods

Suvankar Banerjee, Sandip Kumar Baidya,
Nilanjan Adhikari, and Tarun Jha

CONTENTS

ABSTRACT

In this chapter, the overall aspects of 3D-QSAR methodologies related to drug design and discovery are highlighted. The implication of the most popular widely applied field-based 3D-QSAR approaches, such as comparative molecular field analysis (CoMFA) and comparative molecular similarity indices analysis (CoMSIA), as well as their methodologies, including their basis, field-based molecular interaction energy calculation, advantages, and disadvantages, are discussed in detail. In addition, other 3D-QSAR techniques and their implications (such as GRID, MSA,

DOI: 10.1201/9781003303282-3

GRIND, RSA, SOMFA, GERM, VolSurf, Compass, CoSA, CoRIA, COMBINE, etc.) in drug design and discovery processes are highlighted in detail.

Keywords: 3D-QSAR; CoMFA; CoMSIA; Topomer CoMFA

2.1 INTRODUCTION

Quantitative structure-activity relationship (QSAR) methodologies have been applied in chemoinformatics over many years to tally the structural and physico-chemical properties of bioactive compounds with their biological efficacy [1–4]. Fundamentally, QSAR techniques correlate and identify the relationship between the structural variance of a set of molecules and their biological efficacy. From a simpler perspective, QSAR methodologies help to identify the effect of structural variance/similarities (quantifiable) of a group of compounds with their biological activity through statistical models/methods. The QSAR technique can be grouped into various classes depending upon the calculation method of the independent variables, such as 0D-, 1D-, 2D, 3D, 4D, 5D, and 6D as well as 7D-QSAR methods [1, 2]. Among these various QSAR classes, the 2D and 3D-QSAR methodologies are the most frequently used QSAR techniques. In this chapter, a brief history of QSAR and 3D-QSAR method development and popular 3D-QSAR methods like comparative molecular field analysis (CoMFA), comparative molecular similarity indices analysis (CoMSIA), and Topomer CoMFA methods are discussed while providing a glimpse of other 3D-QSAR techniques that are used to correlate the 3D features of bioactive compounds with their biological responses.

2.2 HISTORY/ORIGIN OF 3D-QSAR STUDY

The concept of quantitatively correlating attributes of small bioactive molecules with their biological responses can be first found in the study of Crum-Brown and Fraser in 1868 [5]. The preliminary concept of modern QSAR methodologies was proposed in the work of Corwin Hansch and Toshio Fujita in 1964 [6]. Their works have been recognized as Hansch analysis followed by Free-Wilson analysis [7]. Modern QSAR approaches are advanced and sophisticated derivatives of the aforementioned ideas that evolved through time and technology. A brief history of the earlier events of the development of the QSAR technique is depicted in Figure 2.1 [3, 5–22].

The first concept of the 3D-QSAR technique was proposed by Cramer and co-workers in 1983 and was developed in 1988 [22]. Besides the 2D- and 3D-QSAR approaches, other higher multidimensional QSAR approaches have also been developed (such as 4D-QSAR, 5D-QSAR, etc.), which are not more than an advanced modification of the common QSAR techniques.

The first 3D-QSAR technique was suggested as the dynamic lattice-oriented molecular modeling system (DYLOMMS) in the work of Wise and Cramer in 1983 [20]. The DYLOMMS utilizes the principal component analysis (PCA)-mediated extraction of vector values of the molecular interaction fields (MIFs) to correlate them with the biological activity of the molecules. In 1985, Goodford provided

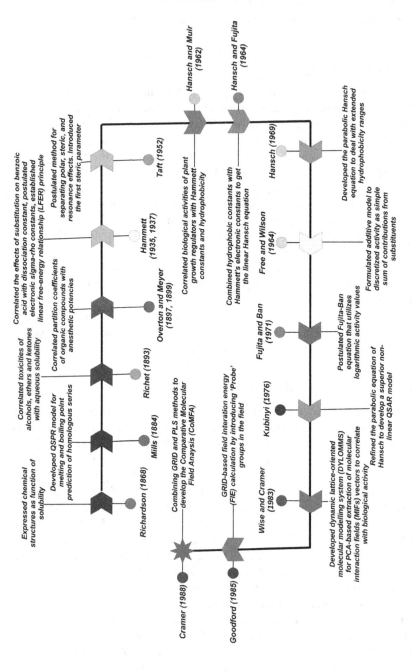

FIGURE 2.1 A schematic representation of the history of QSAR technology development.

another "GRID"-based approach to calculate the field interaction energy (FIE) by introducing "Probe" groups in the field [21]. Later, in 1988, by combining the GRID and partial least square (PLS) methods, Cramer and co-workers developed the 3D-QSAR technique, which is today popular with the name "comparative molecular field analysis (CoMFA)" [22].

2.3 COMPARATIVE MOLECULAR FIELD ANALYSIS

CoMFA is one of the prime 3D-QSAR techniques for performing the QSAR study of bioactive molecule studies. CoMFA is an alignment-dependent ligand-based 3D-QSAR technique that mainly deals with the steric and electrostatic fields of molecules in the 3D space. As discussed earlier, the CoMFA method was first introduced in the work of Cramer and co-workers [22]. CoMFA employs a 3D lattice-based field calculation of molecular energies and correlates them with their biological activity.

In their study, Cramer et al. [22] demonstrated that the four crucial aspects of performing the CoMFA method are as follows:

a. Steric and electrostatic field-based representation of small molecules via 3D-lattice intersection sampling.
b. "Fit field" technique for the mutual alignment of molecules through minimum root mean square (RMS)-based field differences.
c. PLS-based cross-validation-mediated analysis of the 3D data of aligned molecules for likelihood and predictable validation.
d. Graphical representation of the outcomes as field-based contour maps around the aligned ligands/molecules into the 3D space.

In CoMFA, the Lennard-Jones equation **2.1** is used to calculate the van der Waals steric field, whereas the Coulombic equation **2.2** is applied to estimate the electrostatic field inside the 3D lattice. The van der Waals steric values are calculated using the standard Tripos Force Field, where the Gasteiger–Marsili method calculates the atomic charges [1, 23, 24].

$$V_{LJ} = 4\varepsilon\left[\left(\frac{\sigma}{r}\right)^{12} - \left(\frac{\sigma}{r}\right)^{6}\right] = \varepsilon\left[\left(\frac{r_m}{r}\right)^{12} - \left(\frac{r_m}{r}\right)^{6}\right] \tag{2.1}$$

In equation **2.1**, ε refers to the potential well depth, σ indicates the distance value at which the interparticle potential is zero, r_m is the distance at which the potential is maximum, and r symbolizes the interparticle distance

$$E = \left[\frac{q_1 q_2}{4\pi\varepsilon r}\right] \tag{2.2}$$

In equation **2.2**, ε indicates the dielectric constant for the medium, Q_1, and Q_2 are the point charges at the distance r.

Also, 2Å grid intersection spacing is used inside the 3D lattice. Besides, the molecules/ligands are on a common scaffold of the molecules. Now, for calculating steric and electrostatic energies, different "probes" are introduced at each intersection of the 3D lattice. Additionally, to eliminate the singularities depicted by the Lennard and Coulombic potentials, an energy cut-off value of ± 30 kcal/mol is settled for the calculated energies. Now, each of the introduced probes with specific charge and hybridization experiences a steric repulsion greater than the cut-off values used for PLS-based analysis. One of the benefits of this study is like all the procured energy values that have been used as descriptors, they all bear the same units (kcal/mol), therefore avoiding the necessity of descriptor auto-scaling. The PLS analysis of the data is represented as correlation equations along with latent variables (LVs). Finally, the graphical representation of the CoMFA study is visualized using 3D-coefficient contour maps [1–3, 22].

2.3.1 CoMFA Methodology

The steps that are involved in the CoMFA methodologies are shown in Figure 2.2 and as well as described below:

i) The molecular structures of the compounds (2D) are sketched and converted into their respective 3D structures.

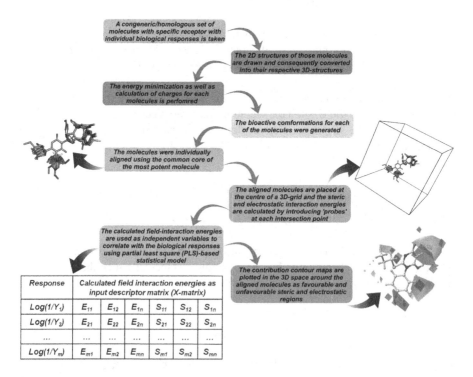

FIGURE 2.2   A schematic representation of CoMFA methodology.

ii) The molecules are subjected to energy minimization followed by charge calculation.

iii) The molecules are aligned on the common scaffold manually or with the help of different automated techniques.

iv) After the molecular alignment, the superimposed compounds are taken at the center of a 3D lattice with a grid interaction distance of 2Å.

v) In the 3D space, the van der Waals steric fields are estimated with the help of the Lennard-Jones equation **2.1**, whereas the Coulombic interactions equation **2.2** is used to calculate the electrostatic field inside the 3D lattice.

vi) With the calculation of the molecular fields, the probes with specific hybridization and charges are introduced into each intersection present in the lattice.

vii) After that, the interaction energy values are calculated at each intersection to generate a set of descriptors that will serve as the independent parameters for the model building and correlate with the biological responses of the set of molecules.

viii) For CoMFA, the PLS-based technique is used to extract and identify the important features and their significance/influence on biological activity in a linear fashion.

ix) For the visualization of the model outcomes, the results from the PLS analysis are visualized graphically as contours. Here, the coefficients from the PLS model are represented by 3D coefficient contour maps around the superimposed molecules inside the 3D lattice in a different color (generally, the green-yellow and blue-red color combinations are used to illustrate the favorable and unfavorable field areas for steric and electrostatic field coefficients, respectively).

x) Besides that, the performance of the CoMFA analysis is carried out by calculating the correlation coefficient (R/R^2) values of the independent variables and the biological responses from the constructed PLS model. Here, external validation may also be carried out on an external set of molecules with the help of the developed PLS model by calculating the externally cross-validated squared correlation coefficient (R^2_{Ext-CV}/R^2_{Pred}) values to adjudicate the reliability and predictive capability of the CoMFA model.

2.3.2 ADVANTAGES AND DISADVANTAGES OF CoMFA

From the first use of the CoMFA method, it has been primarily applied in medicinal chemistry and other related fields because of its high interpretability and capability to identify the importance of specific fields (i.e., steric and electrostatic) near bioactive molecules. These are important for receptor-ligand interactions and the ability to design newer bioactive compounds. The advantages and drawbacks of CoMFA are mentioned below:

i) The CoMFA method is relatively facile for almost any set of molecules that are aligned on a common substructure present in those molecules.

ii) It deals with two fundamental yet crucial molecular fields (i.e., steric and electrostatic fields) that have an important role in the receptor-ligand interactions for the bioactive molecules.

iii) The interactive 3D visualization of the CoMFA study helps to scrutinize the importance of a specific group of aligned molecules depending on the CoMFA-generated 3D-coefficient-contour map with different color coding.

iv) Each of the CoMFA parameters represents the interaction energy of the entire molecule.

v) As CoMFA provides an interactive visualization of the outcomes around the ligands/aligned molecules in 3D space, the interpretation of the outcomes is extremely easy.

vi) Only a few inputs like the 3D structure of molecules, alignment rule, and the lattice description of the molecule are required. These yield the model predictions, model performance summary, and important field contributions that can be visualized graphically as 3D coefficient contour maps.

Apart from the advantages, CoMFA also has some important limitations that are discussed below:

i) CoMFA is an alignment-dependent 3D-QSAR approach where the mutual alignment of the ligands plays a quite crucial role in field energy calculation, model development, and 3D contour visualization. A set of compounds with some common scaffold can be used for CoMFA, but with a set of ligands with high structural diversity, molecular alignment can be quite an important issue that can affect the study's outcome.

ii) Utilization of too many variables, such as the step size, type of probe atoms, the overall orientation of molecules, and lattice placement.

iii) The use of cut-off limits for interaction energy inside the 3D lattice.

iv) Suitable for *in vitro* data.

v) Hydrophobicity is not well-quantified.

vi) Flaws in the potential energy function.

vii) Improbability in molecule and variable selection.

viii) The presence of a low signal-to-noise ratio because of unnecessary field values.

2.3.3 Factors Affecting the Performance and Outcome of CoMFA

Although CoMFA is quite useful to correlate the molecular interaction fields with their biological responses, there are quite a few variables/factors that can influence the performance and outcomes of CoMFA.

2.3.3.1 Diversity of Molecules and Molecular Alignment

As the molecular alignment of the set of molecules is crucial for CoMFA studies, a CoMFA study is preferable for molecules of congeneric series. More diversity in the common scaffold of a series of ligands can provide deviated results from the actual improper outcome. Several processes/techniques can be adopted for molecular alignment, such as:

- *Atomic overlapping-based alignment*
  This molecular alignment method is based on the atom-to-atom pairing between the molecules and is also popular as a pharmacophore-based technique. This is a quite famous method of molecular alignment that requires a common substructure and aligns the molecules based on the common structure present in the molecules. It can provide the best mapping of the preselected atoms based on their positions.
- *Alignment based on the binding site*
  This method may be employed by superimposing the active site/active site residues interacting with the ligand of a protein. This method of alignment is supposed to be more feasible because of its increased degree of freedom despite having problems in conformational analysis.
- *Pseudo-field/field-based alignment*
  For this technique, the molecules are superimposed based on calculated interaction field energy present between two molecules where similarities of molecular surface and electrostatic energy can be used for this type of molecular alignment.
- *Multiple conformer-based alignments*
  This method is applicable for situations where the ligand may bind to the receptor in multiple conformations or for an unknown ligand with a reasonable amount of flexibility and/or degree of freedom. For example, a 3D-QSAR method like Compass or Topomer CoMFA [25, 26]. These methods are used for the interactive determination of the best bioactive conformation selection and the optimal alignment from a set of initial poses of molecules.

2.3.3.2 Biological Activity/Data of the Molecules

Similar to other QSAR methodologies, the more accurate and precise biological data of a set of ligands is important for creating a good CoMFA model. There is more than one condition that is required to be maintained for a good CoMFA model:

- All the molecules subjected to the CoMFA study must be congeneric in nature.
- All the ligands should have similar methods/mechanisms of action.
- The biological response of all the molecules should obviously be tested using the same protocol.
- The biological activities should be correlated with their binding affinity.
- The biological responses must be in the same unit of measurement (e.g., K_i, IC_{50}, EC_{50}, LD_{50}), and symmetrical activity distribution throughout the set is preferable.
- The variation in the biological activity of the molecules should be as much as possible.

2.3.3.3 3D Ligand-Structure Optimization

The structural representation of the initial molecules is an important subject of concern for 3D-QSAR studies such as CoMFA. In this scenario, both computation and experimental approaches may be utilized to obtain the initial conformation of molecules that are subjected to CoMFA [1, 3].

For the experimental approach, crystal-bound ligands can be used for confirmation detection. This will experimentally determine the protein-bound ligand structure of a molecule with proper biological conformation. The crystal structure can be accessed from databases like the protein data bank [27], the Cambridge Crystallographic Data Center [28], and so on.

Apart from that, computationally, the 3D structures of the desired molecules can be generated by several different processes, such as:

- Manually drawing the 3D structure of the molecule using an interactive 3D graphic interface from an existing fragment library.
- Numerically, the structures can be generated from quantum mechanics (QM) or molecular mechanics (MM) and distance geometry with the help of mathematical techniques.
- By using automatic methods that can be employed to create 3D molecular structure databases.

Also, when one of the 3D molecular structure generations is completed, structural optimization of the 3D structure can be performed by conformational energy minimization to refine structural geometries. This can be achieved through the following methods [1, 3]:

- *Molecular mechanics*
  This method is fast and accurate, although it does not precisely require electronic motion. It can be used for a larger molecular structure, such as proteins/enzymes.
- *Ab initio/quantum mechanics*
  Due to its consideration of 3D electronic distribution around the nuclei, this type of method is highly precise, time-consuming, computationally intensive, and is not used for macromolecular structures.
- *Semi-empirical*
  This type of method generally relies on quantum mechanics that attempt to address the low accuracy and slow speed of the quantum mechanical methods by avoiding some factors such as atomic ionization energies and molecular dipole moments. These methods, therefore, use approximations.

Typically, in this method, the geometry optimization of the molecules is performed by molecular mechanics, where the atomic charges are calculated by ab initio or the empirical method. This method of structural refinement is fast and can be used for large molecules that may provide accurate outcomes for the molecules that have similarities with the molecules used for parameterization [1, 3].

2.3.3.4 Conformational Analysis of Molecules

The confirmation of the bioactive molecules is one of the important factors for accurate model generation. The molecules with single bonds (one or more) can exist in different conformations, which are known as rotamers or conformers. Therefore, several rotamers can exist in the biological system for a specific molecule. Hence, analysis of the structural conformations is a crucial factor for 3D-QSAR studies like CoMFA. Thus, to search and analyze the conformation of molecules that will be subjected to the CoMFA study, the following methods can be adopted:

- *Systemic/grid search*
    This method is capable of producing all possible conformations of a molecule systematically, which varies in each of the torsion angles by increments while keeping the bond lengths and angles fixed for a molecule.
- *Random search*
    This method can produce a set of conformations for a molecule by arbitrarily and repetitively changing the Cartesian coordinates or the bond angle, bond length, and torsion/dihedral angles of the molecules while taking the starting geometry under consideration.
- *Monte Carlo*:
    This method simulates the dynamic behavior of a molecule to generate different conformations via making random changes in the molecular structure, comparing the energy of the conformation with the previous one, and taking aspects of the results if a unique conformation is found.
- *Molecular dynamics*
    This method utilizes Newton's second law (force = mass × acceleration) to perform a time-dependent simulation of molecules and acquire the conformational changes and movement of a molecule in a molecular system. The yields of the trajectory of the molecular movement elucidate the position and velocity of the atoms in the molecular system that varies with time.
- *Simulated annealing*
    This method uses heating a molecular system to overcome high energy barriers under the consideration of high temperature, which, after equilibrating via molecular dynamics for some time, is cooled down gradually to process low-energy conformations according to Boltzmann distribution.
- *Distance geometry algorithm*
    This method forms constraints in a distance matrix by generating a random set of coordinates through random distance selection within each pair of upper and lower bounds, which are used to create energetically viable structural conformations for a molecule.
- *Evolutionary and/or genetic algorithm*
    This process utilizes the biological evaluation process where a pool/population of a possible solution is created at the primary stage. Therefore, the solution with the best fitness score is crossed over and mutated over time, which propagates the good properties down the generations to deliver a better solution as new molecular conformers/conformations.

2.3.3.5 Biological Conformation Determination of Molecules

A bioactive conformer of a molecule symbolizes the conformation of a molecule that is formed during the ligand-protein interaction to provide an experimental biological activity. The intra-molecular forces between the atom of a molecule and the inter-molecular forces between the molecule and the surrounding environment govern bioactive conformation. Therefore, as 3D-QSAR studies, like CoMFA, correlate the biological response of a molecule along with its 3D conformation, the reliability of the CoMFA study is dependent on the bioactive conformation of the molecules. The estimation of the bioactive conformation of the molecules can be performed both experimentally as well as computationally:

- *X-ray crystallographic data of target-bound bioactive molecules*

  X-ray crystallography is a method that can elucidate a precise 3D structure of macromolecules (e.g., proteins). The crystallographic data of biological macromolecules contains a bioactive molecule bound to them, which can easily provide the bioactive conformation of that ligand molecule, which can be used for 3D-QSAR studies. However, some of the disadvantages associated with this method are:
  - To acquire the crystallographic data of a protein molecule, the macromolecule is required to be crystallized where the crystallizing media formation may not be similar to the physiological conditions.
  - Structural distortion of molecules can occur during crystal packing.
  - Because of the occlusion of the active site and crystal stability, the diffusion of substrate or other bioactive molecules into the crystals is frequently not possible.
  - For the crystallographic data, there is the possibility of the presence of errors during ligand-structure determination.
  - In protein-bound structures, the determination of the positions of the hydrogen atoms can be deceptive.
  - The unavailability of a crystal-bound conformer for all the molecules is a major concern, where the determination of bioactive conformation for all the molecules from a set is quite time-consuming. On the other hand, determining the bioactive conformation of the rest of the molecules from one or more crystal-bound conformations for a molecular set may not provide precise results.
- *NMR spectroscopy*

  This method is used to elucidate the 3D structural data in solution and can be the technique of choice for cases where there is a failure to crystallize the molecule via experimental means. As for the membrane-bound receptors and other receptors, those are yet to be isolated because of the stability, resolution, and other issues. The salient features/attributes of these processes are:
  - As no crystallization of protein is needed for this process, the protein conformation is unaffected by the packing forces of the crystal environment.

- The conditions for the solution, such as ionic strength, substrate, pH, and temperature, can be customized to correlate with the physiological conditions.
- The process applies to smaller molecules, which consumes less time.
- The position of the hydrogen atoms of compounds can be resolved.
- The conformation obtained through NMR can be dissimilar to the one procured from the experimental method and may or may not represent the receptor-bound conformation.
- It is possible to acquire crucial dynamic information regarding the molecular motion of ligands from this method.
- The presence of apolar/non-polar solvents in the solution may lead to overestimated hydrogen bonding.

Theoretically, the 3D structure and spatial information regarding the bioactive conformation of molecules can be collected by employing knowledge-based approaches such as homology modeling, where the primary amino acid sequence of new/unknown proteins can be constructed and compared to the known sequences of structurally similar proteins available in the database, such as RCSB PDB [27].

Also, other methods, such as molecular docking analysis of the molecules at the active site of the protein and molecular dynamic (MD) simulation of protein-ligand complexes, can elucidate or predict the bioactive conformation of molecules.

2.3.3.6 Molecular Interaction Energy Field Calculation

For CoMFA, the estimation of molecular interaction energy fields is a crucial step for independent variable (descriptor) generation. Therefore, as we can recapitulate, for CoMFA, alignment/superimposed molecular structures are located at the center of a 3D lattice with grid intersections and probe introduction for interaction energy calculation [3, 22, 29, 30]. Thus, several factors need to be addressed while calculating interaction energies, such as:

- The position of the grid box has a crucial effect on the statistical evaluation of the CoMFA model, specifically for the number of components present in the PLS model. Hence, typically, the elementary models for CoMFA are developed at diverse locations to identify the best position inside the grid.
- The grid spacing for the 3D lattice is generally 2Å and is inversely proportional to the precision of the calculations. Hence, if the grid spacing is decreased, the exhaustiveness of the calculations is increased, and vice-versa.
- The size of the grid box is also a crucial factor in influencing the outcomes of the CoMFA study. Generally, the grid box size is 3–4Å larger compared with the total surface of the aligned molecules. Therefore, Coulombic electrostatic, as well as van der Waals steric interaction, consists of a long range, and a larger grid box may be preferable.
- The "probes" are one crucial part of the CoMFA interaction energy calculation inside the lattice, which can be small molecules such as water or groups

like the methyl group with specific charge and hybridization. Typically, the electrostatic energies are calculated using the incorporation of H^+ probes, whereas carbon atoms with sp^3 hybridization, 1.53Å effective radius, and a charge of 1.0 are used for steric energy calculation. Therefore, changes in the introduced probes can affect the calculation of interaction energies, thus affecting the outcome of CoMFA studies.

- The CoMFA technique utilizes the Lennard-Jones and Coulombic equations to estimate the steric and electrostatic field interactions, respectively. This potential displays singularity at atomic positions to avoid such singularity; an energy cut-off value ($\pm$ 30 kcal/mol) is used for interaction energy calculation.

- A forcefield can be defined as the combination of bond lengths, dihedral angles, interatomic distance, bond angles with coordinates, and other molecular features empirically fitting the potential energy surface. Primary forces like electrostatic, steric, hydrophobic, and hydrogen bonding interactions are mainly observed during receptor-ligand interactions, where the hydrogen bonding and electrostatic interactions are responsible for ligand-receptor specificity, and hydrophobic and steric interaction delivers binding strength.

2.4 COMPARATIVE MOLECULAR SIMILARITY INDICES ANALYSIS

CoMSIA is another grid and field-interaction-based 3D-QSAR technique quite similar to the CoMFA method. Unlike the CoMFA technique, five different similarity fields, steric, electrostatic, hydrophobic, hydrogen bond donor, and hydrogen bond acceptor fields, are examined for the superimposed set of molecules at regular grid spacing points inside the 3D lattice [1–3, 31, 32].

For the CoMFA methodology, the potential energy at specific distance grid intersection points is used for mapping the gradual changes in the interaction energies of aligned molecules, but in the CoMFA method, the entropic parameters are crucial for the binding affinity of ligands with a specific protein not considered [31, 32]. Also, CoMFA has a few problems, such as:

- The step proximity of the Lennard-Jones potential to the van der Waals surface leads to a drastic change in the potential energy expressed at the grid point near the molecular surface.

- The use of Coulombic and Lennard-Jones potential depicts singularity at the atomic position. To circumvent such a problem and to avoid a large value, arbitrary cut-off values for interaction energy are used; the potential evaluation is limited in the regions outside the molecules. Because of the variation in the potential and slope, the cut-off values are exceeded for different terms and different molecular distances [33], which requires ability settings for the simulation evaluation of two molecular fields. Therefore, loss of information may occur in the processes.

Therefore, in CoMSIA, the calculation of similarity indices fields is introduced to overcome the abovementioned problems to describe the differences between the superimposed molecules. These similarity indices are estimated for each superimposed molecule by introducing a common probe at each of the grid interaction points. Also, unlike CoMFA, Gaussian-type functions are used to calculate the interactions. As the Gaussian potentials are devoid of singularities, in CoMSIA, no energy cutoff values are required for the calculation. In this process, five different properties, such as hydrophobic, electrostatic, steric, hydrogen bond donor and hydrogen bond acceptor capabilities, which are crucial and fundamental factors for binding affinity, are calculated as field similarity indices. Similar to the CoMFA method, the PLS-based analysis is also performed to establish the correlation between the molecular similarity indices and the biological responses of the molecules. The step-by-step methodology is also quite similar (Figure 2.3) to that of the CoMFA study.

2.4.1 THE METHODOLOGY OF CoMSIA

i) In the interceptive step, conformations are generated for the set of molecules that will be subjected to CoMSIA.

ii) Energy minimization and calculation of charges are performed for the molecules. This calculation of the partial atomic charges can be done with the help of the Gasteiger–Huckle method, dipole charges, Mulliken analysis, Voronoi deformation density, and other density-derived chemical and electrostatic methods.

iii) Thereafter, the molecules are superimposed on the conformation of the common scaffold of the most potent molecule from the series as the template.

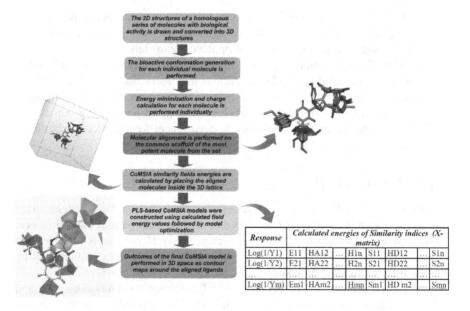

The 2D structures of a homologous series of molecules with biological activity is drawn and converted into 3D structures

The bioactive conformation generation for each individual molecule is performed

Energy minimization and charge calculation for each molecule is performed individually

Molecular alignment is performed on the common scaffold of the most potent molecule from the set

CoMSIA similarity fields energies are calculated by placing the aligned molecules inside the 3D lattice

PLS-based CoMSIA models were constructed using calculated field energy values followed by model optimization

Outcomes of the final CoMSIA model is performed in 3D space as contour maps around the aligned ligands

Response	Calculated energies of Similarity indices (X-matrix)							
Log(1/Y1)	E11	HA12	...	H1n	S11	HD12	...	S1n
Log(1/Y2)	E21	HA22	...	H2n	S21	HD22	...	S2n
...	...	...	...	...	...	...	...	...
Log(1/Ym)	Em1	HAm2	...	Hmn	Sm1	HD m2	...	Smn

FIGURE 2.3 A schematic representation of CoMSIA methodology.

iv) Then, the five physiochemical properties are calculated for each of the aligned molecules by introducing a common probe with a unit (value = 1) radius (Å) and hydrophobicity and hydrogen bond donor-acceptor properties. Here, the grid size can be extended by 2Å in all directions far from the total molecular dimension.

v) After calculating the molecular fields, the PLS-based technique is utilized to develop the 3D-QSAR model to correlate the calculated field interaction energies with the biological responses.

vi) Finally, after the development of the valid PLS model, the field contributions are visualized via interactive coefficient contour maps around the superimposed ligands, characterized by favorable and unfavorable regions for each of the properties that are quite similar to that of the CoMFA output visualization.

2.4.2 THE ADVANTAGES OF CoMSIA

i) CoMSIA involves other physiochemical parameters (i.e., hydrophobic, hydrogen bond donor, and acceptor features) from the conventional steric and electrostatic parameters used for CoMFA. This provides an in-depth analysis of the important field contribution to protein-ligand binding.

ii) The influences of the solvent entropic information can also be considered in CoMSIA by hydrophobic probes.

iii) The use of "Gaussian distribution of similarity indices" is beneficial for avoiding undesirable alterations in the grid-based atom-probe interactions inside the 3D lattice.

iv) In CoMSIA, the selection of similarity probes is not restricted to the steric and electrostatic parameters but can also be used for hydrogen bonding (donor and acceptor) as well as hydrophobic parameters.

v) In CoMFA, the contour map only highlights the areas where the aligned molecules depicted favorable and unfavorable interactions with a probable receptor environment. Again, the contour map from CoMSIA highlights those spaces around the aligned molecules where a particular group of a molecule has favorable or unfavorable occurrences for a particular physiochemical property [1–3, 31, 32].

2.5 TOPOMER CoMFA

A topomer is generally a set of structures originating from a native molecular structure and is obtained by changing the different coordinates of a molecule while preserving the backbone covalent bonds undisrupted [34]. Hence, the topomer can be considered as a pool of different structural conformations of a molecule generated by altering the coordinates while keeping the backbone covalent bonds intact.

Molecular alignment is one of the essential processes for developing good and reliable CoMFA models. Also, it is assumed that the optimal CoMFA alignment for ligands can be achieved by aligning the ligands using their receptor-bound conformation. This type of alignment can produce an excellent CoMFA model for congeneric series and can produce higher predictive accuracy [35–38]. In the absence of such protein-bound ligand conformation, one must choose from the variety of available molecular alignment techniques. This can lead to better statistical outcomes for the CoMFA model in comparison with the actual conformations [35, 39–42]. CoMFA can passively filter lists of molecule structures, whereas building those lists of conformers is an exhaustive task. Moreover, solving the alignment-related issue for the structure of each molecule is necessary [35]. This kind of speculative task can be easily done and evaluated with the help of the universal "topomer" methodology to generate a structural fragment alignment [35, 43]. This topomer technology can provide an absolute orientation of any fragments by superimposing the common scaffold [35]. A 3D-standardized model can be developed via the rule-based adjustment of chirality and acyclic bond torsion, where aligned 3D-topomer structures should be used for the study.

The topomer CoMFA is a combination of the "topomer" method, and the CoMFA technique can be utilized for alignment-independent 3D-QSAR model development, library screening, and rapid lead optimization [22, 35].

2.5.1 THE METHODOLOGY OF TOPOMER CoMFA

The method of topomer CoMFA [26, 35] is as follows:

i) The molecules having experimental biological activities are taken in uncharged form for all the ionizable groups while ignoring the stereoisomerism.

ii) The molecules are minimized, and the charge calculation is carried out with the help of available methods (such as the Gasteiger–Marsili method).

iii) Two different fragment groups are denoted (R_1 and R_2) for the side chain fragments present in the molecules.

iv) Topomer alignment is applied to each of the molecular fragments.

v) After that, sp^3 hybridized probes are introduced to calculate the field interaction energy for each fragment. This will provide the descriptor/continuous variables for PLS analysis. Here, unlike the CoMFA method, two CoMFA columns should be required for each of the R groups (R_1 and R_2).

vi) Thereafter, the PLS technique is utilized to match the interaction energies with the biological activities in the form of a statistical model.

vii) Finally, the outcomes are interactively visualized inside the 3D space in the form of contribution contour maps around the fragments separately for each of the denoted R groups (R_1 and R_2).

2.5.2 THE ADVANTAGES OF TOPOMER CoMFA

i) As topomer CoMFA is an alignment-independent 3D-QSAR study [26], optimum molecular alignment for a diverse set of molecules with a minimum common core may be achievable to perform the 3D-QSAR analysis.

TABLE 2.1

Available 3D-QSAR Methodologies not Including CoMFA, CoMSIA, and Topomer CoMFA Studies

Sl. No.	Technique	Description	Reference
1	GRID	GRID is a 3D-QSAR technique similar to CoMFA that computes non-bonded/non-covalent interactions using probe groups and principal component analysis.	[21]
2	MSA	Molecular shape analysis (MSA) is a ligand-based 3D-QSAR technique that involves molecular conformational analysis using the Hansch approach and is associated with the characterization, representation, and manipulation of molecular shape.	[44]
3	GRIND	This method utilizes the molecular interaction field (MIF) spatial distribution of molecules encoded into *grid-*independent descriptors (GRIND) to correlate them with the biological responses.	[1, 3, 45]
4	RSA	Receptor surface analysis (RSA) is a method useful for where the 3D structure of the receptor is unknown. This process employs the genetic function approximation (GFA) or PLS technique to correlate the surface properties as interaction energies (surface point energies) with biological responses.	[46]
5	SOMFA	Self-organizing molecular field analysis (SOMFA) is a method similar to CoMFA that correlates electrostatic potential values calculated at each grid point from the master grid with the logarithmic biological activity values.	[47]
6	GERM	Genetically evolved receptor modeling (GERM) is a 3D-QSAR technique to develop a 3D-macromolecular model based on the alignment of bioactive conformers. This method utilizes the genetic algorithm (GA) function to generate possible conformers at the receptor active site and calculates interaction energies to correlate them with biological potency.	[48]
7	MQSM	Molecular quantum similarity measures (MQSM) utilize the electronic density function vectors as continuous variables.	[49]
8	AFMoC	Adaptation of the fields for molecular comparison (AFMoC) is also known as the reverse/inverted CoMFA method. In this method, the receptor protein-specific potential field calculation is done at the binding site of the protein, which is used to predict the binding affinity.	[50]
9	VFA	Voronoi field analysis (VFA) divides the aligned molecules in the 3D space to assign the Voronoi polyhedra. It calculates the potential and electrostatic energies to correlate them with biological responses via PLS model development.	[51]
10	HIFA	Hint interaction field analysis is an alignment-independent 3D-QSAR technique for empirical hydrophobic interaction calculation.	[52]

(Continued)

TABLE 2.1 (CONTINUED)

Available 3D-QSAR Methodologies not Including CoMFA, CoMSIA, and Topomer CoMFA Studies

Sl. No.	Technique	Description	Reference
11	CoMMA	Comparative molecular moment analysis (CoMMA) is another alignment-independent 3D-QSAR technique that utilizes the distribution of mass, second-order shape moments, and charge distributions. This method is a molecular conformation-sensitive technique like CoMFA.	[53]
12	VolSurf	This method introduces specific probes in the 3D grid where the descriptors are calculated based on the 3D contour volume or surfaces from the resulting lattices.	[54]
13	Compass	This method of the 3D-QSAR technique allows automatic conformation selection and molecular alignment, where a set of feature values is used to represent the molecules. Also, this method uses three physicochemical features, steric, hydrogen bond donor, and acceptors, to construct a neural network-based model for correlating them with the biological responses.	[25]
14	CoSA	Comparative spectral analysis (CoSA) is a method that employs molecular spectroscopic techniques for 3D descriptor generation and uses molecular spectra to predict biological potency.	[55]
15	HASL	Hypothetical active site lattice (HASL) is an inverse grid-based 3D-QSAR method that depicts the molecular shape of molecules as a set of grid points at the active site of the receptor.	[56]
16	COMBINE	Comparative binding energy analysis (COMBINE) is a 3D-QSAR technique that utilizes the theory of free binding energy that can be correlated with the energy component subset obtained from the bound and unbound forms of ligands and proteins. The steric and electrostatic non-bonded energies are calculated in all the pairs of protein residues and ligand fragments with the help of a molecular mechanics forcefield. Here, the PLS technique is used to correlate the biological responses with the biological potency of molecules.	[57, 58]
17	CoRIA	Comparative residue interaction analysis (CoRIA) is another 3D-QSAR method that involves thermodynamic events associated with ligand binding at the active site of the receptor protein. This method utilizes non-bonded interaction energies like steric and electrostatic interaction energies between the protein residues and the ligand molecule, as well as other physicochemical properties such as molar refractivity, lipophilicity, molecular surface area, strain energy, molecular volume, JURS descriptors, and so on to correlate with the biological activity of molecules via a genetic variant of the PLS (G/PLS) technique.	[59]

(Continued)

TABLE 2.1   (CONTINUED)

Available 3D-QSAR Methodologies not Including CoMFA, CoMSIA, and Topomer CoMFA Studies

Sl. No.	Technique	Description	Reference
18	CoMASA	Comparative molecular active site analysis (CoMASA) is an alignment-dependent 3D-QSAR method that, instead of using lattice points like CoMFA, uses the continuous removal of atoms that are proximal to each other while replacing them with pseudo atoms until the distance between the atoms/pseudo atoms becomes greater than the threshold value of 0.75 Å. Then, the calculated interaction energies are correlated with the biological responses via the PLS technique.	[60]
19	CoMPIA	Comparative molecular/pseudo receptor interaction analysis is another 3D-QSAR method that utilizes nine different hybrid atoms/probes and distributes them at each of the 3D lattices using the GA method. Also, the calculated interaction energies are correlated with the biological potencies with the help of PLS analysis.	[61]

ii) For alignment-dependent studies like CoMFA and CoMSIA, a molecular alignment is a necessary approach for model development, and the method of alignment may interfere with the model outcomes. On the other hand, this method allows for circumventing such an alignment process by using topomer generation.

iii) Topomer CoMFA depicts the contour maps around the side chain fragments from the R_1 and R_2 groups as favorable and unfavorable contour maps. This can help to identify the important effects of specific side-chain fragments of a molecule as well as the substitutions present at the different R groups on the biological response of the molecule.

iv) Topomer CoMFA is a comparatively fast and less time-consuming method that does not demand conventional process time management.

Over time, with the advancement of technology, various other 3D-QSAR techniques and techniques have been constructed (Table 2.1). These popular methods can be used diversely in QSAR-related drug discovery and development processes.

2.6 SUMMARY

In this chapter, the detailed descriptions and the techniques, along with the advantages and disadvantages of the widely accepted 3D-QSAR methodologies (mainly CoMFA, CoMSIA, and Topomer CoMFA), have been discussed in detail. Additionally, the other available 3D-QSAR methodologies have been mentioned. All these 3D-QSAR methodologies can be applied successfully for designing potential drug candidates, lead identification, lead modification, and the screening of drug-like candidates.

REFERENCES

[1]. Roy K, Kar S, Das RN. *Understanding the basics of QSAR for applications in pharmaceutical sciences and risk assessment.* Academic Press, New York, 2015.

[2]. Madhavan T. A review of 3D-QSAR in drug design. *J Chosun Nat Sci* 2012;5(1):1–5.

[3]. Verma J, Khedkar VM, Coutinho EC. 3D-QSAR in drug design - A review. *Curr Top Med Chem* 2010;10(1):95–115.

[4]. Rasulev B. Recent developments in 3D QSAR and molecular docking studies of organic and nanostructures. In: *Handbook of Computational Chemistry*, 2016, p. 2133.

[5]. Brown AC, Fraser TR. On the connection between chemical constitution and physiological action; with special reference to the physiological action of the salts of the ammonium bases derived from strychnia, Brucia, Thebaia, Codeia, Morphia, and Nicotia. *J Anat Physiol* 1868;2(2):224–242.

[6]. Hansch C, Fujita T. p-σ-π Analysis. A method for the correlation of biological activity and chemical structure. *J Am Chem Soc* 1964;86(8):1616–1626.

[7]. Free SM Jr, Wilson JW. A mathematical contribution to structure-activity studies. *J Med Chem* 1964;7:395–399.

[8]. Richardson BJ. Physiological research on alcohols. *Med Times Gaz* 1868;2:703–706.

[9]. Mills EJ. On melting point and boiling point as related to composition. *Philos Mag* 1884;17:173–187.

[10]. Richet C. On the relationship between the toxicity and the physical properties of substances. *Compt. Rendus Seances Soc Biol* 1893;9:775–776.

[11]. Overton E. Osmotic properties of cells in the bearing on toxicology and pharmacology. *Z Phys Chem* 1897;22:189–209.

[12]. Meyer H. On the theory of alcohol narcosis I. Which property of anesthetics gives them their narcotic activity? *Arch Exp Pathol Pharmakol* 1899;42:109–118.

[13]. Hammett LP. Some relations between reaction rates and equilibrium constants. *Chem Rev* 1935;17(1):125–136.

[14]. Hammett LP. The effect of structure upon the reactions of organic compounds benzene derivatives. *J Am Chem Soc* 1937;59:96–103.

[15]. Taft RW. Polar and steric substituent constants for aliphatic and o- benzoate groups from rates of esterification and hydrolysis of esters 1. *J Am Chem Soc* 1952;74:3120–3128.

[16]. Hansch C, Maloney PP, Fujita T, et al. Correlation of biological activity of phenoxyacetic acids with Hammett substituent constants and partition coefficients. *Nature* 1962;194:178–180.

[17]. Hansch C. Quantitative approach to biochemical structure-activity relationships. *Acc Chem Res* 1969;2(8):232–239.

[18]. Fujita T, Ban T. Structure-activity study of phenethylamines as substrates of biosynthetic enzymes of sympathetic transmitters. *J Med Chem* 1971;14(2):148–152.

[19]. Kubinyi H. Quantitative structure-activity relationships. IV. Non-linear dependence of biological activity on hydrophobic character: A new model. *Arzneim Forsch* 1976;26(11):1991–1997.

[20]. Wise M, Cramer RD, Smith DM, et al. *In Quantitative Approaches to Drug Design*, Dearden JC, Ed. Elsevier: Amsterdam, 1983; p. 145. Wise M. In *Molecular Graphics and Drug Design*; Burgen ASV, Roberts GCK, Tute MS, Elsevier: New York, 1986, pp. 183–194. Cramer RD, 111; Bunce JD. In *QSAR in Drug Design and Toxicology*; Hadzi D, Jerman-Blazic B, Eds.; Elsevier: New York, 1987, p. 3.

[21]. Goodford PJ. A computational procedure for determining energetically favorable binding sites on biologically important macromolecules. *J Med Chem* 1985;28(7):849–857.

[22]. Cramer RD, Patterson DE, Bunce JD. Comparative molecular field analysis (CoMFA). 1. Effect of shape on binding of steroids to carrier proteins. *J Am Chem Soc* 1988;110(18):5959–5967.

[23]. Vinter JG, Davis A, Saunders MR. Strategic approaches to drug design. I. An integrated software framework for molecular modelling. *J Comput Aid Mol Des* 1987;1(1):31–51.

[24]. Gasteiger J, Marsili M. Iterative partial equalization of orbital electronegativity-a rapid access to atomic charges. *Tetrahedron* 1980;36(22):3219–3228.

[25]. Jain AN, Koile K, Chapman D. Compass: Predicting biological activities from molecular surface properties. Performance comparisons on a steroid benchmark. *J Med Chem* 1994;37(15):2315–2327.

[26]. Amin SA, Adhikari N, Gayen S, et al. First report on the structural exploration and prediction of new BPTES analogs as glutaminase inhibitors. *J Mol Struct* 2017;1143:49–64.

[27]. https://www.rcsb.org/ as accessed in April 2022.

[28]. https://www.ccdc.cam.ac.uk/ as accessed in April 2022.

[29]. Kim KH. Comparative molecular field analysis (CoMFA). In: Dean PM, Ed. *Molecular Similarity in Drug Design*. Blackie Academic & Professional, Glasgow, 1995, pp. 291–331.

[30]. Norinder U. Recent progress in CoMFA methodology and related techniques. In: Kubinyi H, Folkers G, Martin YC, Eds. *3D QSAR in Drug Design - Recent Advances*. Kluwer Academic Publishers, New York, 1998, Vol. 3, pp. 24–39.

[31]. Klebe G, Abraham U, Mietzner T. Molecular similarity indices in a comparative analysis (CoMSIA) of drug molecules to correlate and predict their biological activity. *J Med Chem* 1994;37(24):4130–4146.

[32]. Klebe G. Comparative molecular similarity indices analysis: CoMSIA. In Hugo Kubinyi, Gerd Folkers, and Yvonne C. Martin, Eds. *3D QSAR in drug design*. Springer, Dordrecht, 1998, pp. 87–104.

[33]. Folkers G, Merz A, Rognan D. CoMFA: Scope and limitations. In Kubinyi H, Ed. *3D QSAR in drug design*. ESCOM, Leiden, The Netherlands, 1993, pp. 583–618.

[34]. Debe DA, Carlson MJ, Goddard WA 3rd. The topomer-sampling model of protein folding. *Proc Natl Acad Sci U S A* 1999;96(6):2596–2601.

[35]. Cramer RD. Topomer CoMFA: A design methodology for rapid lead optimization. *J Med Chem* 2003;46(3):374–388.

[36]. Kubinyi H, Folkers G, Martin YC, Eds. *3D-QSAR in drug design: Volume 2: Ligand-protein interactions and molecular similarity*. Springer Science & Business Media, Dordrecht, the Netherlands, 1998.

[37]. Bursi R, Grootenhuis PD. Comparative molecular field analysis and energy interaction studies of thrombin-inhibitor complexes. *J Comput Aid Mol Des* 1999;13(3):221–232.

[38]. So SS, Karplus M. Evaluation of designed ligands by a multiple screening method: Application to glycogen phosphorylase inhibitors constructed with a variety of approaches. *J Comput Aid Mol Des* 2001;15(7):613–647.

[39]. Klebe G, Mietzner T, Weber F. Different approaches toward an automatic structural alignment of drug molecules: Applications to sterol mimics, thrombin and thermolysin inhibitors. *J Comput Aid Mol Des* 1994;8(6):751–778.

[40]. Oprea TI, Waller CL, Marshall GR. Three-dimensional quantitative structure-activity relationship of human immunodeficiency virus (I) protease inhibitors. 2. Predictive power using limited exploration of alternate binding modes. *J Med Chem* 1994;37(14):2206–2215.

[41]. DePriest SA, Mayer D, Naylor CB, et al. 3D-QSAR of angiotensin-converting enzyme and thermolysin inhibitors: A comparison of CoMFA models based on deduced and experimentally determined active site geometries. *J Am Chem Soc* 1993;115(13):5372–5384.

[42]. Muegge I, Podlogar BL. 3D-Quantitative structure activity relationships of biphenyl carboxylic acid MMP-3 inhibitors: Exploring automated docking as alignment method. *Quant Struct Act Relat* 2001;20(3):215–222.

[43]. Cramer RD, Clark RD, Patterson DE, et al. Bioisosterism as a molecular diversity descriptor: Steric fields of single "topomeric" conformers. *J Med Chem* 1996;39(16):3060–3069.

[44]. Hopfinger AJ. A QSAR investigation of dihydrofolate reductase inhibition by Baker triazines based upon molecular shape analysis. *J Am Chem Soc* 1980;102(24):7196–7206.

[45]. Ermondi G, Caron G. GRIND-based 3D-QSAR to predict inhibitory activity for similar enzymes, OSC and SHC. *Eur J Med Chem* 2008;43(7):1462–1468.

[46]. Hahn M. Receptor surface models. 1. Definition and construction. *J Med Chem* 1995;38(12):2080–2090.

[47]. Robinson DD, Winn PJ, Lyne PD, et al. Self-organizing molecular field analysis: A tool for structure-activity studies. *J Med Chem* 1999;42(4):573–583.

[48]. Walters DE, Hinds RM. Genetically evolved receptor models: A computational approach to construction of receptor models. *J Med Chem* 1994;37(16):2527–2536.

[49]. Amat L, Robert D, Besalú E, et al. Molecular quantum similarity measures tuned 3D QSAR: An antitumoral family validation study. *J Chem Inf Comput Sci* 1998;38(4):624–631.

[50]. Silber K, Heidler P, Kurz T, et al. AFMoC enhances predictivity of 3D QSAR: A case study with DOXP-reductoisomerase. *J Med Chem* 2005;48(10):3547–3563.

[51]. Chuman H, Karasawa M, Fujita T. A novel three-dimensional QSAR procedure: Voronoi field analysis. *Quant Struct Act Relat* 1998;17(04):313–326.

[52]. Semus SF. A novel hydropathic intermolecular field analysis (HIFA) for the prediction of ligand-receptor binding affinities. *Med Chem Res* 1999;9(7–8):535–547.

[53]. Silverman BD, Platt DE. Comparative molecular moment analysis (CoMMA): 3D-QSAR without molecular superposition. *J Med Chem* 1996;39(11):2129–2140.

[54]. Crivori P, Cruciani G, Carrupt PA, et al. Predicting blood-brain barrier permeation from three-dimensional molecular structure. *J Med Chem* 2000;43(11):2204–2216.

[55]. Asikainen A, Ruuskanen J, Tuppurainen K. Spectroscopic QSAR methods and self-organizing molecular field analysis for relating molecular structure and estrogenic activity. *J Chem Inf Comput Sci* 2003;43(6):1974–1981.

[56]. Doweyko AM. The hypothetical active site lattice. An approach to modelling active sites from data on inhibitor molecules. *J Med Chem* 1988;31(7):1396–1406.

[57]. Ortiz AR, Pisabarro MT, Gago F, Wade RC. Prediction of drug binding affinities by comparative binding energy analysis. *J Med Chem* 1995;38(14):2681–2691.

[58]. Lushington GH, Guo JX, Wang JL. Whither combine? New opportunities for receptor-based QSAR. *Curr Med Chem* 2007;14(17):1863–1877.

[59]. Datar PA, Khedkar SA, Malde AK, Coutinho EC. Comparative residue interaction analysis (CoRIA): A 3D-QSAR approach to explore the binding contributions of active site residues with ligands. *J Comput Aid Mol Des* 2006;20(6):343–360.

[60]. Kotani T, Higashiura K. Comparative molecular active site analysis (CoMASA). 1. An approach to rapid evaluation of 3D QSAR. *J Med Chem* 2004;47(11):2732–2742.

[61]. Zhou P, Tong J, Tian F, Li Z. A novel comparative molecule/pseudo receptor interaction analysis. *Chin Sci Bull* 2006;51(15):1824–1829.

3 Other Modeling Approaches

Pharmacophore Mapping, Molecular Docking, and Molecular Dynamic Simulation Studies

Sk. Abdul Amin, Shovanlal Gayen,
Sanjib Das, and Tarun Jha

CONTENTS

DOI: 10.1201/9781003303282-4

ABSTRACT

In this chapter, the application of other molecular modeling techniques (namely ligand- and structure-based pharmacophore mapping followed by virtual screening as well as molecular docking and molecular dynamics simulation) in drug design and discovery are discussed in detail. Currently, such types of molecular modeling studies not only strengthen conventional QSAR and related drug designing strategies but also offer a new avenue in the binding mode of interaction analysis followed by the screening of appropriate drug molecules from databases and proper pharmacophoric features of ligands/molecules to get relevant ideas regarding structures and functions for designing potential and effective bioactive compounds.

Keywords: Pharmacophore; Molecular docking; Molecular dynamic (MD) simulation; Virtual screening

3.1 INTRODUCTION

Traditional drug discovery in the pharmaceutical industry in the early 1960s was mainly devoted to screening natural and synthetic compounds against a particular biological endpoint [1, 2]. Once a potential drug/drug-like molecule was chosen from thousands of natural and synthetic molecules by a tedious approach, medicinal chemists could then synthesize hundreds of related molecules (derivatives or analogs) to find the safest and most effective molecule [3]. Hence, the costs and risks related to this technique have become gigantic. A drastic change in the traditional drug design process was observed in the 1960s, and several notable works published in the 1960s led to a paradigm shift [1]. Since then, rational drug design (RDD) paradigms have gained attention to design new chemical entities and optimize chemical structures for better biological activity [4]. In the early 1980s, advances in molecular biology, protein crystallography, and computational chemistry greatly advanced RDD paradigms to increase the accuracy of binding affinity predictions. Now, rational drug discovery has become highly interdisciplinary, with rapidly evolving high throughput screening (HTS), combinatorial chemistry technologies, and computer-aided drug design (CADD) strategies successfully contributing [5–7]. Numerous CADD applications are utilized at almost early phases of drug discovery cascades [8, 9]. Thus, CADD can be described as a method to enhance the drug discovery process [10, 11]. It allows better engagement in experiments and reduces the cost and time to find new drugs. CADD comprises (i) *in silico* design and prediction of novel compounds by making the drug discovery and development process faster, (ii) identifying and optimizing new compounds with the aid of a computational approach, and (iii) eliminating molecules with unwanted features and selecting candidates with more chances for success.

Pharmacophore-based approaches presently are an integral part of many CADD workflows (Figure 3.1) [12–14] and have been extensively employed for many assignments, such as *de novo* design, virtual screening, and lead optimization [15–17]. The pharmacophore model may be generated from receptor- and ligand-based techniques (Figure 3.1) [18–20].

Similarly, molecular docking [21–23] and molecular dynamic (MD) simulations allow an understanding of the 3D binding mode of a provided molecule at the binding site of a macromolecule (protein/DNA). The binding affinity can also be predicted quantitatively through a docking score, and the stability of the protein-ligand complex is judged by proper MD simulation studies [24–27]. More interestingly, pharmacophore-dependent virtual screening, when combined with docking analyses, provides a great chance of acceptability [28–30].

This chapter focuses on the pharmacophore, docking, and MD concepts and their applications in the modern CADD approach. The chapter is divided into two definite parts. The first part briefly introduces the pharmacophore concept followed by explaining the most common nonbonded interaction types, their depiction as pharmacophoric features, and the importance of pharmacophore modeling. The second section is dedicated to molecular docking and MD simulations. Finally, this chapter will finish with a discussion and conclusions related to the future direction of the field.

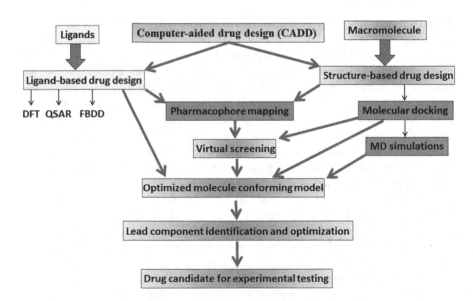

FIGURE 3.1 Computer-aided drug discovery (CADD) workflows: based on the available structural information, a structure- or ligand-based approach is selected for drug design. After the successful finding of lead molecules, several cycles of lead optimization result in one or more drug-like molecules. Since this chapter is dedicated to pharmacophore mapping, molecular docking, and molecular dynamic (MD) simulation, these boxes are highlighted in light gray.

3.2 PHARMACOPHORE MAPPING: AN OVERVIEW

The word "pharmacophore" is from the Latin words "pharmakon" (meaning drug) and "phoros" (meaning carrier/carrying) [18, 31]. In the 1900s, a Nobel laureate German physician and scientist, Paul Ehrlich, coined the term "pharmacophore" as "a molecular framework that carries the essential features responsible for a drug's biological activity" [32, 33]. Later in the 1960s, Kier, a pioneer of QSAR, modified Ehrlich's concept by stating that a drug should contain (i) "those atomic characters appropriate for the necessary drug-receptor interaction phenomena" and (ii) "the proper spatial disposition of these characters required to bring about the required sequential interaction with the receptor" [34–36]. Peter Gund, in 1977, included "molecular recognition" and again defined "pharmacophore" as "a set of structural features in a molecule that is recognized at a receptor site and is responsible for that molecule's biological activity" [37]. Later, Fischer stated that a biological substrate (i.e., ligand) is "recognized" by the enzyme, protein, or receptor by forming a supra-molecular complex.

To date, the IUPAC definition of pharmacophore can be considered the most particular [38]. IUPAC denotes pharmacophore as "an ensemble of steric and electronic features that is necessary to ensure the optimal supramolecular interactions with a specific biological target and trigger (or block) its biological response" [38].

3.2.1 PHARMACOPHORE MODEL AND PHARMACOPHORE FINGERPRINT

The basic concept of ligand-based design methods lies in the hypothesis that at least one (potential) binding partner is called a "binder" [39]. The descriptors (2D parameters like *logP, molar refectory, Tanimoto index*, etc.) of the binder are estimated, which may assist as a search template to identify numerous newer binding partners by application of the prototype "similar molecules should bind similarly." Approaches like a simple search of the substructure, similarity, and/or pharmacophore models can be used [39].

Pharmacophore rendition denoted a compound to a number of features (points) at the 3D level (Figure 3.2). A pharmacophore fingerprint typically annotates a compound as a distinctive data string. All probable three-point or four-point sets (rarely five-point) of pharmacophore features are illustrated for every ligand (Figure 3.2). The distance between the feature points is computed in bonds or by distance-binning when utilizing 3D fingerprints [40]. The resulting fingerprint is a string explaining the frequency of each probable combination at pre-explained positions in the string (Figure 3.2). Various variants of pharmacophore fingerprints have been designed and are often utilized. Such a pharmacophore fingerprint may also be applied for the analysis of the similarity among compounds or pool of molecules. Moreover, a fingerprint model may be employed to judge the common elements of active molecules to find the essential characteristics of the particular endpoint [40].

The pharmacophore model comprises a few characters assembled in a particular 3D pattern. Typically, every feature is presented as a sphere with a radius controlling the tolerance on the variation from the exact location (Figure 3.2).

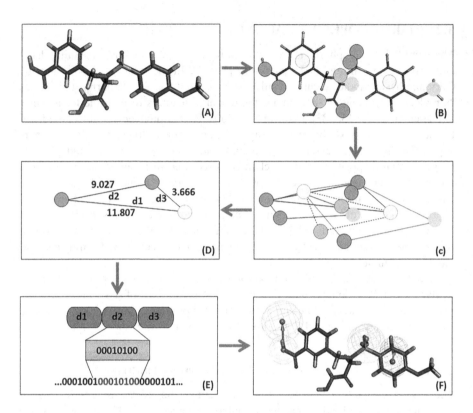

FIGURE 3.2 Pharmacophore fingerprints. (A) A conformer of the ligand; (B) pharmacophore fingerprint is the representation of the ligand; (C) possible molecular interaction features into a string; (D) a selected combination; (E) calculation and the frequency of occurrence is stored in a string; (F) final pharmacophore model with features hydrogen bond acceptor (HBA, dark gray), ring aromatic (RA, light gray).

3.2.2 A SHORT TRIP TO THE PHARMACOPHORIC FEATURES

A pharmacophore model (hypothesis) must be (i) specific to extract active from inactive molecules, (ii) universal enough to pinpoint ligands as novel/new candidates, and (iii) capable of correlating huge molecular libraries in an instinctive way [41]. However, selectivity is a prime concern in the validation of pharmacophores. Hence, feature elucidations are common requirements to be substituted from exploring universal chemical functionality to illustrate definite functional groups. The common viewpoint is to generate a model from definite ligands by including or excluding descriptive chemical features. This approach is to represent the specific mode of interaction.

Scientists already proposed a simple layer model to offer a referral to these features easily [41]. This describes the levels of universality and specificity of chemical features. Table 3.1 shows a classification of abstraction layers of chemical features in which a higher level corresponds to lower specificity and, thus, higher universality.

3.2.2.1 Automated Perception of Chemical Features

The chemical features in Table 3.1 are classified into hydrogen bond interactions (layer 3 features), charge interactions, and lipophilic interactions (level 4 features). The layer 4 features are presented by vectors, while layer 3 features are designated as points with a tolerance radius structuring a sphere. Figure 3.3 highlights the chemical feature definitions designated in Daylight Smiles Arbitrary Target Specification (SMARTS) notation.

3.2.2.2 Basic Interactions and Representation of Pharmacophoric Features

The widely acquired conception of drug-receptor interaction is dependent on "induced fit," which considers conformational alterations of receptors influenced by flexible ligands. Depending on different ligand-receptor interactions, pharmacophoric features are assigned as hydrophobic (HYP), ring aromatic (RA), hydrogen bond acceptor (HBA), hydrogen bond donor (HBD), cationic (or positive ionizable, P), and anionic (or negative ionizable, N) as highlighted in Table 3.2. Pharmacophore modeling software supports metal interactions (for metalloenzymes) like Zn-binding domains. Unlike features, the shape of a ligand is also a prime component for ligand-receptor interaction.

3.2.3 PHARMACOPHORE ELUCIDATION

Pharmacophore models are mainly formed in three different ways. Data availability, data quality, and computational resources are key factors in selecting a particular

TABLE 3.1
Abstraction Layers of Chemical Features

Layer	Classification	Specificity	Universality	Example
1	Molecular graph descriptor (atom, bond) with geometric constraint	Very high	Very low	A phenol group facing a parallel benzenoid system within 2–4 Å
2	Molecular graph descriptor (atom, bond) without geometric constraint	High	Low	A phenol group
3	Chemical functionality (hydrogen bond donor, acceptor) with geometric constraint	Low	High	HBA vector, including an acceptor point as well as a projected donor point; aromatic ring including a ring plane
4	Chemical functionality (positive ionizable area, lipophilic contact) without geometric constraint	Very low	Very high	HBA without the projected point; lipophilic group

	HBA	HBD	PI	NI
Inclusion patterns	{[O,S]}{#1} {N}{#1} C{F}	{[N,O,S;X1,X2]}	{[NX3]}([CX4])([CX4,#1])[CX4,#1] {N}=[CX3]({[N;H1,H2]})[! N] N=[CX3]({[NH1]}){[NH1]} {[+,+2,+3;! $(*[−,−2,−3])]}	[S,P](={O})(={O}){[OH]} [S,C,P](={O}){[OH]} {c}1{n}{n}{n}{n}1 {[−,−2,−3;! $(*[+,+2,+3])]}
Exclusion patterns	c1nnnn1	[−,−2,−3]		

FIGURE 3.3   The SMARTS syntax.

TABLE 3.2

Summary of the Pharmacophoric Feature Types and Their Interactions Typically Observed in Biological Systems

Feature type	Interaction type(s)	Geometrical representation	Structural examples
Hydrophobic (H or HY)	Hydrophobic contact	Sphere	Alkyl groups, ALICYCLES, Weakly or nonpolar aromatic rings, halogen substituents
Aromatic (RA)	π-stacking, cation-π	Plane or sphere	Any aromatic ring
Hydrogen bond acceptor (HBA)	Hydrogen bonding	Vector or sphere	Amines, carboxylates, ketones, alcohols, fluorine substituents
Hydrogen bond donor (HBD)	Hydrogen bonding	Vector or sphere	Amines, amides, alcohols
Positive ionizable (PI)	Ionic, cation-π	Sphere	Ammonium ion, metal cations
Negative ionizable (NI)	Ionic	Sphere	Carboxylates

pharmacophore approach. One can create a pharmacophore model manually. It is also possible to generate a pharmacophore model in an automated technique starting from the structure of one or multiple ligands. This type of pharmacophore model generation from ligand structures can be stated as ligand-based pharmacophore mapping; 3D-pharmacophore modeling software is listed in Table 3.3.

Another way to deduce a pharmacophore model from the 3D structure of the target receptor is called the receptor-based pharmacophore model (also called the structure-based pharmacophore model). The techniques for pharmacophore modeling and their important features are described in the following sections.

TABLE 3.3

3D-Pharmacophore Modeling Software, Their Components, and the Availability of Free Academic Licenses

Software	Source[a]	Input	Identification methods
Catalyst	www.3ds.com/products -services/biovia/products/ molecular-modeling -simulation/biovia-discovery -studio/pharmacophore/	Ligand, complex, apo	Substructure pattern, feature, molecular field
FLAP	www.moldiscovery.com/ software/flap/	Ligand, complex, apo	Molecular field
Forge	www.cresset-group.com/about /news/forge-design-released/	Ligand	Molecular field
LigandScout	https://ligandscout.software .informer.com/	Ligand, complex, apo	Substructure pattern, feature, molecular field
MOE	www.chemcomp.com/ Products.htm	Ligand, complex, apo	Substructure pattern, feature, molecular field
Pharao	https://github.com/gertthijs/ pharao	Ligand	Substructure pattern
PharmaGist	https://bioinfo3d.cs.tau.ac.il/ PharmaGist/php.php	Ligand	Substructure pattern, feature
Pharmer	http://smoothdock.ccbb.pitt .edu/pharmer/	Ligand, complex	Substructure pattern, feature
PharmMapper	www.lilab-ecust.cn/ pharmmapper/	Ligand	Substructure pattern, feature
PHASE	www.schrodinger.com/ products/phase	Ligand, complex, apo	Substructure pattern, feature, molecular field

[a] Accessed April 2022.

3.2.3.1 Manually Created Pharmacophore Models

Manual creation is the simplest manner to construct pharmacophore models. It depends on information related to known prime features and/or the molecular features of a set of active molecules. Nowadays, this method is generally left to computer-aided techniques. Manual association has moved toward the refining of the model, while the model is automatically constructed through specified software.

3.2.3.2 Ligand-Based Pharmacophore Models

Regarding the general point of view, ligand-based pharmacophore modeling is the best option when no information related to the 3D structure of the target (receptor/ protein) is unknown, but a number of active ligands are available. It is good practice to split the ligand data into two sets, a training and an assessment (test) set, to validate the generated pharmacophore query when multiple active ligands (and inactive derivatives) are known. The general workflow of ligand-based pharmacophore model generation is depicted in Figure 3.4.

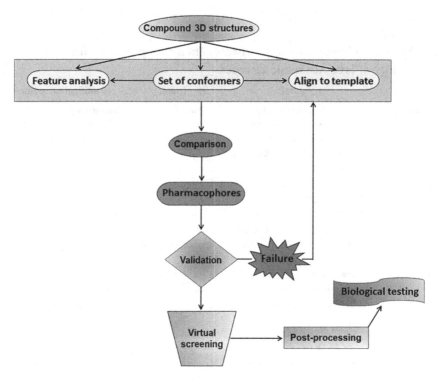

FIGURE 3.4   Overall workflow of ligand-based pharmacophore model generation.

3.2.3.3 Receptor-Based Pharmacophore Models

The accessibility of 3D information about a ligand-receptor complex offers a considerable chance for producing high-quality and robust pharmacophore models. A thorough binding site analysis recognizes potential interaction points and interactions of interest through several available methods. A typical receptor-based pharmacophore model is shown in Figure 3.5.

Grid-based techniques such as GRID probe the binding site at discrete points by applying small molecules or functional groups. Interaction energies between probe compounds and the receptor atoms are estimated, resulting in molecular interaction fields (MIF). These fields may be utilized to identify energetically favorable and unfavorable regions for specific ligand-receptor interactions that help place a correct pharmacophoric feature or aid in ligand design and optimization.

A crucial source for these complexes, for example, derived from NMR-spectroscopy or X-ray crystallography, produces the Protein Data Bank (PDB). A lot of macromolecular structures are collected in this online repository of PDB [42]. Pharmacophore modeling software, namely Discovery Studio [43] and LigandScout [44], also deliver tools to develop pharmacophore models depending on the topology of the binding site and in the absence of a ligand. So far, we have already described the different methods of pharmacophore model generations. Based on how much is

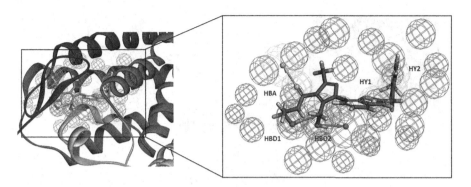

FIGURE 3.5   A receptor-based pharmacophore model.

TABLE 3.4
Different Situations for the Pharmacophore Search

Protein/ligand	No	Yes
No	Situation I: Not possible	Situation II: Ligand-based pharmacophore
Yes	Situation III: Structure-based pharmacophore	Situation IV: Ligand-based pharmacophore Structure-based pharmacophore

---

known about the ligands and particular protein targets, various options are available to build such a query. Table 3.4 shows the four different situations depending on the availability of the ligands and particular protein targets.

(A) Situation I. This situation occurs when both the ligand and protein structure information are not available (Table 3.4). In this case, pharmacophore-based virtual screening is not feasible, hence, experimental screening is a way to screen a database.

(B) Situation II. The second option is the presence of active ligands, but the protein structure is not known (or some information is missing). In this case, a ligand-based virtual screening approach can be used.

(C) Situation III. The most demanding option is when only a protein structure is accessible.

(D) Situation IV. The best circumstance is when binding ligand and structural knowledge are present.

3.2.4 PHARMACOPHORE-BASED VIRTUAL SCREENING

Pharmacophore models serve as an effective search filter to screen molecules with desired stereo-electronic features. This is a prevalent basis for the construction of

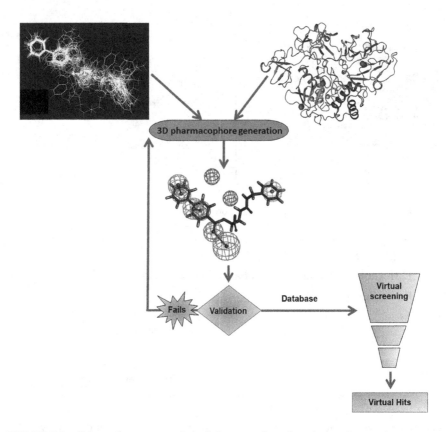

FIGURE 3.6   Schematic representation of pharmacophore-based virtual screening.

pharmacophore models. Nowadays, pharmacophore-based virtual screening is a
well-accepted powerful and fast search tool. Initially, virtual screening is carried out
by pharmacophore model (query) generation that most likely encrypts the necessary
3D orientation of the required interaction pattern. This generated model is then used
to screen and reclaim a set of initial hit molecules from databases (Figure 3.6).

This search retrieves molecules either similar to the pharmacophore features or
completely different scaffolds, as the pharmacophore features of the model developed may map to various structural properties of the functional groups of molecules.
Then, the high-scored and better-fitted molecules to the pharmacophore model are
collected as hits. Hence, the pharmacophore query process dramatically reduces,
obviously in a scientific way, the number of database compounds.

3.3 MOLECULAR DOCKING STUDY

Drug interactions with the target protein are a handshake where both try to fit some-
what to accommodate the other. Molecular docking is a powerful tool for understanding protein-ligand interactions [45]. Currently, molecular docking studies have
become a regular practice tool in various steps of drug design processes [46]. In

protein-ligand docking, a candidate ligand, a target of interest, and a strategy to evaluate binding interaction poses are generally required. The overall workflow of molecular docking is depicted in Figure 3.7.

The candidate ligand in molecular docking study may be a small molecule, DNA, peptide, or sometimes protein. The RSCB PDB is the prime source of protein structures from which these can be retrieved for molecular docking study [47]. Currently, in the RSCB PDB (www.rcsb.org/), there are more than 62,000 PDB entries of protein-ligand complexes, of which about 60,000 were solved by X-ray and about 1,700 by NMR methods. Numerous commercial/open-source molecular docking algorithms have been found that successfully predict protein-ligand poses and calculate binding energies. A list of protein-ligand docking tools is shown in Table 3.5. A list of protein-peptide and protein-protein docking tools is provided in Table 3.6.

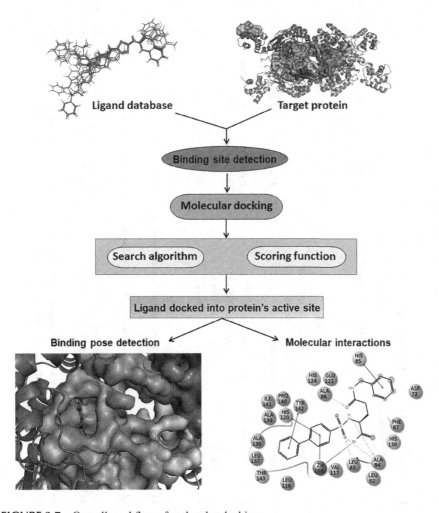

FIGURE 3.7 Overall workflow of molecular docking.

TABLE 3.5

List of Protein-Ligand Docking Software/Tools

Sl	Software/tools	Source[a]	Method	Types
1	3D-Dock Suite	www.sbg.bio.ic.ac.uk/docking/index.html	Fourier correlation algorithm, self-consistent mean field optimization procedure, single distance constraint empirically derived pair potential	PLI
2	ArgusLab	www.arguslab.com	Genetic algorithm and ArgusDock	PLI
3	AutoDock	http://autodock.scripps.edu/	Lamarckian genetic algorithm	PLI
4	BiGGER	www.cqfb.fct.unl.pt/	Soft docking	PLI
5	ClusPro	https://cluspro.org/	Ten most populated low energy clusters, iRMSD > 9 Å	Automatic docking web servers
6	Dock Vision	http://dockvision.com/	Hybrid evolutionary algorithm	PLI
7	DOT	www.sdsc.edu/CCMS/DOT/	Fast Fourier transforms	PLI
8	FlexX	www.biosolveit.de/FlexX/	Sequential importance sampling (SIS)-algorithm	PLI
9	FRED	www.eyesopen.com/fred	Directed docking with smiles arbitrary target specification (SMARTS) patterns	PLI
10	Gold	www.ccdc.cam.ac.uk/	Genetic algorithm	PLI
11	GRAMM-X	http://vakser.compbio.ku.edu/resources/gramm/grammx/	Up to 300 lowest energy conformations	Automatic docking web servers
12	HADDOCK	https://wenmr.science.uu.nl/haddock2.4/	Fully flexible for interacting residues of peptide and protein	Automatic docking web servers
13	HADDOCK	www.nmr.chem.uu.nl/haddock/	Uses ambiguous interaction restraints of NMR	PLI
14	HDOCK	http://hdock.phys.hust.edu.cn/	Top 100 lowest energy clusters, iRMSD> 5 Å	Automatic docking web servers
15	Hex	www.loria.fr/ritchied/hex/	Similar to conventional fast Fourier transform	PLI
16	InterPred	http://bioinfo.ifm.liu.se/inter/interpred/	No conformational search (template-based)	Automatic docking web servers

(Continued)

TABLE 3.5 (CONTINUED)
List of Protein–Ligand Docking Software/Tools

Sl	Software/tools	Source[a]	Method	Types
17	LZerD	https://lzerd.kiharalab.org/	Up to 50,000 generated geometries	Automatic docking web servers
18	MDockPP	https://zougrouptoolkit.missouri.edu/MDockPP/	Up to 3,000 generated geometries; clustering cutoff adjustable	Automatic docking web servers
19	PatchDock	http://bioinfo3d.cs.tau.ac.il/PatchDock/	Up to 100 top-ranking candidates; clustering cutoff adjustable	Automatic docking web servers
20	pyDockWEB	http://life.bsc.es/servlet/pydock	Top 100 lowest energy conformations	Automatic docking web servers
21	rDock	www.ysbl.york.ac.uk/rDock	Weighted sum of intermolecular, ligand intramolecular, site intramolecular, and external restraint terms	PLI
22	RosettaDock	http://rosettadock.graylab.jhu.edu	1000 decoys can be downloaded	Automatic docking web servers
23	Surflex-Dock	www.tripos.com/	Hammerhead docking system	PLI
24	ZDOCK	https://zdock.umassmed.edu/	Top 10 lowest energy conformations; possibility to retrieve top 500	Automatic docking web servers

[a] Accessed April 2022; PLI, protein–ligand interactions.

TABLE 3.6

List of Protein-Peptide and Protein-Protein Docking Software/Tools

Sl	Software/tools	Source[a]	Method
1	ClusPro PeptiDock	https://peptidock.cluspro.org/	Fast Fourier transform-based docking method, clustering by structure scoring, and CAPRI peptide docking criteria
2	DOCK	http://dock.compbio.ucsf.edu/	Geometric matching algorithm
3	DynaDock	Not available to the public	Combined optimized potential molecular dynamics (OPMD) with a soft-core potential
4	GalaxyPepDock	http://galaxy.seoklab.org/pepdock	Use similarity search (known template structures) as scaffolds for prediction
5	GRAMM	http://vakser.bioinformatics.ku.edu/main/resources _gramm.php	Empirical approach
6	HPEPDOCK	http://huanglab.phys.hust.edu.cn/hpepdock/	Ensemble peptide conformation by MODPEP
7	ICM-Docking	www.molsoft.com/docking.html	Flexible docking
8	PBRpredict-Suite	http://cs.uno.edu/~{}tamjid/Software/PBRpredict/p brpredict-suite.zip	Integrated six machine learning algorithms (model stacking)
9	pepATTRACT	http://bioserv.rpbs.univ-parisdiderot.fr/services/ pepATTRACT/	Rigid body peptide docking within the binding pocket
10	PepComposer	https://cassandra.med.uniroma1.it/pepcomposer/ webserver/pepcomposer.php	Motif similarity search to defined binding interfaces from monomeric protein databases PepX (http://pepx.switchlab.org)
11	PepCrawler	http://bioinfo3d.cs.tau.ac.il/PepCrawler	Rapidly exploring random tree algorithm
12	PepSite 2.0	http://pepsite2.russelllab.org	Coarse-grained peptide orientation by spatial position-specific scoring matrix (S-PSSM)
13	Rosetta FlexPepDock	http://flexpepdock.furmanlab.cs.huji.ac.il	Rosetta energy function-based clustering and scoring
14	Situs	http://situs.biomachina.org/index.html	Correlation-based rigid body docking and density filtering, ARD
15	SPRINT-Str	http://sparks-lab.org/server/SPRINT-Str	Use SVM with optimized parameters

[a] Accessed April 2022

Since its inception 50 years ago, protein-ligand docking has been used successfully in a variety of real-world situations, including the subsequent approval of new medications developed with the aid of structure-based drug design. These new medications include enzyme inhibitors, receptor antagonists and agonists, and ion channel blockers. The area is developing swiftly with approximations that offer a better balance between accuracy and computing cost as the practical applications of molecular models expand as a result of the ongoing gains in computational power. Future work on these projects will surely result in many more fascinating applications.

3.3.1 STAGES OF MOLECULAR DOCKING STUDY

Molecular docking is mainly composed of two stages: (1) sampling and (2) scoring function (Figure 3.8) [48]. The sampling process effectively searches the conformational space narrated by the free energy landscape. The scoring function associates a score to each predicted pose from the free energy landscape [22, 49, 50]. The scoring function enables the association of the native bound conformation to the global minimum of the energy hypersurface.

3.3.1.1 Sampling

Kuntz et al. [51] devised the very first molecular docking algorithm in the 1980s. A series of spheres were used to approximate the receptor's surface clefts, while another set of spheres was used to estimate the ligand's volume. The best steric overlap between the binding site and receptor spheres was sought, with no regard for conformational mobility. According to Nussinov and coworkers' classification of docking methods, depending on the degrees of flexibility of compounds involved in the computation, this method is associated with the group of fully rigid docking procedures (Figure 3.8) [52]. Any docking software, as previously stated, requires protein-ligand sampling algorithms to produce appropriate ligand poses. Ligand sampling algorithms are critical for achieving ligand posture and active site

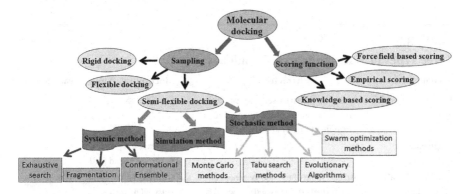

FIGURE 3.8 Schematic representation of the stages of molecular docking: (1) sampling and (2) scoring function.

placement. These algorithms are classified into three types: systematic search algorithms, shape-matching algorithms, and stochastic algorithms.

3.3.1.1.1 Rigid Docking Study

In rigid docking, both the ligand and the protein are rigid components, and only the three translational and three rotational degrees of freedom are taken into account during sampling [48]. This approach is related to the "lock-key" binding model. It is mostly utilized in protein-protein docking when the number of conformational degrees of freedom is very large to sample. In general, the binding site and ligand are estimated by "hot" points in these approaches, and the superposition of matching points is assessed [53].

3.3.1.1.2 Semi-Flexible Docking Study

In a semi-flexible docking study, the ligand is the only flexible molecule, while the protein is rigid. Apart from the six translational and rotational degrees of freedom, the ligand's structural degrees of freedom are sampled. These approaches presume that a protein's stable conformation corresponds to the one capable of recognizing the ligands to be docked [48]. As previously stated, this assumption is not always validated.

3.3.1.1.2.1 Systematic Search Techniques

Systematic search deals with a set of discretized values that are linked with each degree of freedom. All coordinate values are investigated in a combinatorial manner [54]. Systematic search techniques can be clubbed into three types (Table 3.7).

3.3.1.1.2.2 Stochastic Methods

In stochastic methods, the values of the degrees of freedom of the system are changed randomly rather than systematically. The rapidity of stochastic algorithms is a benefit since they might potentially locate the best solution very quickly. However, stochastic approaches have the limitation of not ensuring a thorough search of the

---

TABLE 3.7

Three Types of Systemic Search Techniques

Search type	Characteristic	Incorporated by software/tool
Exhaustive search	Search in the strict sense since all the rotatable bonds of the ligands are examined in a systematic way	• Glide [55, 56]
Fragmentation		• FlexX [57] • Hammerhead [58]
Conformational Ensemble	An ensemble of previously generated conformers of the ligand is docked to the target	• FLOG [59] • EUDOC [60] • MS-DOCK [61]

conformational space, which means the true solution may be overlooked. Increasing the number of iterations may help to partially fix the problem of lack of convergence [22]. Table 3.8 outlines the well-known stochastic algorithms.

3.3.1.1.3 Flexible Docking Study

Based on the hypothesis that both the ligand and the protein are flexible counterparts, flexible docking studies contend that proteins are not passive, rigid entities during binding. Many methods for flexible docking have been developed over time, some based on the induced fit binding model and others on conformational selection [48].

The potential energy surface is a function of several coordinates thanks to the numerous degrees of freedom that flexible docking provides. As a result, the computational capacity needed for docking calculations is increased, although sampling and scoring should be adjusted to provide an appropriate balance of accuracy and speed [48]. In fact, the effectiveness of a virtual screening campaign involving millions of molecules is based on how quickly docking calculations are completed. The creation of a unique algorithm that can thoroughly search the phase space without sacrificing velocity has thus advanced.

3.3.1.2 Scoring Functions

In the pool of poses generated by the sampling engine, scoring functions serve as a pose selector, segregating putative valid, binding modes and binders from nonbinders. Scoring functions are depicted in Table 3.9.

TABLE 3.8
The Most Famous Stochastic Algorithms

Algorithms	Characteristic	Incorporated by software/tool
Monte Carlo (MC) methods	Metropolis MC algorithm, which introduces an acceptance criterion in the evolution of the docking search	• AutoDock [62, 63] • ICM [64] • QXP [65] • MCDOCK [66] • AutoDock Vina [67] • ROSETTALIGAND [68]
Tabu search methods		• PRO_LEADS [69] • PSI-DOCK [70]
Evolutionary algorithms (EA)	Based on the idea of biological evolution, with the most famous genetic algorithms (GAs). The concept of the gene, chromosome, mutation, and crossover is borrowed from biology.	• GOLD [71, 72] • AutoDock 3 AND 4 (which implement a different version of GA, the Lamarckian GA) [73] • PSI-DOCK [70] • rDock [74]
Swarm optimization (SO) methods	These methods take inspiration from swarm behavior	• PLANTS [75] • SODOCK [76] • pso@autodock [77]

TABLE 3.9
Three Types of Scoring Functions

Scoring functions	Characteristic	Incorporated by software/tool
Forcefield based	Forcefield is a molecular mechanics concept that approximates the potential energy of a system composed of bonded (intramolecular) and nonbonded (intermolecular) components. Nonbonded components are generally taken into account in molecular docking, with presumably the addition of ligand-bonded terms, particularly torsional components. It also includes the solvation terms (Brooijmans and Kuntz, 2003).	• GoldScore [78] • AutoDock [73] (improved as a semiempirical version in AutoDock4 [79]) • GBVI/WSA [80]
Empirical	These functions are the sum of various empirical energy terms such as van der Waals, hydrogen bonds, electrostatic, entropy, desolvation, hydrophobicity, etc., which are weighted by coefficients optimized to reproduce binding affinity data of a training set by least squares fitting (Huang and Zou, 2010).	• LUDI [81]; GlideScore [55, 56] • ChemScore [82] • PLANTSCHEMPLP [75]
Knowledge-based	These approaches assume that statistically more explored ligand-protein contacts are associated with favorable interactions.	• DrugScore [83] • GOLD/ASP [84]

Another technique is to combine multiple scoring functions to achieve what is known as consensus scoring [85]. Furthermore, novel scoring functions, such as interaction fingerprints and attempts with quantum mechanical scores, have also been devised using machine learning technology [86].

3.3.2 PROTEIN-PROTEIN DOCKING

Understanding pathophysiology and drug discovery needs the exploration of protein-protein interaction (PPI) networks [87–91]. As a result, in terms of computational biophysics and structural biology, the protein-protein docking challenge is a hot topic. Generally, estimating the 3D structure of a protein-protein complex is more demanding than estimating the structure of a single protein.

Because there are more and more protein structures that are known, especially in light of structural genomics, effective computational algorithms to predict protein interactions are essential. Docking offers resources for fundamental studies of protein interactions and a structural basis for medication creation. Using the individual protein structures, a procedure known as protein-protein docking can be used to infer the structure of a complex. Docking technology is based on the idea of steric and physicochemical complementarity at the protein-protein interface.

Additionally, *in silico*, PPI prediction methods based on tertiary structure have been devised using two common approaches: *de novo* protein docking and template matching with known protein structures.

3.3.3 FRAGMENT-BASED DOCKING

Molecular docking may also be an excellent tool in the context of fragment-based drug design (FBDD). Fragment-based docking is demanding for several reasons, including incorrect binding modes, an increased chance of false positives, and problematic scoring compared with a full ligand [92–96]. Hence, there is a chance to explore the evaluation criteria of fragment docking and the development of fragment-specific approaches.

3.3.4 INVERSE DOCKING

Inverse docking (also known as target fishing) is a relatively new means of determining and validating potential target(s) of the active compound. It could also be used to anticipate negative side effects like toxicity [97–98]. With the heightened focus on drug repurposing in recent decades, molecular inverse docking has become a popular tool for predicting a molecule's possible protein targets. In fact, inverse docking has a number of advantages, including early monitoring of drug side effects and toxicity [99]. Nonetheless, various studies have been conducted to see if this strategy is feasible.

3.3.5 NANOPARTICLE DOCKING

Currently, nanotechnology demonstrates tremendous possibilities and useful solicitation as well as a potential hazard to human health [100]. In this condition, the therapeutical and toxicological effects of investigated nanoparticles (NPs) can be predicted by molecular docking [100–102]. Nanoparticle docking should be employed to study the binding of different types of nanoparticles with proteins and nucleic acids. The application of molecular docking techniques to explore the mechanism of NPs is still relatively new.

3.4 MOLECULAR DYNAMICS SIMULATIONS

MD simulations have become a cornerstone of many drug discovery programs, from hit identification to lead optimization and far beyond [103, 104]. MD simulations have quite a substantial effect not just on drug development but also on molecular biology. It analyses the time-resolved motion of proteins and other biomolecules by preserving the movements of macromolecules in full atomic detail while maintaining a good temporal resolution. The visualization of MD trajectories offers a rapid and instinctive comprehension of dynamics and function (Figure 3.9) [105]. It can generate a plethora of information regarding protein and ligand interactions and dynamic structural information on biomacromolecules [106]. This knowledge is crucial for establishing the target's structure-function relationship and the fundamentals of protein-ligand interactions, as well as for directing drug development and design approaches (Figure 3.9).

As a result, MD simulations have been extensively and reliably used in all stages of current drug discovery research [107]. Based on a general model of the physics driving interatomic interactions, it also predicts how each atom in a protein or other molecular system would move over time [108]. These simulations are capable of capturing a wide range of key biomolecular processes, such as conformational change, ligand binding, and protein folding. At femtosecond temporal resolution, it can reveal the positions of all atoms [109]. Moreover, such simulations may also anticipate how biomolecules will respond to perturbations such as mutation, phosphorylation, protonation, or the addition or removal of a ligand at the atomic level [105].

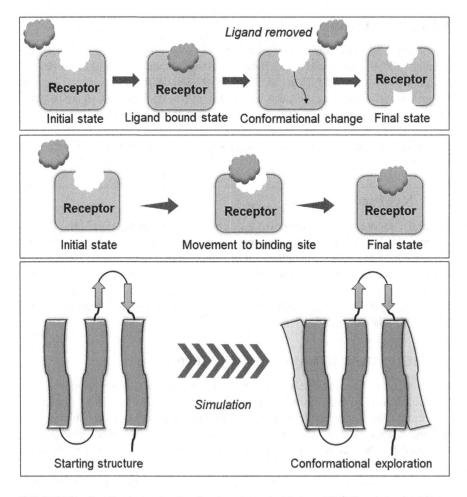

FIGURE 3.9 Applications of molecular dynamics simulations. This illustration highlights some of the most common applications of MD simulations.

3.4.1 ANALYSIS OF THE INTERFACE DYNAMICS

Several tools developed to process all-atom MD trajectories are now accessible. These tools are intended to identify changes in covalent (intra) and noncovalent (inter) contacts, as well as changes in the inherent dynamics of the biomolecular complex. These analysis tools are usually included in the simulation package used to construct the relevant MD trajectory. For example, a large number of gmx scripts in GROMACS allow users to calculate changes in interfacial backbone-related variables (such as dihedral angles), salt bridges, hydrogen bonds, particular interfacial distances, interfacial water molecules, buried surface area, and RMSDs/RMSFs. Visual Molecular Dynamics (VMD) is the analysis package for NAMD, while CPPTRAJ/PYTRAJ is the package for AMBER (Amber Tools). All of these tools can work with any ensemble file (recorded in the PDB format) in addition to their internal formats. Gmx and CPPTRAJ are command-line-based programs, VMD is a GUI-based tool, and PYTRAJ is a Python front-end of the CPPTRAJ package that runs on a Jupyter notebook with the NGL viewer molecular visualization option.

3.5 ADVANCE APPROACHES

Structure-based pharmacophore models built from a single 3D coordinate set obtained from X-ray structures may or may not contain several features due to the crystal-specific packing of ligand-receptor complexes. One way to solve this problem is to use multiple crystal structures of active ligand complexes for the same purpose. Each ligand interaction is recognized and bound to a more accurate pharmacophore hypothesis. However, this strategy is limited to ligand-target complexes for which multiple crystal structures are known and each ligand must have the same binding mechanism. Performing MD simulations of the system under study is another way to generate various accurate sets of atomic coordinates without being limited by the availability of multiple experimental structures. The vast amount of data collected can be used in a variety of ways for pharmacophore modeling and pharmacophore-based virtual screening.

3.5.1 APPROACHES EMPLOYING THE 3D PHARMACOPHORE CONCEPT WITH MOLECULAR DOCKING AND MD SIMULATIONS

The docking method provides new mechanistic insights into protein-ligand binding mechanisms and studies the effects of protein mutations on ligand binding by providing mutational cues that enable robust survival of drug-resistant pathogens. The field is advancing rapidly as continued improvements in computational power expand the practical application of molecular models, offering a better compromise between accuracy and computational cost. These efforts will undoubtedly lead to many more compelling applications in the future. Table 3.10 shows some approaches employing the 3D pharmacophore concept with molecular docking and MD simulations.

TABLE 3.10

Advanced Approaches Employing the 3D Pharmacophore Concept with Molecular Docking and MD Simulations

Approach	Characteristic features	Reference
Hot-spots-guided receptor-based pharmacophores (HS-Pharm)	It allows the prioritization of cavity atoms that should be targeted for ligand binding by training machine learning algorithms with atom-based fingerprints of known ligand-binding pockets.	[110]
Pharmacophore-based interaction fingerprint (Pharm-IF)	Support vector machine and random forest are trained on pharmacophoric fingerprints to rank the docking poses.	[111]
Hydration-site restricted pharmacophore (HSRP)	It reduces the number of pharmacophore features by identifying hydration sites on the protein surface, whose water molecules suffer unfavorable thermodynamic properties as calculated by MD simulations.	[112]
Site-identification by ligand competitive saturation (SILCS) assisted pharmacophore modeling (SILCS-Pharm)	It considers protein flexibility and desolvation effects by using full MD simulations to determine 3D maps of the functional group-affinity patterns on a target receptor.	[113]
Dynamic pharmacophores (Dynophore)	A combination of static three-dimensional pharmacophores and molecular dynamics-based conformational sampling	[114]
Molecular dynamics shared pharmacophore (MYSHAPE)	Construction of a pharmacophore model that exploits information derived from multiple short MD simulations using different molecules within the binding pocket of the target.	[115]
Common hits approach	Three-dimensional pharmacophore models from MD simulations are grouped according to interaction patterns and used for parallel screening.	[116]
Water pharmacophore (WP)	Generation of 3D pharmacophores based on thermodynamic properties of hydration sites.	[117]
Grids of pharmacophore interaction fields (GRAIL)	It is a grid-based approach for the identification of interaction sites and the power of the pharmacophore concept. This approach depicts MIFs on the pharmacophore level in MD simulations.	[118]
AutoDock Bias	It provides cosolvent-based pharmacophores to bias docking algorithms toward hotspots of probe molecule binding for improving virtual screening performance.	[119]
PyRod	It offers structure-based screening campaigns by providing easy-to-interpret dynamic molecular interaction fields (dMIFs) and purely protein-based pharmacophores solely based on tracing water molecules in MD simulations.	[120]
DeepSite	The convolutional neural network is trained on pharmacophoric descriptors to detect cavities, predict binding affinities, and design new molecules	[121]
Pharmmaker	Cosolvent simulations are analyzed to generate 3D pharmacophores for virtual screening.	[122]

3.5.2 INTEGRATED PHARMACOPHORE AND DOCKING-BASED VIRTUAL SCREENING

Pharmacophore-based virtual screening was described earlier in this chapter. Since the pharmacophore model (query) is used to filter and retrieve the initial set of hits from a large database, this search uses the pharmacophore model as a feature of the pharmacophore model. Molecules with either similar features to the cophore or completely different scaffolds are obtained. It maps to multiple structures that can be elements of the compound's functional groups (Figure 3.10). Molecules with higher scores and better fit to the pharmacophore model are then collected as hits. This requires further investigation with different modeling approaches. For example, the highest-scoring perfect match compounds found in a pharmacophore-based screen can be docked into the putative binding pocket of a specific target of interest to reduce the number of active hits. This approach is also called docking-based virtual screening. Furthermore, the stability of the ligand-receptor complex can be confirmed by MD simulations (Figure 3.10). Therefore, the combination of pharmacophore and docking-based virtual screening followed by MD simulation has proven to be a powerful approach to incorporate all available information into computational hit identification (Figure 3.10).

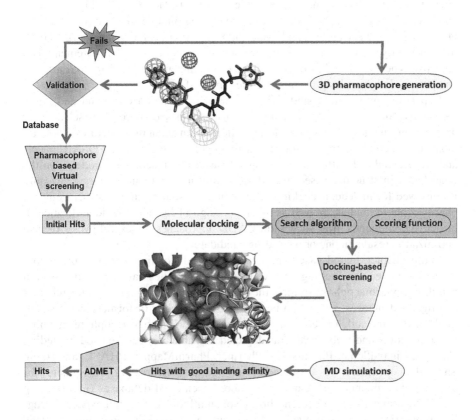

FIGURE 3.10 Schematic representation of integrated pharmacophore and docking-based virtual screening.

3.6 SUMMARY

In pharmaceutical research, CADD is regarded as an excellent tool that is highly accurate and saves time and money. Ligand-based or structure-based drug design approaches are chosen for drug design, depending on the availability of structural information on the ligand and target (receptor or macromolecule). Ligand-based drug design examines information about small molecule (ligand) structures and their associated activities using quantitative structure-activity relationship (QSAR) models or summarizes using ligand-based pharmacophore models. Structure-based drug discovery, on the other hand, uses information about target structures for molecular docking, MD simulation studies, structure-based pharmacophore models, and *de novo* design of ligands. Identification of bioactive compounds after a successful CADD approach, and several cycles of lead optimization, result in one or more drug candidates.

A bioactive compound (or drug molecule/candidate) acts in a milieu of labyrinthine with numerous potential interaction associates. Every single component of the body, from sugars, proteins, nucleic acids, lipids, and metabolites to other small molecules, all inherently interact with a drug molecule. Perhaps, in many cases, these unwanted interactions augment undesirable side effects. Hence, it should be the main objective to design a drug molecule with the desired binding to one or more targets of interest (broad selectivity) and avoid the interaction of undesirable targets (narrow selectivity). It is a continual drug development challenge. The aforementioned objective is accomplished through trial and error, but some rational approaches, like computer-aided drug design, can guide the tuning of selectivity.

Depending on the accessibility of structural information on ligand and target (receptor or macromolecule), a ligand- or structure-based approach is selected for drug design. In ligand-based drug design, information about the structures of a small molecule (ligand) and their associated activity can be studied using QSAR models and/or encapsulated with the aid of ligand-based pharmacophore models. On the other hand, in structure-based drug design, information about the target structure is employed for molecular docking, MD simulation studies, and/or structure-based pharmacophore models, as well as *de novo* design of ligands. The identification of bioactive compounds after successful CADD approaches of several cycles of lead optimization results in one or more drug candidates.

In this chapter, ligand-based and structure-based techniques of pharmacophore modeling, molecular docking, and MD simulation studies have been discussed in detail. For pharmacophore studies, the availability of coordinate files for receptor and ligand structures, which can be obtained in a variety of formats such as .sdf, .mol2, .pdb, and .cif, is necessary. A large number of pharmacophore mapping programs/tools and web servers (as depicted in Table 3.3) can be used, including Catalyst, LigandScout, PharmaGist, Pharmer, PharmMapper, PHASE, and so on. Similarly, coordinate files for receptor and ligand structures are prerequisites for docking experiments. One can also explore specialized databases (i.e., Binding DB, ZINC database) from which libraries of small molecules with expected drug-like properties can be retrieved. A large number of docking programs and web servers can be used (as depicted in Tables 3.5 and 3.6), including GOLD, GLIDE, AutoDock, AutoDock Vina, and so on. Analysis of docking results can be done by programs for visualization, such as PyMOL (https://pymol.org/2/), UCSF Chimera (www.cgl.ucsf.edu/chimera/), BIOVIA Discovery Studio Visualizer (https://discover.3ds.com/discovery-studio-visualizer-download), and VMD (www.ks.uiuc.edu/Research/vmd/). In the case of MD simulations, an initial coordinate file containing the atomic coordinates of the ligand-receptor complex is required. Programs for MD simulations of biomolecules include AMBER (https://ambermd.org/), CHARMM (www.charmm.org/), GROMACS (www.gromacs.org/), and NAMD (www.ks.uiuc.edu/Research/namd/) (Table 3.11). Trajectory analysis can be done with tools described in Table 3.12.

The purpose of this chapter was to provide an overview of the pharmacophore concept and its application in modern computational drug design. The first section of the chapter described the details of pharmacophore modeling. The second section described molecular docking and MD simulations. We concluded with some discussion and comments on future directions in this area. This study provides a basic idea for the rational design of novel/new scaffolds. Ligand-based predictive models can be developed to extract information about the characteristic structural features required for ligand-receptor interactions. MD simulation analysis in 3D pharmacophore model building, followed by molecular docking and virtual screening of available databases, appears more meaningful and time-saving.

TABLE 3.11
List of MD Software/Tool(s)

Sl	Software	Source[a]	Features
1	Amber	https://ambermd.org/	A biomolecular simulation program developed in the 1970s
2	Desmond	www.schrodinger.com/products/desmond	High-speed molecular dynamics simulations of biological systems
3	Gromacs	www.gromacs.org/	Molecular dynamics package is mainly designed for simulations of proteins, lipids, and nucleic acids.
4	Molecular operating environment (MOE)	www.chemcomp.com/Products.htm	A popular molecular dynamics tool
5	NAMD	https://www.ks.uiuc.edu/Research/namd/	Molecular dynamics code designed for high-performance simulation of large biomolecular systems
6	Yasara dynamics	www.yasara.org/	Molecular graphics, modeling, and simulation programs for Windows, Linux, MacOS, and Android developed since 1993

[a]Accessed April 2022.

TABLE 3.12

List of the Described MD Analysis Tools That Can Be Used to Dissect Interface Dynamics

Tool	Characteristic	Source[a]
GROMACS	Includes many tools for preparing, running, and analyzing molecular dynamics simulations.	https://manual.gromacs.org/documentation/2021/reference-manual/analysis.html
gRINN interface	A software for residue interaction energy-based analysis of protein MD simulation trajectories. Facilitate the analysis of interfaces of a wide range of biomolecular complexes.	https://grinn.readthedocs.io/en/latest/ https://github.com/JoaoRodrigues/interfacea/tree/master
MDAnalysis	An object-oriented Python library to analyze trajectories from molecular dynamics simulations	www.mdanalysis.org
MD-TASK	to analyze molecular dynamics trajectories. Residue interaction network (RIN) analysis, perturbation response scanning (PRS), and dynamic cross-correlation.	https://md-task.readthedocs.io/
MDTraj	Extensive analysis functions, including those that compute bonds, angles, dihedrals, hydrogen bonds, secondary structure, and NMR observables.	www.mdtraj.org/1.9.5/index.html
ProDy	Protein structural dynamics analysis. It is designed as a flexible and responsive API suitable for interactive usage and application development.	http://prody.csb.pitt.edu/
ProLIF	Designed to generate interaction fingerprints for complexes made of ligands, protein, DNA, or RNA Molecules extracted from molecular dynamics trajectories, docking simulations, and experimental structures.	https://github.com/chemosim-lab/ProLIF
PYTRAJ/CPPTRAJ	Support > 50 types of analysis, support parallel processing, able to handle many files at the same time, and able to handle very large trajectories.	https://amber-md.github.io/pytraj/latest/index.html
VMD	Molecular visualization program for displaying, animating, and analyzing large biomolecular systems using 3D graphics and built-in scripting.	www.ks.uiuc.edu/Research/vmd/

[a] Accessed April 2022.

REFERENCES

[1]. Muratov EN, Bajorath J, Sheridan RP, et al. QSAR without borders. *Chem Soc Rev* 2020;49(11):3525–3564.

[2]. Dias DA, Urban S, Roessner U. A historical overview of natural products in drug discovery. *Metabolites* 2012;2(2):303–336.

[3]. Lombardino JG, Lowe JA 3rd. The role of the medicinal chemist in drug discovery– Then and now. *Nat Rev Drug Discov* 2004;3(10):853–862.

[4]. Hughes JP, Rees S, Kalindjian SB, et al. Principles of early drug discovery. *Br J Pharmacol* 2011;162(6):1239–1249.

[5]. Bajorath J. Integration of virtual and high-throughput screening. *Nat Rev Drug Discov* 2002;1(11):882–894.

[6]. Kiriiri GK, Njogu PM, Mwangi AN. Exploring different approaches to improve the success of drug discovery and development projects: A review. *Futur J Pharm Sci* 2020;6(11):27.

[7]. Shaker B, Ahmad S, Lee J, et al. In silico methods and tools for drug discovery. *Comput Biol Med* 2021;137:104851.

[8]. Kato Y, Hamada S, Goto H. Validation study of QSAR/DNN models using the competition datasets. *Mol Inform* 2020;39(1–2):e1900154.

[9]. Sliwoski G, Kothiwale S, Meiler J, et al. Computational methods in drug discovery. *Pharmacol Rev* 2013;66(1):334–395.

[10]. Amin SA, Adhikari N, Jha T, et al. First molecular modeling report on novel aryl-pyrimidine kynurenine monooxygenase inhibitors through multi-QSAR analysis against Huntington's disease: A proposal to chemists! *Bioorg Med Chem Lett* 2016;26(23):5712–5718.

[11]. Radaeva M, Dong X, Cherkasov A. The use of methods of computer-aided drug discovery in the development of topoisomerase II inhibitors: Applications and future directions. *J Chem Inf Model* 2020;60(8):3703–3721.

[12]. Amin SA, Jha T. Fight against novel coronavirus: A perspective of medicinal chemists. *Eur J Med Chem* 2020;201:112559.

[13]. Amin SA, Adhikari N, Gayen S, et al. Reliable structural information for rational design of benzoxazole type potential cholesteryl ester transfer protein (CETP) inhibitors through multiple validated modeling techniques. *J Biomol Struct Dyn* 2019;37(17):4528–4541.

[14]. Amin SA, Gayen S. Modelling the cytotoxic activity of pyrazolo-triazole hybrids using descriptors calculated from the open source tool "PaDEL-descriptor." *J Taibah Univ Sci* 2016;10(6):896–905.

[15]. Halder AK, Saha A, Jha T. The role of 3D pharmacophore mapping based virtual screening for identification of novel anticancer agents: An overview. *Curr Top Med Chem* 2013;13(9):1098–1126.

[16]. Macalino SJ, Gosu V, Hong S, et al. Role of computer-aided drug design in modern drug discovery. *Arch Pharm Res* 2015;38(9):1686–1701.

[17]. Choudhury C, Sastry GN. Pharmacophore modelling and screening: Concepts, recent developments and applications in rational drug design. In C. Gopi Mohan, Ed. *Structural bioinformatics: Applications in preclinical drug discovery process.* Springer, Cham, 2019, pp. 25–53.

[18]. Seidel T, Schuetz DA, Garon A, et al. The pharmacophore concept and its applications in computer-aided drug design. *Prog Chem Org Nat Prod* 2019;110:99–141.

[19]. Voet A, Zhang KY. Pharmacophore modelling as a virtual screening tool for the discovery of small molecule protein-protein interaction inhibitors. *Curr Pharm Des* 2012;18(30):4586–4598.

[20]. Yang SY. Pharmacophore modeling and applications in drug discovery: Challenges and recent advances. *Drug Discov Today* 2010;15(11–12):444–450.

[21]. Guedes IA, de Magalhães CS, Dardenne LE. Receptor-ligand molecular docking. *Biophys Rev* 2014;6(1):75–87.

[22]. Huang SY, Zou X. Advances and challenges in protein-ligand docking. *Int J Mol Sci* 2010;11(8):3016–3034.

[23]. Kontoyianni M. Docking and virtual screening in drug discovery. In Iulia M. Lazar, Maria Kontoyianni, and Alexandru C. Lazar, Eds., *Proteomics for drug discovery.* Humana Press, New York, 2017, pp. 255–266.

[24]. Cournia Z, Allen B, Sherman W. Relative binding free energy calculations in drug discovery: Recent advances and practical considerations. *J Chem Inf Model* 2017;57(12):2911–2937.

[25]. Lin X, Li X, Lin X. A review on applications of computational methods in drug screening and design. *Molecules* 2020;25(6):1375.

[26]. Amin SA, Banerjee S, Singh S, et al. First structure-activity relationship analysis of SARS-CoV-2 virus main protease (Mpro) inhibitors: An endeavor on COVID-19 drug discovery. *Mol Divers* 2021;25(3):1827–1838.

[27]. Maia EHB, Assis LC, de Oliveira TA, et al. Structure-based virtual screening: From classical to artificial intelligence. *Front Chem* 2020;8:343.

[28]. Kaserer T, Beck KR, Akram M, et al. Pharmacophore models and pharmacophore-based virtual screening: Concepts and applications exemplified on hydroxysteroid dehydrogenases. *Molecules* 2015;20(12):22799–22832.

[29]. Kutlushina A, Khakimova A, Madzhidov T, et al. Ligand-based pharmacophore modeling using novel 3d pharmacophore signatures. *Molecules* 2018;23(12):3094.

[30]. Scior T, Bender A, Tresadern G, et al. Recognizing pitfalls in virtual screening: A critical review. *J Chem Inf Model* 2012;52(4):867–881.

[31]. Güner OF, Bowen JP. Setting the record straight: The origin of the pharmacophore concept. *J Chem Inf Model* 2014;54(5):1269–1283.

[32]. Ehrlich P. Über den jetzigen Stand der Chemotherapie. *Ber Dtsch Chem Ges* 1909;42(1):17–47.

[33]. Ehrlich P. Über die constitution des diphtheriegiftes. *Dtsch Wochschr* 1898;24(38):597–600.

[34]. Kier LB. Molecular orbital calculation of preferred conformations of acetylcholine, muscarine, and muscarone. *Mol Pharmacol* 1967;3(5):487–494.

[35]. Kier LB. *Molecular orbital theory in drug research; Medicinal chemistry-A series of monographs.* Academic Press, New York, 1971, Vol. 10.

[36]. Kier LB. Receptor mapping using molecular orbital theory. In James Frederic Danielli, J. F. Moran, and D. J. Triggle, Eds., *Fundamental concepts in drug-receptor interactions.* Academic Press, New York, 1970, pp. 15–46.

[37]. Gund P. Three-dimensional pharmacophoric pattern searching. *In* Hahn FE, Ed. *Progress in molecular and subcellular biology.* Springer-Verlag, Berlin, 1977; Vol. 11, pp. 117–143.

[38]. Wermuth C-G, Ganellin CR, Lindberg P, et al. Glossary of terms used in medicinal chemistry (IUPAC recommendations 1998). *Pure Appl Chem* 1998;70(5):1129–1143.

[39]. Yu W, MacKerell AD Jr. Computer-aided drug design methods. *Methods Mol Biol* 2017;1520:85–106.

[40]. Qing X, Lee XY, De Raeymaecker J, et al. Pharmacophore modeling: Advances, limitations, and current utility in drug discovery. *J Recep LiG Chan Res* 2014;7:81–92.

[41]. Wolber G, Kosara R. Pharmacophores from macromolecular complexes with LigandScout. *In* Langer T, Hoffmann RD, Eds. *Pharmacophores and Pharmacophore Searches.* Wiley-VCH Verlag GmbH & Co. KGaA, Weinheim, 2006, pp. 131–150.

[42]. Berman HM, Westbrook J, Feng Z, et al. The Protein Data Bank. *Nucleic Acids Res* 2000;28(1):235–242.

[43]. Dassault Systèmes BIOVIA. *Discovery studio modeling environment.* Dassault Systèmes, San Diego, 2022.

[44]. Wolber G, Langer T. LigandScout: 3-D pharmacophores derived from protein-bound ligands and their use as virtual screening filters. *J Chem Inf Model* 2005;45(1):160–169.

[45]. Kalyaanamoorthy S, Chen YP. Structure-based drug design to augment hit discovery. *Drug Discov Today* 2011;16(17–18):831–839.

[46]. Tripathi A, Bankaitis VA. Molecular docking: From lock and key to combination lock. *J Mol Med Clin Appl* 2017;2(1): 10.16966/2575-0305.106.

[47]. Burley SK, Berman HM, Christie C, et al. RCSB protein data bank: Sustaining a living digital data resource that enables breakthroughs in scientific research and biomedical education. *Protein Sci* 2018;27(1):316–330.

[48]. Salmaso V, Moro S. Bridging Molecular docking to molecular dynamics in exploring ligand-protein recognition process: An overview. *Front Pharmacol* 2018;9:923.

[49]. Abagyan R, Totrov M. High-throughput docking for lead generation. *Curr Opin Chem Biol* 2001;5(4):375–382.

[50]. Kitchen DB, Decornez H, Furr JR, et al. Docking and scoring in virtual screening for drug discovery: Methods and applications. *Nat Rev Drug Discov* 2004;3(11):935–949.

[51]. Kuntz ID, Blaney JM, Oatley SJ, et al. A geometric approach to macromolecule-ligand interactions. *J Mol Biol* 1982;161(2):269–288.

[52]. Halperin I, Ma B, Wolfson H, et al. Principles of docking: An overview of search algorithms and a guide to scoring functions. *Proteins* 2002;47(4):409–443.

[53]. Taylor RD, Jewsbury PJ, Essex JW. A review of protein-small molecule docking methods. *J Comput Aid Mol Des* 2002;16(3):151–166.

[54]. Brooijmans N, Kuntz ID. Molecular recognition and docking algorithms. *Annu Rev Biophys Biomol Struct* 2003;32(1):335–373.

[55]. Friesner RA, Banks JL, Murphy RB, et al. Glide: A new approach for rapid, accurate docking and scoring. 1. Method and assessment of docking accuracy. *J Med Chem* 2004;47(7):1739–1749.

[56]. Halgren TA, Murphy RB, Friesner RA, et al. Glide: A new approach for rapid, accurate docking and scoring. 2. Enrichment factors in database screening. *J Med Chem* 2004;47(7):1750–1759.

[57]. Rarey M, Kramer B, Lengauer T, et al. A fast flexible docking method using an incremental construction algorithm. *J Mol Biol* 1996;261(3):470–489.

[58]. Welch W, Ruppert J, Jain AN. Hammerhead: Fast, fully automated docking of flexible ligands to protein binding sites. *Chem Biol* 1996;3(6):449–462.

[59]. Miller MD, Kearsley SK, Underwood DJ, et al. FLOG: A system to select 'quasi-flexible' ligands complementary to a receptor of known three-dimensional structure. *J Comput Aid Mol Des* 1994;8(2):153–174.

[60]. Pang YP, Perola E, Xu K, et al. EUDOC: A computer program for identification of drug interaction sites in macromolecules and drug leads from chemical databases. *J Comput Chem* 2001;22(15):1750–1771.

[61]. Sauton N, Lagorce D, Villoutreix BO, et al. MS-DOCK: Accurate multiple conformation generator and rigid docking protocol for multi-step virtual ligand screening. *BMC Bioinformatics* 2008;9(1):184.

[62]. Gohlke H, Hendlich M, Klebe G. Knowledge-based scoring function to predict protein-ligand interactions. *J Mol Biol* 2000;295(2):337–356.

[63]. Morris GM, Goodsell DS, Huey R, et al. Distributed automated docking of flexible ligands to proteins: Parallel applications of AutoDock 2.4. *J Comput Aid Mol Des* 1996;10(2):293–304.

[64]. Abagyan R, Totrov M, Kuznetsov D. ICM? A new method for protein modeling and design: Applications to docking and structure prediction from the distorted native conformation. *J Comput Chem* 1994;15(5):488–506.

[65]. McMartin C, Bohacek RS. QXP: Powerful, rapid computer algorithms for structure-based drug design. *J Comput Aid Mol Des* 1997;11(4):333–344.

[66]. Liu M, Wang S. MCDOCK: A Monte Carlo simulation approach to the molecular docking problem. *J Comput Aid Mol Des* 1999;13(5):435–451.

[67]. Trott O, Olson AJ. AutoDock Vina: Improving the speed and accuracy of docking with a new scoring function, efficient optimization, and multithreading. *J Comput Chem* 2010;31(2):455–461.

[68]. Meiler J, Baker D. Rosettaligand: Protein-small molecule docking with full side-chain flexibility. *Proteins* 2006;65(3):538–548.

[69]. Baxter CA, Murray CW, Clark DE, et al. Flexible docking using tabu search and an empirical estimate of binding affinity. *Proteins* 1998;33(3):367–382.

[70]. Pei J, Wang Q, Liu Z, et al. PSI-DOCK: Towards highly efficient and accurate flexible ligand docking. *Proteins* 2006;62(4):934–946.

[71]. Jones G, Willett P, Glen RC. Molecular recognition of receptor sites using a genetic algorithm with a description of desolvation. *J Mol Biol* 1995;245(1):43–53.

[72]. Jones G, Willett P, Glen RC, et al. Development and validation of a genetic algorithm for flexible docking. *J Mol Biol* 1997;267(3):727–748.

[73]. Morris GM, Goodsell DS, Halliday RS, et al. Automated docking using a Lamarckian genetic algorithm and an empirical binding free energy function. *J Comput Chem* 1998;19(14):1639–1662.

[74]. Ruiz-Carmona S, Alvarez-Garcia D, Foloppe N, et al. rDock: A fast, versatile and open source program for docking ligands to proteins and nucleic acids. *PLOS Comput Biol* 2014;10(4):e1003571.

[75]. Korb O, Stützle T, Exner TE. PLANTS: Application of ant colony optimization to structure-based drug design. *In* Dorigo M, Gambardella LM, Birattari M, Martinoli A, Poli R, Stützle T, Eds. *Ant colony optimization and swarm intelligence.* Springer, Berlin; Heidelberg, 2006, pp. 247–258.

[76]. Chen HM, Liu BF, Huang HL, et al. Sodock: Swarm optimization for highly flexible protein-ligand docking. *J Comput Chem* 2007;28(2):612–623.

[77]. Namasivayam V, Günther R. pso@autodock: A fast flexible molecular docking program based on Swarm intelligence. *Chem Biol Drug Des* 2007;70(6):475–484.

[78]. Verdonk ML, Cole JC, Hartshorn MJ, et al. Improved protein-ligand docking using gold. *Proteins* 2003;52(4):609–623.

[79]. Huey R, Morris GM, Olson AJ, et al. A semiempirical free energy force field with charge-based desolvation. *J Comput Chem* 2007;28(6):1145–1152.

[80]. Corbeil CR, Williams CI, Labute P. Variability in docking success rates due to dataset preparation. *J Comput Aid Mol Des* 2012;26(6):775–786.

[81]. Böhm HJ. The development of a simple empirical scoring function to estimate the binding constant for a protein-ligand complex of known three-dimensional structure. *J Comput Aid Mol Des* 1994;8(3):243–256.

[82]. Eldridge MD, Murray CW, et al. Empirical scoring functions: I. The development of a fast empirical scoring function to estimate the binding affinity of ligands in receptor complexes. *J Comput Aid Mol Des* 1997;11(5):425–445.

[83]. Velec HFG, Gohlke H, Klebe G. DrugScore(CSD)-knowledge based scoring function derived from small molecule crystal data with superior recognition rate of near-native ligand poses and better affinity prediction. *J Med Chem.* 2005;48(20):6296–6303.

[84]. Mooij WT, Verdonk ML. General and targeted statistical potentials for protein-ligand interactions. *Proteins* 2005;61(2):272–287.

[85]. Charifson PS, Corkery JJ, Murcko MA, et al. Consensus scoring: A method for obtaining improved hit rates from docking databases of three-dimensional structures into proteins. *J Med Chem* 1999;42(25):5100–5109.

[86]. Yuriev E, Holien J, Ramsland PA. Improvements, trends, and new ideas in molecular docking: 2012–2013 in review. *J Mol Recognit* 2015;28(10):581–604.

[87]. Andreani J, Guerois R. Evolution of protein interactions: from interactomes to interfaces. *Arch Biochem Biophys* 2014;554:65–75.

[88]. Ohue M, Matsuzaki Y, Shimoda T, et al. Highly precise protein-protein interaction prediction based on consensus between template-based and de novo docking methods. *BMC Proc* 2013;7;S6.

[89]. Ohue M, Matsuzaki Y, Uchikoga N, et al. Megadock: An all-to-all protein-protein interaction prediction system using tertiary structure data. *Protein Pept Lett* 2014;21(8):766–778.

[90]. Shin WH, Christoffer CW, Kihara D. In silico structure-based approaches to discover protein-protein interaction-targeting drugs. *Methods* 2017;131:22–32.

[91]. Vakser IA. Protein-protein docking: From interaction to interactome. *Biophys J* 2014;21(8):1785–1793.

[92]. Bian Y, Xie XS. Computational fragment-based drug design: Current trends, strategies, and applications. *AAPS J* 2018;20(3):59.

[93]. Fukunishi Y. Post processing of protein-compound docking for fragment-based drug discovery (FBDD): In-silico structure-based drug screening and ligand-binding pose prediction. *Curr Top Med Chem* 2010;10(6):680–694.

[94]. Konteatis ZD. In silico fragment-based drug design. *Expert Opin Drug Discov* 2010;5(11):1047–1065.

[95]. Mortier J, Rakers C, Frederick R, et al. Computational tools for in silico fragment-based drug design. *Curr Top Med Chem* 2012;12(17):1935–1943.

[96]. Rachman M, Piticchio S, Majewski M, et al. Fragment-to-lead tailored in silico design. *Drug Discov Today Technol* 2021;40:44–57.

[97]. Ban F, Hu L, Zhou XH, et al. Inverse molecular docking reveals a novel function of thymol: Inhibition of fat deposition induced by high-dose glucose in Caenorhabditis elegans. *Food Sci Nutr* 2021;9(8):4243–4253.

[98]. Jukič M, Kores K, Janežič D, et al. Repurposing of drugs for SARS-CoV-2 using inverse docking fingerprints. *Front Chem* 2021;9:757826.

[99]. Ma Z, Zou X. MDock: A suite for molecular inverse docking and target prediction. *Methods Mol Biol* 2021;2266:313–322.

[100]. Wasukan N, Kuno M, Maniratanachote R. Molecular docking as a promising predictive model for silver nanoparticle-mediated inhibition of cytochrome P450 enzymes. *J Chem Inf Model* 2019;59(21):5126–5134.

[101]. Ranjan S, Dasgupta N, Sudandiradoss C, et al. Titanium dioxide nanoparticle-protein interaction explained by docking approach. *Int J Nanomedicine* 2018;13(T-NANO 2014 Abstracts):47–50.

[102]. Abdelsattar AS, Dawoud A, Helal MA. Interaction of nanoparticles with biological macromolecules: A review of molecular docking studies. *Nanotoxicology* 2021;15(1):66–95.

[103]. Parrill AL, Reddy MR. Rational drug design. *In* Parrill AL, Reddy MR, Eds. *Novel methodology and practical applications.* American Chemical Society.

[104]. Sussman JL, Silman I. Computational studies on cholinesterases: Strengthening our understanding of the integration of structure, dynamics and function. *Neuropharmacology* 2020;179:108265.

[105]. Hollingsworth SA, Dror RO. Molecular dynamics simulation for all. *Neuron* 2018;99(6):1129–1143.

[106]. Adcock SA, McCammon JA. Molecular dynamics: Survey of methods for simulating the activity of proteins. *Chem Rev* 2006;106(5):1589–1615.

[107]. Liu X, Shi D, Zhou S, et al. Molecular dynamics simulations and novel drug discovery. *Expert Opin Drug Discov* 2018;13(1):23–37.

[108]. Karplus M, McCammon JA. Molecular dynamics simulations of biomolecules. *Nat Struct Biol* 2002;9(9):646–652.

[109]. Hildebrand PW, Rose AS, Tiemann JKS. Bringing Molecular Dynamics simulation data into view. *Trends Biochem Sci* 2019;44(11):902–913.

[110]. Barillari C, Marcou G, Rognan D. Hot-spots-guided receptor-based pharmacophores (HS-Pharm): A knowledge-based approach to identify ligand-anchoring atoms in protein cavities and prioritize structure-based pharmacophores. *J Chem Inf Model* 2008;48(7):1396–1410.

[111]. Sato T, Honma T, Yokoyama S. Combining machine learning and pharmacophore-based interaction fingerprint for in silico screening. *J Chem Inf Model* 2010;50(1):170–185.

[112]. Hu B, Lill MA. Protein pharmacophore selection using hydration-site analysis. *J Chem Inf Model* 2012;52(4):1046–1060.

[113]. Yu W, Lakkaraju SK, Raman EP, et al. Site-identification by ligand competitive saturation (SILCS) assisted pharmacophore modeling. *J Comput Aid Mol Des* 2014;28(5):491–507.

[114]. Bock A, Bermudez M, Krebs F, et al. Ligand binding ensembles determine graded agonist efficacies at a G protein-coupled receptor. *J Biol Chem* 2016;291(31):16375–16389.

[115]. Perricone U, Wieder M, Seidel T, et al. A molecular dynamics-shared pharmacophore approach to boost early-enrichment virtual screening: A case study on peroxisome proliferator-activated receptor α. *ChemMedChem* 2017;12(16):1399–1407.

[116]. Wieder M, Garon A, Perricone U, et al. Common hits approach: Combining pharmacophore modeling and molecular dynamics simulations. *J Chem Inf Model* 2017;57(2):365–385.

[117]. Jung SW, Kim M, Ramsey S, et al. Water pharmacophore: Designing ligands using molecular dynamics simulations with water. *Sci Rep* 2018;8(1):10400.

[118]. Schuetz DA, Seidel T, Garon A, et al. GRAIL: GRids of pharmacophore interaction fieLds. *J Chem Theor Comput* 2018;14(9):4958–4970.

[119]. Arcon JP, Modenutti CP, Avendaño D, et al. AutoDock Bias: Improving binding mode prediction and virtual screening using known protein-ligand interactions. *Bioinformatics* 2019;35(19):3836–3838.

[120]. Schaller D, Pach S, Wolber G. PyRod: Tracing water molecules in molecular dynamics simulations. *J Chem Inf Model* 2019;59(6):2818–2829.

[121]. Jiménez J, Doerr S, Martínez-Rosell G, et al. DeepSite: Protein-binding site predictor using 3D-convolutional neural networks. *Bioinformatics* 2017;33(19):3036–3042.

[122]. Lee JY, Krieger JM, Li H, et al. Pharmmaker: Pharmacophore modeling and hit identification based on druggability simulations. *Protein Sci* 2020;29(1):76–86.

Part B

Matrix Metalloproteinases
and Their Inhibitors

4 Collagenases and Their Inhibitors

Sandip Kumar Baidya, Suvankar Banerjee,
Nilanjan Adhikari, and Tarun Jha

CONTENTS

ABSTRACT

This chapter includes a detailed overview of each of the collagenases, namely collagenase-1 (also known as MMP-1), collagenase-2 (also known as MMP-8), and collagenase-3 (also known as MMP-13). All of these collagenases have a solid track record of regulating several serious disease problems, namely various cancers, cardiovascular illnesses, and inflammatory disease conditions, including osteoarthritis and rheumatoid arthritis. Moreover, both pharmaceutical corporations and research and academic organizations have developed a significant number of new molecules with crucial inhibitory activity against collagenases. Unfortunately, these molecules have shown adverse effects despite exhibiting promising outcomes. In this chapter, detailed knowledge about the key structural features of existing collagenase inhibitors can be found, and with the help of drug design strategies, a novel class of collagenase inhibitors may be identified. Therefore, this chapter will be useful for

DOI: 10.1201/9781003303282-6

scientists researching the mechanisms involved in designing and discovering new drugs that target collagenases.

Keywords: Collagenases; Hydroxamates; Carboxylic acid; Thiol and mercaptosulfide; Phosphonates; Compounds with other ZBGs

4.1 INTRODUCTION

Matrix metalloproteinases (MMPs) are a group of Zn^{2+}-dependent endopeptidase enzymes that are associated with the degradation of the extracellular matrix (ECM). These MMPs are excreted in the body from various proinflammatory cells and connective tissues, namely osteoblasts, fibroblasts, endothelial cells, neutrophils, lymphocytes, and macrophages [1–4]. The family of MMPs can be grouped into five different subclasses known as collagenases (comprising MMP-1, MMP-8, MMP-13, and MMP-18), gelatinases (comprising MMP-2 and MMP-9), stromelysins (comprising MMP-3, MMP-10, and MMP-11), matrilysins (comprising MMP-7 and MMP-26), membrane-type MMPs (comprising MMP-14, MMP-15, MMP-16, MMP-17, MMP-24, and MMP-25), and other types of MMPs (comprising MMP-12, MMP-19, MMP-20, MMP-21, MMP-22, MMP-23, MMP-27, and MMP-28) [1, 2]. Among these various MMPs, collagenases (MMP-1, MMP-8, MMP-13, and MMP-18) mainly assist in the degradation of collagen. Because of the unique capability to break down the collagen triple helix, these collagenases allow the uncoiling of the collagen chain, eventually leading to its degradation by other MMPs [2, 5].

4.2 STRUCTURAL OVERVIEW OF COLLAGENASES

As far as the structure of collagenases is concerned, all of them display a structural resemblance to each other. Collagenases consist of (a) the N-terminal signal sequence, (b) a pro-peptide domain, (c) the zinc and calcium ion-containing catalytic domain, and (d) the C-terminal hemopexin domain (Figure 4.1A).

The C-terminal hemopexin domain can be found in almost all the MMP isoforms except MMP-7 and MMP-26 [2, 6]. The catalytic domain of the collagenases comprises two Ca^{2+} ions, one structural Zn^{2+} ion, and a catalytic Zn^{2+} ion at the active site. The active site of the collagenase is highly conserved and has a conserved active site amino acid sequence motif (HEXXHXXGXXH) coordinated with the catalytic Zn^{2+} ion where the glutamic acid residue is associated with the catalytic function of the enzyme [2, 7–9]. The inhibitor-bound crystal structures of MMP-1 (PDB ID: 1CGL), MMP-8 (PDB ID: 1ZS0), and MMP-13 (PDB ID: 1FM1) are represented in Figure 4.1 [10].

4.3 PATHOPHYSIOLOGY AND COLLAGENASES

Among the four collagenases discovered (MMP-1, MMP-8, MMP-13, and MMP-18), no significant correlations between MMP-18 (collagenase-4) and pathophysiological conditions have been explored to date. However, the rest of the major collagenase isoforms, such as MMP-1 (collagenase-1), MMP-8 (collagenase-2), and MMP-13 (collagenase-3), are well-established to be associated with a wide array of diseases and pathophysiological conditions (Figure 4.2).

Regarding the contributions of MMP-1 (collagenase-1) in different pathophysiological conditions, MMP-1 enzymatic efficacy is found to be highly correlated with disease conditions like cardiovascular disorders [11, 12], chronic obstructive

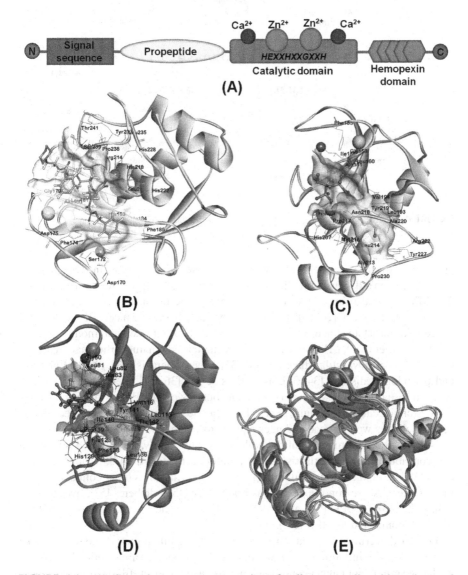

FIGURE 4.1 (A) General cartoon representation of collagenases; ligand-bound crystal structure of (B) MMP-1 (PDB ID: 1CGL); (C) MMP-8 (PDB ID: 1ZS0); (D) MMP-13 (PDB ID: 1FM1); (E) Superimposed structure of collagenases (MMP-1: gray; MMP-8: light gray; and MMP-13: dark gray).

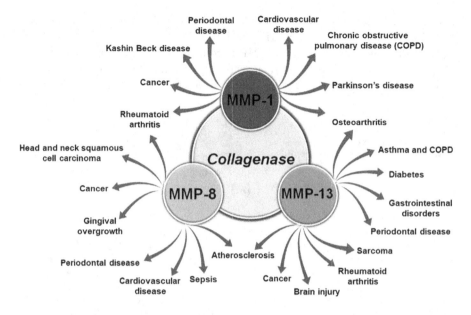

FIGURE 4.2 Role of collagenases in various disease conditions.

pulmonary disease (COPD) [13], periodontal diseases [14], Kashin-Beck disease [15], Parkinson's disease [16], rheumatoid arthritis [17, 18], and osteoarthritis [19, 20]. MMP-1 is also involved with several neoplastic or cancerous conditions that include breast cancer [21–23], tongue cancer [24], bladder cancer [25], colorectal cancer [26], prostate cancer [27], and esophageal squamous cell carcinoma [28].

On the other hand, MMP-8 is correlated with diseases, namely rheumatoid arthritis [29, 30], cardiovascular disorders [31, 32], atherosclerosis [33], gingival growth, and periodontal disease [34, 35], as well as sepsis [36, 37]. Nevertheless, various types of research disclosed the crucial contributions of MMP-8 in multiple cancers such as breast cancer [38], lung cancer [39], gastric cancer [40], and colorectal cancers [41, 42], as well as head and neck squamous cell carcinoma [43, 44].

Notably, the final member of the collagenase sub-family, i.e., MMP-13, is also a key contributor to osteoarthritis and rheumatoid arthritis [45–47], periodontal diseases [48, 49], and cardiovascular disorders [50], similar to its other collagenase siblings. Other disease conditions such as brain injury [51], diabetes [52], liver fibrosis [53], asthma and COPD [54], atherosclerosis [55, 56], and keratoacanthoma [57] are also well-connected to MMP-13 activity.

Due to the crucial association of MMP-13 with inflammatory conditions like arthritis [45–47], inflammatory bowel disease [58], and ulcerative colitis [59, 60], as well as several major cancer conditions such as gastric cancer [61, 62], thyroid cancer [63], prostate cancer [64], lung cancer [65], bladder cancer [66], colorectal cancer [67, 68], breast cancer [69, 70], head and neck cancer [71, 72], and non-small cell lung cancer [73], MMP-13 has become a valuable target for potential drug development and discovery. In addition, several other neoplastic conditions such as hepatocellular carcinoma [74], squamous cell carcinoma [75], eyelid basal carcinoma [76], tumor angiogenesis [77], malignant peripheral nerve sheath tumor [78], melanoma [79], cutaneous malignant melanoma [80], fibrosarcoma [81], osteosarcoma [82], chondrosarcoma [83, 84], glioma [85, 86], and nasopharyngeal carcinoma [87] are also highly correlated with the activity of MMP-13.

4.4 POTENT MMP INHIBITORS TESTED CLINICALLY

As far as several potent MMP inhibitors (MMPIs) [88–97] are concerned, these have been studied extensively in different phases of clinical evaluation for the last three decades (Figure 4.3). Many research activities have been conducted and are continuing. This may inspire the acceleration of developing and discovering newer MMPIs for effectively managing diseases associated with MMPs.

4.5 COLLAGENASE INHIBITORS

It is manifested clearly that collagenases perform vital roles and subsequently function in the progression of several cancers. Therefore, collagenase inhibitors may be a fruitful remedy to resist various cancers. As these collagenases are Zn^{2+}-dependent MMPs, inhibitors comprising diverse zinc binding groups (ZBGs) may be utilized to design potent compounds for anticancer therapy. Several compounds possessing various ZBGs are shown in the following sections.

4.5.1 Hydroxamate-Based Inhibitors

Scientists from Pfizer Central Research [98] reported that succinimide-based hydroxamates were promising MMP-1 inhibitors. Compound **4.11** (Figure 4.4) was the strongest MMP-1 inhibitor (IC_{50} = 150 nM).

The same group of scientists from Pfizer [99] again reported some pyrrolidine-based MMP-13 inhibitors. Compound **4.12** (Figure 4.4) was the most efficacious MMP-13 inhibitor (IC_{50} = 7 nM) selective over other MMPs. A further study by Pfizer Scientists [100] led to the developing of some 2-oxo-imidazolidine-4-carboxylic acid hydroxamates as potential MMPIs. Compound **4.13** (Figure 4.4) was the most promising MMP-13 inhibitor (IC_{50} = 3 nM), which was highly selective over gelatinases, and sparing MMP-3 and MMP-1.

Letavic et al. [101] reported some piperazine-based dual inhibitors of MMP-13 and TACE. Some of them were potent and selective MMP-13 inhibitors over TACE. Compound **4.14** (Figure 4.4) was the most potent MMP-13 inhibitor (IC_{50} = 3 nM), showing selectivity over TACE and sparing MMP-1. A series of pyran-based sulfonamide hydroxamic acids were reported by Reiter et al. [102]. Compounds **4.15** and **4.16** (Figure 4.4) were highly efficacious but non-selective MMP-13 inhibitors. Although these (compounds **4.15** and **4.16**) displayed moderate bioavailability in rats and dogs, patients with osteoarthritis reported musculoskeletal symptoms (MSS) while taking these drugs for four to six weeks.

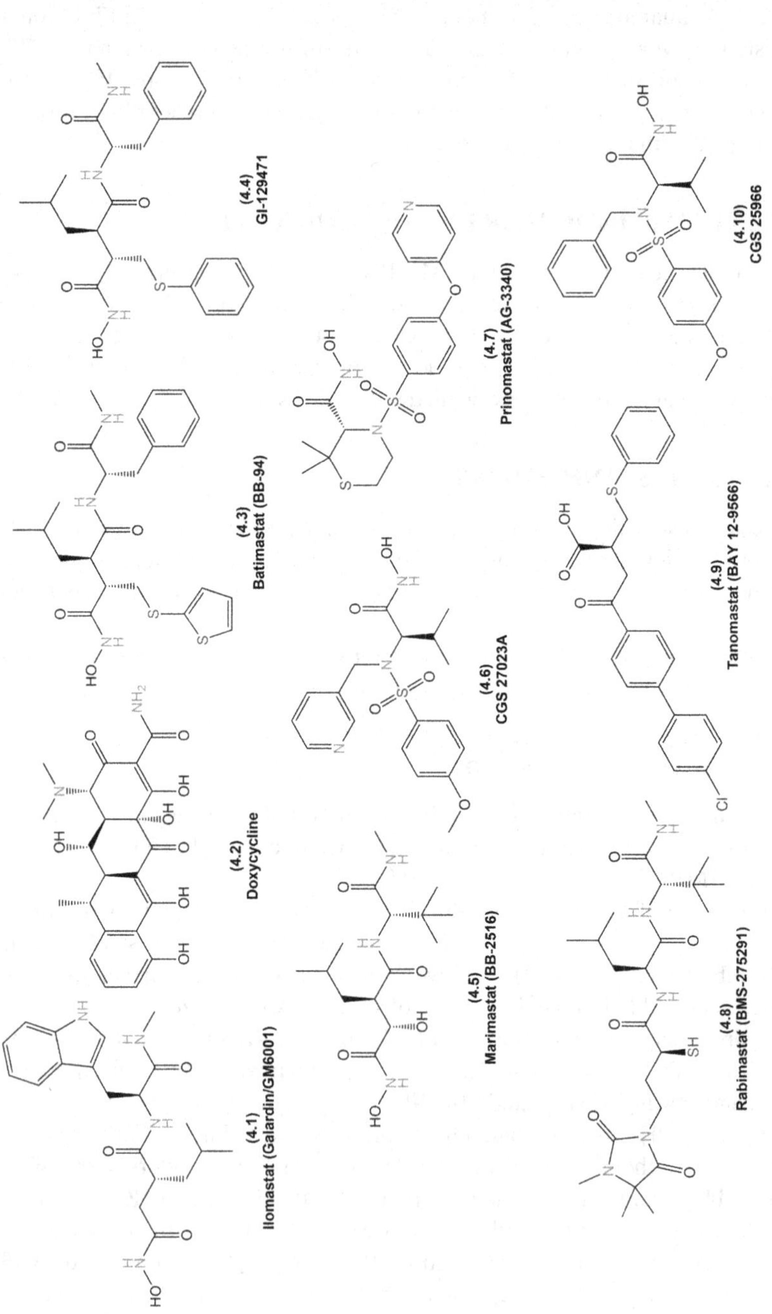

FIGURE 4.3 Potential MMPIs evaluated in various clinical studies (compounds **4.1**–**4.10**).

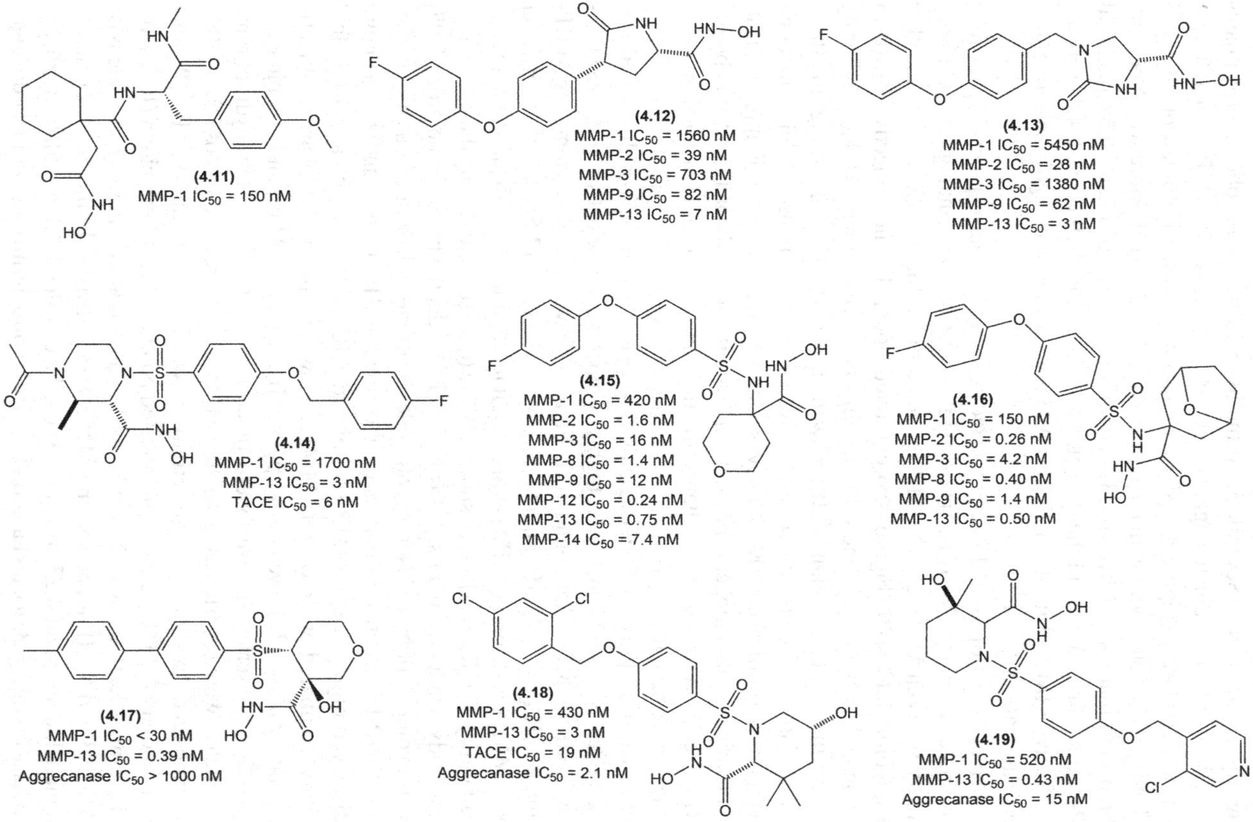

(4.11)
MMP-1 IC$_{50}$ = 150 nM

(4.12)
MMP-1 IC$_{50}$ = 1560 nM
MMP-2 IC$_{50}$ = 39 nM
MMP-3 IC$_{50}$ = 703 nM
MMP-9 IC$_{50}$ = 82 nM
MMP-13 IC$_{50}$ = 7 nM

(4.13)
MMP-1 IC$_{50}$ = 5450 nM
MMP-2 IC$_{50}$ = 28 nM
MMP-3 IC$_{50}$ = 1380 nM
MMP-9 IC$_{50}$ = 62 nM
MMP-13 IC$_{50}$ = 3 nM

(4.14)
MMP-1 IC$_{50}$ = 1700 nM
MMP-13 IC$_{50}$ = 3 nM
TACE IC$_{50}$ = 6 nM

(4.15)
MMP-1 IC$_{50}$ = 420 nM
MMP-2 IC$_{50}$ = 1.6 nM
MMP-3 IC$_{50}$ = 16 nM
MMP-8 IC$_{50}$ = 1.4 nM
MMP-9 IC$_{50}$ = 12 nM
MMP-12 IC$_{50}$ = 0.24 nM
MMP-13 IC$_{50}$ = 0.75 nM
MMP-14 IC$_{50}$ = 7.4 nM

(4.16)
MMP-1 IC$_{50}$ = 150 nM
MMP-2 IC$_{50}$ = 0.26 nM
MMP-3 IC$_{50}$ = 4.2 nM
MMP-8 IC$_{50}$ = 0.40 nM
MMP-9 IC$_{50}$ = 1.4 nM
MMP-13 IC$_{50}$ = 0.50 nM

(4.17)
MMP-1 IC$_{50}$ < 30 nM
MMP-13 IC$_{50}$ = 0.39 nM
Aggrecanase IC$_{50}$ > 1000 nM

(4.18)
MMP-1 IC$_{50}$ = 430 nM
MMP-13 IC$_{50}$ = 3 nM
TACE IC$_{50}$ = 19 nM
Aggrecanase IC$_{50}$ = 2.1 nM

(4.19)
MMP-1 IC$_{50}$ = 520 nM
MMP-13 IC$_{50}$ = 0.43 nM
Aggrecanase IC$_{50}$ = 15 nM

FIGURE 4.4 Some hydroxamate-based potential collagenase inhibitors (compounds **4.11–4.19**).

Several 3-hydroxy-4-arylsulfonyltetrahydropyranyl-3-hydroxamic acids were established as potent inhibitors of both MMP-13 and aggrecanase, sparing MMP-1 [103]. Compound **4.17** (Figure 4.4) was the best MMP-13 inhibitor ($IC_{50} = 0.39$ nM) among these inhibitors. Several 3,3-dimethyl-5-hydroxypipecolic hydroxamates were synthesized and evaluated against aggrecanase, MMP-1, MMP-13, and TACE [104]. Compound **4.18** (Figure 4.4) showed maximum MMP-13 inhibition ($IC_{50} = 3$ nM), having good selectivity with respect to TACE and MMP-1. Moreover, Noe et al. [105] reported that some 3-hydroxy-3-methylpipecolic hydroxamates have potential MMP-13 and aggrecanase inhibitory activity. Compound **4.19** (Figure 4.4) was the most effective MMP-13 inhibitor ($IC_{50} = 0.43$ nM), which was highly selective over aggrecanases and MMP-1.

Becker et al. [106] from Pfizer reported a set of β- and α-piperidine-sulfone hydroxamates as potent MMPIs. Interestingly, most of these analogs exerted non-selectivity between MMP-2 and MMP-13, maintaining higher selectivity over other MMPs. Compound **4.20** (Figure 4.5) exhibited potent but non-selective MMP-13 inhibition ($IC_{50} = 0.40$ nM) and a higher selectivity than other MMPs. Regarding pharmacokinetics, it (compound **4.20**) showed an excellent C_{max} of 281 mg/ml after 6 hr of administration in rats. In a corneal neovascularisation mouse model, compound **4.20** (Figure 4.5) inhibited 50% of neovascularization at a dose of 50 mpk, indicating its promising antiangiogenic property. In combination with paclitaxel, compound **4.20** (Figure 4.5) was found to enhance the median survival time of mice by about 46.7 days, indicating its ability to inhibit tumor growth.

Kolodziej et al. [107] at Pfizer disclosed a series of phenylpiperidine α-sulfone hydroxamates as orally bioavailable, highly competent, and selective MMP-13 inhibitors over other MMPs. Compound **4.21** (Figure 4.5) was the most promising MMP-13 inhibitor ($IC_{50} = 0.42$ nM), maintaining a minimum of 12.5-fold selectivity over different MMPs and sparing MMP-1 and -14. It (compound **4.21**) exhibited moderate bioavailability (20.70%) and a very short half-life ($t_{1/2} = 0.24$ hr) during the pharmacokinetics study conducted in rats. A further study conducted by the same group [108] led to the evolution of N-aryl isonipecotamide α-sulfone hydroxamates as highly efficacious MMP-13-selective inhibitors over various MMPs. Compound **4.22** (Figure 4.5) displayed highly potent MMP-13 inhibition ($IC_{50} = 9$ nM) with at least 41-fold selectivity compared with various MMPs. However, in the rat pharmacokinetic model, compound **4.22** showed a very poor half-life ($t_{1/2} = 0.83$ hr) and oral bioavailability (4.2%). A series of α-sulfone-α-piperidine, as well as α-tetrahydropyranyl hydroxamates, were reported as promising MMPIs by the researchers of Pfizer [109]. Many compounds exhibited non-selectivity between MMP-13 and MMP-2. Among these, compound **4.23** (Figure 4.5) manifested potent MMP-13 inhibition ($IC_{50} < 0.1$ nM), but non-selectivity with MMP-2 and MMP-9, maintaining higher selectivity over MMP-3 and MMP-8 and sparing MMP-1 and MMP-7. In the rat pharmacokinetics model, compound **4.23** (Figure 4.5) produced effective bioavailability (68%), a good half-life ($t_{1/2} = 3$ hr), and a good C_{max} (> 20,000 ng/ml) after 6 hr of dosing.

Some α-sulfone hydroxamates were also produced as selective MMP-13 inhibitors [110]. Among these, compound **4.24** (Figure 4.5) displayed the most potent MMP-13 inhibition ($K_i = 0.13$ nM) with an intense selectivity over other MMPs. In the rat

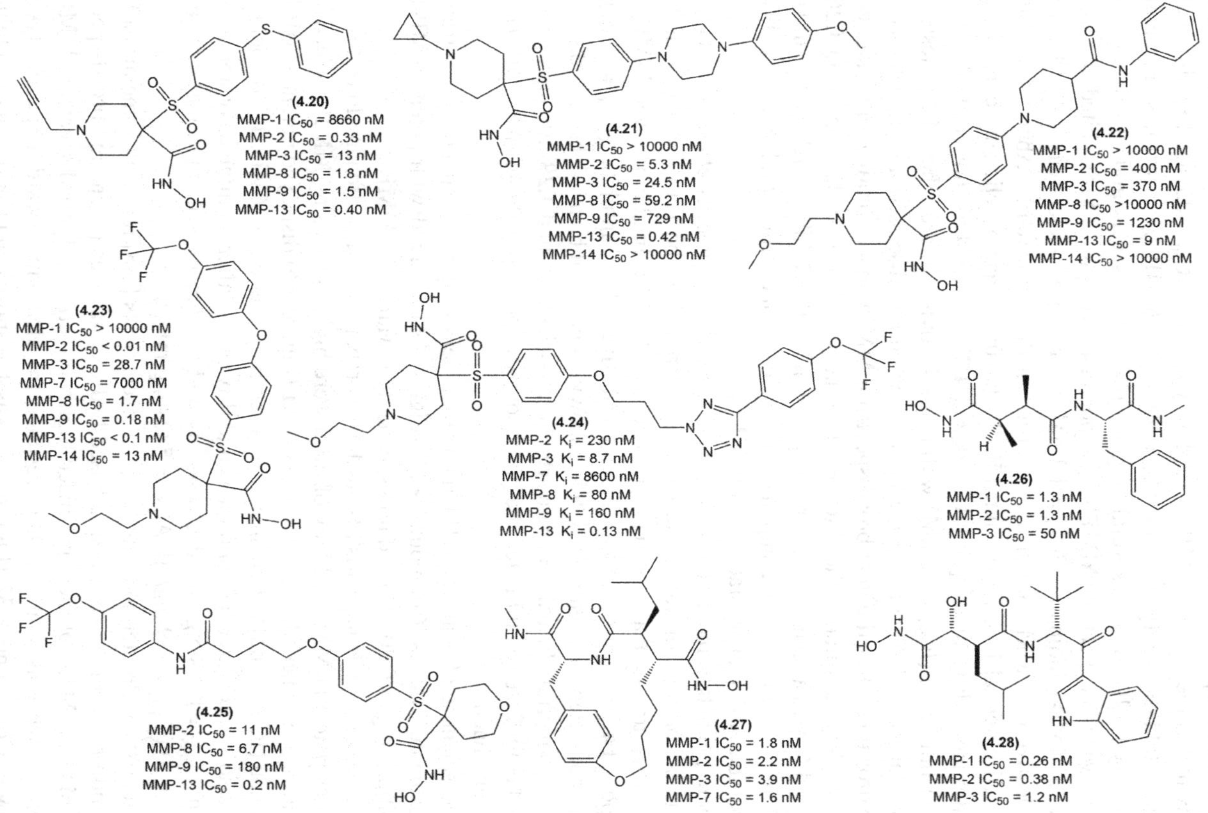

(4.22)

MMP-1 IC_{50} > 10000 nM
MMP-2 IC_{50} = 400 nM
MMP-3 IC_{50} = 370 nM
MMP-8 IC_{50} >10000 nM
MMP-9 IC_{50} = 1230 nM
MMP-13 IC_{50} = 9 nM
MMP-14 IC_{50} > 10000 nM

(4.26)

MMP-1 IC_{50} = 1.3 nM
MMP-2 IC_{50} = 1.3 nM
MMP-3 IC_{50} = 50 nM

(4.28)

MMP-1 IC_{50} = 0.26 nM
MMP-2 IC_{50} = 0.38 nM
MMP-3 IC_{50} = 1.2 nM

(4.21)

MMP-1 IC_{50} > 10000 nM
MMP-2 IC_{50} = 5.3 nM
MMP-3 IC_{50} = 24.5 nM
MMP-8 IC_{50} = 59.2 nM
MMP-9 IC_{50} = 729 nM
MMP-13 IC_{50} = 0.42 nM
MMP-14 IC_{50} > 10000 nM

(4.24)

MMP-2 K_i = 230 nM
MMP-3 K_i = 8.7 nM
MMP-7 K_i = 8600 nM
MMP-8 K_i = 80 nM
MMP-9 K_i = 160 nM
MMP-13 K_i = 0.13 nM

(4.27)

MMP-1 IC_{50} = 1.8 nM
MMP-2 IC_{50} = 2.2 nM
MMP-3 IC_{50} = 3.9 nM
MMP-7 IC_{50} = 1.6 nM

(4.20)

MMP-1 IC_{50} = 8660 nM
MMP-2 IC_{50} = 0.33 nM
MMP-3 IC_{50} = 13 nM
MMP-8 IC_{50} = 1.8 nM
MMP-9 IC_{50} = 1.5 nM
MMP-13 IC_{50} = 0.40 nM

(4.23)

MMP-1 IC_{50} > 10000 nM
MMP-2 IC_{50} < 0.01 nM
MMP-3 IC_{50} = 28.7 nM
MMP-7 IC_{50} = 7000 nM
MMP-8 IC_{50} = 1.7 nM
MMP-9 IC_{50} = 0.18 nM
MMP-13 IC_{50} < 0.1 nM
MMP-14 IC_{50} = 13 nM

(4.25)

MMP-2 IC_{50} = 11 nM
MMP-8 IC_{50} = 6.7 nM
MMP-9 IC_{50} = 180 nM
MMP-13 IC_{50} = 0.2 nM

FIGURE 4.5 Another set of hydroxamate-based potential collagenase inhibitors (compounds **4.20–4.28**).

pharmacokinetic model, it (compound **4.24**) exhibited good bioavailability (26%), including a good C_{max} (1400 ng/ml) and a half-life ($t_{1/2}$ = 1.3 hr). The research work by Fobian and co-workers [111] at Pfizer led to the disclosure of a set of α-sulfone hydroxamates as potential and selective MMP-13 inhibitors. Compound **4.25** (Figure 4.5) exhibited the highest MMP-13 inhibitory activity (IC_{50} = 0.2 nM), retaining at least a 33-fold selectivity over MMP-2, MMP-8, and MMP-9. Researchers of Abbott Laboratory [112] disclosed several C_α gem disubstituted succinimide hydroxamates as effective broad-spectrum MMPIs. Compound **4.26** (Figure 4.5) exhibited the most effective MMP-1 inhibition (IC_{50} = 1.3 nM), showing non-selectivity with MMP-2 but selective over MMP-3. Further extension of their research by Abbott scientists produced potential broad-spectrum MMPIs having a macrocyclic ring containing succinimide hydroxamates [113]. Compound **4.27** (Figure 4.5) showed the highest MMP-1 inhibition (IC_{50} = 1.8 nM) with non-selectivity toward other MMPs tested. The researchers of Abbott, in their subsequent study, disclosed a series of succi-nyl hydroxamate-based potent broad-spectrum MMPIs incorporating an arylamino ketone moiety substituting the C-terminal amino acid amides [114]. Compound **4.28** (Figure 4.5) was a highly potent broad-spectrum MMP-1 inhibitor (IC_{50} = 0.26 nM). At 10 mg/kg per oral dose, compound **4.28** resulted in excellent oral bioavailability comparable with marimastat (compound **4.5**).

Some phenylglycine-based hydroxamates were delineated as effective collage-nase inhibitors by Hirayama and co-workers from Kanebo [115]. Many of these compounds unveiled a potential and selective MMP-1 inhibition over MMP-9. Compound **4.29** (Figure 4.6) was the most effective MMP-1 inhibitor (IC_{50} = 3 nM), having non-selectivity with MMP-9 but showing good oral bioavailability and solu-bility (0.05 mg/ml). In a rat adjuvant arthritis model, compound **4.29** (100 mg/kg p.o. twice/day for 20 days) inhibited the hind foot paw swelling, although it was inferior to indomethacin.

The scientist of Kanebo [116] reported a series of potential broad-spectrum hydroxamate MMPIs. Compound **4.30** (Figure 4.6) emerged with potent MMP-1 inhibition (IC_{50} = 0.20 nM) and non-specificity toward other MMPs.

The researchers from British Biotech [117] reported some sulfonamido hydroxa-mates as potential MMPIs. Many of them were highly promising MMP-1-selective inhibitors over other MMPs. Compound **4.31** (Figure 4.6) displayed potent MMP-1 inhibition (IC_{50} = 6 nM), showing higher selectivity over other MMPs. It (compound **4.31**) also showed excellent oral bioavailability in rats after 30 minutes of adminis-tration (C_{max} = 171.8 mg/ml, AUC = 662 ng/ml.hr) compared with marimastat (com-pound **4.5**) (C_{max} = 139 mg/ml, AUC = 582.4 ng/ml.hr).

Scientists at Procter and Gamble Pharmaceuticals [118] reported some arylsul-fonamido thiazepine and thiazine-based hydroxamates as potent and broad-spec-trum MMPIs. Many of them produced highly effective and broad-spectrum MMP inhibition, whereas some of them resulted in selectivity toward a specific type of MMP. Compound **4.32** (Figure 4.6) was the most potent collagenase inhibi-tor (MMP-1 IC_{50} = 0.8 nM and MMP-13 IC_{50} = 0.9 nM), showing non-selectiv-ity toward other MMPs. Pikul and co-workers [119] from Procter and Gamble Pharmaceuticals reported several phosphinamide-based hydroxamates as potent

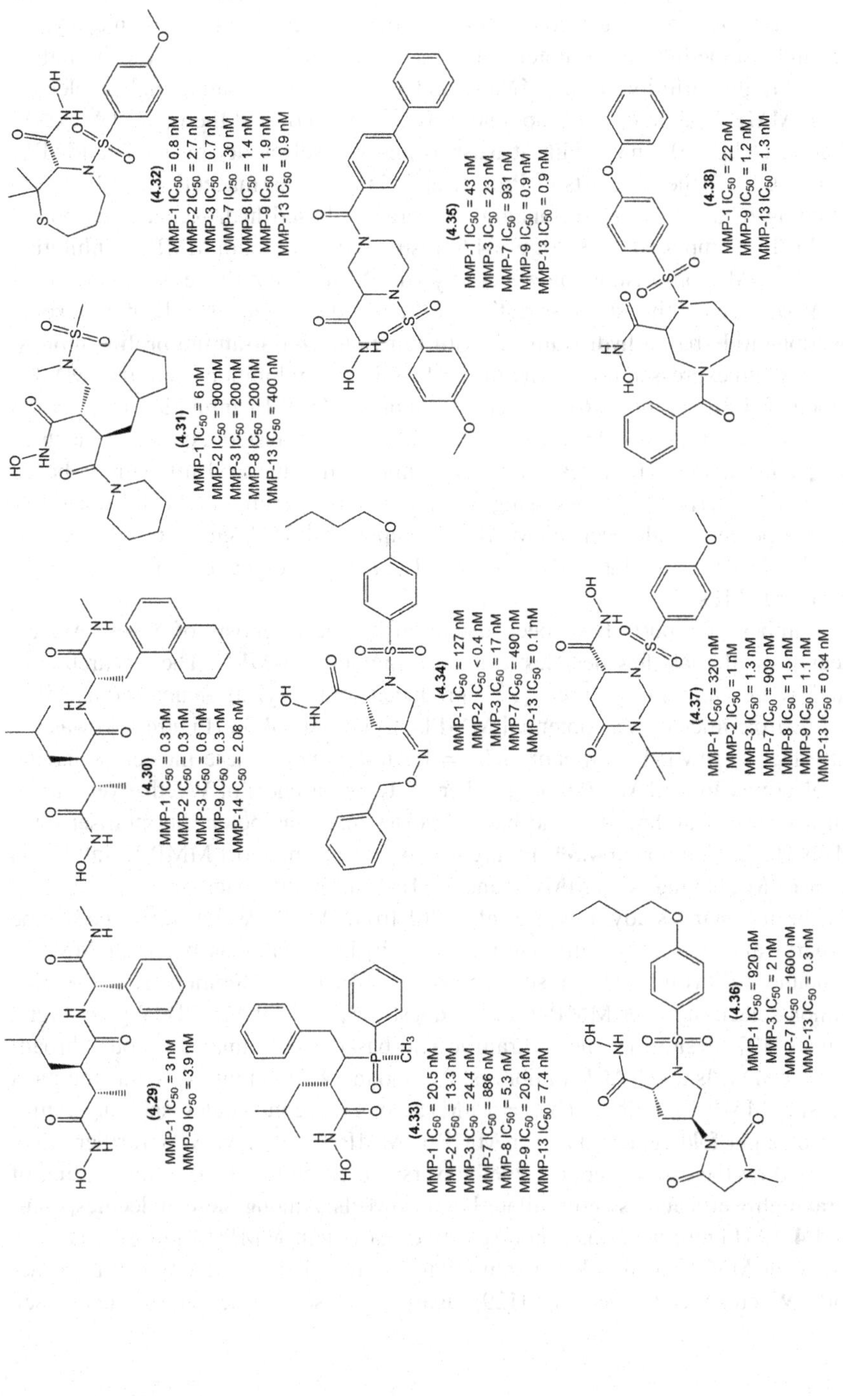

(4.32)
MMP-1 IC$_{50}$ = 0.8 nM
MMP-2 IC$_{50}$ = 2.7 nM
MMP-3 IC$_{50}$ = 0.7 nM
MMP-7 IC$_{50}$ = 30 nM
MMP-8 IC$_{50}$ = 1.4 nM
MMP-9 IC$_{50}$ = 1.9 nM
MMP-13 IC$_{50}$ = 0.9 nM

(4.31)
MMP-1 IC$_{50}$ = 6 nM
MMP-2 IC$_{50}$ = 900 nM
MMP-3 IC$_{50}$ = 200 nM
MMP-8 IC$_{50}$ = 200 nM
MMP-13 IC$_{50}$ = 400 nM

(4.35)
MMP-1 IC$_{50}$ = 43 nM
MMP-3 IC$_{50}$ = 23 nM
MMP-7 IC$_{50}$ = 931 nM
MMP-9 IC$_{50}$ = 0.9 nM
MMP-13 IC$_{50}$ = 0.9 nM

(4.38)
MMP-1 IC$_{50}$ = 22 nM
MMP-9 IC$_{50}$ = 1.2 nM
MMP-13 IC$_{50}$ = 1.3 nM

(4.30)
MMP-1 IC$_{50}$ = 0.3 nM
MMP-2 IC$_{50}$ = 0.3 nM
MMP-3 IC$_{50}$ = 0.6 nM
MMP-9 IC$_{50}$ = 0.3 nM
MMP-14 IC$_{50}$ = 2.08 nM

(4.34)
MMP-1 IC$_{50}$ = 127 nM
MMP-2 IC$_{50}$ < 0.4 nM
MMP-3 IC$_{50}$ = 17 nM
MMP-7 IC$_{50}$ = 490 nM
MMP-13 IC$_{50}$ = 0.1 nM

(4.37)
MMP-1 IC$_{50}$ = 320 nM
MMP-2 IC$_{50}$ = 1 nM
MMP-3 IC$_{50}$ = 1.3 nM
MMP-7 IC$_{50}$ = 909 nM
MMP-8 IC$_{50}$ = 1.5 nM
MMP-9 IC$_{50}$ = 1.1 nM
MMP-13 IC$_{50}$ = 0.34 nM

(4.29)
MMP-1 IC$_{50}$ = 3 nM
MMP-9 IC$_{50}$ = 3.9 nM

(4.33)
MMP-1 IC$_{50}$ = 20.5 nM
MMP-2 IC$_{50}$ = 13.3 nM
MMP-3 IC$_{50}$ = 24.4 nM
MMP-7 IC$_{50}$ = 886 nM
MMP-8 IC$_{50}$ = 5.3 nM
MMP-9 IC$_{50}$ = 20.6 nM
MMP-13 IC$_{50}$ = 7.4 nM

(4.36)
MMP-1 IC$_{50}$ = 920 nM
MMP-3 IC$_{50}$ = 2 nM
MMP-7 IC$_{50}$ = 1600 nM
MMP-13 IC$_{50}$ = 0.3 nM

FIGURE 4.6 Various hydroxamate-based potential collagenase inhibitors (compounds **4.29**–**4.38**).

MMPIs. Compound **4.33** (Figure 4.6) was a potent MMPI showing good inhibition against MMP-8 (IC_{50} = 5.3 nM), MMP-13 (IC_{50} = 7.4 nM), and MMP-1 (IC_{50} = 20.5 nM).

Cheng et al. [120] from Procter and Gamble reported a series of arylsulfonamido proline-based hydroxamates comprising various moieties, namely oxime, hydrazone, and exomethylene, as potent broad-spectrum MMPIs. All these inhibitors produced higher affinity toward MMP-2 and MMP-13, maintaining higher selectivity over MMP-1, -3, and -7. Compound **4.34** (Figure 4.6) had the highest MMP-13 inhibition (IC_{50} = 0.1 nM) with at least a four-fold selectivity over other MMPs. Further study by the scientists of Procter and Gamble Pharmaceuticals [121] led to the finding of a set of arylsulfonamido piperazine-based hydroxamates as potential MMPIs. Compound **4.35** (Figure 4.6) resulted in maximum MMP-13 inhibition (IC_{50} = 0.9 nM) comprising non-selectivity with MMP-9 but higher selectivity over other MMPs. In another study, scientists of Procter and Gamble [122] reported some arylsulfonamide-based hydroxamates with functionalized 4-amino proline moiety. Many of them expressed potent and MMP-13-selective inhibition over other MMPs. Compound **4.36** (Figure 4.6) showed the highest MMP-13 inhibition (IC_{50} = 0.3 nM) with at least a six-fold selectivity over other MMPs tested. Again, scientists at Procter and Gamble [123] designed and synthesized some arylsulfonamide-based hydroxamate derivatives possessing 6-oxohexahydropyridine and 1,4-diazepine moiety as potent broad-spectrum MMPIs. Compound **4.37** (Figure 4.6) was the best promising MMP-13 inhibitor (IC_{50} = 0.34 nM), having at least a three-fold selectivity over other MMPs.

A number of reports have been disclosed by the scientists of Wyeth-Ayerest Research for the last few decades to identify potential MMPIs. The research conducted by Levin and co-workers [124] produced some arylsulfonamido diazepine-based hydroxamic acids as potential MMPIs. Compound **4.38** (Figure 4.6) was the most effective MMP-13 inhibitor (IC_{50} = 1.3 nM) among these molecules having non-selectivity toward MMP-9. In another study, researchers of Wyeth-Ayerst identified a series of anthranilic acid-based hydroxamates as potent but non-selective MMPIs [125]. Compound **4.39** (Figure 4.7) produced the most MMP-13 inhibition (IC_{50} = 1 nM), having good MMP-9 and MMP-1 inhibitory potency.

In the following study, Levin et al. [126] from Wyeth-Ayerst introduced some heteroaryl and cycloalkyl sulfonamide-based hydroxamates as potential MMPIs. Compound **4.40** (Figure 4.7) resulted in potent MMP-13 inhibition (IC_{50} = 8 nM) with non-selectivity over MMP-9. In the quest for potential MMPIs, Wyeth-Ayerst scientists [127] designed some anthranilic acid-based hydroxamates as potent broad-spectrum MMPIs and TACE inhibitors. Compound **4.41** (Figure 4.7) was the most promising MMP-13 inhibitor (IC_{50} = 1 nM) among these molecules, showing a minimum of eight-fold selectivity over MMP-1, MMP-9, and TACE. A further study conducted by the researchers of Wyeth-Ayerst Research [128] led to the finding of several highly efficacious anthranilate-based MMPIs. Among these molecules, compound **4.42** (Figure 4.7) was a non-selective but potent MMP-13 inhibitor (IC_{50} = 1 nM) over MMP-9 with a lower inhibition toward MMP-1 and TACE. In another report, Wyeth-Ayerst scientists [129] again disclosed some anthranilate-based

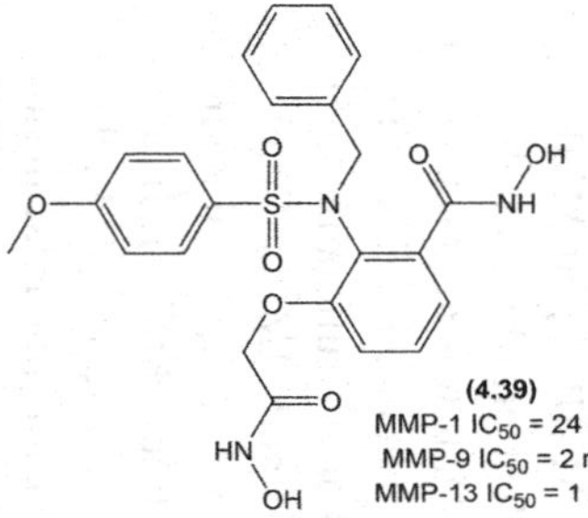

(4.39)
MMP-1 IC$_{50}$ = 24 nM
MMP-9 IC$_{50}$ = 2 nM
MMP-13 IC$_{50}$ = 1 nM

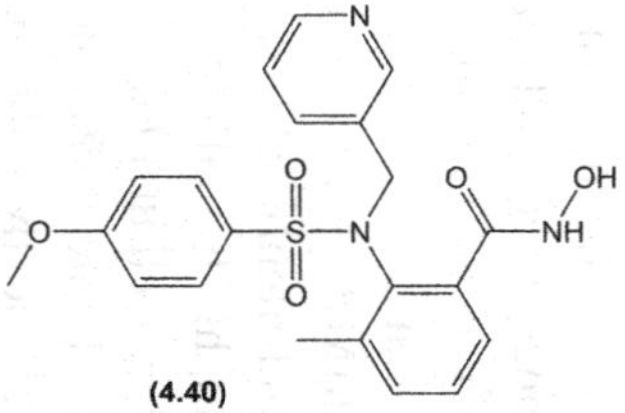

(4.40)
MMP-1 IC$_{50}$ = 143 nM
MMP-9 IC$_{50}$ = 5 nM
MMP-13 IC$_{50}$ = 8 nM

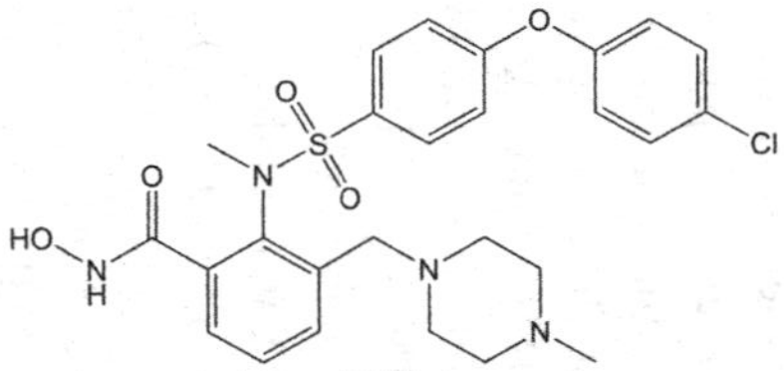

(4.41)
MMP-1 IC$_{50}$ = 155 nM
MMP-9 IC$_{50}$ = 1 nM
MMP-13 IC$_{50}$ = 0.8 nM
TACE IC$_{50}$ = 122 nM

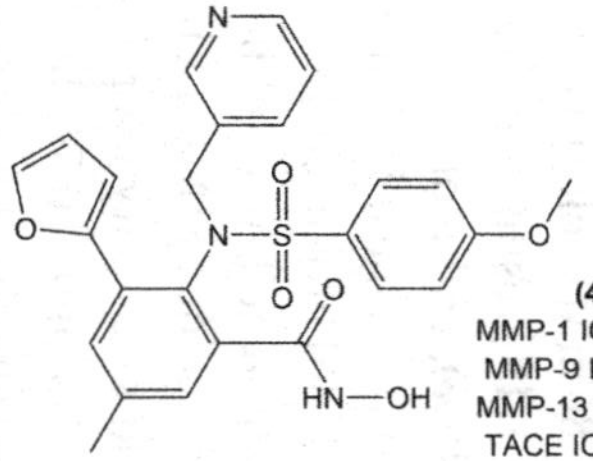

(4.42)
MMP-1 IC$_{50}$ = 18 nM
MMP-9 IC$_{50}$ = 8 nM
MMP-13 IC$_{50}$ = 1 nM
TACE IC$_{50}$ = 61 nM

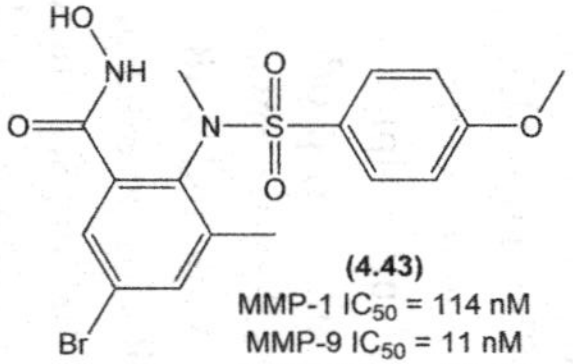

(4.43)
MMP-1 IC$_{50}$ = 114 nM
MMP-9 IC$_{50}$ = 11 nM
MMP-13 IC$_{50}$ = 21 nM
TACE IC$_{50}$ = 32 nM

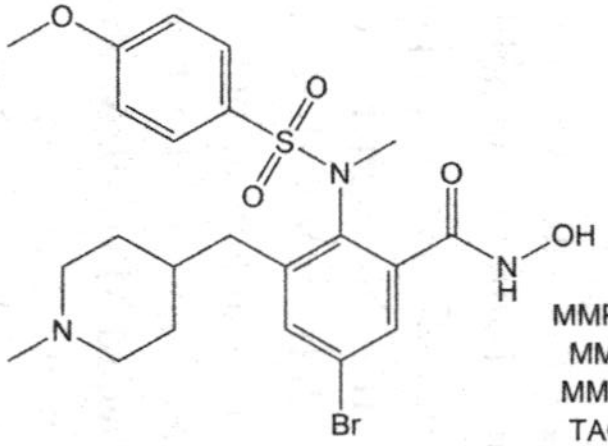

(4.44)
MMP-1 IC$_{50}$ = 194 nM
MMP-9 IC$_{50}$ = 2 nM
MMP-13 IC$_{50}$ = 5 nM
TACE IC$_{50}$ = 26 nM

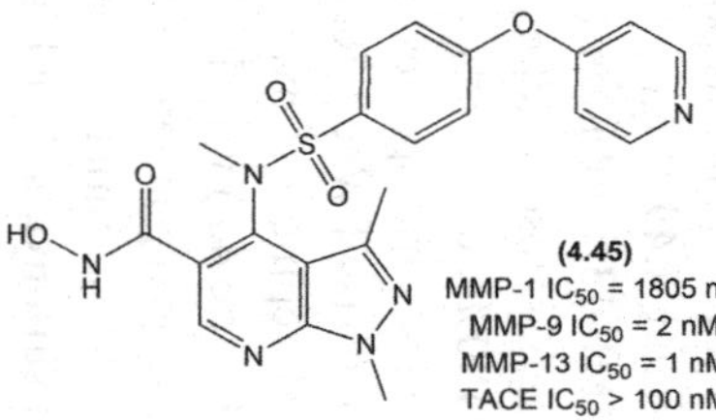

(4.45)
MMP-1 IC$_{50}$ = 1805 nM
MMP-9 IC$_{50}$ = 2 nM
MMP-13 IC$_{50}$ = 1 nM
TACE IC$_{50}$ > 100 nM

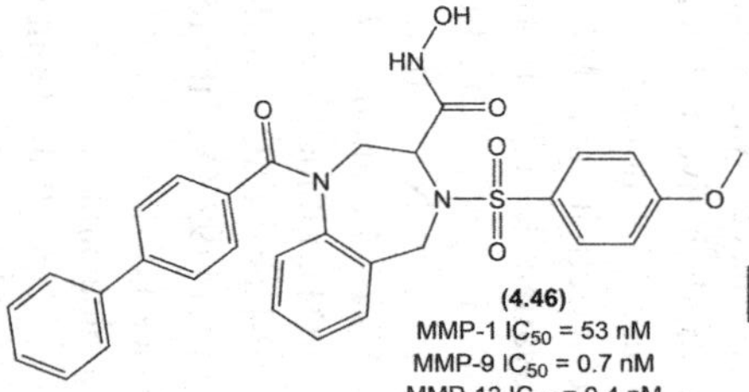

(4.46)
MMP-1 IC$_{50}$ = 53 nM
MMP-9 IC$_{50}$ = 0.7 nM
MMP-13 IC$_{50}$ = 0.4 nM
TACE IC$_{50}$ = 199 nM

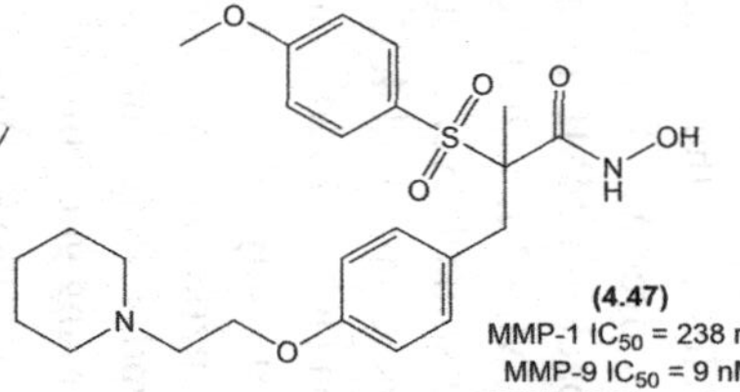

(4.47)
MMP-1 IC$_{50}$ = 238 nM
MMP-9 IC$_{50}$ = 9 nM
MMP-13 IC$_{50}$ = 1 nM
TACE IC$_{50}$ = 41 nM

FIGURE 4.7 Some other hydroxamate-based potential collagenase inhibitors (compounds **4.39–4.47**).

sulfonamide hydroxamates as potent MMPIs and TACE inhibitors. Compound **4.43** (Figure 4.7) showed potent broad-spectrum MMP-13 inhibition (IC_{50} = 21 nM) having non-selectivity toward MMP-9 and MMP-1, as well as TACE. In continuation of their research, another series of anthranilate-based sulfonamide hydroxamates were disclosed by the scientists of Wyeth-Ayerst [130] as potent and selective TACE inhibitors over MMPs. However, compound **4.44** (Figure 4.7) resulted in potent broad-spectrum MMP-13 inhibition (IC_{50} = 5 nM) having good inhibition against MMP-9, MMP-1, and TACE. Zask et al. [131] of Wyeth-Ayerst Research again designed some bicyclic heteroaryl hydroxamic acids as potent MMPIs and TACE inhibitors. Compound **4.45** (Figure 4.7) produced potent but non-selective MMP-13 inhibition (IC_{50} = 1 nM) with MMP-9 but higher selectivity over MMP-1 and TACE. In another study, Nelson et al. [132] from Wyeth Research reported some arylsulfonamido benzodiazepine-based hydroxamates as potent MMPIs and TACE inhibitors. Compound **4.46** (Figure 4.7) was the most effective MMP-13 inhibitor (IC_{50} = 0.4 nM), showing good inhibition toward MMP-9, MMP-1, and TACE.

The scientists of Wyeth Research further reported a series of α-sulfonyl hydroxamates as orally active and potent inhibitors of MMPs and TACE [133]. Compound **4.47** (Figure 4.7) showed potent MMP-13 inhibition (IC_{50} = 1 nM) with at least a nine-fold selectivity over MMP-9 and sparing MMP-1 and TACE. Furthermore, the oral bioavailability of compound **4.47** (Figure 4.7) in the rat model was excellent (81%) with a $t_{1/2}$ of 1.5 hr. In the following study, the Wyeth researchers reported [134] a series of N-substituted 4-arylsulfonylpiperidine-4 hydroxamates as orally active MMPIs. Compound **4.48** (Figure 4.8) produced potent MMP-13 inhibition (IC_{50} = 1 nM), although it was non-selective toward MMP-9 and highly selective over MMP-1 and TACE. Although compound **4.48** was found highly bound to the plasma protein (99%) of the rat, rabbit, dog, and human, it absorbed well in all these four species (10–25 mg/kg). In rats and dogs, compound **4.48** exhibited 55% and 47% oral bioavailability, respectively, and was found to be metabolically stable in these four species (rabbit<monkey<dog<rat<human).

The scientists of Wyeth Research further reported [135] some acyclic sulfonamide hydroxamates as potent TACE-selective inhibitors over MMP-1, -9, and -13. Compound **4.49** (Figure 4.8) explored potent TACE inhibition (IC_{50} = 10 nM), and MMP-13 inhibition (IC_{50} = 86 nM) selective over MMP-9, and MMP-1. At a 10 mg/kg dose, it (compound **4.49**) resulted in excellent oral bioavailability in mice (100%), dogs (75%), rats (46%), and monkeys (17%). It was also found to be stable in several species' liver microsomes, including humans. Further study by the scientists of Wyeth Research [136] produced a series of arylsulfonamido-based benzodiazepine hydroxamates as potent TACE inhibitors and MMPIs. Compound **4.50** (Figure 4.8) was the best efficacious MMP-13 inhibitor (IC_{50} = 7 nM) in this series, showing at least a five-fold selectivity over TACE and MMP-1. In another report, the scientists of Wyeth Research [137] disclosed a series of 4-alkyloxy phenyl sulfonyl, sulfinyl, and sulfonyl alkyl hydroxamates as potential inhibitors of TACE and MMPs. Compound **4.51** (Figure 4.8) exhibited the highest MMP-13 inhibition (IC_{50} = 2 nM) with at least a five-fold selectivity over MMP-1, MMP-9, and TACE. Zask et al. [138] explored a set of thiazepine and diazepine-based

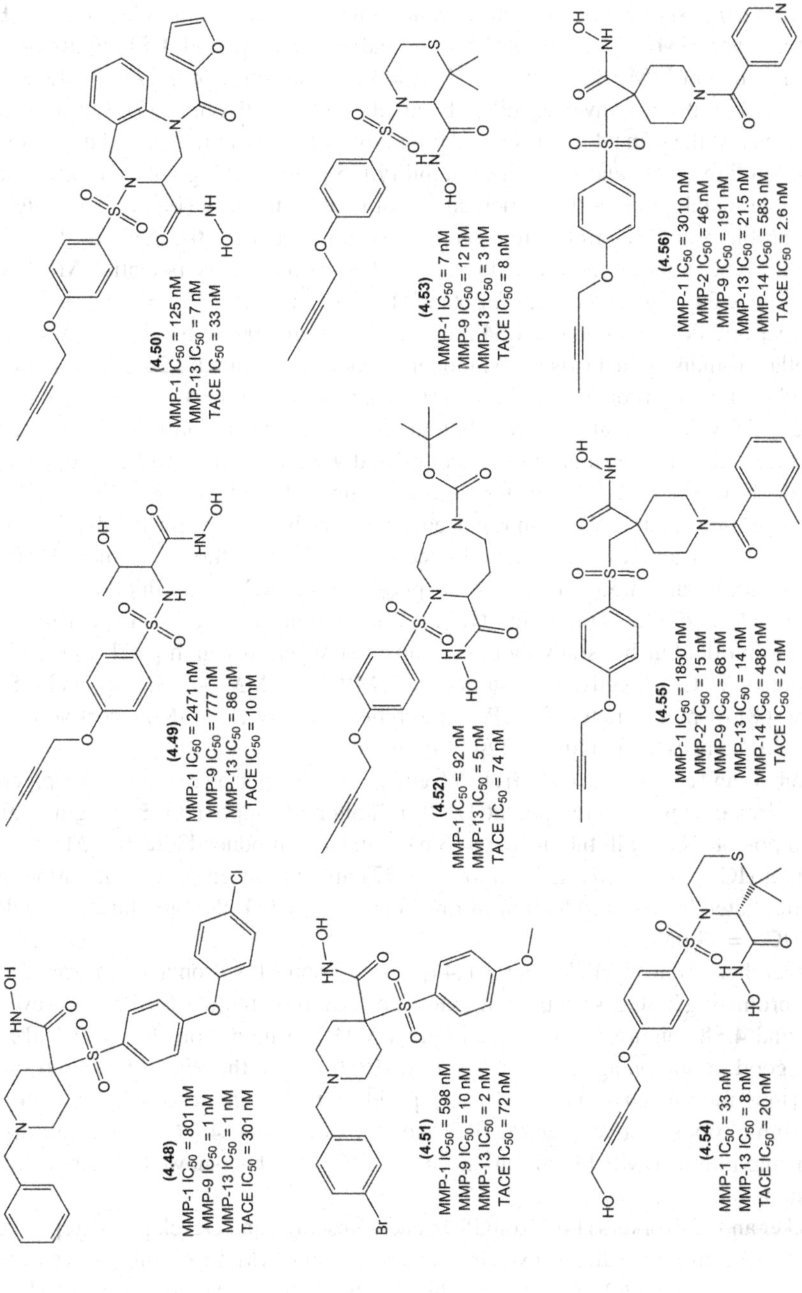

(4.50)
MMP-1 IC$_{50}$ = 125 nM
MMP-13 IC$_{50}$ = 7 nM
TACE IC$_{50}$ = 33 nM

(4.53)
MMP-1 IC$_{50}$ = 7 nM
MMP-9 IC$_{50}$ = 12 nM
MMP-13 IC$_{50}$ = 3 nM
TACE IC$_{50}$ = 8 nM

(4.56)
MMP-1 IC$_{50}$ = 3010 nM
MMP-2 IC$_{50}$ = 46 nM
MMP-9 IC$_{50}$ = 191 nM
MMP-13 IC$_{50}$ = 21.5 nM
MMP-14 IC$_{50}$ = 583 nM
TACE IC$_{50}$ = 2.6 nM

(4.49)
MMP-1 IC$_{50}$ = 2471 nM
MMP-9 IC$_{50}$ = 777 nM
MMP-13 IC$_{50}$ = 86 nM
TACE IC$_{50}$ = 10 nM

(4.52)
MMP-1 IC$_{50}$ = 92 nM
MMP-13 IC$_{50}$ = 5 nM
TACE IC$_{50}$ = 74 nM

(4.55)
MMP-1 IC$_{50}$ = 1850 nM
MMP-2 IC$_{50}$ = 15 nM
MMP-9 IC$_{50}$ = 68 nM
MMP-13 IC$_{50}$ = 14 nM
MMP-14 IC$_{50}$ = 488 nM
TACE IC$_{50}$ = 2 nM

(4.48)
MMP-1 IC$_{50}$ = 801 nM
MMP-9 IC$_{50}$ = 1 nM
MMP-13 IC$_{50}$ = 1 nM
TACE IC$_{50}$ = 301 nM

(4.51)
MMP-1 IC$_{50}$ = 598 nM
MMP-9 IC$_{50}$ = 10 nM
MMP-13 IC$_{50}$ = 2 nM
TACE IC$_{50}$ = 72 nM

(4.54)
MMP-1 IC$_{50}$ = 33 nM
MMP-13 IC$_{50}$ = 8 nM
TACE IC$_{50}$ = 20 nM

FIGURE 4.8 Another set of hydroxamate-based potential collagenase inhibitors (compounds **4.48–4.56**).

TACE inhibitors and MMPIs. Compound **4.52** (Figure 4.8) was the most effective MMP-13 inhibitor (IC_{50} = 5 nM), being highly selective over MMP-1 and TACE.

Levin et al. [139] from Wyeth Research disclosed some arylsulfonamide hydroxamates bearing six-membered heterocyclic rings as potent and selective TACE inhibitors over MMPs (such as MMP-1, -9, and -13). Compound **4.53** (Figure 4.8) resulted in potent MMP-13 inhibition (IC_{50} = 3 nM) selective over TACE, MMP-1, and MMP-9. It also displayed excellent bioavailability in DBA mice (71%) at 10 mg/kg, whereas, at the same dose, it showed poor bioavailability in the rat and dog. High protein binding (40%) and moderate solubility (75 µg/ml), along with a production of multiple metabolites in liver microsomes of compound **4.53** (Figure 4.8), might lead to problems in designing potent agents in rheumatoid arthritis. Levin et al. [140] explored some thiomorpholine sulfonamide hydroxamates as potential MMPIs. Compound **4.54** (Figure 4.8) was a potent MMP-13 inhibitor (IC_{50} = 8 nM). At 10 mg/kg per oral dose, compound **4.54** reduced more than 50% clinical severity score in a collagen-induced arthritis (CIA) model in mice. Compound **4.54** also inhibited LPS-induced TNF production (IC_{50} = 300 nM). Compound **4.54** was permeable in Caco-2 cells, was not highly protein-bound, and improved solubility in gastric and intestinal fluids. At a 10 mg/kg dose, compound **4.54** was found to be moderately bioavailable in mice (24%) and dogs (36%) compared with rats (8%). The scientist of Wyeth research [141] again reported a series of butynyloxyphenyl β-sulphone piperidine hydroxamates as potent and selective TACE inhibitors over other MMPs. However, compound **4.55** (Figure 4.8) displayed potent MMP-13 inhibition (IC_{50} = 14 nM) and good TACE inhibition (IC_{50} = 2 nM) along with a broad spectrum of MMP inhibition. Further study by the scientists of Wyeth research [142] resulted in some potent TACE-selective inhibitors over MMP-2 and MMP-13. Compound **4.56** (Figure 4.8) displayed potent MMP-13 inhibition (IC_{50} = 21. 5 nM) selective over other MMPs but exhibited higher TACE inhibition.

Lombart and co-workers [143] from Wyeth Research reported a series of 3,3-piperidine hydroxamates as highly potent TACE inhibitors. Compound **4.57** (Figure 4.9) showed potent TACE inhibition (IC_{50} = 3 nM) and also produced effective MMP-13 inhibition (IC_{50} = 470 nM). It (compound **4.57**) also produced potent inhibition of LPS-stimulated TNF-α production in raw cells (IC_{50} = 0.3 µM) and human whole blood (IC_{50} = 13 µM).

Researchers from Wyeth Research [144] reported some β-sulfonyl hydroxamate as highly promising TACE-selective inhibitors compared with other MMPs. However, compound **4.58** (Figure 4.9) exhibited potent MMP-13 inhibition (IC_{50} = 2.4 nM), having good inhibition against TACE and MMP-2. Again, the Wyeth Research scientist [145] introduced some α-sulfone piperidine hydroxamates as highly potent TACE inhibitors selective over MMP-2 and -13. Compound **4.59** (Figure 4.9) displayed maximum MMP-13 inhibition (IC_{50} = 57 nM) but showed better TACE inhibition.

Becker and co-workers [146] from Pharmacia Research and Development reported a series of α-amino-β-sulfone hydroxamates as potent MMP-13 inhibitors sparing MMP-1. Compound **4.60** (Figure 4.9) exhibited the highest MMP-13 inhibition (IC_{50} = 0.2 nM) with a 450-fold selectivity over MMP-1. At an oral dose of 20 mpk in

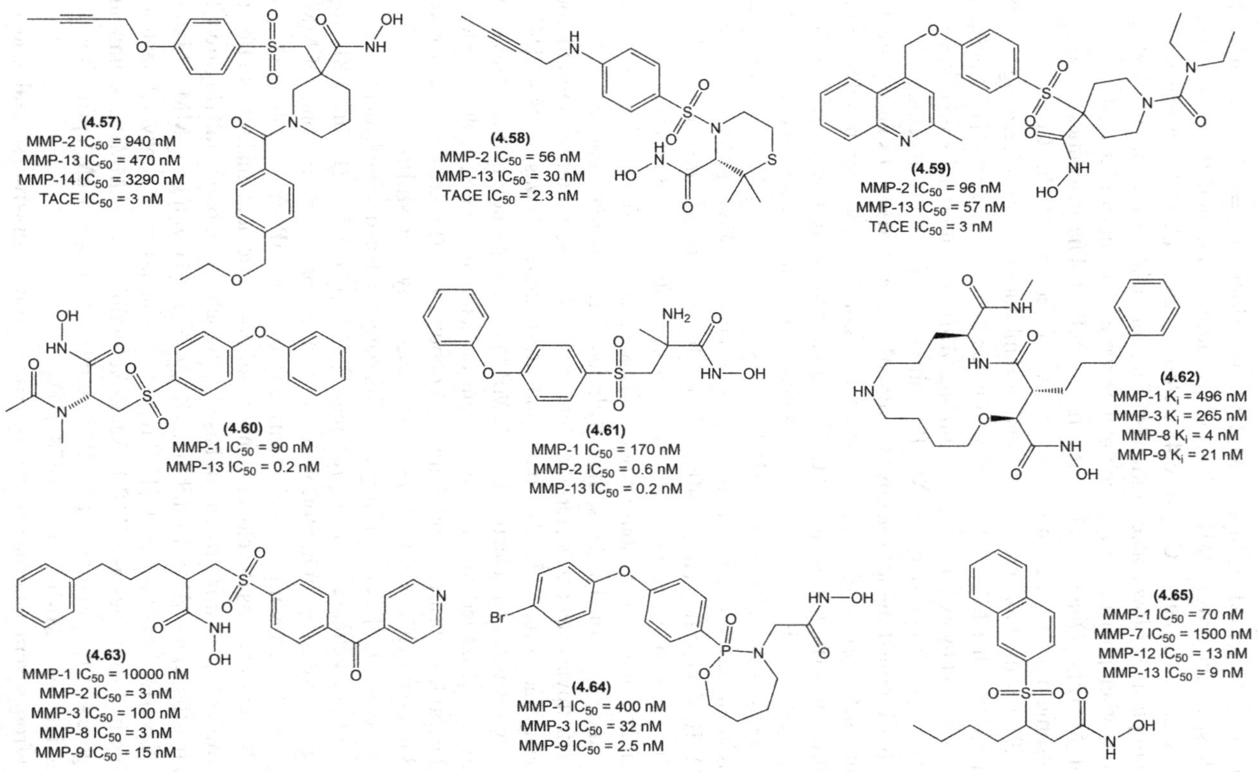

FIGURE 4.9 Different hydroxamate-based potential collagenase inhibitors (compounds **4.57**–**4.65**).

rats, it displayed a C_{max} of 2.45 µg/ml, indicating good oral absorption properties. Further study by the same group of researchers [147] identified a series of α-alkyl-α-amino-β-sulfone hydroxamates as potential MMPIs sparing MMP-1. Compound **4.61** (Figure 4.9) yielded the highest MMP-13 inhibition (IC_{50}= 0.2 nM), comprising three-fold selectivity over MMP-2. During oral administration in the rat at a 20 mpk dose, it exhibited a higher C_{max} of 6.43 µg/ml, whereas all of these MMPIs were retained in plasma at low concentration (<15 mg/ml) after 6 hr of administration.

Several other pharmaceutical companies were also motivated to design some potential MMPIs. Duan et al. [148] from DuPont Pharmaceuticals Company reported some macrocyclic amine derivatives as effective MMPIs. Compound **4.62** (Figure 4.9) was the most promising MMP-8 inhibitor (K_i = 4 nM), having a higher selectivity over other MMPs. Scientists from Celltech Chiroscience [149] designed some arylsulfonyl hydroxamates as promising MMPIs. Compound **4.63** (Figure 4.9) explored potent but non-selective MMP-8 inhibition (IC_{50} = 3 nM) compared with MMP-2 but retained higher selectivity over MMP-3 and MMP-9 sparing MMP-1. Compound **4.63** also resulted in a significant plasma level (300 mg/ml) during oral administration (10 mg/kg) in rats. In the B16F10 melanoma mouse model, compound **4.63** displayed 80% inhibition, which was better than marimastat (compound **4.5**).

The scientists of LEO Pharma [150] disclosed a set of cyclic phosphinamides and phosphonamides as efficacious MMPIs. Compound **4.64** (Figure 4.9) showed potent MMP-1 inhibition (IC_{50} = 400 nM) and had a better affinity toward MMP-3 and MMP-9. It also exhibited 48% tumor growth inhibition in HT1080 cells *in vivo* in the human fibrosarcoma mouse model. The scientist of Hoffmann-La Roche [151] reported some β-sulfonyl and β-sulfinyl hydroxamates as potent inhibitors of *E. Coli* peptide deformylase as antibacterial agents. Some of these inhibitors showed good inhibition against several MMPs. Compound **4.65** (Figure 4.9) was a potent MMP-13 inhibitor, but it was non-selective over MMP-12. Further study by the same group of researchers [152] led to the development of heteroaryl-based hydroxamates as potential peptide deformylase inhibitors. Compound **4.66** (Figure 4.10) was a potent MMP-13 inhibitor (IC_{50} = 460 nM) showing selectivity over MMP-12.

Durham et al. [153] from Eli Lilly and Company produced some hydantoin-based inhibitors of aggrecanase-1 and aggrecanase-2. Compound **4.67** (Figure 4.10) was a nonspecific aggrecanase inhibitor, which was also a promising inhibitor of MMP-13 (IC_{50} = 1 nM), showing non-selectivity over other MMPs. Takahashi et al. [154] of Ono Pharmaceuticals developed some γ-aminobutyric acid analogs as effective MMPIs through an *in silico* fragment-based approach. Compound **4.68** (Figure 4.10) resulted in efficacious MMP-1 inhibition (IC_{50} = 530 nM) with good MMP-2 inhibition. At Novartis, Tommasi et al. [155] reported some potent 2-naphylsulfonamide-containing hydroxamates as MMP-13-selective inhibitors over MMP-2. Compound **4.69** (Figure 4.10) showed potent MMP-13 inhibition (IC_{50} = 1 nM), providing 178-fold selectivity over MMP-2 (IC_{50} = 178 nM).

Apart from several pharmaceutical companies, researchers from several academic and research institutes were also devoted to designing and discovering potential MMPIs. A set of arysulfonyl hydroxamates was disclosed as highly potent broad-spectrum MMPIs by Hanessian and co-workers from Université de Montréal [156].

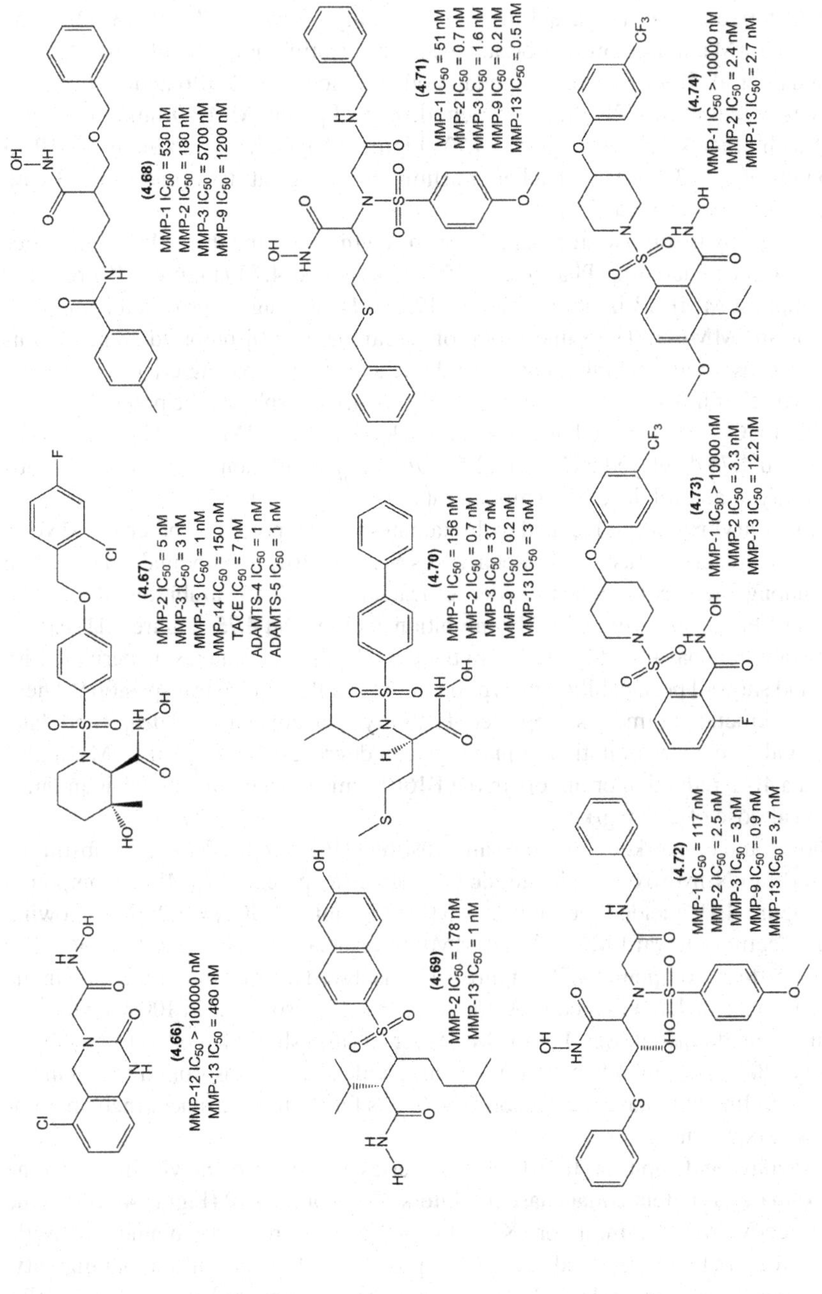

(4.66)
MMP-12 IC_{50} > 100000 nM
MMP-13 IC_{50} = 460 nM

(4.67)
MMP-2 IC_{50} = 5 nM
MMP-3 IC_{50} = 3 nM
MMP-13 IC_{50} = 1 nM
MMP-14 IC_{50} = 150 nM
TACE IC_{50} = 7 nM
ADAMTS-4 IC_{50} = 1 nM
ADAMTS-5 IC_{50} = 1 nM

(4.68)
MMP-1 IC_{50} = 530 nM
MMP-2 IC_{50} = 180 nM
MMP-3 IC_{50} = 5700 nM
MMP-9 IC_{50} = 1200 nM

(4.69)
MMP-2 IC_{50} = 178 nM
MMP-13 IC_{50} = 1 nM

(4.70)
MMP-1 IC_{50} = 156 nM
MMP-2 IC_{50} = 0.7 nM
MMP-3 IC_{50} = 37 nM
MMP-9 IC_{50} = 0.2 nM
MMP-13 IC_{50} = 3 nM

(4.71)
MMP-1 IC_{50} = 51 nM
MMP-2 IC_{50} = 0.7 nM
MMP-3 IC_{50} = 1.6 nM
MMP-9 IC_{50} = 0.2 nM
MMP-13 IC_{50} = 0.5 nM

(4.72)
MMP-1 IC_{50} = 117 nM
MMP-2 IC_{50} = 2.5 nM
MMP-3 IC_{50} = 3 nM
MMP-9 IC_{50} = 0.9 nM
MMP-13 IC_{50} = 3.7 nM

(4.73)
MMP-1 IC_{50} > 10000 nM
MMP-2 IC_{50} = 3.3 nM
MMP-13 IC_{50} = 12.2 nM

(4.74)
MMP-1 IC_{50} > 10000 nM
MMP-2 IC_{50} = 2.4 nM
MMP-13 IC_{50} = 2.7 nM

FIGURE 4.10 A set of hydroxamate-based potential collagenase inhibitors (compounds **4.66–4.74**).

Compound **4.70** (Figure 4.10) was the maximum effective MMP-13 inhibitor (IC_{50} = 3 nM), exerting higher potency toward other MMPs.

Further study by the same group of researchers led to the identification of a set of arylsulfonyl homocysteine hydroxamates as potent and broad-spectrum MMPIs [157]. Compound **4.71** (Figure 4.10) yielded highly efficacious MMP-13 inhibition (IC_{50} = 0.5 nM), maintaining a broad spectrum of inhibition toward other MMPs. Hanessian et al. [158] further designed another series of arylsulfonamide hydroxamates as potential MMPIs. Most of them displayed potent MMP-9 inhibition compared with other MMPs. Compound **4.72** (Figure 4.10) showed maximum MMP-13 inhibition (IC_{50} = 3.7 nM) with a better affinity toward gelatinases and MMP-3 with higher selectivity over MMP-1.

Some arylhydroxamate sulfonamides were synthesized and their MMP inhibitory activity was evaluated by Pharmacia [159]. Compound **4.73** (Figure 4.10) resulted in the highest MMP-13 inhibition (IC_{50} = 12.2 nM), although it provided better efficacy toward MMP-2. The same group of researchers [160] reported some sulfonamide hydroxamates having an aryl backbone as MMP-1-sparing effective MMP-2 and MMP-13 inhibitors. Compound **4.74** (Figure 4.10) displayed the potent MMP-13 inhibition (IC_{50} = 2.7 nM), but it was non-selective over MMP-2 (IC_{50} = 2.4 nM). Compound **4.74** displayed a C_{max} of 22.5 µg/ml, a $t_{1/2}$ of 1.9 hours, and 32% oral bioavailability at an oral dose of 20 mpk in rats.

Some 3-aryloxy propionic acid hydroxamates were reported as potential MMPIs by the researchers of Institut de Recherches Servier [161]. Compound **4.75** (Figure 4.11) among these compounds yielded efficacious MMP-13 inhibition (IC_{50} = 0.6 nM) and a broad spectrum of MMP inhibition. Compound **4.75** (Figure 4.11) exhibited metabolic bioavailability of 42% in the Caco2 cell line monolayers permeability assay and showed permeability absorption of 96% in the *in vivo* transposition. These pharmacokinetic parameters supported its ability to become a good drug candidate. Along with excellent inhibition of proteoglycan degradation (IC_{50} = 0.1 µM), it also yielded a 40% reduction of tumors in the B16F10 mice melanoma model at an intraperitoneal dose of 200 mg/kg.

Chollet and co-workers from the same institute [162] reported some α-substituted 3-bisarylthio N-hydroxy propionamide derivatives as potential MMPIs. Compound **4.76** (Figure 4.11) yielded the highest MMP-13 inhibition (IC_{50} = 1.2 nM), showing better selectivity toward MMP-2 and MMP-9, respectively. Not only that, at a 200 mg/kg i.p. dose, compound **4.76** (Figure 4.11) displayed a 55% tumor reduction in the B16F10 mouse melanoma model. At the same dose, it also reduced 100% metastasis in tumors of diameter over 1 mm. Moreover, it also showed moderate metabolic stability (20%) in human hepatic microsomes and excellent absorption (92%) in the Caco-2 cell line monolayer permeability study as far as the pharmacokinetic parameters were concerned.

Scozzafava and Supuran [163] disclosed a series of N-4-nitrobenzylsulfonylglycine hydroxamates as potent collagenase inhibitors. Compound **4.77** (Figure 4.11) was the most effective MMP-8 inhibitor (K_i = 0.1 nM) among these compounds. Rossello and co-workers [164] disclosed several N-*i*-propoxy-N-biphenylsulfonyl-aminobutyl hydroxamates as potent MMP-2-selective inhibitors compared with other MMPs.

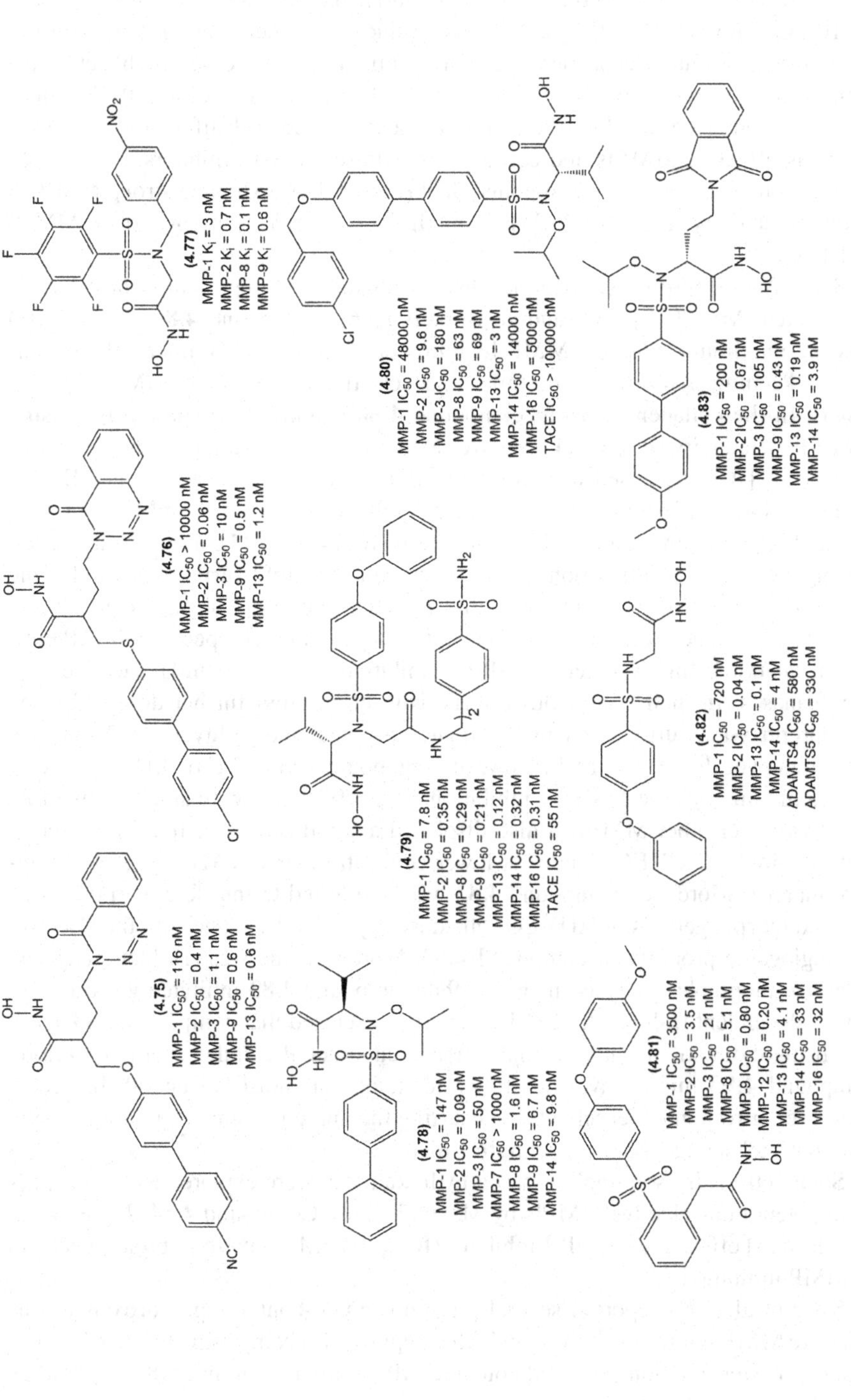

FIGURE 4.11 Several potential hydroxamate-based collagenase inhibitors (compounds **4.75–4.83**).

(4.77)
MMP-1 K_i = 3 nM
MMP-2 K_i = 0.7 nM
MMP-8 K_i = 0.1 nM
MMP-9 K_i = 0.6 nM

(4.80)
MMP-1 IC_{50} = 48000 nM
MMP-2 IC_{50} = 9.6 nM
MMP-3 IC_{50} = 180 nM
MMP-8 IC_{50} = 63 nM
MMP-9 IC_{50} = 69 nM
MMP-13 IC_{50} = 3 nM
MMP-14 IC_{50} = 14000 nM
MMP-16 IC_{50} = 5000 nM
TACE IC_{50} > 100000 nM

(4.83)
MMP-1 IC_{50} = 200 nM
MMP-2 IC_{50} = 0.67 nM
MMP-3 IC_{50} = 105 nM
MMP-9 IC_{50} = 0.43 nM
MMP-13 IC_{50} = 0.19 nM
MMP-14 IC_{50} = 3.9 nM

(4.76)
MMP-1 IC_{50} > 10000 nM
MMP-2 IC_{50} = 0.06 nM
MMP-3 IC_{50} = 10 nM
MMP-9 IC_{50} = 0.5 nM
MMP-13 IC_{50} = 1.2 nM

(4.79)
MMP-1 IC_{50} = 7.8 nM
MMP-2 IC_{50} = 0.35 nM
MMP-8 IC_{50} = 0.29 nM
MMP-9 IC_{50} = 0.21 nM
MMP-13 IC_{50} = 0.12 nM
MMP-14 IC_{50} = 0.32 nM
MMP-16 IC_{50} = 0.31 nM
TACE IC_{50} = 55 nM

(4.82)
MMP-1 IC_{50} = 720 nM
MMP-2 IC_{50} = 0.04 nM
MMP-13 IC_{50} = 0.1 nM
MMP-14 IC_{50} = 4 nM
ADAMTS4 IC_{50} = 580 nM
ADAMTS5 IC_{50} = 330 nM

(4.75)
MMP-1 IC_{50} = 116 nM
MMP-2 IC_{50} = 0.4 nM
MMP-3 IC_{50} = 1.1 nM
MMP-9 IC_{50} = 0.6 nM
MMP-13 IC_{50} = 0.6 nM

(4.78)
MMP-1 IC_{50} = 147 nM
MMP-2 IC_{50} = 0.09 nM
MMP-3 IC_{50} = 50 nM
MMP-7 IC_{50} > 1000 nM
MMP-8 IC_{50} = 1.6 nM
MMP-9 IC_{50} = 6.7 nM
MMP-14 IC_{50} = 9.8 nM

(4.81)
MMP-1 IC_{50} = 3500 nM
MMP-2 IC_{50} = 3.5 nM
MMP-3 IC_{50} = 21 nM
MMP-8 IC_{50} = 5.1 nM
MMP-9 IC_{50} = 0.80 nM
MMP-12 IC_{50} = 0.20 nM
MMP-13 IC_{50} = 4.1 nM
MMP-14 IC_{50} = 33 nM
MMP-16 IC_{50} = 32 nM

Although compound **4.78** (Figure 4.11) exhibited potential MMP-2 inhibition, it also produced good MMP-8 inhibition (IC_{50} = 1.6 nM), maintaining selectivity over other MMPs. Compound **4.78** (Figure 4.11) also reduced the chemoinvasion of HUVEC cells to cross the matrigel barrier. Therefore, it might be considered a highly effective antiangiogenic agent to inhibit the chemoinvasive effects of HUVEC cells. Marques and co-workers [165] disclosed some iminodiacetyl-based arylsulfonamide hydroxamates as effective MMPIs and carbonic anhydrases (CAs) inhibitors. Apart from being a potent CA inhibitor, compound **4.79** (Figure 4.11) exhibited strong MMP-13 inhibitory activity (IC_{50} = 0.12 nM), maintaining some selectivity over other MMPs and TACE.

Some N-O-isopropyl sulfonamide hydroxamates were reported as broad-spectrum potent MMPIs by Nuti and co-workers [166]. Compound **4.80** (Figure 4.11) was the maximum effective MMP-13 inhibitor (IC_{50} = 3 nM) among these molecules, keeping a minimum of three-fold selectivity over other MMPs sparing TACE. In the collagenase assay, compound **4.80** (Figure 4.11) showed promising MMP-13 selectivity (IC_{50} = 1.4 nM) over MMP-1 (IC_{50} = 15 µM). In another study, Nuti et al. [167] disclosed a set of arylsulfone hydroxamates as potent MMPIs. Compound **4.81** (Figure 4.11) in this series exhibited the most potent MMP-13 inhibition (IC_{50} = 4.1 nM) and MMP-8 inhibition (IC_{50} = 5.1 nM), although it exerted the highest MMP-12 inhibition. Nuti and co-workers [168] further explored some arylsulfonamido hydroxamates as highly effective inhibitors of aggrecanases and MMPs. Compound **4.82** (Figure 4.11) resulted in potent broad-spectrum MMP inhibition, including highly potent MMP-13 inhibition (IC_{50} = 0.1 nM) selective over aggrecanases. In their continuous efforts, Nuti et al. [169] further designed some N-isopropoxy-arylsulfonamide hydroxamates as potent and highly MMP-2-selective inhibitors over different MMPs. However, compound **4.83** (Figure 4.11) resulted in the maximum effective MMP-13 inhibition (IC_{50} = 0.19 nM) with at least a two-fold selectivity over other MMPs. It also displayed a significant reduction in migration and invasion of HUVEC *in vitro* at lower concentrations (1 nM) in a dose-dependent manner. Moreover, compound **4.83** was also found to interfere with the FBS-induced morphogenesis of HUVEC cells dose dependently, suggesting the effective antiangiogenic property of compound **4.83**. Moreover, the western blot study and gelatin zymography analysis suggested that compound **4.83** inhibited gelatinase in a dose-dependent fashion. An MTT assay also disclosed that compound **4.83** was a promising cytotoxic agent that might induce endothelial cellular death. Therefore, compound **4.83** might have the ability to induce apoptosis in endothelial cells. Moreover, it responded excellently in exerting the antiangiogenic response in the *in vivo* matrigel sponge assay model in the mice.

Some tetrahydroisoquinoline-based hydroxamates were explored as broad-spectrum potent non-selective MMPIs by Ma et al. [170]. Compound **4.84** (Figure 4.12) was the most efficacious MMP-1 inhibitor (IC_{50} = 41 nM), showing a broad spectrum of MMP inhibition.

Sawa et al. [171] reported several phosphonamide-containing hydroxamates as effective MMP inhibitors. Compound **4.85** (Figure 4.12) comprising the 3, 3, 3-trifluoropropyl ester function exhibited potent MMP-1 inhibitory activity (K_i = 6.23 nM),

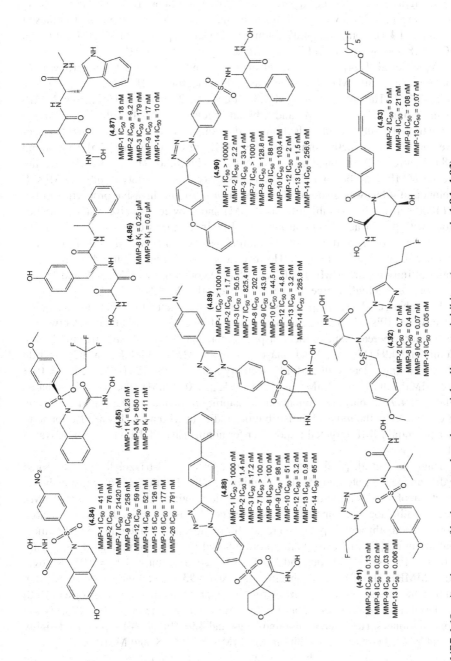

FIGURE 4.12 Another set of hydroxamate-based potential collagenase inhibitors (compounds 4.84–4.93).

sparing MMP-3 and MMP-9. Some oxal hydroxamic acids were reported as potential inhibitors of neutrophil collagenase by Krumme and Tschesche [172]. Compound **4.86** (Figure 4.12) was the most potent MMP-8 inhibitor ($K_i = 0.25$ µM) among these molecules. Moroy et al. [173] synthesized and evaluated analogs of ilomastat (compound **4.1**). Compound **4.87** (Figure 4.12) yielded promising MMP-1 inhibition ($IC_{50} = 18$ nM) with good inhibitory efficacy against other MMPs.

Zapico et al. [174] reported a set of potent and selective α-tetrahydropyranyl-containing arylsulfonyl hydroxamates as highly effective MMP-2-selective inhibitors over MMP-9. However, compound **4.88** (Figure 4.12) exhibited efficacious MMP-13 inhibition ($IC_{50} = 0.9$ nM) and a broad spectrum of MMP inhibitory activity. Some triazolyl-substituted arylsulfonyl hydroxamates were explored as highly effective and MMP-2-selective inhibitors over MMP-9 by Fabre et al. [175]. Compound **4.89** (Figure 4.12) exhibited promising MMP-13 inhibition ($IC_{50} = 3.2$ nM), having greater MMP-2 inhibition and a higher selectivity over a variety of other MMPs. It (compound **4.89**) was also found to exhibit *in vitro* anti-invasive properties in the HT1080 cell line (37% inhibition at 10 µM) and showed effective water solubility along with good Caco-2 cellular permeability. In another study, Zapico et al. [176] reported a set of arylsulfonamide-containing hydroxamates with triazole function as efficacious gelatinase inhibitors. However, compound **4.90** (Figure 4.12) provided better affinity toward MMP-13 ($IC_{50} = 1.5$ nM) compared with MMP-2 and MMP-12, along with a high degree of selectivity over other MMPs.

Hugenberg et al. [177] reported some triazole-substituted hydroxamates as highly effective MMPIs. Many of these compounds exhibited potency but non-selectivity to each other, whereas some of them displayed potent and MMP-9-selective inhibition. Compound **4.91** (Figure 4.12) displayed promising MMP-13 inhibition ($IC_{50} = 0.006$ nM), retaining at least a three-fold selectivity over other MMPs (MMP-2 $IC_{50} = 0.13$ nM, MMP-8 $IC_{50} = 0.02$ nM, and MMP-9 $IC_{50} = 0.03$ nM). The radio fluorinated analog of **4.91** displayed excellent serum stability *in vitro* as well as rapid clearance, as evidenced by the *in vivo* biodistribution studies in wild mice. It was also found to be a potential MMP-targeted radiotracer for noninvasive PET-imaging for activated MMPs *in vivo*.

Hugenberg et al. [178] further reported a set of 1,2,3-triazolylethyl substituted hydroxamates as potential MMPIs. Compound **4.92** (Figure 4.12) displayed a broad spectrum of MMP inhibition with good inhibition against MMP-13 ($IC_{50} = 0.05$ nM). The ^{18}F-radiolabeled compound **4.92** showed good serum stability. It was also cleared from the body through hepatic and renal elimination, as evaluated in C57/BL6 mice. Kalinin et al. [179] reported some proline-based MMPIs. Compound **4.93** (Figure 4.12) was the most efficacious and MMP-13-selective inhibitor ($IC_{50} = 0.07$ nM) over other MMPs. The [18F] radiolabeled compound **4.93** showed metabolic stability in human and mouse serum *in vitro*. A further report by Kalinin and co-workers [180] disclosed a set of proline-containing hydroxamates as zinc-dependent deacetylase LpxC inhibitors. However, compounds **4.94** and **4.95** (Figure 4.13) produced highly potent MMP-13-selective inhibition over MMP-2, MMP-8, and MMP-9.

A set of arylsulfonamide hydroxamates was reported as effective broad-spectrum MMPIs by Wagner and co-workers [181]. Compound **4.96** (**Figure 4.13**) exerted a

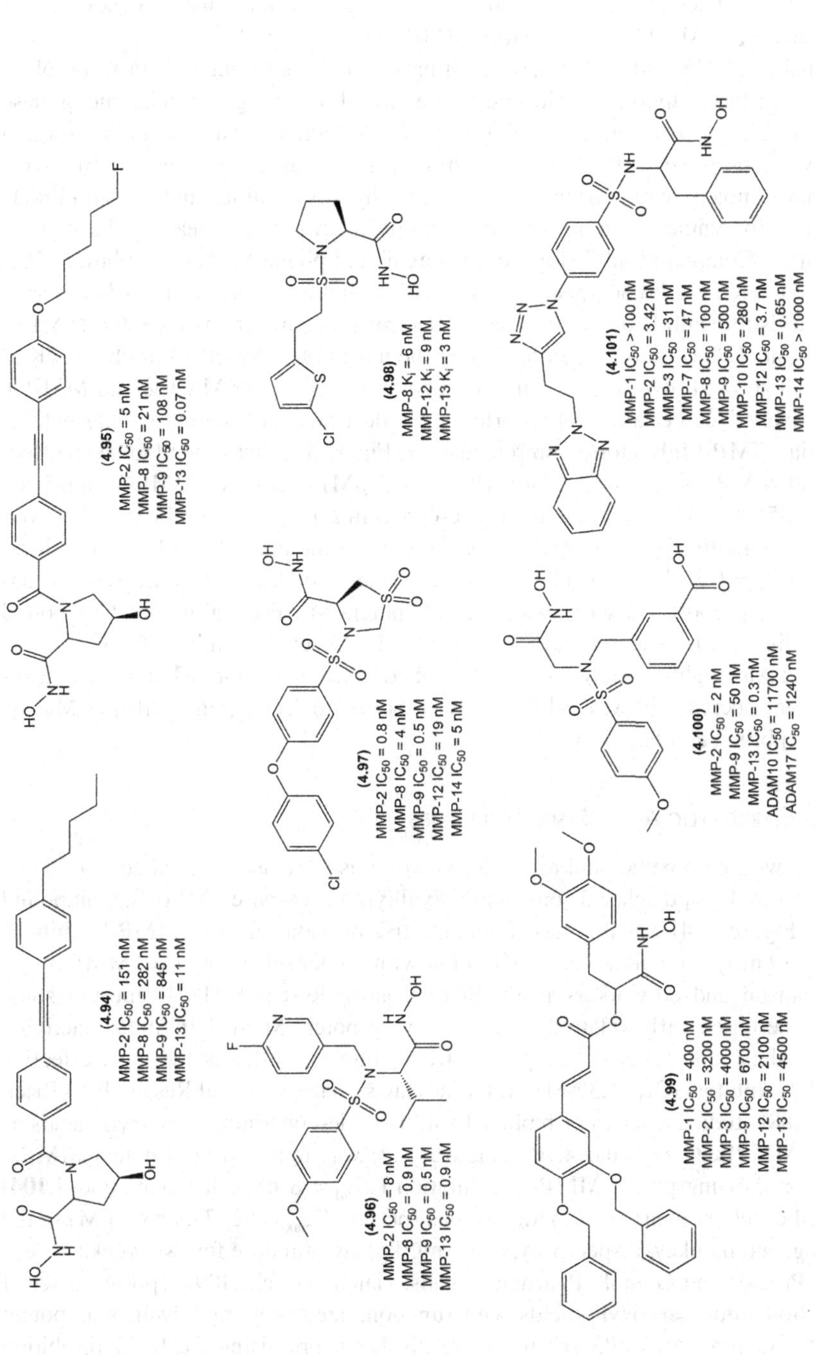

(4.94)
MMP-2 IC_{50} = 151 nM
MMP-8 IC_{50} = 282 nM
MMP-9 IC_{50} = 845 nM
MMP-13 IC_{50} = 11 nM

(4.95)
MMP-2 IC_{50} = 5 nM
MMP-8 IC_{50} = 21 nM
MMP-9 IC_{50} = 108 nM
MMP-13 IC_{50} = 0.07 nM

(4.96)
MMP-2 IC_{50} = 8 nM
MMP-8 IC_{50} = 0.9 nM
MMP-9 IC_{50} = 0.5 nM
MMP-13 IC_{50} = 0.9 nM

(4.97)
MMP-2 IC_{50} = 0.8 nM
MMP-8 IC_{50} = 4 nM
MMP-9 IC_{50} = 0.5 nM
MMP-12 IC_{50} = 19 nM
MMP-14 IC_{50} = 5 nM

(4.98)
MMP-8 K_i = 6 nM
MMP-12 K_i = 9 nM
MMP-13 K_i = 3 nM

(4.99)
MMP-1 IC_{50} = 400 nM
MMP-2 IC_{50} = 3200 nM
MMP-3 IC_{50} = 4000 nM
MMP-9 IC_{50} = 6700 nM
MMP-12 IC_{50} = 2100 nM
MMP-13 IC_{50} = 4500 nM

(4.100)
MMP-2 IC_{50} = 2 nM
MMP-9 IC_{50} = 50 nM
MMP-13 IC_{50} = 0.3 nM
ADAM10 IC_{50} = 11700 nM
ADAM17 IC_{50} = 1240 nM

(4.101)
MMP-1 IC_{50} > 100 nM
MMP-2 IC_{50} = 3.42 nM
MMP-3 IC_{50} = 31 nM
MMP-7 IC_{50} = 47 nM
MMP-8 IC_{50} = 100 nM
MMP-9 IC_{50} = 500 nM
MMP-10 IC_{50} = 280 nM
MMP-12 IC_{50} = 3.7 nM
MMP-13 IC_{50} = 0.65 nM
MMP-14 IC_{50} > 1000 nM

FIGURE 4.13 Various potential hydroxamate-based collagenase inhibitors (compounds **4.94–4.101**).

potent broad-spectrum of MMP inhibition, having good inhibitory potency against collagenases (MMP-13 $IC_{50} = 0.9$ nM, MMP-8 $IC_{50} = 0.9$ nM).

Topai et al. [182] identified new gelatinase inhibitors through an *in silico* pharmacophore-based approach, followed by the virtual screening method. Among these new scaffolds, pyroglutamate analog produced effective gelatinase inhibition and thus was a promising hit. Bioisosteric modification was done to replace the pyroglutamate moiety with proline, thiazolidine, hydroxyproline, and thiazolidinone functions to synthesize some arylsulfonamide hydroxamates bearing these functionalities. Compound **4.97** (Figure 4.13) exhibited potent MMP-8 inhibition (IC_{50} = 4 nM), having a broad spectrum of MMP inhibition. Mori et al. [183] reported some arylsulfonamide derivatives having hydroxamate moiety as potential MMPIs. Compound **4.98** (Figure 4.13) was among the most potent MMP-13 inhibitors (K_i = 3 nM). It showed two-fold and three-fold better efficacy over MMP-8 and MMP-9, respectively. Yuan et al. [184] reported some derivatives of methyl rosmarinate as potential MMP-1 inhibitors. Compound **4.99** (Figure 4.13) was found to be an effective and MMP-1-selective inhibitor ($IC_{50} = 0.4$ µM) over other MMPs. Ramsbeck et al. [185] designed some hydroxamate-containing meprin-β inhibitors. However, compound **4.100** (Figure 4.13) exhibited highly potent and MMP-13-selective inhibition ($IC_{50} = 0.3$ nM) over other metalloenzymes tested. Recently, Zapico and co-workers [82] reported a set of water-soluble potent MMP-13 inhibitors. Compound **4.101** (Figure 4.13) was the most effective MMP-13-selective inhibitor ($IC_{50} = 0.65$ nM) and was highly selective over other MMPs. Compound **4.101** showed a dose-dependent decrease of MMP-13 activity in human osteosarcoma cell line MG-63 (51% inhibition at 50 nM).

4.5.2 CARBOXYLIC ACID-BASED INHIBITORS

MMPIs with carboxylic acid as the ZBG were also extensively studied. At Glaxo, Brown et al. [186] disclosed some (carboxyalkyl) amino-based MMPIs. Compound **4.102** (Figure 4.14) was the maximum effective but non-selective MMP-1 inhibitor ($IC_{50} = 19$ nM) compared with MMP-9 but with higher selectivity over MMP-3.

Robinson and co-workers from Pfizer Central Research [187] reported some glutamine-based carboxylate derivatives having potent MMP-1 inhibitory activity. Among these compounds, Compound **4.103** (Figure 4.14) was the most effective MMP-1 inhibitor ($IC_{50} = 23$ nM). At Parke-Davis Pharmaceutical Research, O'Brien et al. [188] studied a series of biphenyl sulfonamide-containing carboxylic acids as potent MMPIs. Compound **4.104** (Figure 4.14) was found to be a potent MMP-2 inhibitor showing potent MMP-13 inhibition ($IC_{50} = 8$ nM). It (compound **4.104**) showed excellent pharmacokinetic profiles (plasma $C_{max} = 62$, 73, and 7 µM) in the rat, dog, and monkey, respectively, at a 3 mg/kg/day oral dose for two weeks.

At Procter and Gamble Pharmaceuticals, Natchus et al. [189] reported a set of arylsulfonamido carboxylic acids with functionalized propargylglycines as potent MMPIs. Compound **4.105** (Figure 4.14) displayed promising MMP-13 inhibition ($IC_{50} = 21$ nM) but exhibited greater affinity toward MMP-2 and sparing MMP-1 and MMP-3. Regarding *in vivo* pharmacokinetics, it (compound **4.105**) was highly soluble

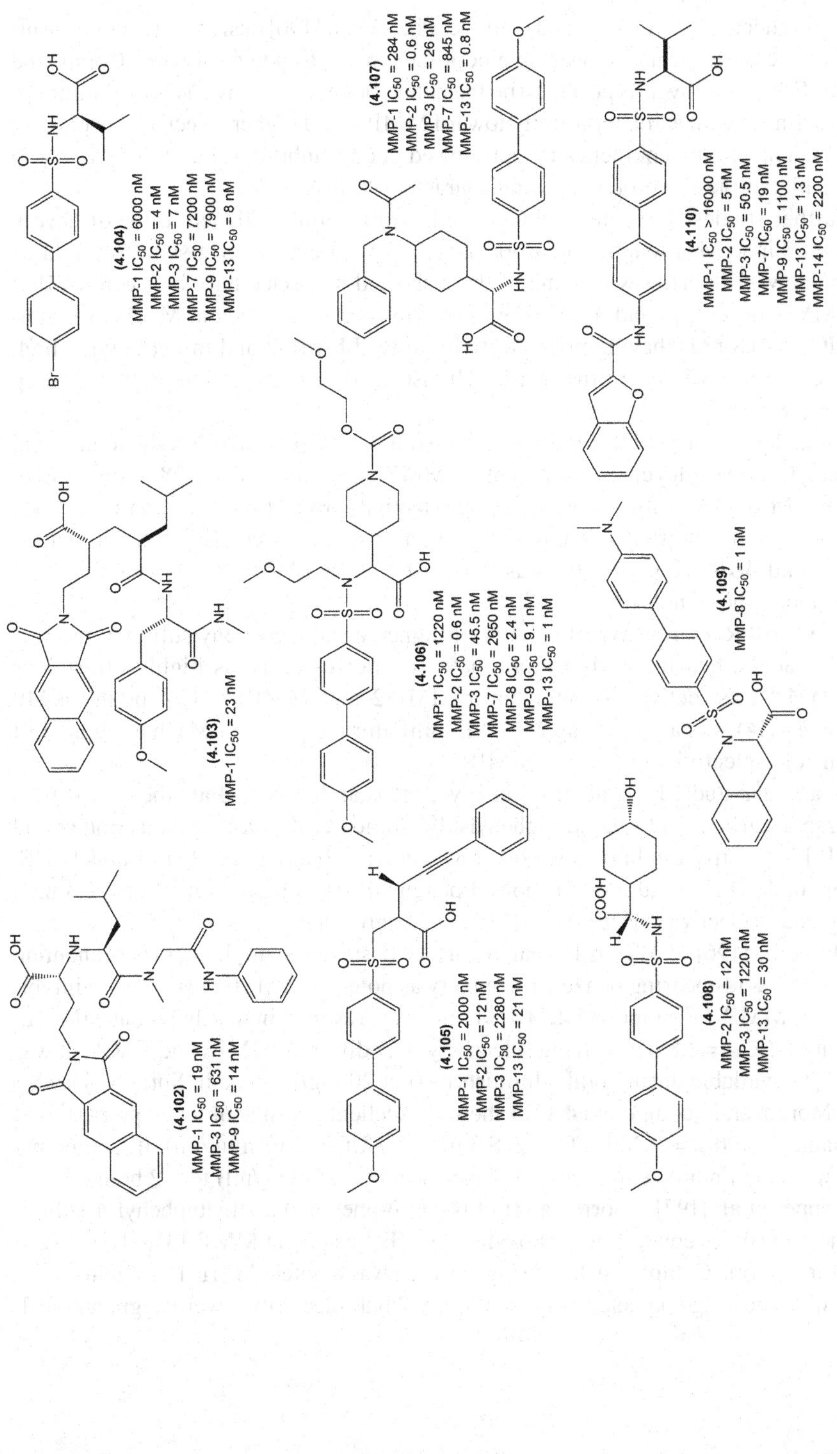

FIGURE 4.14 Carboxylic acid-based potential collagenase inhibitors (compounds **4.102–4.110**).

(151 mg/ml) and highly plasma protein-bound (96.2%) in rats. It also displayed moderate bioavailability (49%) and a shorter half-life ($t_{1/2}$ = 1.7 hr). High water solubility, as well as serum protein binding character (>90%), might be difficult to overcome for such a type of inhibitor.

In another study at Procter and Gamble, Pikul et al. [190] designed a set of arylsulfonamide carboxylic acids, bearing piperidine moiety, as potent MMPIs. Compound **4.106** (Figure 4.14) was reported to be the potent but non-selective MMP-13 inhibitor (IC_{50} = 1 nM) with a greater affinity toward MMP-2 and higher selectivity over other MMPs. The pharmacokinetics model showed good solubility (11.09 mg/ml at pH 7) with a higher plasma protein binding character (90.7%).

Further studies at Procter and Gamble by Tullis et al. [191] led to the discovery of some biphenylsulfonamido carboxylic acids with cyclohexylglycine scaffold as potential MMPIs. However, some of them showed non-selectivity between MMP-2 and MMP-13. Compound **4.107** (Figure 4.14) was the most potent MMP-13 inhibitor (IC_{50} = 0.8 nM), having non-selectivity toward MMP-2 and maintaining a high degree of selectivity over other MMPs. It also showed high plasma protein binding ability (98.5%).

Hudlicky et al. [192] reported some functionalized cyclohexylglycines and α-methylcyclohexylgycines as potential MMPIs. Compound **4.108** showed dual MMP-2/MMP-13 inhibition having good selectivity over MMP-3. Matter et al. [193] disclosed some tetrahydroisoquinoline-3-carboxylate-based MMP-8 inhibitors. Compound **4.109** (Figure 4.14) was the most effective MMP-8 inhibitor (IC_{50} = 1 nM) among these molecules.

At Wyeth Research, Wu et al. [194] designed a set of biphenylsulfonamido carboxylic acids, bearing carboxamide heterocyclic functions as highly efficacious and MMP-13-selective inhibitors over MMP-2 and MMP-14. Compound **4.110** (**Figure 4.14**) was a promising MMP-13 inhibitor (IC_{50} = 1.3 nM), having at least a four-fold selectivity over other MMPs.

In another study, Li et al. [195] at Wyeth Research reported another set of benzofuran 2-carboxamido-based biphenylsulfonamido carboxylic acids as potent and MMP-13-selective inhibitors over other MMPs as well as aggrecanase-1 and TACE. Compound **4.111** (Figure 4.15) showed potent MMP-13 inhibition (IC_{50} = 2.3 nM) and greater selectivity over other MMPs and aggrecanase-1.

Hu et al. [196] at Wyeth Research further designed some biphenylsulfonamido carboxylic acids bearing benzofuran moiety as potent and MMP-13-selective inhibitors over MMP-2. Compound **4.112** (Figure 4.15) resulted in highly potent MMP-13 inhibition (IC_{50} = 1.8 nM) having selectivity over different MMPs and TACE. It was 100% bioavailable during oral administration at 20 mg/kg dose in Sprague-Dawley rats. Moreover, it (compound **4.112**) showed excellent pharmacokinetic properties at the same dose ($t_{1/2}$ = 3.28 hr, C_{max} = 8.3 μg/ml, AUC = 65.7 h μg/ml). It (compound **4.112**) also maintained an excellent plasma level (>1,000 ng/ml) for 12 hours.

Hopper et al. [197] reported a set of (4-keto)-phenoxy) methylbiphenyl-4-sulfonamide derivatives containing carboxylic acid ZBG as potent MMP-13 and aggrecanase-1 inhibitors. Compound **4.113** (Figure 4.15) was a potent MMP-13 inhibitor (IC_{50} = 1.1 nM) showing non-selectivity over MMP-2 but selectivity toward aggrecanase-1.

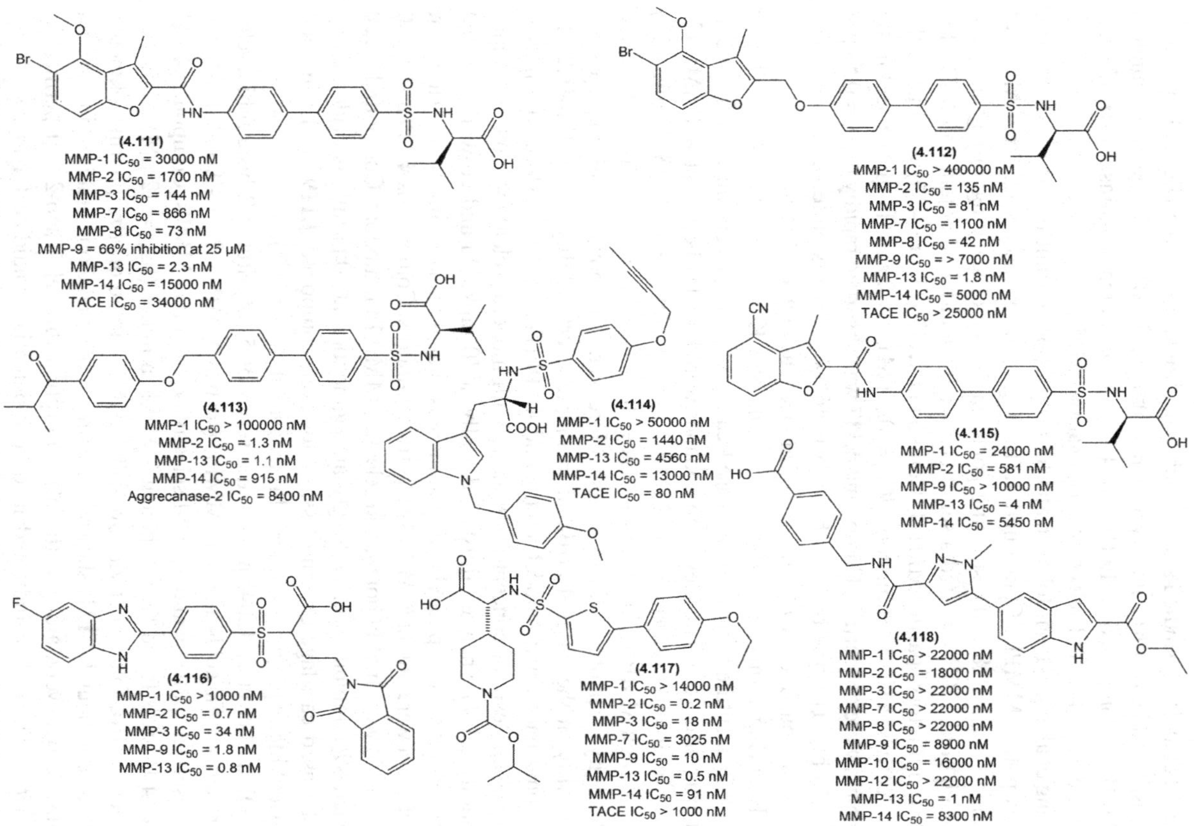

(4.111)
MMP-1 IC$_{50}$ = 30000 nM
MMP-2 IC$_{50}$ = 1700 nM
MMP-3 IC$_{50}$ = 144 nM
MMP-7 IC$_{50}$ = 866 nM
MMP-8 IC$_{50}$ = 73 nM
MMP-9 = 66% inhibition at 25 μM
MMP-13 IC$_{50}$ = 2.3 nM
MMP-14 IC$_{50}$ = 15000 nM
TACE IC$_{50}$ = 34000 nM

(4.112)
MMP-1 IC$_{50}$ > 400000 nM
MMP-2 IC$_{50}$ = 135 nM
MMP-3 IC$_{50}$ = 81 nM
MMP-7 IC$_{50}$ = 1100 nM
MMP-8 IC$_{50}$ = 42 nM
MMP-9 IC$_{50}$ = > 7000 nM
MMP-13 IC$_{50}$ = 1.8 nM
MMP-14 IC$_{50}$ = 5000 nM
TACE IC$_{50}$ > 25000 nM

(4.113)
MMP-1 IC$_{50}$ > 100000 nM
MMP-2 IC$_{50}$ = 1.3 nM
MMP-13 IC$_{50}$ = 1.1 nM
MMP-14 IC$_{50}$ = 915 nM
Aggrecanase-2 IC$_{50}$ = 8400 nM

(4.114)
MMP-1 IC$_{50}$ > 50000 nM
MMP-2 IC$_{50}$ = 1440 nM
MMP-13 IC$_{50}$ = 4560 nM
MMP-14 IC$_{50}$ = 13000 nM
TACE IC$_{50}$ = 80 nM

(4.115)
MMP-1 IC$_{50}$ = 24000 nM
MMP-2 IC$_{50}$ = 581 nM
MMP-9 IC$_{50}$ > 10000 nM
MMP-13 IC$_{50}$ = 4 nM
MMP-14 IC$_{50}$ = 5450 nM

(4.116)
MMP-1 IC$_{50}$ = 1000 nM
MMP-2 IC$_{50}$ = 0.7 nM
MMP-3 IC$_{50}$ = 34 nM
MMP-9 IC$_{50}$ = 1.8 nM
MMP-13 IC$_{50}$ = 0.8 nM

(4.117)
MMP-1 IC$_{50}$ > 14000 nM
MMP-2 IC$_{50}$ = 0.2 nM
MMP-3 IC$_{50}$ = 18 nM
MMP-7 IC$_{50}$ = 3025 nM
MMP-9 IC$_{50}$ = 10 nM
MMP-13 IC$_{50}$ = 0.5 nM
MMP-14 IC$_{50}$ = 91 nM
TACE IC$_{50}$ = 1000 nM

(4.118)
MMP-1 IC$_{50}$ > 22000 nM
MMP-2 IC$_{50}$ = 18000 nM
MMP-3 IC$_{50}$ > 22000 nM
MMP-7 IC$_{50}$ > 22000 nM
MMP-8 IC$_{50}$ > 22000 nM
MMP-9 IC$_{50}$ = 8900 nM
MMP-10 IC$_{50}$ = 16000 nM
MMP-12 IC$_{50}$ > 22000 nM
MMP-13 IC$_{50}$ = 1 nM
MMP-14 IC$_{50}$ = 8300 nM

FIGURE 4.15 Another set of carboxylic acid-based potential collagenase inhibitors (compounds **4.111–4.118**).

Park et al. [198] reported a set of tryptophan sulfonamides as highly potent TACE inhibitors. Among these compounds, compound **4.114** (Figure 4.15), though showing highly potent TACE inhibition, also displayed potent broad-spectrum MMP inhibition with effective MMP-13 inhibition (IC_{50} = 4.56 μM). In another study at Wyeth, Li et al. [199] studied a set of biphenylsulfonamide carboxylic acids having 3, 4-disubstituted benzofuran moiety as potent and highly MMP-13-selective inhibitors over MMP-2. Compound **4.115** (Figure 4.15) showed potency against MMP-13 (IC_{50} = 4 nM) having 145-fold selectivity over various MMPs.

Zhang et al. [200] from Johnson and Johnson reported some α-sulfonyl carboxylic acids as potent MMPIs. Compound **4.116** (Figure 4.15) disclosed potent MMP-13 inhibition (IC_{50} = 0.8 nM), showing good inhibitory efficacy against gelatinases. Monovich et al. [201] reported a set of carboxylic acid-based potent and MMP-13-selective inhibitors sparing MMP-1. Compound **4.117** (Figure 4.15) was one of the most effective MMP-13 inhibitors (IC_{50} = 0.5 nM). As far as the pharmacokinetic parameters were concerned, Compound **4.117** was absorbed rapidly (C_{max} = 0.58 μg/ ml at 0.56 hr). The oral bioavailability was 46.6%, which is quite appreciable. The half-life was found to be 7 hr and the clearance was high (112 ml/min/kg).

At Boehringer Ingelheim Pharmaceuticals and Karos Pharmaceuticals, Taylor et al. [202] identified some indole-based carboxylic acid esters through fragment-based drug discovery. These ester compounds were found to be potent and MMP-13-selective inhibitors compared with MMP-2 and -14. Compound **4.118** (Figure 4.15) displayed high MMP-13 inhibitory potency (IC_{50} = 1 nM) along with a high degree of selectivity over other MMPs tested. Moreover, it responded with high passive permeability in the parallel artificial membrane permeability assay (PAMPA). In the rat pharmacokinetic model, compound **4.118** (Figure 4.15) exhibited a micro-molar plasma level of concentration along with moderate clearance and good bio-availability (39%) when administrated orally at 10 mpk. Hu and co-workers [203] tried to design some biphenyl sulfonamide-based aggrecanases inhibitors. However, most of them were potent MMP-13-selective inhibitors. Compounds **4.119** and **4.120** (Figure 4.16) were highly potent and selective MMP-13 inhibitors. Compound **4.120** exhibited 87% inhibition of proteoglycan degradation at 10 μg/ml, as evidenced by the cell-based cartilage explants assay. However, compound **4.119** displayed good pharmacokinetic properties ($t_{1/2}$ = 6 hr; bioavailability = 23%).

Le Diguarher et al. [204] produced a series of 5-substituted 2-bisarylthiocyclo-pentane carboxylic acids as potent MMPIs (such as MMP-1, -2, -3, -9, and -13). Some of them showed potency and MMP-1 selectivity over other MMPs. Compound **4.121** (Figure 4.16) was found to be a potent MMP-1 inhibitor (IC_{50} = 12 μM), maintaining at least a five-fold selectivity over other MMPs. In an *in vitro* pharmacokinetics model, it (compound **4.121**) showed 74% and 100% metabolic stability in rats and humans, respectively, along with 95% absorption through Caco-2 cell permeability *in vitro*. These data indicated it to be a potential candidate for *in vivo* study. Compound **4.121** (Figure 4.16) significantly reduced metastasis in the B16F10 mouse melanoma model (>60% at 200 mg/kg IP) and was also found to reduce the tumor size by 1 mm diameter (100%). It also exhibited potential *in vivo* pharmacokinetics parameters in mice (C_{max} = 40 μg/ml, $t_{1/2}$ = 3.4 hr at 5 mg/kg dose i.v.).

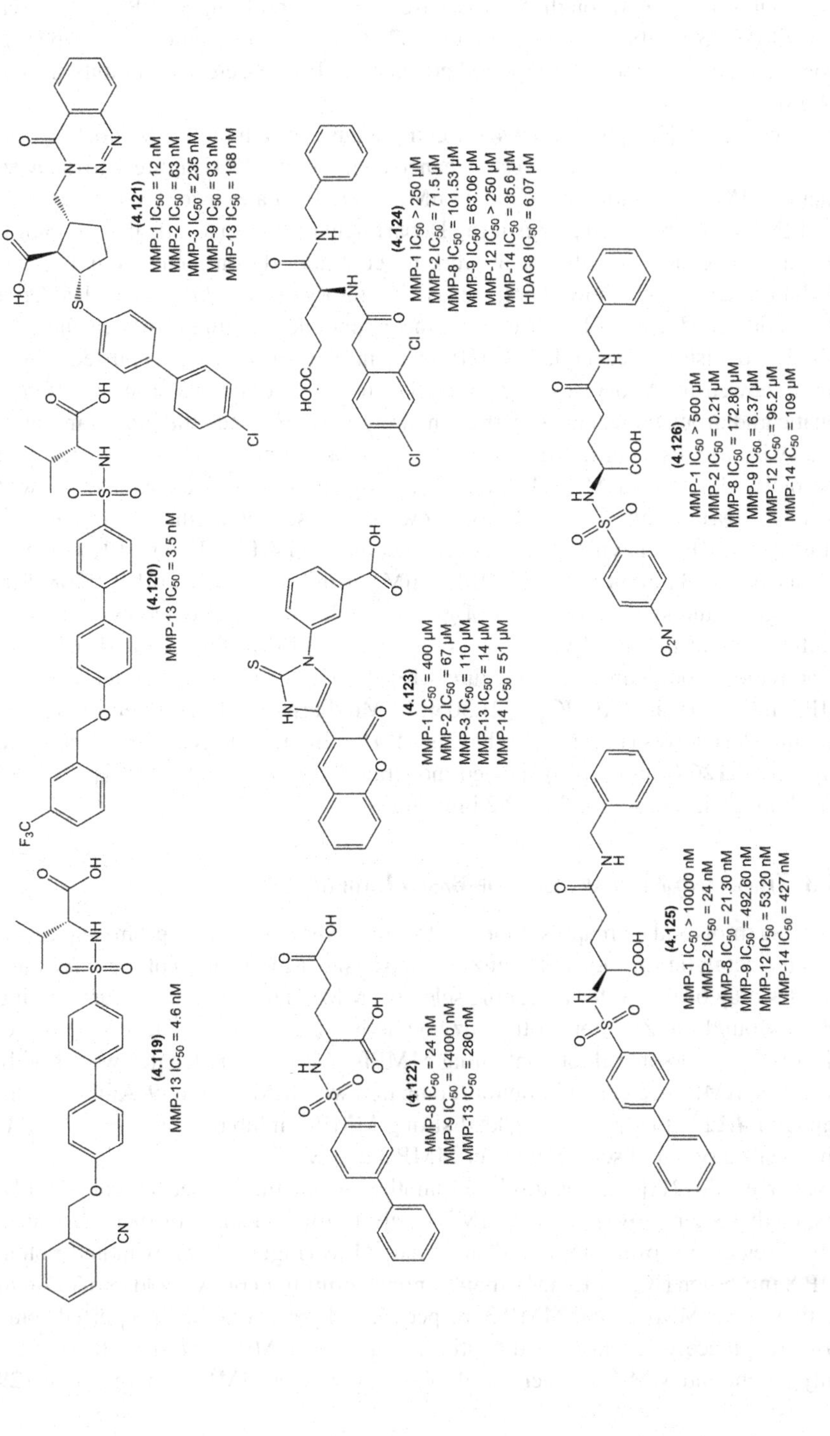

(4.121)
MMP-1 IC$_{50}$ = 12 nM
MMP-2 IC$_{50}$ = 63 nM
MMP-3 IC$_{50}$ = 235 nM
MMP-9 IC$_{50}$ = 93 nM
MMP-13 IC$_{50}$ = 168 nM

(4.124)
MMP-1 IC$_{50}$ > 250 µM
MMP-2 IC$_{50}$ = 71.5 µM
MMP-8 IC$_{50}$ = 101.53 µM
MMP-9 IC$_{50}$ = 63.06 µM
MMP-12 IC$_{50}$ > 250 µM
MMP-14 IC$_{50}$ = 85.6 µM
HDAC8 IC$_{50}$ = 6.07 µM

(4.120)
MMP-13 IC$_{50}$ = 3.5 nM

(4.126)
MMP-1 IC$_{50}$ > 500 µM
MMP-2 IC$_{50}$ = 0.21 µM
MMP-8 IC$_{50}$ = 172.80 µM
MMP-9 IC$_{50}$ = 6.37 µM
MMP-12 IC$_{50}$ = 95.2 µM
MMP-14 IC$_{50}$ = 109 µM

(4.123)
MMP-1 IC$_{50}$ = 400 µM
MMP-2 IC$_{50}$ = 67 µM
MMP-3 IC$_{50}$ = 110 µM
MMP-13 IC$_{50}$ = 14 µM
MMP-14 IC$_{50}$ = 51 µM

(4.119)
MMP-13 IC$_{50}$ = 4.6 nM

(4.122)
MMP-8 IC$_{50}$ = 24 nM
MMP-9 IC$_{50}$ = 14000 nM
MMP-13 IC$_{50}$ = 280 nM

(4.125)
MMP-1 IC$_{50}$ > 10000 nM
MMP-2 IC$_{50}$ = 24 nM
MMP-8 IC$_{50}$ = 21.30 nM
MMP-9 IC$_{50}$ = 492.60 nM
MMP-12 IC$_{50}$ = 53.20 nM
MMP-14 IC$_{50}$ = 427 nM

FIGURE 4.16 Another set of carboxylic acid-based potential collagenase inhibitors (compounds **4.119–4.126**).

Nakai and co-workers [205] from Scripps Research Institute performed a high throughput screening through activity-based protein profiling (ABPP) to screen potent MMP-13 inhibitors. Compound **4.122** (Figure 4.16), containing a biphenyl sulfonyl glutamic acid moiety, explored potent and MMP-8-selective inhibition (IC$_{50}$ = 24 nM).

La Pietra et al. [206] identified some compounds through molecular docking followed by virtual screening. The best-screened compound **4.123** (Figure 4.16) showed moderate MMP-13 inhibition (IC$_{50}$ = 14 µM) and at least a four-fold selectivity over other MMPs. Our research group at the Department of Pharmaceutical Technology, Jadavpur University, has also been working continuously on some isoglutamines and glutamines, which showed collagenase inhibitory activity [207–209]. Halder et al. [207] designed a set of L(+)-isoglutamine compounds (Figure 4.16) bearing dual MMP-2 and histone deacetylase 8 (HDAC8) inhibitory activities. Fourteen compounds showed inhibitory activities on collagenase-2 over collagenase-1. Different aliphatic and aromatic residue substitutions were made to check the important interactions with MMPs. As the bulky aromatic P1' substitutions increase the activity of these molecules toward MMP-8, these L(+)-isoglutamine derivatives also showed moderate MMP-8 inhibitory activity. However, these compounds were inactive against the MMP-1 enzyme. The best active compound **4.124** (Figure 4.16) showed moderate MMP-8 inhibition (IC$_{50}$ = 101.53 µM). Adhikari and co-workers [208] further designed and synthesized a set of glutamine derivatives and screened initially for inhibitions of MMPs. Twelve compounds showed MMP-8 over MMP-1 inhibitory activities. Compound **4.125** (Figure 4.16) showed the most significant result for MMP-8 inhibitory activity (IC$_{50}$ = 21.30 nM). Mukherjee et al. [209] reported some glutamine derivatives (Figure 4.16) having MMP inhibitory activity. The best active compound **4.126** (Figure 4.16) showed moderate MMP-8 inhibition (IC$_{50}$ = 172.80 µM), although it was a good MMP-2 inhibitor.

4.5.3 THIOL AND MERCAPTOSULFIDE-BASED INHIBITORS

Regarding thiols and mercaptosulfides, both ZBGs were found to be promising chelators of the catalytic Zn^{2+} ion at the enzyme active site. Modification of these mercaptosulfides may be useful for designing selective MMPIs targeted to the surrounding pockets around the Zn^{2+} ion in the enzyme active site. At Chiroscience, Baxter et al. [210] designed some thiol-containing MMPIs. All these molecules were highly efficacious MMP-8-selective inhibitors compared with MMP-3 and -9. Among them, compound **4.127** (Figure 4.17) yielded strong MMP-8 inhibition (IC$_{50}$ = 0.05 µM) with at least a two-fold selectivity over MMP-3 and -9.

Baxter et al. [211] further disclosed another set of thiol-based potent MMPIs. Some of these derivatives exerted MMP-8 selectivity, and some of them displayed MMP-9 selectivity over MMP-3. Compound **4.128** (Figure 4.17) exhibited potent MMP-8 inhibition (IC$_{50}$ = 15 nM), maintaining a minimum of two-fold and 285-fold selectivity over MMP-9 and MMP-3, respectively. Lynas et al. [212] reported some N-α-mercaptoacetyl containing dipeptides as potent MMPIs. Most of them were highly potent and MMP-8-selective inhibitors over other MMPs. Compound **4.129**

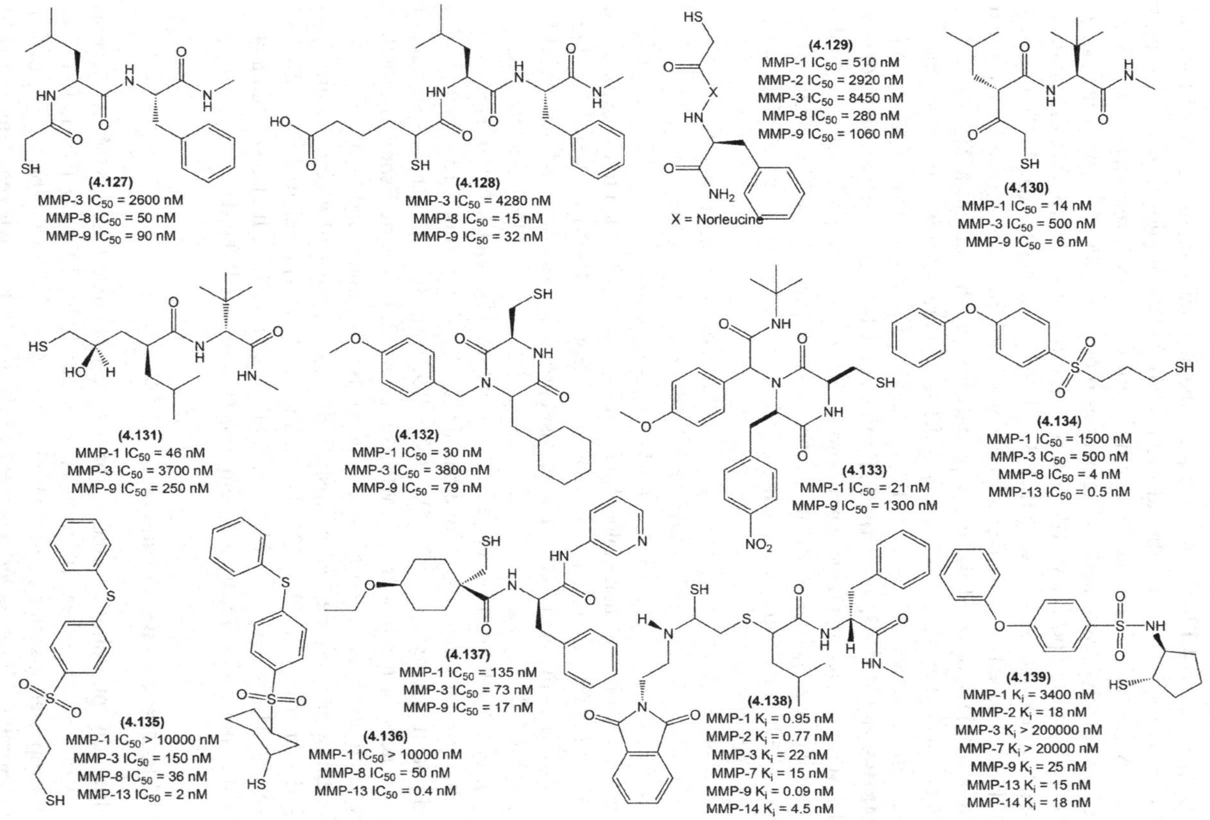

FIGURE 4.17 Thiol and mercaptosulfide-based potential collagenase inhibitors (compounds **4.127–4.139**).

(4.130)
MMP-1 IC_{50} = 14 nM
MMP-3 IC_{50} = 500 nM
MMP-9 IC_{50} = 6 nM

(4.134)
MMP-1 IC_{50} = 1500 nM
MMP-3 IC_{50} = 500 nM
MMP-8 IC_{50} = 4 nM
MMP-13 IC_{50} = 0.5 nM

(4.139)
MMP-1 K_i = 3400 nM
MMP-2 K_i = 18 nM
MMP-3 K_i > 200000 nM
MMP-7 K_i > 20000 nM
MMP-9 K_i = 25 nM
MMP-13 K_i = 15 nM
MMP-14 K_i = 18 nM

(4.129)
MMP-1 IC_{50} = 510 nM
MMP-2 IC_{50} = 2920 nM
MMP-3 IC_{50} = 8450 nM
MMP-8 IC_{50} = 280 nM
MMP-9 IC_{50} = 1060 nM

X = Norleucine

(4.133)
MMP-1 IC_{50} = 21 nM
MMP-9 IC_{50} = 1300 nM

(4.138)
MMP-1 K_i = 0.95 nM
MMP-2 K_i = 0.77 nM
MMP-3 K_i = 22 nM
MMP-7 K_i = 15 nM
MMP-9 K_i = 0.09 nM
MMP-14 K_i = 4.5 nM

(4.128)
MMP-3 IC_{50} = 4280 nM
MMP-8 IC_{50} = 15 nM
MMP-9 IC_{50} = 32 nM

(4.132)
MMP-1 IC_{50} = 30 nM
MMP-3 IC_{50} = 3800 nM
MMP-9 IC_{50} = 79 nM

(4.137)
MMP-1 IC_{50} = 135 nM
MMP-3 IC_{50} = 73 nM
MMP-9 IC_{50} = 17 nM

(4.136)
MMP-1 IC_{50} > 10000 nM
MMP-8 IC_{50} = 50 nM
MMP-13 IC_{50} = 0.4 nM

(4.127)
MMP-3 IC_{50} = 2600 nM
MMP-8 IC_{50} = 50 nM
MMP-9 IC_{50} = 90 nM

(4.131)
MMP-1 IC_{50} = 46 nM
MMP-3 IC_{50} = 3700 nM
MMP-9 IC_{50} = 250 nM

(4.135)
MMP-1 IC_{50} > 10000 nM
MMP-3 IC_{50} = 150 nM
MMP-8 IC_{50} = 36 nM
MMP-13 IC_{50} = 2 nM

(Figure 4.17) resulted in promising MMP-8 inhibition (IC_{50} = 280 nM), maintaining selectivity over other MMPs.

The joint venture of Affimax and Wyeth-Ayrest Research led Campbell et al. [213] to discover malonyl α-mercaptoketones and α-mercaptoalcohols as potential MMPIs. Compound **4.130** (Figure 4.17) was the maximum effective MMP-1 inhibitor (IC_{50} = 14 nM) along with a broad-spectrum of MMP inhibition. In another study at Wyeth-Ayrest and Affymax Research, Levin et al. [214] reported some succinyl mercaptoalcohols and mercaptoketones as promising MMPIs. Compound **4.131** (Figure 4.17) was the potent MMP-1-selective inhibitor (IC_{50} = 46 nM), maintaining at least a five-fold selectivity over MMP-3 and -9. In Affimax Research, Szardenings et al. [215] developed a set of diketopiperazine-containing thiol derivatives as potent inhibitors of MMPs. All of these compounds were highly potent MMP-1-selective inhibitors over other MMPs. Compound **4.132** (Figure 4.17) was the best MMP-1 inhibitor of this series (IC_{50} = 30 nM) along with 2.6-fold and 126.6-fold selectivity over MMP-9 and MMP-3, respectively. Further study by Szardenings et al. [216] produced several diketopiperazine-based thiol analogs as potent collagenase-1 inhibitors selective over gelatinase-B and stromelysin. Compound **4.133** (Figure 4.17) exhibited the highest collagenase-1 inhibition (IC_{50} = 21 nM), having 62-fold selectivity over gelatinase-B.

Freskos et al. [217] reported some γ-sulfone thiols as potent MMP-13-selective inhibitors. Compounds **4.134** and **4.135** (Figure 4.17) were promising MMP-13-selective inhibitors (IC_{50} of 0.5 nM and 2 nM, respectively) over other MMPs tested. Further modification of such molecules by Freskos et al. [218] led to the exploration of compound **4.136** (Figure 4.17), which was a potent MMP-13-selective inhibitor (IC_{50} = 0.4 nM). Fink et al. [219] at Novartis reported a series of thiol-based MMPIs. Compound **4.137** (Figure 4.17) was the most efficacious MMP-1 inhibitor (IC_{50} = 135 nM), but it exhibited better affinity toward MMP-3 and MMP-9. Hurst et al. [220] reported some mercaptosulfide-based MMPIs. Compound **4.138** (Figure 4.17) showed potent affinity toward MMP-1 (K_i = 0.95 nM), having a broad spectrum of inhibitory activity toward other MMPs. Jin et al. [221] reported some pyrrolidine mercaptosulfide, 2-mercapto cyclopentane arylsulfonamide, and 3-mercapto-4-arylsulfonamide pyrrolidines as promising MMPIs. Compound **4.139** (Figure 4.17) exhibited non-selective MMP-13 inhibition (K_i = 15 nM) compared with MMP-2, MMP-9, and MMP-14 sparing MMP-1, MMP-3, and MMP-7. It also showed a 40% reduction of human mesenchymal stem cells (hMSCs) at 100 μM.

4.5.4 PHOSPHONATE-BASED INHIBITORS

Regarding the phosphonate and carbamoylphosphonate-based MMPIs, several studies were conducted in different laboratories [222, 223]. At Pfizer, Reiter et al. [224] reported a series of phosphinic acids as potential inhibitors of MMP-1 and -13. Some of these molecules were MMP-1 selective, whereas some showed selectivity over MMP-13. Compound **4.140** (Figure 4.18) displayed strong MMP-13 inhibition (IC_{50} = 14 nM) with 49-fold and 85-fold selectivity over MMP-1 and -3, respectively.

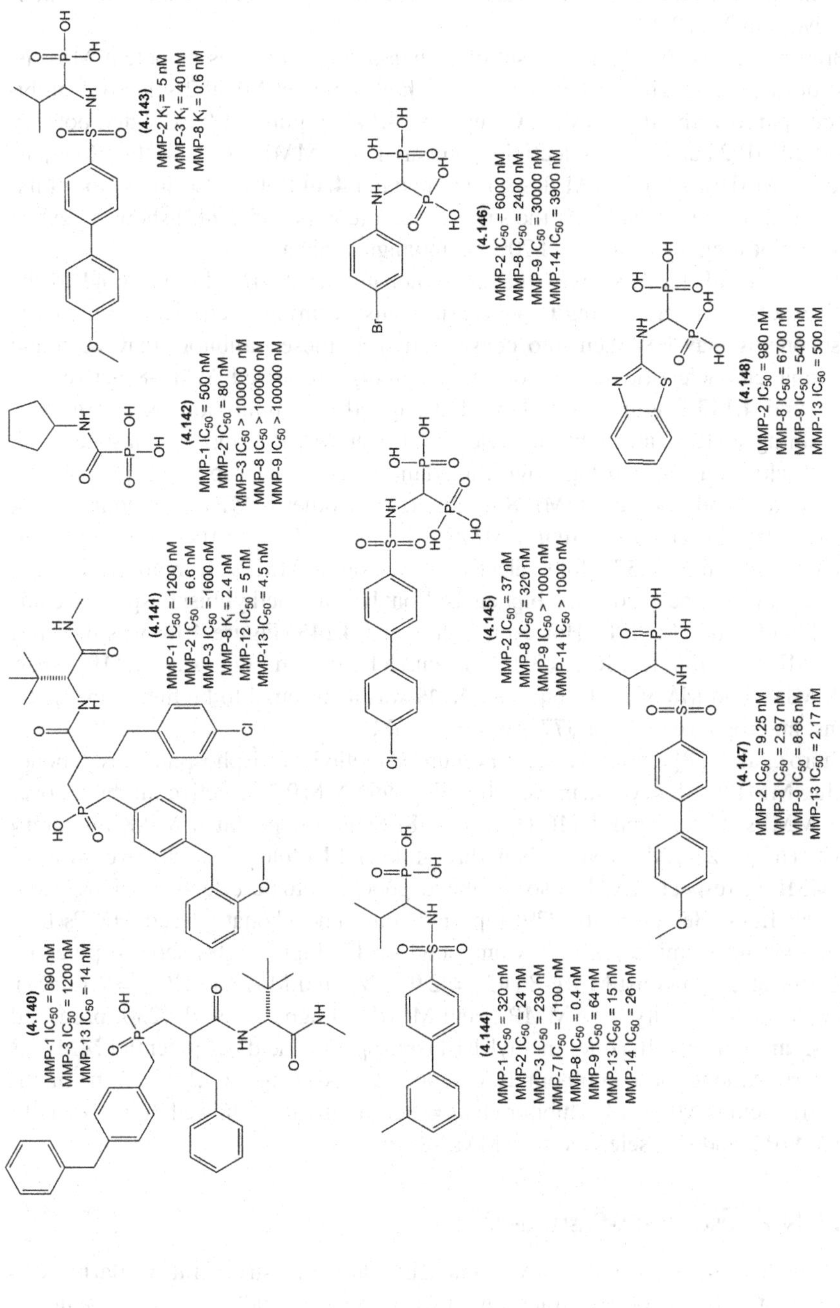

FIGURE 4.18 Phosphonate-based potential collagenase inhibitors (compounds **4.140–4.148**).

(4.143)
MMP-2 K_i = 5 nM
MMP-3 K_i = 40 nM
MMP-8 K_i = 0.6 nM

(4.142)
MMP-1 IC_{50} = 500 nM
MMP-2 IC_{50} = 80 nM
MMP-3 IC_{50} > 100000 nM
MMP-8 IC_{50} > 100000 nM
MMP-9 IC_{50} > 100000 nM

(4.146)
MMP-2 IC_{50} = 6000 nM
MMP-8 IC_{50} = 2400 nM
MMP-9 IC_{50} = 30000 nM
MMP-14 IC_{50} = 3900 nM

(4.148)
MMP-2 IC_{50} = 980 nM
MMP-8 IC_{50} = 6700 nM
MMP-9 IC_{50} = 5400 nM
MMP-13 IC_{50} = 500 nM

(4.141)
MMP-1 IC_{50} = 1200 nM
MMP-2 IC_{50} = 6.6 nM
MMP-3 IC_{50} = 1600 nM
MMP-8 K_i = 2.4 nM
MMP-12 IC_{50} = 5 nM
MMP-13 IC_{50} = 4.5 nM

(4.145)
MMP-2 IC_{50} = 37 nM
MMP-8 IC_{50} = 320 nM
MMP-9 IC_{50} > 1000 nM
MMP-14 IC_{50} > 1000 nM

(4.140)
MMP-1 IC_{50} = 690 nM
MMP-3 IC_{50} = 1200 nM
MMP-13 IC_{50} = 14 nM

(4.147)
MMP-2 IC_{50} = 9.25 nM
MMP-8 IC_{50} = 2.97 nM
MMP-9 IC_{50} = 8.85 nM
MMP-13 IC_{50} = 2.17 nM

(4.144)
MMP-1 IC_{50} = 320 nM
MMP-2 IC_{50} = 24 nM
MMP-3 IC_{50} = 230 nM
MMP-7 IC_{50} = 1100 nM
MMP-8 IC_{50} = 0.4 nM
MMP-9 IC_{50} = 64 nM
MMP-13 IC_{50} = 15 nM
MMP-14 IC_{50} = 26 nM

A further study by Reiter et al. [225] produced some phosphinic acid-containing MMP-13 inhibitors, having some activity against MMP-1 and -3 as well. Compound **4.141** (Figure 4.18) was found to be highly effective against MMP-13 (IC_{50} = 4.5 nM) and 267-fold and 356-fold selectivity over MMP-1 and -3, respectively, but non-selective over MMP-2.

Breuer et al. [226] reported a set of carbamoylphosphonates as potent MMPIs. Most of these belonging to this series were highly potent MMP-2-selective inhibitors compared with other MMPs. Compound **4.142** (Figure 4.18) exhibited potency against MMP-2 but six-fold selectivity compared with MMP-1 (IC_{50} = 500 nM) sparing other MMPs. At a 50 µM dose, it (compound **4.142**) was also found to inhibit 65% of tumor cell invasion. At the same dose, it (compound **4.142**) showed 72% of inhibition of lung metastasis and 70% of antiangiogenic activity.

Pochetti et al. [222] showed that phosphonate-based MMPIs may bind to the MMP-8 active site employing two oxygen atoms, forming a tetrahedral geometry. Phosphonates may be taken into consideration as these inhibitors may be found to exhibit characteristic interaction at the highly conserved MMP-8 active site. Compound **4.143** (Figure 4.18) showed strong MMP-8 inhibition (K_i = 0.6 nM), maintaining at least an eight-fold selectivity over MMP-2 and -3. Biasone et al. [223] disclosed a set of α-biphenylsulfonylamino 2-methylpropyl phosphonates as highly potent and selective MMP-8 inhibitors over other MMPs. Compound **4.144** (Figure 4.18) displayed maximum MMP-8 inhibition (IC_{50} = 0.4 nM) and maintained a minimum of 37.5-fold selectivity over other MMPs. Rubino et al. [227] designed and synthesized some biphenylsulfonylamino methyl bisphosphonic acids as highly effective MMPIs. However, Compound **4.145** (Figure 4.18) was the most potent MMP-8 inhibitor (IC_{50} = 320 nM) with a better affinity toward MMP-2 sparing MMP-9 and MMP-14. Compound **4.145** was also found to be highly cytotoxic against macrophage cell line J774 (IC_{50} = 1.7 µM).

Tauro et al. [228] reported a set of arylamino methylene bisphosphonates as bone-seeking MMPIs. Most of them were highly potent MMP-2-selective inhibitors over other MMPs. Compound **4.146** (Figure 4.18) exhibited potent MMP-8 inhibitory activity (IC_{50} = 2.4 µM), having about three-fold and 15-fold selectivity over MMP-2 and MMP-9, respectively. It also exhibited good cytotoxic effects in HepG2 and J774 cell lines. Beutel et al. [229] reported some phosphonate-based MMPs having an arylsulfonamide scaffold. Compound **4.147** (Figure 4.18) showed potential inhibitory effects against MMP-8 (IC_{50} = 2.97 nM) and MMP-13 (IC_{50} = 2.17 nM), having some selectivity over MMP-2 and MMP-9. Laghezza et al. [230] produced some (2-aminobenzothiazole)-methyl-1,1-bisphosphonic acids as potential MMP-13 inhibitors. Among these compounds, compound **4.148** (Figure 4.18) was the maximum efficacious MMP-13 inhibitor (IC_{50} = 500 nM), but it showed non-selectivity with MMP-2 and was selective over MMP-8 and MMP-9.

4.5.5 N-Hydroxyurea-Based Inhibitors

The N-hydroxyurea function is a valuable ZBG due to its structural similarity with hydroxamates. It was demonstrated that hydroxamates could have a better potency than their corresponding hydroxyurea analog [231]. As the N-hydroxyurea analogs might be able to acquire a *trans* N1-CO amide bond formation, proper Zn^{2+} coordination may be hindered due to intramolecular hydrogen bond interaction within the ZBG. Thus, substitution at the N3 atom of the N-hydroxyurea moiety was proposed with the methyl group to preclude intramolecular hydrogen bond interaction as well as for the betterment of the Zn^{2+} chelating effect. Comparing the crystal structures of the N-hydroxyurea and the hydroxamate inhibitors with MMP-8, it may be proposed that hydroxamates may form chelate to the Zn^{2+} ion in a bidentate pattern to have a five-membered ring, whereas the N-hydroxyurea forms chelate with the Zn^{2+} ion through the terminal hydroxyl function [232]. The sp^2 hybridization at the N3 atom was found to decrease the flexibility of the ZBG, and the binding conformation may hinder the chelation [231]. Campestre et al. [233] further reported some peptidyl 3-substituted 1-hydroxyureas as potent MMPIs. The (R)-hydroxyurea derivative **4.149** (Figure 4.19) possessed good MMP-8 inhibition (IC_{50} = 70 μM), but it was non-selective over other MMPs. The corresponding (S)-conformer **4.150** (Figure 4.19) was two-fold less effective than the former one (IC_{50} = 150 μM), having non-selectivity over MMP-9.

4.5.6 HYDRAZIDE-BASED INHIBITORS

Hydrazides and sulfonylhydrazides were also found to be effective ZBGs. Being an isostere of hydroxamates, these ZBGs also possess similar types of bidentate metal-chelating abilities, though these hydrazides and sulfonylhydrazides were found to be less effective MMPIs compared with the corresponding hydroxamates. As far as the binding affinity of these ZBGs is concerned, it is an advantage that the compounds possessing these ZBGs may be used to bind into the unprimed and primed side pockets in the enzyme active site [234]. These types of ZBGs may also be capable of

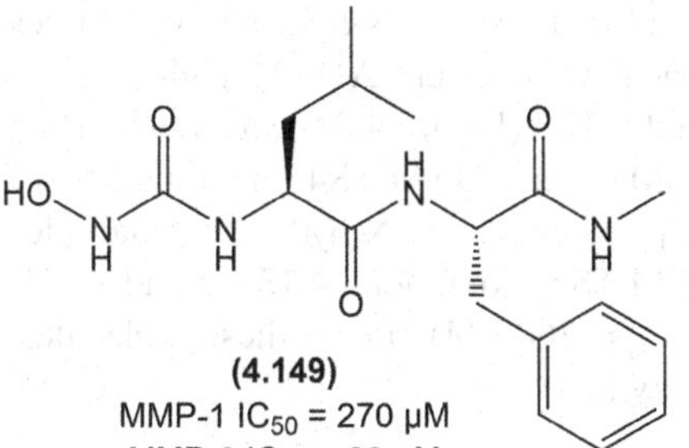

(4.149)
MMP-1 IC_{50} = 270 μM
MMP-2 IC_{50} = 60 μM
MMP-3 IC_{50} > 300 μM
MMP-7 IC_{50} > 300 μM
MMP-8 IC_{50} = 70 μM
MMP-9 IC_{50} = 20 μM

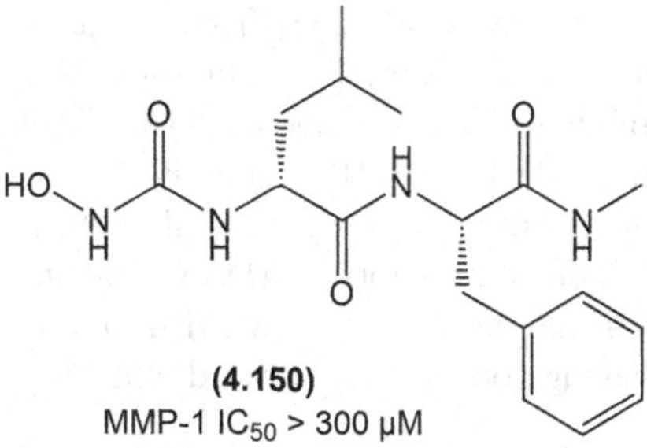

(4.150)
MMP-1 IC_{50} > 300 μM
MMP-2 IC_{50} > 300 μM
MMP-3 IC_{50} > 300 μM
MMP-7 IC_{50} > 300 μM
MMP-8 IC_{50} = 150 μM
MMP-9 IC_{50} = 200 μM

FIGURE 4.19 N-hydroxyurea-based potential collagenase inhibitors (compounds **4.149–4.150**).

forming two hydrogen bonds with the important amino acid residues at the enzyme active site similar to hydroxamates. It was also revealed from the molecular modeling study that the backbone structure of such types of ZBGs may be moved toward the S1', S2', and S2 pockets for proper binding [232]. Augé et al. [235] reported some galardin analogs as inhibitors of MMP-1 and -2. Some of them showed selectivity toward MMP-1. Compound **4.151** (Figure 4.20) was the most effective MMP-1 inhibitor (IC_{50} = 50 nM) among these molecules showing a ten-fold selectivity over MMP-2. In another study, LeDour et al. [234] reported some hydrazide analogs of Ilomastat (**4.1**) as potent MMPIs. Compound **4.152** (Figure 4.20) was the best efficacious MMP-1 inhibitor (IC_{50} = 30 nM) among these compounds and yielded ten-fold better MMP-9 inhibition (IC_{50} = 3 nM).

4.5.7 N-Hydroxyformamide-Based Inhibitors

N-hydroxyformamides were also found to be effective ZBG regarding the inhibition of MMPs. At GlaxoSmithKline, Rabinowitz et al. [236] disclosed a set of N-hydroxyformamides as effective inhibitors of TACE and MMPs. Many of them were selective TACE inhibitors, but some molecules showed greater affinity toward MMP-1. Compound **4.153** (Figure 4.21) was the most effective MMP-1 inhibitor (IC_{50} = 8.1 nM), showing nonselectivity toward MMP-9 but selective inhibition over MMP-3 and TACE.

In another study at Abbott, Wada et al. [237] reported some phenoxyphenyl sulfone N-formylhydroxylamines as highly efficacious and orally bioavailable MMPIs. Compound **4.154** (Figure 4.21) exhibited non-selective gelatinase inhibition with a broad spectrum of collagenase inhibitory activity (MMP-13 IC_{50} = 3.3 nM and MMP-8 IC_{50} = 5 nM). In cynomolgus monkeys, it (compound **4.154**) exhibited excellent pharmacokinetics ($t_{1/2}$ = 16.8 hr, AUC = 53 μM h/L) at a 3 mg/kg dose. Moreover, in the murine synergistic tumor growth model by B16 melanoma, it (compound **4.154**) inhibited 48% of tumor growth.

De Savi et al. [238] from AstraZeneca explored a set of N-hydroxyformamides as potent ADAM-TS4 inhibitors. Most of them were potent ADAM-TS4-selective inhibitors over MMPs and TACE. Compound **4.155** (Figure 4.21) was a potent but non-selective MMP-13 inhibitor (IC_{50} = 1.7 nM) over ADAM-TS4. In another study at AstraZeneca, De Savi et al. [239] further produced some N-hydroxyformamides as potent inhibitors of ADAM-TS4 and ADAM-TS5. Compound **4.156** (Figure 4.21) was the most effective MMP-13 inhibitor (IC_{50} = 260 nM) among these molecules, having good potency toward other metalloenzymes.

4.5.8 Squaric Acid-Based Inhibitors

Onaran et al. [240] developed some squaric acid-based modified hydroxamates containing ZBG as potential MMP-1 inhibitors. During chelating with the Zn^{2+} ion, these types of ZBGs were found to form a six-membered ring, which is different from the five-membered ring of hydroxamates [232]. Thiocarbonyl squaric acids were found to be more effective than precursor carbonyl squaric acid analogs, as

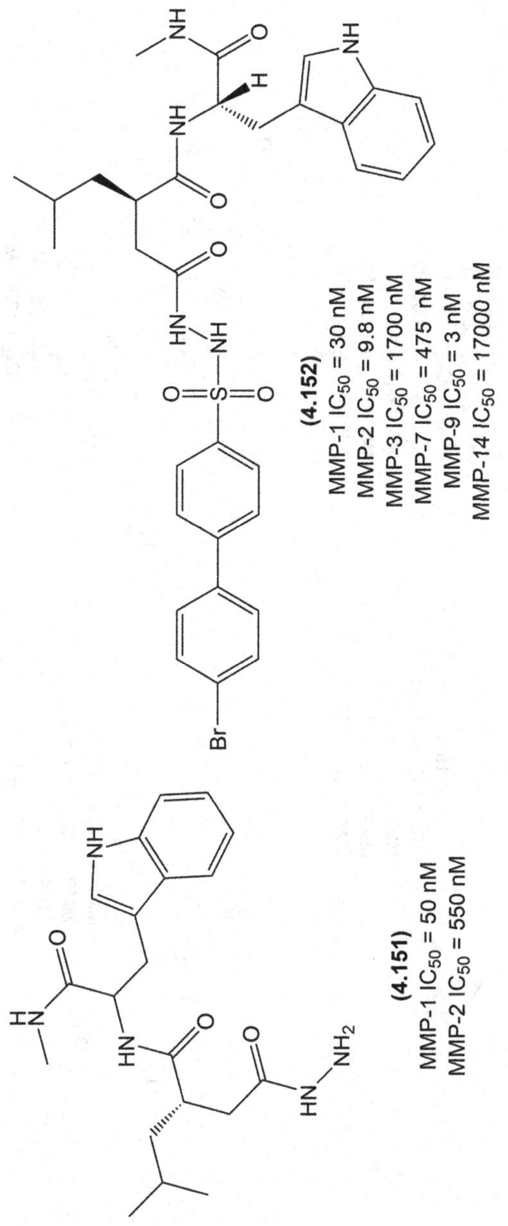

(4.152)

MMP-1 IC_{50} = 30 nM
MMP-2 IC_{50} = 9.8 nM
MMP-3 IC_{50} = 1700 nM
MMP-7 IC_{50} = 475 nM
MMP-9 IC_{50} = 3 nM
MMP-14 IC_{50} = 17000 nM

(4.151)

MMP-1 IC_{50} = 50 nM
MMP-2 IC_{50} = 550 nM

FIGURE 4.20 Hydrazide-based potential collagenase inhibitors (compounds **4.151–4.152**).

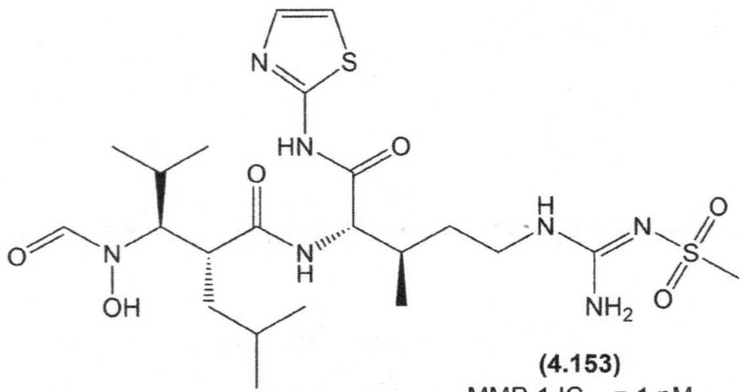

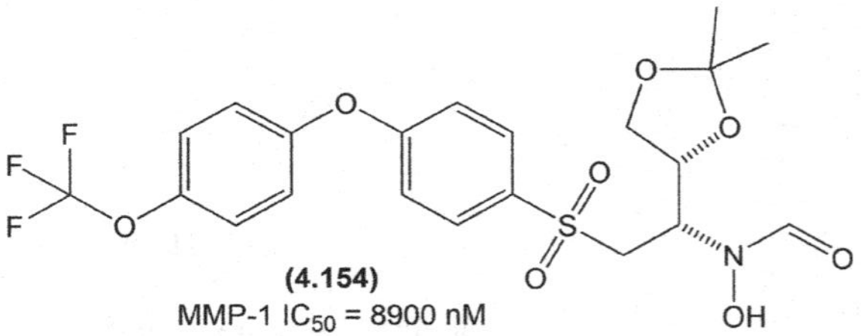

(4.154)
MMP-1 IC_{50} = 8900 nM
MMP-2 IC_{50} = 0.78 nM
MMP-3 IC_{50} = 12 nM
MMP-7 IC_{50} = 11000 nM
MMP-8 IC_{50} = 5 nM
MMP-9 IC_{50} = 0.50 nM
MMP-13 IC_{50} = 3.3 nM

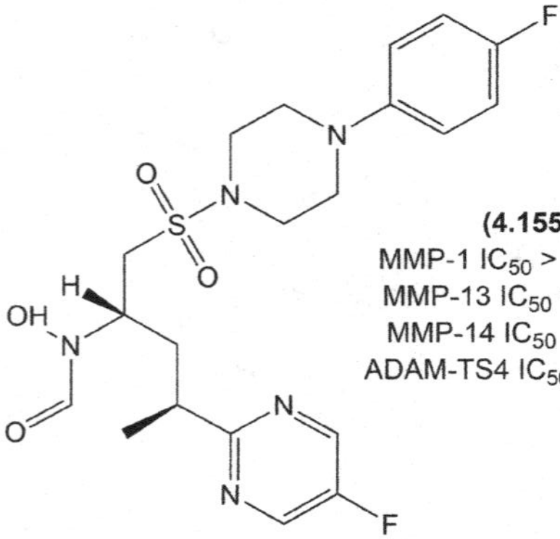

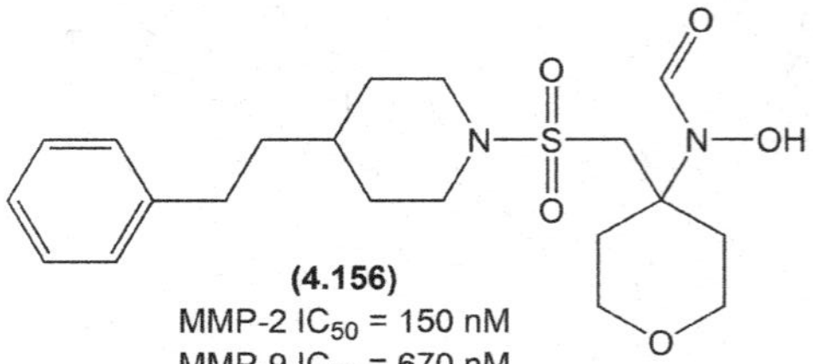

(4.156)
MMP-2 IC_{50} = 150 nM
MMP-9 IC_{50} = 670 nM
MMP-13 IC_{50} = 260 nM
MMP-14 IC_{50} = 1200 nM
ADAM-TS4 IC_{50} = 470 nM
ADAM-TS5 IC_{50} = 1700 nM

(4.153)
MMP-1 IC_{50} = 1 nM
MMP-3 IC_{50} = 49 nM
MMP-9 IC_{50} = 12 nM
TACE IC_{50} = 35 nM

(4.155)
MMP-1 IC_{50} > 1100 nM
MMP-13 IC_{50} = 1.7 nM
MMP-14 IC_{50} = 11 nM
ADAM-TS4 IC_{50} = 1.4 nM

FIGURE 4.21   *N*-hydroxyformamide-based potential collagenase inhibitors (compounds **4.153–4.156**).

evidenced by MMP-1 inhibition [240]. Compound **4.157** (Figure 4.22), a carbonyl squaric acid analog, showed MMP-1 inhibition at an IC_{50} of 270 µM, whereas its corresponding thiocarbonyl analog **4.158** (Figure 4.22) showed an 18-fold improvement in MMP-1 inhibition (IC_{50} = 15 µM).

4.5.9 PYRIMIDINE-2,4,6-TRIONE-BASED INHIBITORS

Nitrogen-based ZBG containing MMPIs like pyrimidine-2,4,6-triones and pyrimidine dione thiones were also explored by several scientists [241–244]. As this class of inhibitors belonged to the barbiturate family, the metabolic features, as well as bioavailability properties, were studied in several FDA-approved barbiturate drugs [241]. Such types of inhibitors may bind to the Zn^{2+} ion through the N3 atom of the barbiturate moiety [242, 244]. The oxygen atom of the carbonyl function adjacent to the nitrogen atom is converted to the enol form as it might obtain stability through dual hydrogen bonding interactions between the enol hydrogen and oxygen atoms of the backbone glutamic acid [242, 244]. The N1 and O6 atoms of the barbiturate ring further stabilize the interaction using hydrogen bonding with the backbone amino acids at the enzyme active site [242, 244].

Blagg et al. [245] designed a set of pyrimidinetrione-containing MMP-13 inhibitors selective over MMP-14. Of them, compound **4.159** (Figure 4.23) was disclosed as a potent MMP-13 inhibitor (IC_{50} = 1 nM) with a higher selectivity over other MMPs. In a pharmacokinetic study in rats, it was noticed to provide a moderate half-life ($t_{1/2}$ = 4 hr), low clearance (0.63 ml/min/kg), and lower volume distribution (0.20 L/kg), but an excellent oral absorption of about 100%.

In another study, Reiter and co-workers [246] at Pfizer reported some highly potent pyrimidinetrione-containing inhibitors of MMP-13 that are highly selective over several other MMPs. Compound **4.160** (Figure 4.23) possessed a high potency for MMP-13 inhibition (IC_{50} = 0.36 nM) and a greater selectivity over other MMPs. At a high dose exposure (100 mg/kg dose for 14 days) in rat plasma (C_{max} = 198 µg/ml, AUC = 3840 µgh/ml), it (compound **4.160**) was found to be well-tolerated. At Pfizer, Freeman-Cook et al. [247] designed a series of spiropyrrolidine pyrimidinetriones as potent MMP-13 inhibitors with high selectivity over other MMPs. Compound **4.161** (Figure 4.23) showed higher MMP-13 inhibitory potency (IC_{50} = 0.12 nM) and a greater selectivity over MMP-2, MMP-8, and MMP-12. Compound

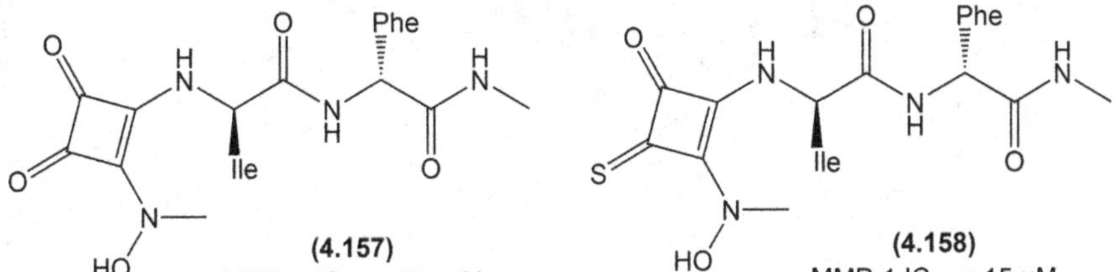

FIGURE 4.22 Squaric acid-based potential collagenase inhibitors (compounds **4.157–4.158**).

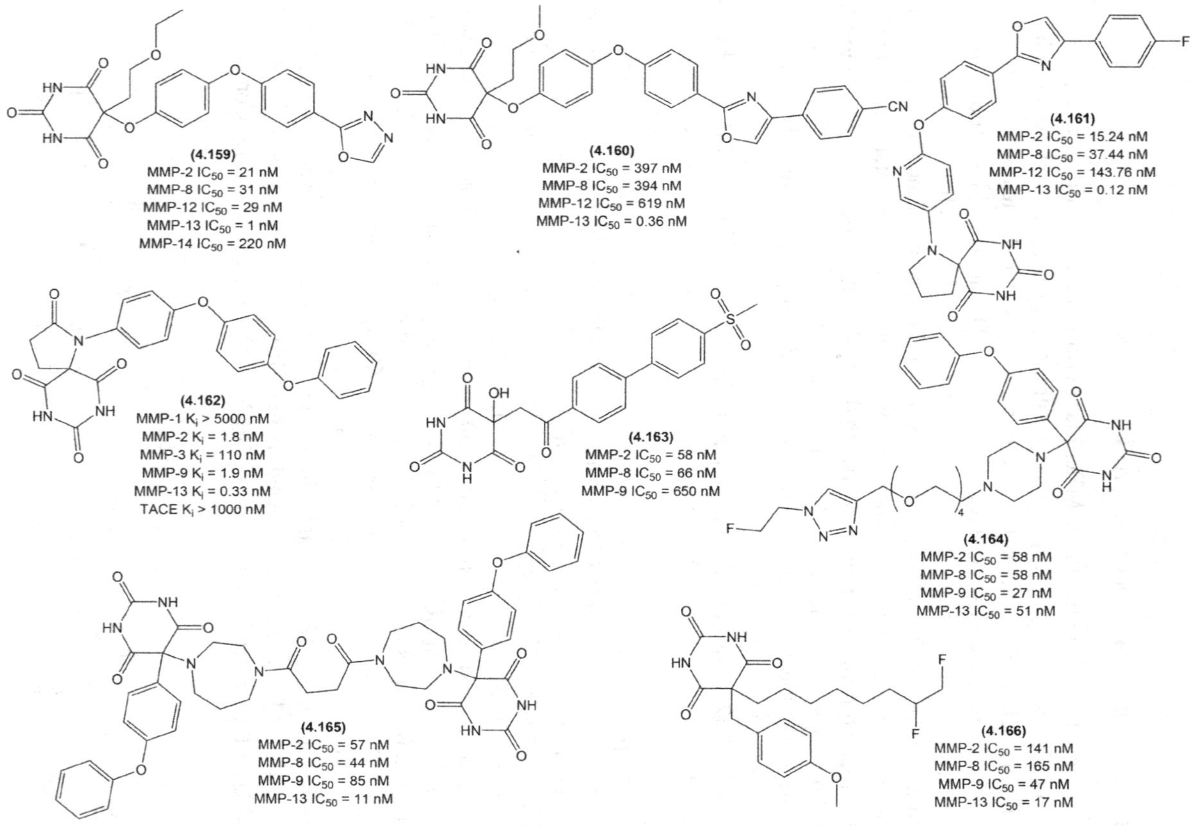

(4.159)
MMP-2 IC$_{50}$ = 21 nM
MMP-8 IC$_{50}$ = 31 nM
MMP-12 IC$_{50}$ = 29 nM
MMP-13 IC$_{50}$ = 1 nM
MMP-14 IC$_{90}$ = 220 nM

(4.160)
MMP-2 IC$_{50}$ = 397 nM
MMP-8 IC$_{50}$ = 394 nM
MMP-12 IC$_{50}$ = 619 nM
MMP-13 IC$_{50}$ = 0.36 nM

(4.161)
MMP-2 IC$_{50}$ = 15.24 nM
MMP-8 IC$_{50}$ = 37.44 nM
MMP-12 IC$_{50}$ = 143.76 nM
MMP-13 IC$_{50}$ = 0.12 nM

(4.162)
MMP-1 K$_i$ > 5000 nM
MMP-2 K$_i$ = 1.8 nM
MMP-3 K$_i$ = 110 nM
MMP-9 K$_i$ = 1.9 nM
MMP-13 K$_i$ = 0.33 nM
TACE K$_i$ > 1000 nM

(4.163)
MMP-2 IC$_{50}$ = 58 nM
MMP-8 IC$_{50}$ = 66 nM
MMP-9 IC$_{50}$ = 650 nM

(4.164)
MMP-2 IC$_{50}$ = 58 nM
MMP-8 IC$_{50}$ = 58 nM
MMP-9 IC$_{50}$ = 27 nM
MMP-13 IC$_{50}$ = 51 nM

(4.165)
MMP-2 IC$_{50}$ = 57 nM
MMP-8 IC$_{50}$ = 44 nM
MMP-9 IC$_{50}$ = 85 nM
MMP-13 IC$_{50}$ = 11 nM

(4.166)
MMP-2 IC$_{50}$ = 141 nM
MMP-8 IC$_{50}$ = 165 nM
MMP-9 IC$_{50}$ = 47 nM
MMP-13 IC$_{50}$ = 17 nM

FIGURE 4.23 Pyrimidine-2,4,6-trione-based potential collagenase inhibitors (compounds **4.159–4.166**).

4.161 was also found to produce an excellent pharmacokinetic profile (volume distribution 1.3 l/kg and $t_{1/2}$ = 4.5 hr).

Kim et al. [248] produced some spirobarbiturates as promising MMP-13 inhibitors. Compound **4.162** (Figure 4.23) was the maximum effective MMP-13 inhibitor (K_i = 0.33 nM) with at least a 5.5-fold selectivity over other MMPs tested. Nicolotti et al. [249] reported a series of 5-hydroxy, 5-substituted-pyrimidine-2,4,6-triones as potential gelatinase inhibitors. Compound **4.163** (Figure 4.23) was the most effective MMP-8 inhibitor (IC_{50} = 66 nM), which was selective over MMP-9 but non-selective toward MMP-2.

Schrigten et al. [250] disclosed some radiofluorinated pyrimidine-2,4,6-trione compounds as MMP-targeted radiotracers that might be visualized noninvasively through positron emission tomography (PET). Compound **4.164** (Figure 4.23) exhibited potent MMP-9 inhibition (IC_{50} = 27 nM) but displayed broad-spectrum collagenase inhibition (MMP-8 IC_{50} = 58 nM, MMP-13 IC_{50} = 51 nM). The ^{18}F-radiolabeled compound **4.164** also resulted in good *in vitro* stability in human serum, whereas no other radiometabolites were observed. It (compound **4.164**) was also found to exhibit rapid clearance characteristics in the adult Balb/c mice, as evidenced by *in vivo* biodistribution studies.

Wang et al. [251] designed some 5-homopiperazine substituted pyrimidinetrions as potential MMPIs. Some of them displayed potent and MMP-13-selective inhibition, and some showed selectivity toward MMP-2. Compound **4.165** (Figure 4.23) was the most promising MMP-13 inhibitor (IC_{50} = 11 nM), having at least a fourfold selectivity over other MMPs. Compound **4.165** also reduced Caco-2 cellular invasion significantly. Erdeljac et al. [252] reported some compounds containing a 1,2-difluoro motif. Compound **4.166** (Figure 4.23) was a highly potent MMP-13-selective inhibitor (IC_{50} = 17 nM) over other MMPs evaluated.

4.5.10 MISCELLANEOUS COLLAGENASE INHIBITORS

Reiter et al. [253] reported some difluoroketones as MMP-13 inhibitors. Compound **4.167** (Figure 4.24) was the maximum effective MMP-13 inhibitor (IC_{50} = 290 nM) among these molecules.

Li and co-workers of Pfizer [254] reported a series of quinazolinone and pyrido [3, 4-*d*] pyrimidine-4-one derivatives as potent and non-zinc binding selective inhibitors. The pyrido [3, 4-*d*] pyrimidine-4-one inhibitor **4.168** (Figure 4.24) exhibited potent MMP-13 inhibition against the catalytic MMP-13 domain and full-length MMP-13 enzyme (IC_{50} = 6.72 nM and 30.5 nM, respectively), but did not show any type of inhibition toward other MMPs. Compound **4.168** displayed moderate bioavailability, clearance, volume distribution, and a half-life of 3.9 hr in rat pharmacokinetic models. Moreover, it (compound **4.168**) was also free from MSS-like adverse effects, which were completely dissimilar from broad-spectrum MMPIs. It also responded negatively in mini-Ames and *in vitro* micronucleus tests. In rat and rabbit models, it (compound **4.168**) did not produce any toxicity *in vivo*.

Schnute et al. [255] from Pfizer further extended their study in designing novel non-zinc binding MMP-13 inhibitors for the treatment of osteoarthritis. They explored a series of (pyridine-4-yl)-2H-tetrazoles as potent MMP-13 inhibitors. Compound **4.169** (Figure 4.24) exhibited potent MMP-13 inhibition ($K_i = 4.4$ nM) and a high degree of selectivity over other MMPs, TACE, and aggrecanases. It also produced excellent oral bioavailability with lower clearance, as evidenced by rat pharmacokinetic studies.

Ruminski et al. [256] reported some methylpyrimidine-4-carboxamide as potent MMP-13 inhibitors. Compound **4.170** (Figure 4.24) was the most potent MMP-13 inhibitor ($K_i = 1.5$ nM). Compound **4.170** was highly orally bioavailable (95%) in rats with low clearance (18.2 ml/min/kg). It was not interfering with CYPs, namely CYP1A2, CYP2C9, CYP2D6, and CYP3A4. Heim-Riether et al. [257] reported a series of non-zinc chelating MMP-13 inhibitors selective over other MMPs. Compound **4.171** (Figure 4.24) was the most potent MMP-13 inhibitor ($IC_{50} = 2$ nM) with a greater selectivity over other MMPs. Gao et al. [258] designed a series of non-zinc chelating MMP-13 inhibitors with a higher selectivity over other MMPs. Compound **4.172** (Figure 4.24) exhibited potent MMP-13 inhibition ($IC_{50} = 5$ nM) with at least a 200-fold selectivity over other MMPs. It (compound **4.172**) showed a

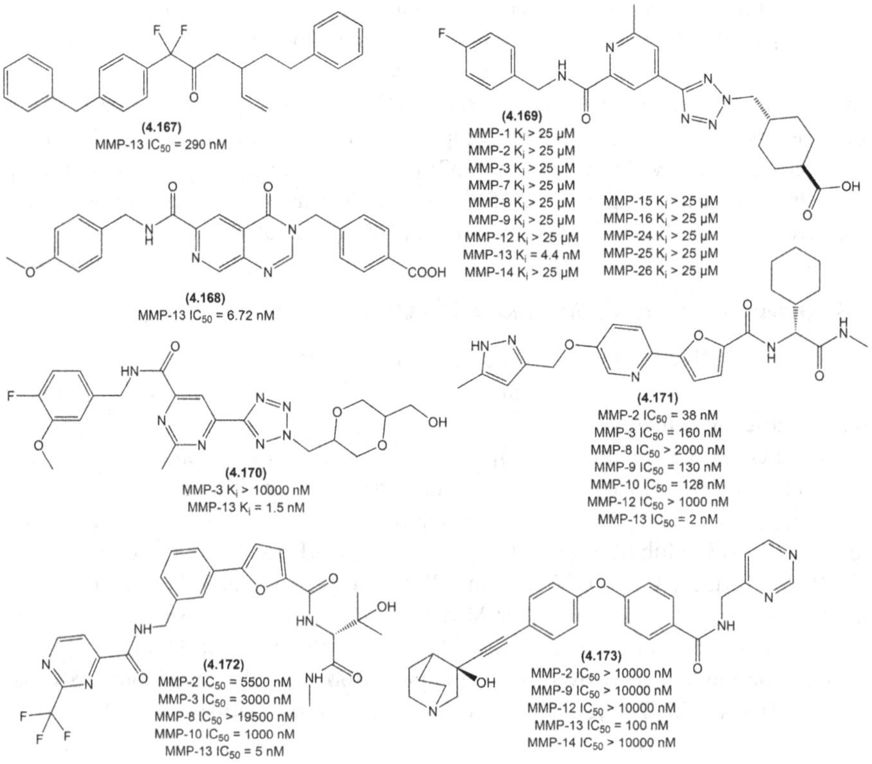

FIGURE 4.24 Potential collagenase inhibitors with diverse structures (compounds **4.167–4.173**).

good pharmacokinetic profile in male SD rats [HLM (%Q_H) = 14, CL (%Q_H = 26), V_{ss} = 0.9 L/kg, $t_{1/2}$ = 0.95 hr).

De Savi and co-workers from AstraZeneca [259] reported a series of non-zinc binding MMP-13 inhibitors. All these inhibitors were highly potent MMP-13-selective inhibitors over other MMPs. Compound **4.173** (Figure 4.24) possessed promising MMP-13 inhibitory activity (IC_{50} = 100 nM) with a greater selectivity over other MMPs. As far as pharmacokinetic studies (ADME and DMPK parameters) were concerned, compound **4.173** fulfilled all the criteria for being the potential lead candidate. In the continuation of optimizing a non-zinc binding lead molecule, De Savi et al. [260] of AstraZeneca further reported some quiniclidine analogs as potent inhibitors of MMPs. During lead optimization, it was found that for some compounds, MMP-13 inhibitory affinity was less than the inhibitory activity for other isoenzymes. Compound **4.174** (Figure 4.25) was the potent MMP-13 inhibitor (IC_{50} = 74 nM) developed as the lead molecule that was highly selective over MMPs as well as ADAMTS-1, -4, and -5. It (compound **4.174**) also exhibited excellent solubility and lower *in vitro* clearance in both human and hepatocyte microsomes. Moreover, it was free from inhibiting all five forms of CYPs. As it contained quinuclidine as a basic function, a phospholipidosis assay was performed. The weak inhibitory profile (EC_{50} > 100 μM) in phospholipidosis assay, as well as the other ADME and DMPK properties suggested that compound **4.174** was the potential non-zinc binding MMP-13 inhibitor.

By using structure-based drug design (SBDD) strategies, Nara et al. [261] designed and synthesized some thieno[2,3-*d*]pyrimidine-2-carboxamide derivatives as potent MMP-13-selective inhibitors. Compound **4.175** (Figure 4.25) was a highly potent MMP-13 inhibitor (IC_{50} = 0.0069 nM) and spared all other MMPs including TACE. It displayed significant pharmacokinetic properties in guinea pigs (AUC = 8,357 ng h/ml; C_{max} = 1,445 ng/ml). It was also found to be orally bioavailable in dogs and monkeys. In another study, Nara and co-workers [262] designed and synthesized some potent MMP-13-selective inhibitors. Compound **4.176** (Figure 4.25) was a highly productive MMP-13 inhibitor (IC_{50} = 0.0039 nM) sparing other MMPs and TACE. The sodium salt of Compound **4.176** displayed favorable oral bioavailability in different animal models (F% in rats, 23; in guinea pigs, 74; in rabbits, 35; in beagle dogs, 58, and cynomolgus monkeys, 45) with a moderate to higher distribution of volume. The toxicity studies conducted on rats showed that no adverse effect was evidenced up to a dose of 200 mg/kg/day. Nara et al. [263] further designed and synthesized a set of fused pyrimidine-2-carboxamide-4-one-containing MMP-13 inhibitors. Compound **4.177** (Figure 4.25) showed excellent MMP-13 inhibition (IC_{50} = 0.071 nM) sparing other MMPs along with TACE. It showed good DMPK properties, i.e., higher stability in rat and human liver microsomes, lower CYP3A4 inhibition, and lower cytotoxicity. However, the oral bioavailability of compound **4.177** in rats was poor, which was probably due to low permeability and solubility as evidenced by a parallel artificial membrane permeability (PAMPA) assay. Nara et al. [264] again developed some highly effective and MMP-13-selective inhibitors containing 1,2,4-triazol-3-yl ZBG moiety through a structure-based drug design (SBDD) approach. Compound **4.178** (Figure 4.25) was the most effective MMP-13 inhibitor (IC_{50} = 0.036 nM) sparing other MMPs and TACE.

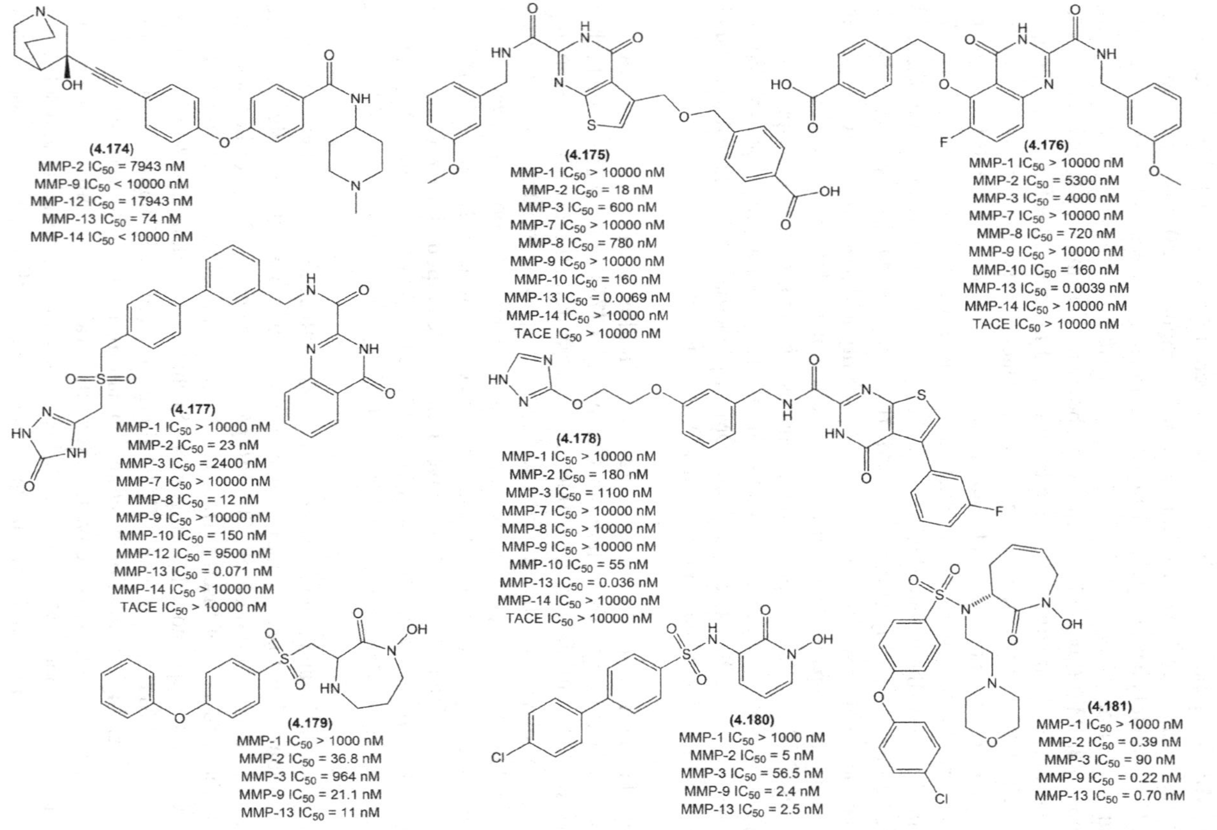

(4.174)
MMP-2 IC_{50} = 7943 nM
MMP-9 IC_{50} < 10000 nM
MMP-12 IC_{50} = 17943 nM
MMP-13 IC_{50} = 74 nM
MMP-14 IC_{50} < 10000 nM

(4.175)
MMP-1 IC_{50} > 10000 nM
MMP-2 IC_{50} = 18 nM
MMP-3 IC_{50} = 600 nM
MMP-7 IC_{50} > 10000 nM
MMP-8 IC_{50} = 780 nM
MMP-9 IC_{50} > 10000 nM
MMP-10 IC_{50} = 160 nM
MMP-13 IC_{50} = 0.0069 nM
MMP-14 IC_{50} > 10000 nM
TACE IC_{50} > 10000 nM

(4.176)
MMP-1 IC_{50} > 10000 nM
MMP-2 IC_{50} = 5300 nM
MMP-3 IC_{50} = 4000 nM
MMP-7 IC_{50} > 10000 nM
MMP-8 IC_{50} = 720 nM
MMP-9 IC_{50} > 10000 nM
MMP-10 IC_{50} = 160 nM
MMP-13 IC_{50} = 0.0039 nM
MMP-14 IC_{50} > 10000 nM
TACE IC_{50} > 10000 nM

(4.177)
MMP-1 IC_{50} > 10000 nM
MMP-2 IC_{50} = 23 nM
MMP-3 IC_{50} = 2400 nM
MMP-7 IC_{50} > 10000 nM
MMP-8 IC_{50} = 12 nM
MMP-9 IC_{50} > 10000 nM
MMP-10 IC_{50} = 150 nM
MMP-12 IC_{50} = 9500 nM
MMP-13 IC_{50} = 0.071 nM
MMP-14 IC_{50} > 10000 nM
TACE IC_{50} > 10000 nM

(4.178)
MMP-1 IC_{50} > 10000 nM
MMP-2 IC_{50} = 180 nM
MMP-3 IC_{50} = 1100 nM
MMP-7 IC_{50} > 10000 nM
MMP-8 IC_{50} > 10000 nM
MMP-9 IC_{50} > 10000 nM
MMP-10 IC_{50} = 55 nM
MMP-13 IC_{50} = 0.036 nM
MMP-14 IC_{50} > 10000 nM
TACE IC_{50} > 10000 nM

(4.179)
MMP-1 IC_{50} > 1000 nM
MMP-2 IC_{50} = 36.8 nM
MMP-3 IC_{50} = 964 nM
MMP-9 IC_{50} = 21.1 nM
MMP-13 IC_{50} = 11 nM

(4.180)
MMP-1 IC_{50} > 1000 nM
MMP-2 IC_{50} = 5 nM
MMP-3 IC_{50} = 56.5 nM
MMP-9 IC_{50} = 2.4 nM
MMP-13 IC_{50} = 2.5 nM

(4.181)
MMP-1 IC_{50} > 1000 nM
MMP-2 IC_{50} = 0.39 nM
MMP-3 IC_{50} = 90 nM
MMP-9 IC_{50} = 0.22 nM
MMP-13 IC_{50} = 0.70 nM

FIGURE 4.25 Various effective collagenase inhibitors with diverse structures (compounds **4.174–4.181**).

Zhang and co-workers [265] from Johnson and Johnson Pharmaceutical Research and Development reported some arylsulfone-based MMPIs containing heterocyclic ZBGs. Compound **4.179** (Figure 4.25) showed good gelatinase inhibition and yielded good inhibition against MMP-13 (IC_{50} = 11 nM). In continuation of their research, Zhang et al. [266] further reported some 1-hydroxy-2-pyridinone-based MMPIs. Compound **4.180** (Figure 4.25) showed good inhibition against gelatinases and potent MMP-13 inhibition (IC_{50} = 2.5 nM). At a 10 mg /kg dose, compound **4.180** resulted in an excellent pharmacokinetic profile with a long half-life ($t_{1/2}$ = 47 hr). Moreover, compound **4.180** exhibited good efficacy in the mouse transient mid-cerebral artery occlusion (tMCAO) model of cerebral ischemia. Wilson et al. [267] from Johnson and Johnson reported some cobactin-T-based MMPIs. Compound **4.181** (Figure 4.25) showed potent broad-spectrum MMP inhibition with good MMP-13 inhibitory potency (IC_{50} = 0.7 nM). At a 0.5 mg/kg IV dose, compound **4.181** showed good pharmacokinetic properties (C_{max} = 4.4 µM, $t_{1/2}$ = 2 hr, AUC = 1831 ng-h/ml, V_{ss} = 1.4 L/kg, CL = 19 ml/min/kg).

Gege et al. [268] from Alantos Pharmaceuticals reported compound **4.182** (Figure 4.26) as a non-zinc chelating, MMP-13-selective inhibitor for the treatment of osteoarthritis. It (compound **4.182**) showed potent and selective MMP-13 inhibition (IC_{50} = 0.03 nM) sparing other MMPs, TACE, and aggrecanase-1. As far as the pharmacokinetic profile of compound **4.182** was concerned, there was no systemic exposure in rats up to 100 mg/kg oral or i.p. dose. The microsomal stability study exerted 95% and 96% unmetabolized products, respectively in rat and human microsomes. Compound **4.182** was found to be safe and tolerable, as evidenced by the pharmacokinetic profile obtained after intra-articular administration. In addition, compound **4.183** (Figure 4.26) also exhibited potent MMP-13 inhibitory activity (IC_{50} = 1.3 nM) sparing MMPs, TACE, and aggrecanase-1.

Deng et al. [269] from GlaxoSmithKline explored a series of small molecule ADAMTS-5 inhibitors. Compound **4.184** (Figure 4.26) displayed potent and selective ADAMTS-5 inhibition and yielded potent MMP-13 inhibition (IC_{50} = 7.9 µM). Johnson et al. [270] showed the binding interaction of compound **4.185** (Figure 4.26) and MMP-13. The phenyl ring of the benzyl ester moiety of inhibitor **4.185** was found to be situated parallel with the His201 plane. The keto function of the ester group was found to be coordinated with the amide moiety of Thr224 for hydrogen bonding. Another carbonyl oxygen atom attached to the heterocyclic moiety of inhibitor **4.185** formed a hydrogen bonding with the amide function of amino acid residues Thr226 and Met232. Both of the benzyl moieties of inhibitor **4.185** were found to be involved in aromatic interactions with Tyr225 and Phe231 amino acid residues. The amino acid Gly227 in the backbone structure helped to open the S1' pocket to accommodate the inhibitor through rational conformation [232]. The crystal structure of inhibitor **4.185** with MMP-13 demonstrated that inhibitor **4.185** binds to the deep S1' pocket without any overlapping with natural substrate-binding space [270]. All these inhibitors (compounds **4.185–4.190**, Figure 4.26) exhibited higher efficacy and selectivity toward MMP-13 than other MMPs. The structural similarity of inhibitors and specific binding interactions at the S1' pocket and variations in shape and size of the S1' pocket throughout the MMPs might be accountable for

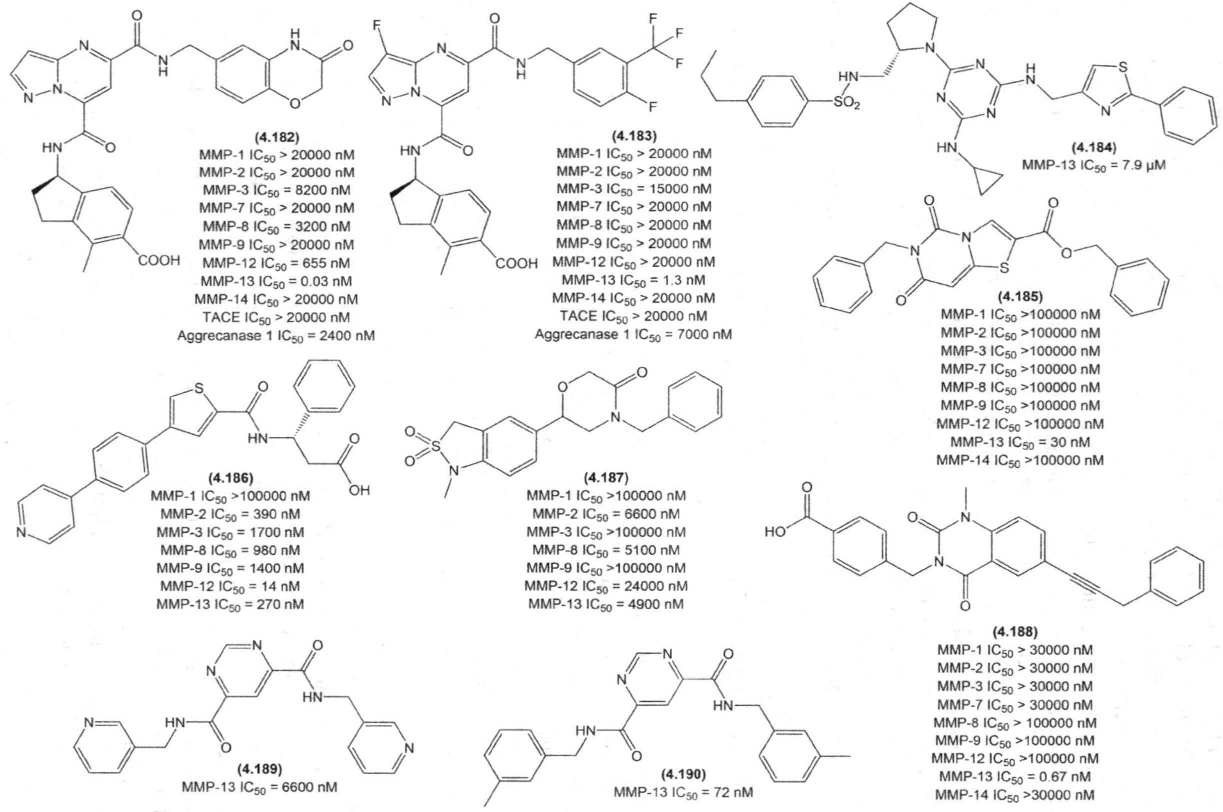

FIGURE 4.26 Another set of potential collagenase inhibitors with diverse structures (compounds **4.182–4.190**).

(4.184)
MMP-13 IC_{50} = 7.9 µM

(4.185)
MMP-1 IC_{50} >100000 nM
MMP-2 IC_{50} > 100000 nM
MMP-3 IC_{50} >100000 nM
MMP-7 IC_{50} >100000 nM
MMP-8 IC_{50} >100000 nM
MMP-9 IC_{50} >100000 nM
MMP-12 IC_{50} >100000 nM
MMP-13 IC_{50} = 30 nM
MMP-14 IC_{50} >100000 nM

(4.188)
MMP-1 IC_{50} > 30000 nM
MMP-2 IC_{50} > 30000 nM
MMP-3 IC_{50} > 30000 nM
MMP-7 IC_{50} > 30000 nM
MMP-8 IC_{50} > 100000 nM
MMP-9 IC_{50} >100000 nM
MMP-12 IC_{50} >100000 nM
MMP-13 IC_{50} = 0.67 nM
MMP-14 IC_{50} >30000 nM

(4.190)
MMP-13 IC_{50} = 72 nM

(4.183)
MMP-1 IC_{50} > 20000 nM
MMP-2 IC_{50} > 20000 nM
MMP-3 IC_{50} = 15000 nM
MMP-7 IC_{50} > 20000 nM
MMP-8 IC_{50} > 20000 nM
MMP-9 IC_{50} > 20000 nM
MMP-12 IC_{50} > 20000 nM
MMP-13 IC_{50} = 1.3 nM
MMP-14 IC_{50} > 20000 nM
TACE IC_{50} = 20000 nM
Aggrecanase 1 IC_{50} = 7000 nM

(4.187)
MMP-1 IC_{50} >100000 nM
MMP-2 IC_{50} = 6600 nM
MMP-3 IC_{50} >100000 nM
MMP-8 IC_{50} = 5100 nM
MMP-9 IC_{50} >100000 nM
MMP-12 IC_{50} = 24000 nM
MMP-13 IC_{50} = 4900 nM

(4.182)
MMP-1 IC_{50} > 20000 nM
MMP-2 IC_{50} > 20000 nM
MMP-3 IC_{50} = 8200 nM
MMP-7 IC_{50} > 20000 nM
MMP-8 IC_{50} = 3200 nM
MMP-9 IC_{50} > 20000 nM
MMP-12 IC_{50} = 655 nM
MMP-13 IC_{50} = 0.03 nM
MMP-14 IC_{50} > 20000 nM
TACE IC_{50} = 20000 nM
Aggrecanase 1 IC_{50} = 2400 nM

(4.186)
MMP-1 IC_{50} >100000 nM
MMP-2 IC_{50} = 390 nM
MMP-3 IC_{50} = 1700 nM
MMP-8 IC_{50} = 980 nM
MMP-9 IC_{50} = 1400 nM
MMP-12 IC_{50} = 14 nM
MMP-13 IC_{50} = 270 nM

(4.189)
MMP-13 IC_{50} = 6600 nM

specific enzyme selectivity. MMP-13 selectivity of these inhibitors over other MMPs is due to their shorter S1′ pocket, which may not be able to orient the longer P1′ substituents directed toward the S1′ pocket. Moreover, the flexibility of the S1′ pocket of MMP-13 was another criterion that might be able to allow specific conformation while binding to the inhibitor that is not relatively assessed in other MMPs.

In the case of inhibitors **4.185** and **4.189** (Figure 4.26), Gly227 and Gly248 amino acid residues rotated relatively along with the conformation of the major chain in the ligand-bound enzyme structure [270, 271]. During rotation, the length of the S1′ pocket was extended to orient the long P1′ group-containing inhibitors. As these glycine residues were not conserved in other MMPs, the conformation of the rotated main chain was not favorable for other residues. Therefore, decreased inhibitor binding affinity might be observed for those MMPs. Similar types of observations were noticed with the crystal structure of MMP-8 and the non-zing binding inhibitors [272]. Hydrophobicity of the non-zinc binding inhibitors might play a crucial role in enzyme-inhibitor interactions, resulting in higher potency and selectivity. However, highly hydrophobic molecules were poorly water-soluble, resulting in less or lower bioavailability. To increase the solubility without hampering potency and selectivity, the solvent-exposed portion of the inhibitors might be modified without any alteration of the hydrophobic core.

Dublanchet and co-workers [273] showed the carboxylic acid function directed toward the solvent-exposed area of the compound might be helpful in enhancing the solubility of the non-zinc binding MMPIs. It was remarkable that the prime reason for the MMP-13 selectivity of inhibitors **4.185** and **4.189** was due to the unique conformation in the S1′ pocket that was not noticed for other MMPs [270, 271]. It was not clear why such a type of MMP-13 selectivity was observed, and no zinc-binding group was present. Comparative studies between non-zinc binding inhibitors as well as an inhibitor that may show both types of conformational alterations toward the MMP-13 S1′ pocket and chelate the Zn^{2+} ion at the active site could provide a detailed insight into the phenomena.

Vidal et al. [274] reported some tetracycline derivatives as effective MMPIs. Compound **4.191** showed a broad spectrum of MMP inhibition with good potency toward MMP-13 (IC_{50} = 4.9 µM). Compound **4.191** (Figure 4.27) effectively inhibited the mRNA expression of MMP-13 more than MMP-3. At 100 µM, compound **4.191** strongly inhibited IL-1β and plasmin-induced collagen degradation by 66%.

Lauer-Fields et al. [275] performed a high throuput screening (HTS) on the MLSCN library of 65,000 compounds to screen 25 MMP-13 inhibitors. Several compounds were found as potent MMP-13-selective inhibitors (**4.192–4.195**, Figure 4.27). As per the report of Nakai et al. [205] from Scripps Research Institute, compounds **4.196** and **4.197** (Figure 4.27) displayed potent and MMP-13-selective inhibition. Vicini et al. [276] reported some benzisothiazolyliminothiazolidine-4-ones as potent MMP-13-selective inhibitors. Compound **4.198** (Figure 4.27) was the most promising MMP-13-selective inhibitor (IC_{50} = 36 nM) sparing MMP-3. Roth et al. [277] reported some exosite-binding MMP-13 inhibitors. Compound **4.199** (Figure 4.27) was the most effective MMP-13 inhibitor (K_i = 800 nM) among these compounds. Marques and co-workers [278] reported some 1-hydroxypiperazine-2,6-diones as

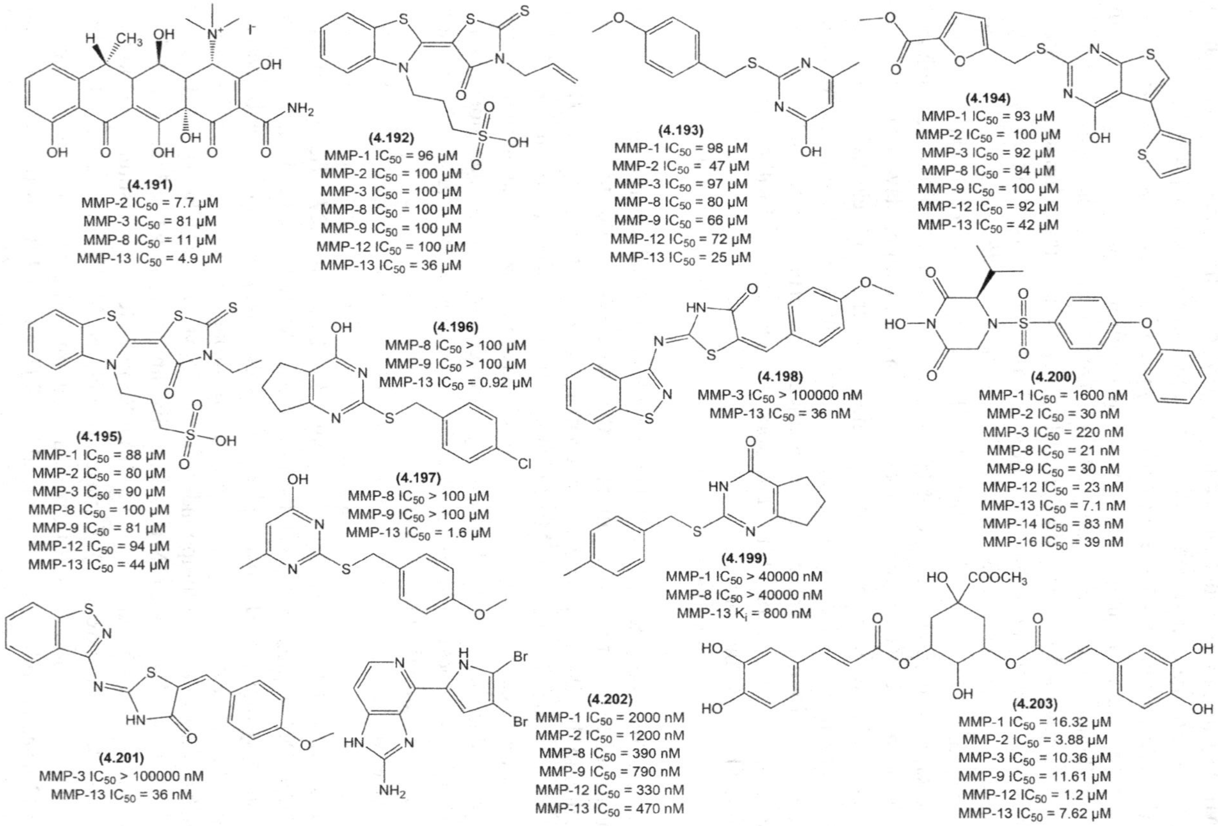

FIGURE 4.27 Different effective collagenase inhibitors with diverse structures (compounds **4.191—4.203**).

(4.194)
MMP-1 IC$_{50}$ = 93 µM
MMP-2 IC$_{50}$ = 100 µM
MMP-3 IC$_{50}$ = 92 µM
MMP-8 IC$_{50}$ = 94 µM
MMP-9 IC$_{50}$ = 100 µM
MMP-12 IC$_{50}$ = 92 µM
MMP-13 IC$_{50}$ = 42 µM

(4.200)
MMP-1 IC$_{50}$ = 1600 nM
MMP-2 IC$_{50}$ = 30 nM
MMP-3 IC$_{50}$ = 220 nM
MMP-8 IC$_{50}$ = 21 nM
MMP-9 IC$_{50}$ = 30 nM
MMP-12 IC$_{50}$ = 23 nM
MMP-13 IC$_{50}$ = 7.1 nM
MMP-14 IC$_{50}$ = 83 nM
MMP-16 IC$_{50}$ = 39 nM

(4.203)
MMP-1 IC$_{50}$ = 16.32 µM
MMP-2 IC$_{50}$ = 3.88 µM
MMP-3 IC$_{50}$ = 10.36 µM
MMP-9 IC$_{50}$ = 11.61 µM
MMP-12 IC$_{50}$ = 1.2 µM
MMP-13 IC$_{50}$ = 7.62 µM

(4.193)
MMP-1 IC$_{50}$ = 98 µM
MMP-2 IC$_{50}$ = 47 µM
MMP-3 IC$_{50}$ = 97 µM
MMP-8 IC$_{50}$ = 80 µM
MMP-9 IC$_{50}$ = 66 µM
MMP-12 IC$_{50}$ = 72 µM
MMP-13 IC$_{50}$ = 25 µM

(4.198)
MMP-3 IC$_{50}$ > 100000 nM
MMP-13 IC$_{50}$ = 36 nM

(4.199)
MMP-1 IC$_{50}$ > 40000 nM
MMP-8 IC$_{50}$ > 40000 nM
MMP-13 K$_i$ = 800 nM

(4.192)
MMP-1 IC$_{50}$ = 96 µM
MMP-2 IC$_{50}$ = 100 µM
MMP-3 IC$_{50}$ = 100 µM
MMP-8 IC$_{50}$ = 100 µM
MMP-9 IC$_{50}$ = 100 µM
MMP-12 IC$_{50}$ = 100 µM
MMP-13 IC$_{50}$ = 36 µM

(4.196)
MMP-8 IC$_{50}$ > 100 µM
MMP-9 IC$_{50}$ > 100 µM
MMP-13 IC$_{50}$ = 0.92 µM

(4.197)
MMP-8 IC$_{50}$ > 100 µM
MMP-9 IC$_{50}$ > 100 µM
MMP-13 IC$_{50}$ = 1.6 µM

(4.202)
MMP-1 IC$_{50}$ = 2000 nM
MMP-2 IC$_{50}$ = 1200 nM
MMP-3 IC$_{50}$ = 390 nM
MMP-8 IC$_{50}$ = 390 nM
MMP-9 IC$_{50}$ = 790 nM
MMP-12 IC$_{50}$ = 330 nM
MMP-13 IC$_{50}$ = 470 nM

(4.191)
MMP-2 IC$_{50}$ = 7.7 µM
MMP-3 IC$_{50}$ = 81 µM
MMP-8 IC$_{50}$ = 11 µM
MMP-13 IC$_{50}$ = 4.9 µM

(4.195)
MMP-1 IC$_{50}$ = 88 µM
MMP-2 IC$_{50}$ = 80 µM
MMP-3 IC$_{50}$ = 90 µM
MMP-8 IC$_{50}$ = 100 µM
MMP-9 IC$_{50}$ = 81 µM
MMP-12 IC$_{50}$ = 94 µM
MMP-13 IC$_{50}$ = 44 µM

(4.201)
MMP-3 IC$_{50}$ > 100000 nM
MMP-13 IC$_{50}$ = 36 nM

potent MMPIs. Many of them exhibited potent and MMP-13-selective inhibition over other MMPs as well as TACE. Compound **4.200** (Figure 4.27) exhibited potent MMP-13 inhibition (IC_{50} = 9.5 nM), maintaining at least a two-fold selectivity over other MMPs as well as TACE. Panico et al. [279] reported some heteroarylimono-4-thiazolidinones as effective inhibitors of cartilage degradation. Compound **4.201** (Figure 4.27) resulted in potent MMP-13 inhibition (IC_{50} = 36 nM) selective over MMP-3. Again, compound **4.201** increased the release of glycosaminoglycans (GAGs) (38%). It also resulted in a moderate effect on NO release.

Shengule et al. [280] reported some ageladine A analogs as potential inhibitors of MMP-2 and MMP-14. Compound **4.202** (Figure 4.27) was an efficacious broad-spectrum MMPI showing good MMP-13 inhibitory efficacy. Compound **4.202** showed potent antiangiogenic activity (IC_{50} = 24 μM) in vascular progenitor cells. Wang et al. [281] screened some natural compounds by using structure-based virtual screening from 4,000 natural compounds and evaluated these against a panel of MMPs. Compound **4.203** (Figure 4.27) showed a broad spectrum of MMP inhibition with good MMP-13 inhibitory efficacy.

Casalini et al. [282] reported some arylsulfone MMPIs. Compound **4.204** (Figure 4.28) showed MMP-2/-13 selective dual inhibition over other MMPs. The ^{18}F-radiolabeled compound showed good efficacy in the U87MG glioblastoma cell line xenograft mice model.

Lu et al. [283] disclosed some 6-oxo-1,6-dihydropyrimidine-2,5-dicarboxamides as effective MMP-13 inhibitors. Compound **4.205** (Figure 4.28) exhibited the most potent MMP-13 inhibitor (IC_{50} = 68 nM), having a minimum of 47-fold selectivity over MMP-3 and MMP-12. Fischer et al. [284] reported some non-zinc binding phthalimide derivatives as potent and selective MMP-13 inhibitors. Compound **4.206** (Figure 4.28) was the most potent MMP-13 inhibitor (IC_{50} = 490 nM) sparing other MMPs.

Crasci et al. [285] reported some 2-benzisothiazlylimino-5-benzylidene-4-thiazo lidinones as protective compounds against cartilage degradation. Compound **4.207** (Figure 4.28) was a highly potent MMP-13 inhibitor (IC_{50} = 158 nM) selective over MMP-3. Compound **4.207** exhibited high antioxidant activity (ORAC value = 1.2 TE/μg), effective NO lowering activity (2/4% decrease), and GAG restoring ability (% increase = 43). Again, compound **4.207** produced good inhibition of NF-κB release (~55%). Lanz and Riedl [286] reported non-zinc binding potent MMP-13 inhibitors through natural product-derived fragments. Compound **4.208** (Figure 4.28) was the most effective MMP-13 inhibitor (IC_{50} = 5.13 nM), and it was found to spare other MMPs.

Agamennone et al. [287] reported some 5-arylisatin-containing potential inhibitors of MMP-13 and MMP-2. All of them were potent and MMP-13-selective inhibitors compared with MMP-2, MMP-8, and MMP-9. Compound **4.209** (Figure 4.28) was the most potent MMP-13 inhibitor (IC_{50} = 2.2 μM), having a greater selectivity over these MMPs.

Hugenberg and co-workers [288] synthesized some N,N'-bis(benzyl)pyrimidine-4,6-dicarboxamide derivatives and radiolabeled with C^{11}, F^{18}, and Ga^{68}. Most of them were highly efficacious MMP-13-selective inhibitors. However, Compound **4.210**

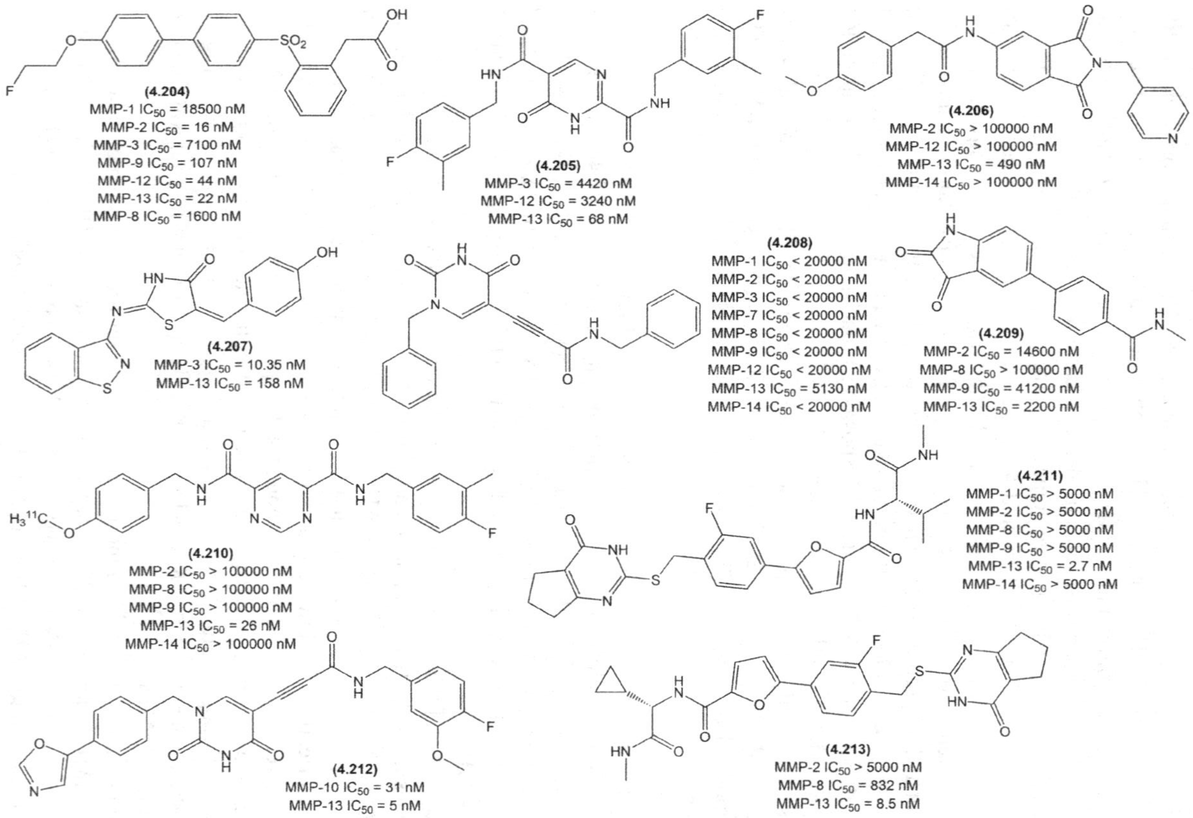

FIGURE 4.28 A set of effective collagenase inhibitors with diverse structures (compounds **4.204**–**4.213**).

(Figure 4.28) was a promising MMP-13 inhibitor (IC_{50} = 26 nM) with at least a three-fold selectivity over other MMPs. The C^{11} methylated compound **4.210** was the most lipophilic radiotracer, which was metabolically stable and well-biodistributed, as evidenced in C57/B16 mice. Choi et al. [289] designed and synthesized some non-zinc chelating MMP-13 inhibitors sparing other MMPs. Compound **4.211** (Figure 4.28) was the maximum effective MMP-13 inhibitor (IC_{50} = 2.7 nM) and was highly selective over other MMPs.

Senn et al. [290] reported a set of non-hydroxamate dual MMP-13/MMP-10 inhibitors. Compound **4.212** (Figure 4.28) was the most potent MMP-13 inhibitor (IC_{50} = 5 nM) with higher selectivity over other MMPs. Fuerst et al. [291] recently designed and synthesized some new MMP-13 inhibitors highly selective over MMP-2 and MMP-8. Compound **4.213** (Figure 4.28) was about 100-fold MMP-13 selective (IC_{50} = 8.5 nM) over MMP-8 (IC_{50} = 832 nM) and spared MMP-2. It also showed enhanced microsomal half-lives (human: 74 min; rat: 13 min; mouse: 31 min). It showed a good permeability coefficient of 21.1 nM/sec. Moreover, Compound **4.213** did not show any CYP3A4 inhibition but displayed excellent pharmacokinetic properties *in vivo*.

El Ashry et al. [292] reported some pyrimidine and 1,2,4-triazole[4,3-*a*]pyrimidine-containing dual MMP-10/MMP-13 inhibitors. Compounds **4.214** and **4.215** (Figure 4.29) showed potent dual inhibition of MMP-10 and MMP-13 selective over MMP-9 and MMP-7. The MTT assay revealed that these compounds exerted promising antiproliferative efficacy against cancer cell lines MDA-MB-231, HepG2, and Caco-2.

Bendele et al. [293], through a retrosynthetic approach, designed compound **4.216** (Figure 4.29), which was an allosteric inhibitor of MMP-13. It was a highly potent MMP-13-selective inhibitor (IC_{50} = 4.8 nM) over other MMPs. Compound **4.216** was a potent disease-modifying osteoarthritis drug (DMOAD) that was chondroprotective when injected intra-articular in the mono-iodoacetic acid (MIA) rat model.

Knapinska and co-workers [294] reported some compounds as highly potent and MMP-13-selective inhibitors over other MMPs (**4.217–4.220**, Figure 4.29). Compounds **4.218** and **4.220**, containing an azetidine ring, showed greater solubility than compounds **4.217** and **4.219** containing an oxetane ring. All these inhibitors had higher half-lives in human microsomes, rat microsomes, and mouse microsomes. A membrane permeability study in the Caco-2 cell line suggested that compounds **4.217**, **4.219**, and **4.220** had medium permeability, whereas compound **4.218** displayed low permeability. All these three inhibitors (**4.217–4.219**) were found to inhibit the collagenolysis at higher concentrations (10 μM or more), whereas compound **4.220** did not inhibit any collagenolysis.

4.6 SUMMARY

In this chapter, the detailed description of all the major collagenases, namely collagenase-1 (MMP-1), collagenase-2 (MMP-8), and collagenase-3 (MMP-13), have been discussed in detail. All these collagenases are well-implicated in the modulation of several major disease conditions, including cancers, cardiovascular diseases, and inflammatory disease conditions such as osteoarthritis and

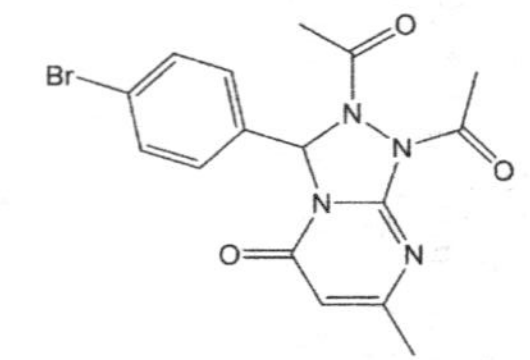

(4.214)

MMP-7 IC$_{50}$ = 711 nM
MMP-9 IC$_{50}$ = 251 nM
MMP-10 IC$_{50}$ = 24 nM
MMP-13 IC$_{50}$ = 460 nM

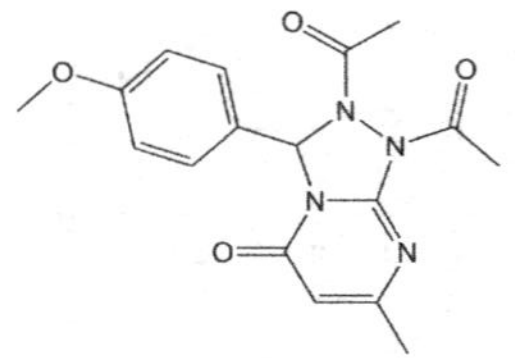

(4.215)

MMP-7 IC$_{50}$ = 397 nM
MMP-9 IC$_{50}$ = 146 nM
MMP-10 IC$_{50}$ = 130 nM
MMP-13 IC$_{50}$ = 294 nM

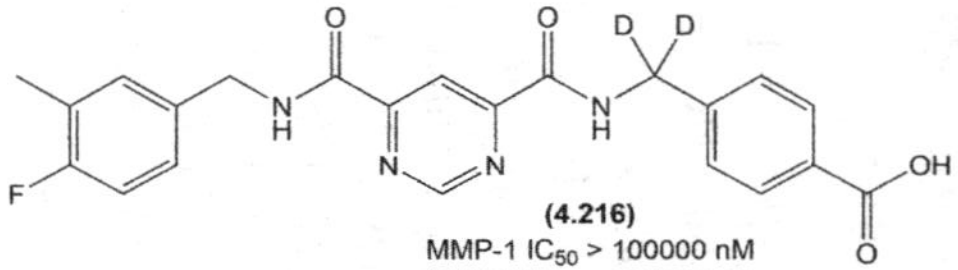

(4.216)

MMP-1 IC$_{50}$ > 100000 nM
MMP-2 IC$_{50}$ > 100000 nM
MMP-3 IC$_{50}$ > 100000 nM
MMP-7 IC$_{50}$ > 100000 nM
MMP-8 IC$_{50}$ = 98000 nM
MMP-9 IC$_{50}$ = 74000 nM
MMP-10 IC$_{50}$ = 1000 nM
MMP-12 IC$_{50}$ > 100000 nM
MMP-13 IC$_{50}$ = 4.8 nM
MMP-14 IC$_{50}$ > 100000 nM

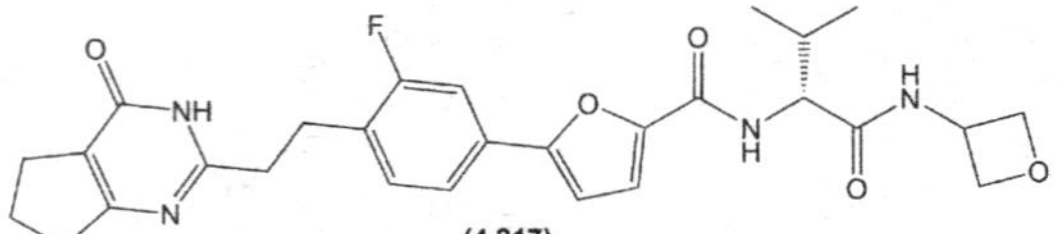

(4.217)

MMP-1 IC$_{50}$ > 5000 nM
MMP-2 IC$_{50}$ > 5000 nM
MMP-8 IC$_{50}$ > 5000 nM
MMP-9 IC$_{50}$ > 5000 nM
MMP-13 K$_i$ = 12.2 nM
MMP-14 IC$_{50}$ > 5000 nM

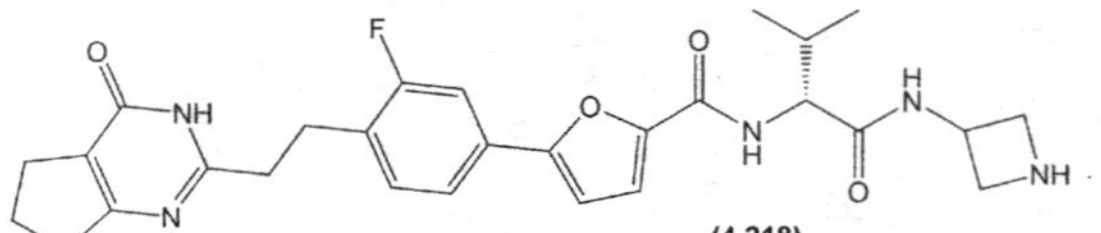

(4.218)

MMP-1 IC$_{50}$ > 5000 nM
MMP-2 IC$_{50}$ > 5000 nM
MMP-8 IC$_{50}$ > 5000 nM
MMP-9 IC$_{50}$ > 5000 nM
MMP-13 K$_i$ = 41.9 nM
MMP-14 IC$_{50}$ > 5000 nM

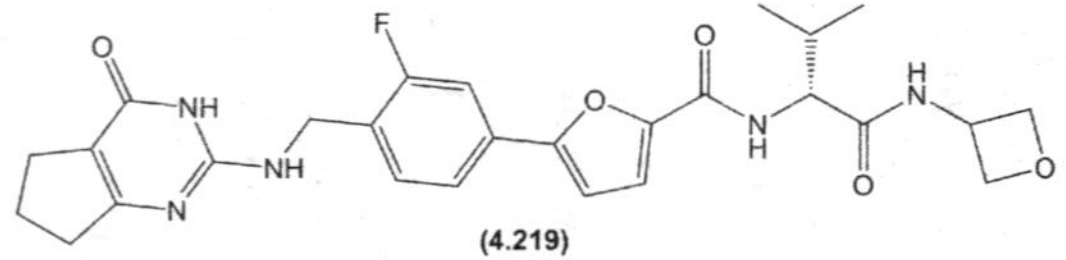

(4.219)

MMP-1 IC$_{50}$ > 5000 nM
MMP-2 IC$_{50}$ > 5000 nM
MMP-8 IC$_{50}$ > 5000 nM
MMP-9 IC$_{50}$ > 5000 nM
MMP-13 K$_i$ = 10.3 nM
MMP-14 IC$_{50}$ > 5000 nM

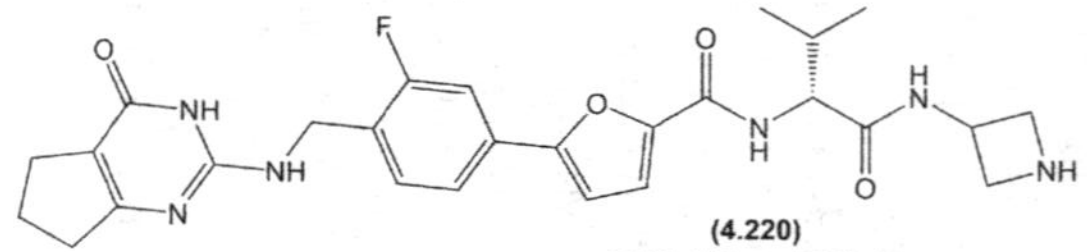

(4.220)

MMP-1 IC$_{50}$ > 5000 nM
MMP-2 IC$_{50}$ > 5000 nM
MMP-8 IC$_{50}$ > 5000 nM
MMP-9 IC$_{50}$ > 5000 nM
MMP-13 K$_i$ = 28.1 nM
MMP-14 IC$_{50}$ > 5000 nM

FIGURE 4.29 Several potential collagenase inhibitors with diverse structures (compounds **4.214–4.220**).

rheumatoid arthritis. Therefore, designing novel potential collagenase inhibitors may be an inevitable approach to combating such life-threatening diseases. A huge number of molecules have been introduced by pharmaceutical companies and research and academic institutions. However, unfortunately, none of them have come to market due to diverse adverse effects despite exhibiting promising outcomes. Still, there are challenges and hopes for accelerating the drug discovery processes related to the novel class of collagenase inhibitors. A novel class of collagenase inhibitors can be identified based on the key structural features of the existing collagenase inhibitors in combination with ligand- and structure-based drug design strategies (LBDD and SBDD). In a nutshell, this chapter provides detailed knowledge about the collagenases and existing collagenase inhibitors. Therefore, it may benefit researchers working in collagenase-related drug design and discovery processes.

REFERENCES

[1]. Mondal S, Adhikari N, Banerjee S, et al. Matrix metalloproteinase-9 (MMP-9) and its inhibitors in cancer: A minireview. *Eur J Med Chem.* 2020;194:112260.

[2]. Yadav MR, Murumkar PR, Zambre VP. Advances in studies on collagenase inhibitors. *Exp Suppl.* 2012;103:83–135.

[3]. Cheng XC, Wang Q, Fang H, et al. Advances in matrix metalloproteinase inhibitors based on pyrrolidine scaffold. *Curr Med Chem.* 2008;15(4):374–385.

[4]. Adhikari N, Amin SA, Jha T. Collagenases and gelatinases and their inhibitors as anticancer agents. In Gupta SP (Ed.), *Cancer-Leading Proteases*, Academic Press, 2020, pp. 265–294.

[5]. Vincenti MP, Brinckerhoff CE. Transcriptional regulation of collagenase (MMP-1, MMP-13) genes in arthritis: Integration of complex signaling pathways for the recruitment of gene-specific transcription factors. *Arthritis Res.* 2002;4(3):157–164.

[6]. Li J, Brick P, O'Hare MC, et al. Structure of full-length porcine synovial collagenase reveals a C-terminal domain containing a calcium-linked, four-bladed beta-propeller. *Structure.* 1995;3(6):541–549.

[7]. Gomis-Rüth FX. Structural aspects of the metzincin clan of metalloendopeptidases. *Mol Biotechnol.* 2003;24(2):157–202.

[8]. Gomis-Rüth FX. Catalytic domain architecture of metzincin metalloproteases. *J Biol Chem.* 2009;284(23):15353–15357.

[9]. Gomis-Rüth FX, Gohlke U, Betz M, et al. The helping hand of collagenase-3 (MMP-13): 2.7 a crystal structure of its C-terminal haemopexin-like domain. *J Mol Biol.* 1996;264(3):556–566. https://www.rcsb.org/. Accessed April 2022.

[10]. RCSB Protein Data Bank. Available at: https://www.rcsb.org.

[11]. Ghaffarzadeh A, Bagheri M, Khadem-Vatani K, et al. Association of MMP-1 (rs1799750)-1607 2G/2G and MMP-3 (rs3025058)-1612 6A/6A genotypes with coronary artery disease risk among Iranian Turks. *J Cardiovasc Pharmacol.* 2019;74(5):420–425.

[12]. Kondapalli MS, Galimudi RK, Gundapaneni KK, et al. MMP-1 circulating levels and promoter polymorphism in risk prediction of coronary artery disease in asymptomatic first degree relatives. *Gene.* 2016;595(1):115–120.

[13]. Geraghty P, Dabo AJ, D'Armiento J. TLR4 protein contributes to cigarette smoke-induced matrix metalloproteinase-1 (MMP-1) expression in chronic obstructive pulmonary disease. *J Biol Chem.* 2011;286(34):30211–30218.

[14]. Popat R, Bhavsar NV, Popat PR. Gingival crevicular fluid levels of matrix metallo-proteinase-1 (MMP-1) and tissue inhibitor of metalloproteinase-1 (TIMP-1) in peri-odontal health and disease. *Singapore Dent J.* 2014;35:59–64.

[15]. Shi X, Lv A, Ma J, et al. Investigation of MMP-1 genetic polymorphisms and pro-tein expression and their effects on the risk of Kashin-Beck disease in the northwest Chinese Han population. *J Orthop Surg Res.* 2016;11(1):64.

[16]. Gupta V, Singh MK, Garg RK, et al. Evaluation of peripheral matrix metalloprotein-ase-1 in Parkinson's disease: A case-control study. *Int J Neurosci.* 2014;124(2):88–92.

[17]. Zhang C, Chen L, Gu Y. Polymorphisms of MMP-1 and MMP-3 and susceptibility to rheumatoid arthritis. A meta-analysis. *Z Rheumatol.* 2015;74(3):258–262.

[18]. Riley GP, Harrall RL, Watson PG, et al. Collagenase (MMP-1) and TIMP-1 in destructive corneal disease associated with rheumatoid arthritis. *Eye (Lond).* 1995;9(6):703–718.

[19]. Liu J, Wang G, Peng Z. Association between the MMP-1-1607 1G/2G polymorphism and osteoarthritis risk: A systematic review and meta-analysis. *Biomed Res Int.* 2020;2020:5190587.

[20]. Liang L, Zhu DP, Guo SS, et al. MMP-1 gene polymorphism in osteoporosis. *Eur Rev Med Pharmacol Sci.* 2019;23(3):67–72.

[21]. Sui J, Huang J, Zhang Y. The *MMP-1* gene rs1799750 polymorphism is associated with breast cancer risk. *Genet Test Mol Biomarkers.* 2021;25(7):496–503.

[22]. Cheng S, Tada M, Hida Y, et al. High MMP-1 mRNA expression is a risk factor for disease-free and overall survivals in patients with invasive breast carcinoma. *J Surg Res.* 2008;146(1):104–109.

[23]. Boström P, Söderström M, Vahlberg T, et al. MMP-1 expression has an independent prognostic value in breast cancer. *BMC Cancer.* 2011;11:348.

[24]. Fan H, Jiang W, Li H, Fang M, et al. MMP-1/2 and TIMP-1/2 expression levels, and the levels of collagenous and elastic fibers correlate with disease progression in a hamster model of tongue cancer. *Oncol Lett.* 2016;11(1):63–68.

[25]. Ay A, Alkanli N, Cevik G. Investigation of the relationship between MMP-1 (–1607 1G/2G), MMP-3 (–1171 5A/6A) gene variations and development of bladder cancer. *Mol Biol Rep.* 2021;48(12):7689–7695.

[26]. Bendardaf R, Buhmeida A, Ristamäki R, et al. MMP-1 (collagenase-1) expres-sion in primary colorectal cancer and its metastases. *Scand J Gastroenterol.* 2007;42(12):1473–1478.

[27]. Zhong WD, Han ZD, He HC, et al. CD147, MMP-1, MMP-2 and MMP-9 protein expression as significant prognostic factors in human prostate cancer. *Oncology.* 2008;75(3–4):230–236.

[28]. Peng HH, Zhang X, Cao PG. MMP-1/PAR-1 signal transduction axis and its prog-nostic impact in esophageal squamous cell carcinoma. *Braz J Med Biol Res.* 2012;45(1):86–92.

[29]. Mattey DL, Nixon NB, Dawes PT. Association of circulating levels of MMP-8 with mortality from respiratory disease in patients with rheumatoid arthritis. *Arthritis Res Ther.* 2012;14(5):R204.

[30]. Tchetverikov I, Lard LR, DeGroot J, et al. Matrix metalloproteinases-3, -8, -9 as markers of disease activity and joint damage progression in early rheumatoid arthri-tis. *Ann Rheum Dis.* 2003;62(11):1094–1099.

[31]. Aquilante CL, Beitelshees AL, Zineh I. Correlates of serum matrix metalloprotein-ase-8 (MMP-8) concentrations in nondiabetic subjects without cardiovascular dis-ease. *Clin Chim Acta.* 2007;379(1–2):48–52.

[32]. Cárcel-Márquez J, Cullell N, Muiño E, et al. Causal effect of MMP-1 (Matrix Metalloproteinase-1), MMP-8, and MMP-12 levels on ischemic stroke: A mendelian randomization study. *Stroke.* 2021;52(7):e316–e320.

[33]. Lenglet S, Mach F, Montecucco F. Role of matrix metalloproteinase-8 in atherosclerosis. *Mediators Inflamm.* 2013;2013:659282.

[34]. Orozco-Páez J, Rodríguez-Cavallo E, Díaz-Caballero A, et al. Quantification of matrix metalloproteinases MMP-8 and MMP-9 in gingival overgrowth. *Saudi Dent J.* 2021;33(5):260–267.

[35]. Romero-Castro NS, Vázquez-Villamar M, Muñoz-Valle JF, et al. Relationship between TNF-α, MMP-8, and MMP-9 levels in gingival crevicular fluid and the subgingival microbiota in periodontal disease. *Odontology.* 2020;108(1):25–33.

[36]. Zhou X, Lu J, Chen D, et al. Matrix metalloproteinase-8 inhibitors mitigate sepsis-induced myocardial injury in rats. *Chin Med J (Engl).* 2014;127(8):1530–1535.

[37]. Sivula M, Hästbacka J, Kuitunen A, et al. Systemic matrix metalloproteinase-8 and tissue inhibitor of metalloproteinases-1 levels in severe sepsis-associated coagulopathy. *Acta Anaesthesiol Scand.* 2015;59(2):176–184.

[38]. Köhrmann A, Kammerer U, Kapp M, et al. Expression of matrix metalloproteinases (MMPs) in primary human breast cancer and breast cancer cell lines: New findings and review of the literature. *BMC Cancer.* 2009;9:188.

[39]. Shen TC, Hsia TC, Chao CY, et al. The contribution of MMP-8 promoter polymorphisms in lung cancer. *Anticancer Res.* 2017;37(7):3563–3567.

[40]. Laitinen A, Hagström J, Mustonen H, et al. Serum MMP-8 and TIMP-1 as prognostic biomarkers in gastric cancer. *Tumour Biol.* 2018;40(9):1010428318799266.

[41]. Sirniö P, Tuomisto A, Tervahartiala T, et al. High-serum MMP-8 levels are associated with decreased survival and systemic inflammation in colorectal cancer. *Br J Cancer.* 2018;119(2):213–219.

[42]. Väyrynen JP, Vornanen J, Tervahartiala T, et al. Serum MMP-8 levels increase in colorectal cancer and correlate with disease course and inflammatory properties of primary tumors. *Int J Cancer.* 2012;131(4):E463–E474.

[43]. Moilanen M, Pirilä E, Grénman R, et al. Expression and regulation of collagenase-2 (MMP-8) in head and neck squamous cell carcinomas. *J Pathol.* 2002;197(1):72–81.

[44]. Åström P, Juurikka K, Hadler-Olsen ES, et al. The interplay of matrix metalloproteinase-8, transforming growth factor-β1 and vascular endothelial growth factor-C cooperatively contributes to the aggressiveness of oral tongue squamous cell carcinoma. *Br J Cancer.* 2017;117(7):1007–1016.

[45]. Burrage PS, Mix KS, Brinckerhoff CE. Matrix metalloproteinases: Role in arthritis. *Front Biosci.* 2006;11:529–543.

[46]. Hu Q, Ecker M. Overview of MMP-13 as a promising target for the treatment of osteoarthritis. *Int J Mol Sci.* 2021;22(4):1742.

[47]. Wan Y, Li W, Liao Z, et al. Selective MMP-13 inhibitors: Promising agents for the therapy of osteoarthritis. *Curr Med Chem.* 2020;27(22):3753–3769.

[48]. Guimaraes-Stabili MR, de Medeiros MC, Rossi D, et al. Silencing matrix metalloproteinase-13 (Mmp-13) reduces inflammatory bone resorption associated with LPS-induced periodontal disease in vivo. *Clin Oral Investig.* 2021;25(5):3161–3172.

[49]. de Aquino SG, Guimaraes MR, Stach-Machado DR, et al. Differential regulation of MMP-13 expression in two models of experimentally induced periodontal disease in rats. *Arch Oral Biol.* 2009;54(7):609–617.

[50]. Zhang CY, Li XH, Zhang T, et al. Hydrogen sulfide suppresses the expression of MMP-8, MMP-13, and TIMP-1 in left ventricles of rats with cardiac volume overload. *Acta Pharmacol Sin.* 2013;34(10):1301–1309.

[51]. Ueno M, Chiba Y, Matsumoto K, et al. Blood-brain barrier damage in vascular dementia. *Neuropathology.* 2016;36(2):115–124.

[52]. Waldron AL, Schroder PA, Bourgon KL, et al. Oxidative stress-dependent MMP-13 activity underlies glucose neurotoxicity. *J Diabetes Complications.* 2018;32(3):249–257.

[53]. Uchinami H, Seki E, Brenner DA, et al. Loss of MMP 13 attenuates murine hepatic injury and fibrosis during cholestasis. *Hepatology.* 2006;44(2):420–429.

[54]. Howell C, Smith JR, Shute JK. Targeting matrix metalloproteinase-13 in bronchial epithelial repair. *Clin Exp Allergy.* 2018;48(9):1214–1221.

[55]. Quillard T, Tesmenitsky Y, Croce K, et al. Selective inhibition of matrix metalloproteinase-13 increases collagen content of established mouse atherosclerosis. *Arterioscler Thromb Vasc Biol.* 2011;31(11):2464–2472.

[56]. Quillard T, Araújo HA, Franck G, et al. Matrix metalloproteinase-13 predominates over matrix metalloproteinase-8 as the functional interstitial collagenase in mouse atheromata. *Arterioscler Thromb Vasc Biol.* 2014;34(6):1179–1186.

[57]. Kuivanen TT, Jeskanen L, Kyllönen L, et al. Transformation-specific matrix metalloproteinases, MMP-7 and MMP-13, are present in epithelial cells of keratoacanthomas. *Mod Pathol.* 2006;19(9):1203–1212.

[58]. Vizoso FJ, González LO, Corte MD, et al. Collagenase-3 (MMP-13) expression by inflamed mucosa in inflammatory bowel disease. *Scand J Gastroenterol.* 2006;41(9):1050–1055.

[59]. Rath T, Roderfeld M, Graf J, et al. Enhanced expression of MMP-7 and MMP-13 in inflammatory bowel disease: A precancerous potential? *Inflamm Bowel Dis.* 2006;12(11):1025–1035.

[60]. Rath T, Roderfeld M, Halwe JM, et al. Cellular sources of MMP-7, MMP-13 and MMP-28 in ulcerative colitis. *Scand J Gastroenterol.* 2010;45(10):1186–1196.

[61]. Sheibani S, Mahmoudian RA, Abbaszadegan MR, et al. Expression analysis of matrix metalloproteinase-13 in human gastric cancer in the presence of Helicobacter Pylori infection. *Cancer Biomark.* 2017;18(4):349–356.

[62]. Elnemr A, Yonemura Y, Bandou E, et al. Expression of collagenase-3 (matrix metalloproteinase-13) in human gastric cancer. *Gastric Cancer.* 2003;6(1):30–38.

[63]. Wang JR, Li XH, Gao XJ, et al. Expression of MMP-13 is associated with invasion and metastasis of papillary thyroid carcinoma. *Eur Rev Med Pharmacol Sci.* 2013;17(4):427–435.

[64]. Wang SW, Tai HC, Tang CH, et al. Melatonin impedes prostate cancer metastasis by suppressing MMP-13 expression. *J Cell Physiol.* 2021;236(5):3979–3990.

[65]. Li Y, Sun B, Zhao X, et al. MMP-2 and MMP-13 affect vasculogenic mimicry formation in large cell lung cancer. *J Cell Mol Med.* 2017;21(12):3741–3751.

[66]. Boström PJ, Ravanti L, Reunanen N, et al. Expression of collagenase-3 (matrix metalloproteinase-13) in transitional-cell carcinoma of the urinary bladder. *Int J Cancer.* 2000;88(3):417–423.

[67]. Yan Q, Yuan Y, Yankui L, et al. The expression and significance of CXCR5 and MMP-13 in colorectal cancer. *Cell Biochem Biophys.* 2015;73(1):253–259.

[68]. Yamada T, Oshima T, Yoshihara K, et al. Overexpression of MMP-13 gene in colorectal cancer with liver metastasis. *Anticancer Res.* 2010;30(7):2693–2699.

[69]. Zhang B, Cao X, Liu Y, et al. Tumor-derived matrix metalloproteinase-13 (MMP-13) correlates with poor prognoses of invasive breast cancer. *BMC Cancer.* 2008;8:83.

[70]. Kotepui M, Punsawad C, Chupeerach C, et al. Differential expression of matrix metalloproteinase-13 in association with invasion of breast cancer. *Contemp Oncol (Pozn).* 2016;20(3):225–228.

[71]. Ansell A, Jerhammar F, Ceder R, et al. Matrix metalloproteinase-7 and -13 expression associate to cisplatin resistance in head and neck cancer cell lines. *Oral Oncol.* 2009;45(10):866–871.

[72]. Luukkaa M, Vihinen P, Kronqvist P, et al. Association between high collagenase-3 expression levels and poor prognosis in patients with head and neck cancer. *Head Neck.* 2006;28(3):225–234.

[73]. Hsu CP, Shen GH, Ko JL. Matrix metalloproteinase-13 expression is associated with bone marrow microinvolvement and prognosis in non-small cell lung cancer. *Lung Cancer.* 2006;52(3):349–357.

[74]. Jin D, Tao J, Li D, et al. Golgi protein 73 activation of MMP-13 promotes hepatocellular carcinoma cell invasion. *Oncotarget.* 2015;6(32):33523–33533.

[75]. Wang H, Li H, Yan Q, et al. Serum matrix metalloproteinase-13 as a diagnostic biomarker for cutaneous squamous cell carcinoma. *BMC Cancer.* 2021;21(1):816.

[76]. Mercuţ IM, Simionescu CE, Stepan AE, et al. The immunoexpression of MMP-1 and MMP-13 in eyelid basal cell carcinoma. *Rom J Morphol Embryol.* 2020;61(4):1221–1226.

[77]. Kudo Y, Iizuka S, Yoshida M, et al. Matrix metalloproteinase-13 (MMP-13) directly and indirectly promotes tumor angiogenesis. *J Biol Chem.* 2012;287(46):38716–38728.

[78]. Holtkamp N, Atallah I, Okuducu AF, et al. MMP-13 and p53 in the progression of malignant peripheral nerve sheath tumors. *Neoplasia.* 2007;9(8):671–677.

[79]. Zhao X, Sun B, Li Y, et al. Dual effects of collagenase-3 on melanoma: Metastasis promotion and disruption of vasculogenic mimicry. *Oncotarget.* 2015;6(11):8890–8899.

[80]. Corte MD, Gonzalez LO, Corte MG, et al. Collagenase-3 (MMP-13) expression in cutaneous malignant melanoma. *Int J Biol Markers.* 2005;20(4):242–248.

[81]. Ala-Aho R, Johansson N, Baker AH, et al. Expression of collagenase-3 (MMP-13) enhances invasion of human fibrosarcoma HT-1080 cells. *Int J Cancer.* 2002;97(3):283–289.

[82]. Zapico JM, Acosta L, Pastor M, et al. Design and synthesis of water-soluble and potent MMP-13 inhibitors with activity in human osteosarcoma cells. *Int J Mol Sci.* 2021;22(18):9976.

[83]. Tang CH, Chen CF, Chen WM, et al. IL-6 increases MMP-13 expression and motility in human chondrosarcoma cells. *J Biol Chem.* 2011;286(13):11056–11066.

[84]. Uría JA, Balbín M, López JM, et al. Collagenase-3 (MMP-13) expression in chondrosarcoma cells and its regulation by basic fibroblast growth factor. *Am J Pathol.* 1998;153(1):91–101.

[85]. Yeh WL, Lu DY, Lee MJ, et al. Leptin induces migration and invasion of glioma cells through MMP-13 production. *Glia.* 2009;57(4):454–464.

[86]. Wang J, Li Y, Wang J, et al. Increased expression of matrix metalloproteinase-13 in glioma is associated with poor overall survival of patients. *Med Oncol.* 2012;29(4):2432–2437.

[87]. Shan Y, You B, Shi S, et al. Hypoxia-induced matrix metalloproteinase-13 expression in exosomes from nasopharyngeal carcinoma enhances metastases. *Cell Death Dis.* 2018;9(3):382.

[88]. Schultz GS, Strelow S, Stern GA, et al. Treatment of alkali-injured rabbit corneas with a synthetic inhibitor of matrix metalloproteinases. *Invest Ophthalmol Vis Sci.* 1992;33(12):3325–3331.

[89]. Suomalainen K, Halinen S, Ingman T, et al. Tetracycline inhibition identifies the cellular sources of collagenase in gingival crevicular fluid in different forms of periodontal diseases. *Drugs Exp Clin Res.* 1992;18(3):99–104.

[90]. Buttle DJ, Handley CJ, Ilic MZ, et al. Inhibition of cartilage proteoglycan release by a specific inactivator of cathepsin B and an inhibitor of matrix metalloproteinases. Evidence for two converging pathways of chondrocyte-mediated proteoglycan degradation. *Arthritis Rheum.* 1993;36(12):1709–1717.

[91]. McGeehan GM, Becherer JD, Bast RC Jr, et al. Regulation of tumour necrosis factor-alpha processing by a metalloproteinase inhibitor. *Nature.* 1994;370(6490):558–561.

[92]. Drummond AH. BB2516: An orally bioavailable matrix metalloproteinase inhibitor with efficacy in animal cancer models. *Proc. Am Assoc Cancer Res.* 1995;36:100.

[93]. O'Byrne EM, Parker DT, Roberts ED, et al. Oral administration of a matrix metalloproteinase inhibitor, CGS 27023A, protects the cartilage proteoglycan matrix in a partial meniscectomy model of osteoarthritis in rabbits. *Inflamm Res.* 1995;44(Supplement 2):S117–S118.

[94]. Santos O, McDermott CD, Daniels RG, et al. Rodent pharmacokinetic and anti-tumor efficacy studies with a series of synthetic inhibitors of matrix metalloproteinases. *Clin Exp Metastasis.* 1997;15(5):499–508.

[95]. Heath EI, Grochow LB. Clinical potential of matrix metalloprotease inhibitors in cancer therapy. *Drugs.* 2000;59(5):1043–1055.

[96]. Gatto C, Rieppi M, Borsotti P, et al. BAY 12-9566, a novel inhibitor of matrix metalloproteinases with antiangiogenic activity. *Clin Cancer Res.* 1999;5(11):3603–3607.

[97]. Zheng QH, Fei X, Liu X, et al. Comparative studies of potential cancer biomarkers carbon-11 labeled MMP inhibitors (S)-2-(4′-[11C]methoxybiphenyl-4-sulfonylamino)-3-methylbutyric acid and N-hydroxy-(R)-2-[[(4′-[11C]methoxyphenyl)sulfonyl]benzylamino]-3-methylbutanamide. *Nucl Med Biol.* 2004;31(1):77–85.

[98]. Robinson RP, Ragan JA, Cronin BJ, et al. Inhibitors of MMP-1: An examination of P1′ Cα gem-disubstitution in the succinamide hydroxamate series. *Bioorg Med Chem Lett.* 1996;6(14):1719–1724.

[99]. Robinson RP, Laird ER, Blake JF, et al. Structure-based design and synthesis of a potent matrix metalloproteinase-13 inhibitor based on a pyrrolidinone scaffold. *J Med Chem.* 2000;43(12):2293–2296.

[100]. Robinson RP, Laird ER, Donahue KM, et al. Design and synthesis of 2-oxo-imidazolidine-4-carboxylic acid hydroxyamides as potent matrix metalloproteinase-13 inhibitors. *Bioorg Med Chem Lett.* 2001;11(9):1211–1213.

[101]. Letavic MA, Barberia JT, Carty TJ, et al. Synthesis and biological activity of piperazine-based dual MMP-13 and TNF-alpha converting enzyme inhibitors. *Bioorg Med Chem Lett.* 2003;13(19):3243–3246.

[102]. Reiter LA, Robinson RP, McClure KF, et al. Pyran-containing sulfonamide hydroxamic acids: Potent MMP inhibitors that spare MMP-1. *Bioorg Med Chem Lett.* 2004;14(13):3389–3395.

[103]. Noe MC, Snow SL, Wolf-Gouveia LA, et al. 3-Hydroxy-4-arylsulfonyltetrahydropyranyl-3-hydroxamic acids are novel inhibitors of MMP-13 and aggrecanase. *Bioorg Med Chem Lett.* 2004;14(18):4727–4730.

[104]. Noe MC, Natarajan V, Snow SL, et al. Discovery of 3,3-dimethyl-5-hydroxypipecolic hydroxamate-based inhibitors of aggrecanase and MMP-13. *Bioorg Med Chem Lett.* 2005;15(11):2808–2811.

[105]. Noe MC, Natarajan V, Snow SL, et al. Discovery of 3-OH-3-methylpipecolic hydroxamates: Potent orally active inhibitors of aggrecanase and MMP-13. *Bioorg Med Chem Lett.* 2005;15(14):3385–3388.

[106]. Becker DP, Villamil CI, Barta TE, et al. Synthesis and structure-activity relationships of beta- and alpha-piperidine sulfone hydroxamic acid matrix metalloproteinase inhibitors with oral antitumor efficacy. *J Med Chem.* 2005;48(21):6713–6730.

[107]. Kolodziej SA, Hockerman SL, Boehm TL, et al. Orally bioavailable dual MMP-1/MMP-14 sparing, MMP-13 selective alpha-sulfone hydroxamates. *Bioorg Med Chem Lett.* 2010;20(12):3557–3560.

[108]. Kolodziej SA, Hockerman SL, DeCrescenzo GA, et al. MMP-13 selective isonipecotamide alpha-sulfone hydroxamates. *Bioorg Med Chem Lett.* 2010;20(12):3561–3564.

[109]. Becker DP, Barta TE, Bedell LJ, et al. Orally active MMP-1 sparing α-tetrahydropyranyl and α-piperidinyl sulfone matrix metalloproteinase (MMP) inhibitors with efficacy in cancer, arthritis, and cardiovascular disease. *J Med Chem.* 2010;53(18):6653–6680.

[110]. Barta TE, Becker DP, Bedell LJ, et al. MMP-13 selective α-sulfone hydroxamates: A survey of P1' heterocyclic amide isosteres. *Bioorg Med Chem Lett.* 2011;21(10):2820–2822.

[111]. Fobian YM, Freskos JN, Barta TE, et al. MMP-13 selective alpha-sulfone hydroxamates: Identification of selective P1' amides. *Bioorg Med Chem Lett.* 2011;21(10):2823–2825.

[112]. Curtin ML, Garland RB, Davidsen SK, et al. Broad spectrum matrix metalloproteinase inhibitors: An examination of succinamide hydroxamate inhibitors with P1 C alpha gem-disubstitution. *Bioorg Med Chem Lett.* 1998;8(12):1443–1448.

[113]. Steinman DH, Curtin ML, Garland RB, et al. The design, synthesis, and structure-activity relationships of a series of macrocyclic MMP inhibitors. *Bioorg Med Chem Lett.* 1998;8(16):2087–2092.

[114]. Sheppard GS, Florjancic AS, Giesler JR, et al. Aryl ketones as novel replacements for the C-terminal amide bond of succinyl hydroxamate MMP inhibitors. *Bioorg Med Chem Lett.* 1998;8(22):3251–3256.

[115]. Hirayama R, Yamamoto M, Tsukida T, et al. Synthesis and biological evaluation of orally active matrix metalloproteinase inhibitors. *Bioorg Med Chem.* 1997;5(4):765–778.

[116]. Yamamoto M, Tsujishita H, Hori N, et al. Inhibition of membrane-type 1 matrix metalloproteinase by hydroxamate inhibitors: An examination of the subsite pocket. *J Med Chem.* 1998;41(8):1209–1217.

[117]. Martin FM, Beckett RP, Bellamy CL, et al. The synthesis and biological evaluation of non-peptidic matrix metalloproteinase inhibitors. *Bioorg Med Chem Lett.* 1999;9(19):2887–2892.

[118]. Almstead NG, Bradley RS, Pikul S, et al. Design, synthesis, and biological evaluation of potent thiazine- and thiazepine-based matrix metalloproteinase inhibitors. *J Med Chem.* 1999;42(22):4547–4562.

[119]. Pikul S, McDow Dunham KL, Almstead NG, et al. Design and synthesis of phosphinamide-based hydroxamic acids as inhibitors of matrix metalloproteinases. *J Med Chem.* 1999;42(1):87–94.

[120]. Cheng M, De B, Almstead NG, et al. Design, synthesis, and biological evaluation of matrix metalloproteinase inhibitors derived from a modified proline scaffold. *J Med Chem.* 1999;42(26):5426–5436.

[121]. Cheng M, De B, Pikul S, et al. Design and synthesis of piperazine-based matrix metalloproteinase inhibitors. *J Med Chem.* 2000;43(3):369–380.

[122]. Natchus MG, Bookland RG, De B, et al. Development of new hydroxamate matrix metalloproteinase inhibitors derived from functionalized 4-aminoprolines. *J Med Chem.* 2000;43(26):4948–4963.

[123]. Pikul S, Dunham KM, Almstead NG, et al. Heterocycle-based MMP inhibitors with P2' substituents. *Bioorg Med Chem Lett.* 2001;11(8):1009–1013.

[124]. Levin JI, DiJoseph JF, Killar LM, et al. The synthesis and biological activity of a novel series of diazepine MMP inhibitors. *Bioorg Med Chem Lett.* 1998;8(19):2657–2662.

[125]. Levin JI, Du MT, DiJoseph JF, et al. The discovery of anthranilic acid-based MMP inhibitors. Part 1: SAR of the 3-position. *Bioorg Med Chem Lett.* 2001;11(2):235–238.

[126]. Levin JI, Gu Y, Nelson FC, et al. Heteroaryl and cycloalkyl sulfonamide hydroxamic acid inhibitors of matrix metalloproteinases. *Bioorg Med Chem Lett.* 2001;11(2):239–242.

[127]. Levin JI, Chen JM, Du MT, et al. The discovery of anthranilic acid-based MMP inhibitors. Part 3: Incorporation of basic amines. *Bioorg Med Chem Lett.* 2001;11(22):2975–2978.

[128]. Levin JI, Chen J, Du M, et al. The discovery of anthranilic acid-based MMP inhibitors. Part 2: SAR of the 5-position and P1(1) groups. *Bioorg Med Chem Lett.* 2001;11(16):2189–2192.

[129]. Chen JM, Jin G, Sung A, et al. Anthranilate sulfonamide hydroxamate TACE inhibitors. Part 1: Structure-based design of novel acetylenic P1′ groups. *Bioorg Med Chem Lett.* 2002;12(8):1195–1198.

[130]. Levin JI, Chen JM, Du MT, et al. Anthranilate sulfonamide hydroxamate TACE inhibitors. Part 2: SAR of the acetylenic P1′ group. *Bioorg Med Chem Lett.* 2002;12(8):1199–1202.

[131]. Zask A, Gu Y, Albright JD, et al. Synthesis and SAR of bicyclic heteroaryl hydroxamic acid MMP and TACE inhibitors. *Bioorg Med Chem Lett.* 2003;13(8):1487–1490.

[132]. Nelson FC, Delos Santos E, Levin JI, et al. Benzodiazepine inhibitors of the MMPs and TACE. *Bioorg Med Chem Lett.* 2002;12(20):2867–2870.

[133]. Aranapakam V, Grosu GT, Davis JM, et al. Synthesis and structure-activity relationship of alpha-sulfonylhydroxamic acids as novel, orally active matrix metalloproteinase inhibitors for the treatment of osteoarthritis. *J Med Chem.* 2003;46(12):2361–2375.

[134]. Aranapakam V, Davis JM, Grosu GT, et al. Synthesis and structure-activity relationship of N-substituted 4-arylsulfonylpiperidine-4-hydroxamic acids as novel, orally active matrix metalloproteinase inhibitors for the treatment of osteoarthritis. *J Med Chem.* 2003;46(12):2376–2396.

[135]. Levin JI, Chen JM, Cheung K, et al. Acetylenic TACE inhibitors. Part 1. SAR of the acyclic sulfonamide hydroxamates. *Bioorg Med Chem Lett.* 2003;13(16):2799–2803.

[136]. Levin JI, Nelson FC, Delos Santos E, et al. Benzodiazepine inhibitors of the MMPs and TACE. Part 2. *Bioorg Med Chem Lett.* 2004;14(16):4147–4151.

[137]. Venkatesan AM, Davis JM, Grosu GT, et al. Synthesis and structure-activity relationships of 4-alkynyloxy phenyl sulfanyl, sulfinyl, and sulfonyl alkyl hydroxamates as tumor necrosis factor-alpha converting enzyme and matrix metalloproteinase inhibitors. *J Med Chem.* 2004;47(25):6255–6269.

[138]. Zask A, Kaplan J, Du X, et al. Synthesis and SAR of diazepine and thiazepine TACE and MMP inhibitors. *Bioorg Med Chem Lett.* 2005;15(6):1641–1645.

[139]. Levin JI, Chen JM, Laakso LM, et al. Acetylenic TACE inhibitors. Part 2: SAR of six-membered cyclic sulfonamide hydroxamates. *Bioorg Med Chem Lett.* 2005;15(19):4345–4349.

[140]. Levin JI, Chen JM, Laakso LM, et al. Acetylenic TACE inhibitors. Part 3: Thiomorpholine sulfonamide hydroxamates. *Bioorg Med Chem Lett.* 2006;16(6):1605–1609.

[141]. Park K, Aplasca A, Du MT, et al. Design and synthesis of butynyloxyphenyl beta-sulfone piperidine hydroxamates as TACE inhibitors. *Bioorg Med Chem Lett.* 2006;16(15):3927–3931.

[142]. Condon JS, Joseph-McCarthy D, Levin JI, et al. Identification of potent and selective TACE inhibitors via the S1 pocket. *Bioorg Med Chem Lett.* 2007;17(1):34–39.

[143]. Lombart HG, Feyfant E, Joseph-McCarthy D, et al. Design and synthesis of 3,3-piperidine hydroxamate analogs as selective TACE inhibitors. *Bioorg Med Chem Lett.* 2007;17(15):4333–4337.

[144]. Huang A, Joseph-McCarthy D, Lovering F, et al. Structure-based design of TACE selective inhibitors: Manipulations in the S1′-S3′ pocket. *Bioorg Med Chem.* 2007;15(18):6170–6181.

[145]. Zhang C, Lovering F, Behnke M, et al. Synthesis and activity of quinolinylmethyl P1′ alpha-sulfone piperidine hydroxamate inhibitors of TACE. *Bioorg Med Chem Lett.* 2009;19(13):3445–3448.

[146]. Becker DP, Barta TE, Bedell L, et al. Alpha-amino-beta-sulphone hydroxamates as potent MMP-13 inhibitors that spare MMP-1. *Bioorg Med Chem Lett.* 2001;11(20):2719–2722.

[147]. Becker DP, DeCrescenzo G, Freskos J, et al. Alpha-alkyl-alpha-amino-beta-sulphone hydroxamates as potent MMP inhibitors that spare MMP-1. *Bioorg Med Chem Lett.* 2001;11(20):2723–2725.

[148]. Duan JJ, Chen L, Xue CB, et al. P1, P2'-linked macrocyclic amine derivatives as matrix metalloproteinase inhibitors. *Bioorg Med Chem Lett.* 1999;9(10):1453–1458.

[149]. Baxter AD, Bhogal R, Bird J, et al. Arylsulphonyl hydroxamic acids: Potent and selective matrix metalloproteinase inhibitors. *Bioorg Med Chem Lett.* 2001;11(11):1465–1468.

[150]. Sørensen MD, Blaehr LK, Christensen MK, et al. Cyclic phosphinamides and phosphonamides, novel series of potent matrix metalloproteinase inhibitors with antitumour activity. *Bioorg Med Chem.* 2003;11(24):5461–5484.

[151]. Apfel C, Banner DW, Bur D, et al. Hydroxamic acid derivatives as potent peptide deformylase inhibitors and antibacterial agents. *J Med Chem.* 2000;43(12):2324–2331.

[152]. Apfel C, Banner DW, Bur D, et al. 2-(2-Oxo-1,4-dihydro-2H-quinazolin-3-yl)- and 2-(2,2-dioxo-1,4-dihydro-2H-2lambda6-benzo[1,2,6]thiadiazin-3-yl)-N-hydroxy-acetamides as potent and selective peptide deformylase inhibitors. *J Med Chem.* 2001;44(12):1847–1852.

[153]. Durham TB, Klimkowski VJ, Rito CJ, et al. Identification of potent and selective hydantoin inhibitors of aggrecanase-1 and aggrecanase-2 that are efficacious in both chemical and surgical models of osteoarthritis. *J Med Chem.* 2014;57(24):10476–10485.

[154]. Takahashi K, Ikura M, Habashita H, et al. Novel matrix metalloproteinase inhibitors: Generation of lead compounds by the in silico fragment-based approach. *Bioorg Med Chem.* 2005;13(14):4527–4543.

[155]. Tommasi RA, Weiler S, McQuire LW, et al. Potent and selective 2-naphthylsulfonamide substituted hydroxamic acid inhibitors of matrix metalloproteinase-13. *Bioorg Med Chem Lett.* 2011;21(21):6440–6445.

[156]. Hanessian S, Bouzbouz S, Boudon A, et al. Picking the S1, S1' and S2' pockets of matrix metalloproteinases. A niche for potent acyclic sulfonamide inhibitors. *Bioorg Med Chem Lett.* 1999;9(12):1691–1696.

[157]. Hanessian S, Moitessier N, Gauchet C, et al. N-Aryl sulfonyl homocysteine hydroxamate inhibitors of matrix metalloproteinases: Further probing of the S(1), S(1)', and S(2)' pockets. *J Med Chem.* 2001;44(19):3066–3073.

[158]. Hanessian S, MacKay DB, Moitessier N. Design and synthesis of matrix metalloproteinase inhibitors guided by molecular modeling. Picking the S(1) pocket using conformationally constrained inhibitors. *J Med Chem.* 2001;44(19):3074–3082.

[159]. Barta TE, Becker DP, Bedell LJ, et al. Synthesis and activity of selective MMP inhibitors with an aryl backbone. *Bioorg Med Chem Lett.* 2000;10(24):2815–2817.

[160]. Barta TE, Becker DP, Bedell LJ, et al. Selective, orally active MMP inhibitors with an aryl backbone. *Bioorg Med Chem Lett.* 2001;11(18):2481–2483.

[161]. Chollet AM, Le Diguarher T, Murray L, et al. General synthesis of alpha-substituted 3-bisaryloxy propionic acid derivatives as specific MMP inhibitors. *Bioorg Med Chem Lett.* 2001;11(3):295–299.

[162]. Chollet AM, Le Diguarher T, Kucharczyk N, et al. Solid-phase synthesis of alpha-substituted 3-bisarylthio N-hydroxy propionamides as specific MMP inhibitors. *Bioorg Med Chem.* 2002;10(3):531–544.

[163]. Scozzafava A, Supuran CT. Protease inhibitors: Synthesis of potent bacterial collagenase and matrix metalloproteinase inhibitors incorporating N-4-nitrobenzylsulfonylglycine hydroxamate moieties. *J Med Chem.* 2000;43(9):1858–1865.

[164]. Rossello A, Nuti E, Carelli P, et al. N-i-propoxy-N-biphenylsulfonylaminobutylhydro xamic acids as potent and selective inhibitors of MMP-2 and MT1-MMP. *Bioorg Med Chem Lett.* 2005;15(5):1321–1326.

[165]. Marques SM, Nuti E, Rossello A, et al. Dual inhibitors of matrix metalloproteinases and carbonic anhydrases: Iminodiacetyl-based hydroxamate-benzenesulfonamide conjugates. *J Med Chem.* 2008;51(24):7968–7979.

[166]. Nuti E, Casalini F, Avramova SI, et al. N-O-isopropyl sulfonamido-based hydroxa-mates: Design, synthesis and biological evaluation of selective matrix metallopro-teinase-13 inhibitors as potential therapeutic agents for osteoarthritis. *J Med Chem.* 2009;52(15):4757–4773.

[167]. Nuti E, Panelli L, Casalini F, et al. Design, synthesis, biological evaluation, and NMR studies of a new series of arylsulfones as selective and potent matrix metal-loproteinase-12 inhibitors. *J Med Chem.* 2009;52(20):6347–6361.

[168]. Nuti E, Santamaria S, Casalini F, et al. Arylsulfonamide inhibitors of aggrecanases as potential therapeutic agents for osteoarthritis: Synthesis and biological evaluation. *Eur J Med Chem.* 2013;62:379–394.

[169]. Nuti E, Cantelmo AR, Gallo C, et al. N-O-isopropyl sulfonamido-based hydroxa-mates as matrix metalloproteinase inhibitors: Hit selection and in vivo antiangio-genic activity. *J Med Chem.* 2015;58(18):7224–7240.

[170]. Ma D, Wu W, Yang G, et al. Tetrahydroisoquinoline based sulfonamide hydroxa-mates as potent matrix metalloproteinase inhibitors. *Bioorg Med Chem Lett.* 2004;14(1):47–50.

[171]. Sawa M, Kondo H, Nishimura S. Encounter with unexpected collagenase-1 selective inhibitor: Switchover of inhibitor binding pocket induced by fluorine atom. *Bioorg Med Chem Lett.* 2002;12(4):581–584.

[172]. Krumme D, Tschesche H. Oxal hydroxamic acid derivatives with inhibitory activity against matrix metalloproteinases. *Bioorg Med Chem Lett.* 2002;12(6):933–936.

[173]. Moroy G, Denhez C, El Mourabit H, et al. Simultaneous presence of unsaturation and long alkyl chain at P'1 of Ilomastat confers selectivity for gelatinase A (MMP-2) over gelatinase B (MMP-9) inhibition as shown by molecular modelling studies. *Bioorg Med Chem.* 2007;15(14):4753–4766.

[174]. Zapico JM, Serra P, García-Sanmartín J, et al. Potent "clicked" MMP-2 inhibi-tors: Synthesis, molecular modeling and biological exploration. *Org Biomol Chem.* 2011;9(12):4587–4599.

[175]. Fabre B, Filipiak K, Zapico JM, et al. Progress towards water-soluble triazole-based selective MMP-2 inhibitors. *Org Biomol Chem.* 2013;11(38):6623–6641.

[176]. Zapico JM, Puckowska A, Filipiak K, et al. Design and synthesis of potent hydroxa-mate inhibitors with increased selectivity within the gelatinase family. *Org Biomol Chem.* 2015;13(1):142–156.

[177]. Hugenberg V, Breyholz HJ, Riemann B, et al. A new class of highly potent matrix metalloproteinase inhibitors based on triazole-substituted hydroxamates: (radio)syn-thesis and in vitro and first in vivo evaluation. *J Med Chem.* 2012;55(10):4714–4727.

[178]. Hugenberg V, Riemann B, Hermann S, et al. Inverse 1,2,3-triazole-1-yl-ethyl sub-stituted hydroxamates as highly potent matrix metalloproteinase inhibitors: (radio) synthesis, in vitro and first in vivo evaluation. *J Med Chem.* 2013;56(17):6858–6870.

[179]. Kalinin DV, Wagner S, Riemann B, et al. Novel potent proline-based metalloprotein-ase inhibitors: Design, (radio)synthesis, and first in vivo evaluation as radiotracers for positron emission tomography. *J Med Chem.* 2016;59(20):9541–9559.

[180]. Kalinin DV, Agoglitta O, Van de Vyver H, et al. Proline-based hydroxamates target-ing the zinc-dependent deacetylase LpxC: Synthesis, antibacterial properties, and docking studies. *Bioorg Med Chem.* 2019;27(10):1997–2018.

[181]. Wagner S, Breyholz HJ, Law MP, et al. Novel fluorinated derivatives of the broad-spectrum MMP inhibitors N-hydroxy-2(R)-[[(4-methoxyphenyl)sulfonyl](benzyl)- and (3-picolyl)-amino]-3-methyl-butanamide as potential tools for the molecular imaging of activated MMPs with PET. *J Med Chem.* 2007;50(23):5752–5764.

[182]. Topai A, Breccia P, Minissi F, et al. In silico scaffold evaluation and solid phase approach to identify new gelatinase inhibitors. *Bioorg Med Chem.* 2012;20(7):2323–2337.

[183]. Mori M, Massaro A, Calderone V, et al. Discovery of a new class of potent MMP inhibitors by structure-based optimization of the arylsulfonamide scaffold. *ACS Med Chem Lett.* 2013;4(6):565–569.

[184]. Yuan H, Lu W, Wang L, et al. Synthesis of derivatives of methyl rosmarinate and their inhibitory activities against matrix metalloproteinase-1 (MMP-1). *Eur J Med Chem.* 2013;62:148–157.

[185]. Ramsbeck D, Hamann A, Schlenzig D, et al. First insight into structure-activity relationships of selective meprin β inhibitors. *Bioorg Med Chem Lett.* 2017;27(11):2428–2431.

[186]. Brown FK, Brown PJ, Bickett DM, et al. Matrix metalloproteinase inhibitors containing a (carboxyalkyl)amino zinc ligand: Modification of the P1 and P2' residues. *J Med Chem.* 1994;37(5):674–688.

[187]. Robinson RP, Cronin BJ, Donahue KM, et al. Inhibitors of MMP-1: An examination of P1' Cα gem-disubstitution in the N-carboxyalkylamine and glutaramide carboxylate series. *Bioorg Med Chem Lett.* 1996;6(14):1725–1730.

[188]. O'Brien PM, Ortwine DF, Pavlovsky AG, et al. Structure-activity relationships and pharmacokinetic analysis for a series of potent, systemically available biphenylsulfonamide matrix metalloproteinase inhibitors. *J Med Chem.* 2000;43(2):156–166.

[189]. Natchus MG, Bookland RG, Laufersweiler MJ, et al. Development of new carboxylic acid-based MMP inhibitors derived from functionalized propargylglycines. *J Med Chem.* 2001;44(7):1060–1071.

[190]. Pikul S, Ohler NE, Ciszewski G, et al. Potent and selective carboxylic acid-based inhibitors of matrix metalloproteinases. *J Med Chem.* 2001;44(16):2499–2502.

[191]. Tullis JS, Laufersweiler MJ, VanRens JC, et al. The development of new carboxylic acid-based MMP inhibitors derived from a cyclohexylglycine scaffold. *Bioorg Med Chem Lett.* 2001;11(15):1975–1979.

[192]. Hudlicky T, Oppong K, Duan C, et al. Chemoenzymatic synthesis of functionalized cyclohexylglycines and alpha-methylcyclohexylglycines via Kazmaier-Claisen rearrangement. *Bioorg Med Chem Lett.* 2001;11(5):627–629.

[193]. Matter H, Schudok M, Schwab W, et al. Tetrahydroisoquinoline-3-carboxylate based matrix-metalloproteinase inhibitors: Design, synthesis and structure-activity relationship. *Bioorg Med Chem.* 2002;10(11):3529–3544.

[194]. Wu J, Rush TS 3rd, Hotchandani R, et al. Identification of potent and selective MMP-13 inhibitors. *Bioorg Med Chem Lett.* 2005;15(18):4105–4109.

[195]. Li J, Rush TS 3rd, Li W, et al. Synthesis and SAR of highly selective MMP-13 inhibitors. *Bioorg Med Chem Lett.* 2005;15(22):4961–4966.

[196]. Hu Y, Xiang JS, DiGrandi MJ, et al. Potent, selective, and orally bioavailable matrix metalloproteinase-13 inhibitors for the treatment of osteoarthritis. *Bioorg Med Chem.* 2005;13(24):6629–6644.

[197]. Hopper DW, Vera MD, How D, et al. Synthesis and biological evaluation of ((4-keto)-phenoxy)methyl biphenyl-4-sulfonamides: A class of potent aggrecanase-1 inhibitors. *Bioorg Med Chem Lett.* 2009;19(9):2487–2491.

[198]. Park K, Gopalsamy A, Aplasca A, et al. Synthesis and activity of tryptophan sulfonamide derivatives as novel non-hydroxamate TNF-alpha converting enzyme (TACE) inhibitors. *Bioorg Med Chem.* 2009;17(11):3857–3865.

[199]. Li W, Hu Y, Li J, et al. 3,4-Disubstituted benzofuran P1' MMP-13 inhibitors: Optimization of selectivity and reduction of protein binding. *Bioorg Med Chem Lett.* 2009;19(16):4546–4550.

[200]. Zhang YM, Fan X, Xiang B, et al. Synthesis and SAR of alpha-sulfonylcarboxylic acids as potent matrix metalloproteinase inhibitors. *Bioorg Med Chem Lett.* 2006;16(12):3096–3100.

[201]. Monovich LG, Tommasi RA, Fujimoto RA, et al. Discovery of potent, selective, and orally active carboxylic acid based inhibitors of matrix metalloproteinase-13. *J Med Chem.* 2009;52(11):3523–3538.

[202]. Taylor SJ, Abeywardane A, Liang S, et al. Fragment-based discovery of indole inhibitors of matrix metalloproteinase-13. *J Med Chem.* 2011;54(23):8174–8187.

[203]. Hu Y, Xing L, Thomason JR, et al. Continued exploration of biphenylsulfonamide scaffold as a platform for aggrecanase-1 inhibition. *Bioorg Med Chem Lett.* 2011;21(22):6800–6803.

[204]. Le Diguarher T, Chollet AM, Bertrand M, et al. Stereospecific synthesis of 5-substituted 2-bisarylthiocyclopentane carboxylic acids as specific matrix metalloproteinase inhibitors. *J Med Chem.* 2003;46(18):3840–3852.

[205]. Nakai R, Salisbury CM, Rosen H, et al. Ranking the selectivity of PubChem screening hits by activity-based protein profiling: MMP-13 as a case study. *Bioorg Med Chem.* 2009;17(3):1101–1108.

[206]. La Pietra V, Marinelli L, Cosconati S, et al. Identification of novel molecular scaffolds for the design of MMP-13 inhibitors: A first round of lead optimization. *Eur J Med Chem.* 2012;47(1):143–152.

[207]. Halder AK, Mallick S, Shikha D, et al. Design of dual MMP-2/HDAC-8 inhibitors by pharmacophore mapping, molecular docking, synthesis and biological activity. *RSC Adv.* 2015;5(88):72373–72386.

[208]. Adhikari N, Halder AK, Mallick S, et al. Robust design of some selective matrix metalloproteinase-2 inhibitors over matrix metalloproteinase-9 through in silico/fragment-based lead identification and de novo lead modification: Syntheses and biological assays. *Bioorg Med Chem.* 2016;24(18):4291–4309.

[209]. Mukherjee A, Adhikari N, Jha T. A pentanoic acid derivative targeting matrix metalloproteinase-2 (MMP-2) induces apoptosis in a chronic myeloid leukemia cell line. *Eur J Med Chem.* 2017;141:37–50.

[210]. Baxter AD, Bird J, Bhogal R, et al. A novel series of matrix metalloproteinase inhibitors for the treatment of inflammatory disorders. *Bioorg Med Chem Lett.* 1997;7(7):897–902.

[211]. Baxter AD, Bhogal R, Bird JB, et al. Mercaptoacyl matrix metalloproteinase inhibitors: The effect of substitution at the mercaptoacyl moiety. *Bioorg Med Chem Lett.* 1997;7(21):2765–2770.

[212]. Lynas JF, Martin SL, Walker B, et al. Solid-phase synthesis and biological screening of N-alpha-mercaptoamide template-based matrix metalloprotease inhibitors. *Comb Chem High Throughput Screen.* 2000;3(1):37–41.

[213]. Campbell DA, Xiao XY, Harris D, et al. Malonyl alpha-mercaptoketones and alpha-mercaptoalcohols, a new class of matrix metalloproteinase inhibitors. *Bioorg Med Chem Lett.* 1998;8(10):1157–1162.

[214]. Levin JI, DiJoseph JF, Killar LM, et al. The asymmetric synthesis and in vitro characterization of succinyl mercaptoalcohol and mercaptoketone inhibitors of matrix metalloproteinases. *Bioorg Med Chem Lett.* 1998;8(10):1163–1168.

[215]. Szardenings AK, Harris D, Lam S, et al. Rational design and combinatorial evaluation of enzyme inhibitor scaffolds: Identification of novel inhibitors of matrix metalloproteinases. *J Med Chem.* 1998;41(13):2194–2200.

[216]. Szardenings AK, Antonenko V, Campbell DA, et al. Identification of highly selective inhibitors of collagenase-1 from combinatorial libraries of diketopiperazines. *J Med Chem.* 1999;42(8):1348–1357.

[217]. Freskos JN, Mischke BV, DeCrescenzo GA, et al. Discovery of a novel series of selective MMP inhibitors: Identification of the gamma-sulfone-thiols. *Bioorg Med Chem Lett.* 1999;9(7):943–948.

[218]. Freskos JN, McDonald JJ, Mischke BV, et al. Synthesis and identification of conformationally constrained selective MMP inhibitors. *Bioorg Med Chem Lett.* 1999;9(13):1757–1760.

[219]. Fink CA, Carlson JE, Boehm C, et al. Design and synthesis of thiol containing inhibitors of matrix metalloproteinases. *Bioorg Med Chem Lett.* 1999;9(2):195–200.

[220]. Hurst DR, Schwartz MA, Jin Y, et al. Inhibition of enzyme activity of and cell-mediated substrate cleavage by membrane type 1 matrix metalloproteinase by newly developed mercaptosulphide inhibitors. *Biochem J.* 2005;392(Pt 3):527–536.

[221]. Jin Y, Roycik MD, Bosco DB, et al. Matrix metalloproteinase inhibitors based on the 3-mercaptopyrrolidine core. *J Med Chem.* 2013;56(11):4357–4373.

[222]. Pochetti G, Gavuzzo E, Campestre C, et al. Structural insight into the stereoselective inhibition of MMP-8 by enantiomeric sulfonamide phosphonates. *J Med Chem.* 2006;49(3):923–931.

[223]. Biasone A, Tortorella P, Campestre C, et al. Alpha-Biphenylsulfonylamino 2-methylpropyl phosphonates: Enantioselective synthesis and selective inhibition of MMPs. *Bioorg Med Chem.* 2007;15(2):791–799.

[224]. Reiter LA, Rizzi JP, Pandit J, et al. Inhibition of MMP-1 and MMP-13 with phosphinic acids that exploit binding in the S2 pocket. *Bioorg Med Chem Lett.* 1999;9(2):127–132.

[225]. Reiter LA, Mitchell PG, Martinelli GJ, et al. Phosphinic acid-based MMP-13 inhibitors that spare MMP-1 and MMP-3. *Bioorg Med Chem Lett.* 2003;13(14):2331–2336.

[226]. Breuer E, Salomon CJ, Katz Y, et al. Carbamoylphosphonates, a new class of in vivo active matrix metalloproteinase inhibitors. 1. Alkyl- and cycloalkylcarbamoylphosphonic acids. *J Med Chem.* 2004;47(11):2826–2832.

[227]. Rubino MT, Agamennone M, Campestre C, et al. Biphenyl sulfonylamino methyl bisphosphonic acids as inhibitors of matrix metalloproteinases and bone resorption. *ChemMedChem.* 2011;6(7):1258–1268.

[228]. Tauro M, Laghezza A, Loiodice F, et al. Arylamino methylene bisphosphonate derivatives as bone seeking matrix metalloproteinase inhibitors. *Bioorg Med Chem.* 2013;21(21):6456–6465.

[229]. Beutel B, Daniliuc CG, Riemann B, et al. Fluorinated matrix metalloproteinases inhibitors—Phosphonate based potential probes for positron emission tomography. *Bioorg Med Chem.* 2016;24(4):902–909.

[230]. Laghezza A, Piemontese L, Brunetti L, et al. (2-Aminobenzothiazole)-methyl-1,1-bisphosphonic acids: Targeting matrix metalloproteinase 13 inhibition to the bone. *Pharmaceuticals (Basel).* 2021;14(2):85.

[231]. Campestre C, Agamennone M, Tortorella P, et al. N-Hydroxyurea as zinc binding group in matrix metalloproteinase inhibition: Mode of binding in a complex with MMP-8. *Bioorg Med Chem Lett.* 2006;16(1):20–24.

[232]. Jacobsen JA, Major Jourden JL, Miller MT, et al. To bind zinc or not to bind zinc: An examination of innovative approaches to improved metalloproteinase inhibition. *Biochim Biophys Acta.* 2010;1803(1):72–94.

[233]. Campestre C, Tortorella P, Agamennone M, et al. Peptidyl 3-substituted 1-hydroxyureas as isosteric analogues of succinylhydroxamate MMP inhibitors. *Eur J Med Chem.* 2008;43(5):1008–1014.

[234]. Ledour G, Moroy G, Rouffet M, et al. Introduction of the 4-(4-bromophenyl)benzene-sulfonyl group to hydrazide analogs of Ilomastat leads to potent gelatinase B (MMP-9) inhibitors with improved selectivity. *Bioorg Med Chem.* 2008;16(18):8745–8759.

[235]. Augé F, Hornebeck W, Decarme M, et al. Improved gelatinase a selectivity by novel zinc binding groups containing galardin derivatives. *Bioorg Med Chem Lett.* 2003;13(10):1783–1786.

[236]. Rabinowitz MH, Andrews RC, Becherer JD, et al. Design of selective and soluble inhibitors of tumor necrosis factor-alpha converting enzyme (TACE). *J Med Chem.* 2001;44(24):4252–4267.

[237]. Wada CK, Holms JH, Curtin ML, et al. Phenoxyphenyl sulfone N-formylhydroxylamines (retrohydroxamates) as potent, selective, orally bioavailable matrix metalloproteinase inhibitors. *J Med Chem.* 2002;45(1):219–232.

[238]. De Savi C, Pape A, Cumming JG, et al. The design and synthesis of novel N-hydroxyformamide inhibitors of ADAM-TS4 for the treatment of osteoarthritis. *Bioorg Med Chem Lett.* 2011;21(5):1376–1381.

[239]. De Savi C, Pape A, Sawyer Y, et al. Orally active achiral N-hydroxyformamide inhibitors of ADAM-TS4 (aggrecanase-1) and ADAM-TS5 (aggrecanase-2) for the treatment of osteoarthritis. *Bioorg Med Chem Lett.* 2011;21(11):3301–3306.

[240]. Onaran MB, Comeau AB, Seto CT. Squaric acid-based peptidic inhibitors of matrix metalloprotease-1. *J Org Chem.* 2005;70(26):10792–10802.

[241]. Grams F, Brandstetter H, D'Alò S, et al. Pyrimidine-2,4,6-triones: A new effective and selective class of matrix metalloproteinase inhibitors. *Biol Chem.* 2001;382(8):1277–1285.

[242]. Brandstetter H, Grams F, Glitz D, et al. The 1.8-A crystal structure of a matrix metalloproteinase 8-barbiturate inhibitor complex reveals a previously unobserved mechanism for collagenase substrate recognition. *J Biol Chem.* 2001;276(20):17405–17412.

[243]. Foley LH, Palermo R, Dunten P, et al. Novel 5,5-disubstitutedpyrimidine-2,4,6-t riones as selective MMP inhibitors. *Bioorg Med Chem Lett.* 2001;11(8):969–972.

[244]. Dunten P, Kammlott U, Crowther R, et al. X-ray structure of a novel matrix metalloproteinase inhibitor complexed to stromelysin. *Protein Sci.* 2001;10(5):923–926.

[245]. Blagg JA, Noe MC, Wolf-Gouveia LA, et al. Potent pyrimidinetrione-based inhibitors of MMP-13 with enhanced selectivity over MMP-14. *Bioorg Med Chem Lett.* 2005;15(7):1807–1810.

[246]. Reiter LA, Freeman-Cook KD, Jones CS, et al. Potent, selective pyrimidinetrione-based inhibitors of MMP-13. *Bioorg Med Chem Lett.* 2006;16(22):5822–5826.

[247]. Freeman-Cook KD, Reiter LA, Noe MC, et al. Potent, selective spiropyrrolidine pyrimidinetrione inhibitors of MMP-13. *Bioorg Med Chem Lett.* 2007;17(23):6529–6534.

[248]. Kim SH, Pudzianowski AT, Leavitt KJ, et al. Structure-based design of potent and selective inhibitors of collagenase-3 (MMP-13). *Bioorg Med Chem Lett.* 2005;15(4):1101–1106.

[249]. Nicolotti O, Catto M, Giangreco I, et al. Design, synthesis and biological evaluation of 5-hydroxy, 5-substituted-pyrimidine-2,4,6-triones as potent inhibitors of gelatinases MMP-2 and MMP-9. *Eur J Med Chem.* 2012;58:368–376.

[250]. Schrigten D, Breyholz HJ, Wagner S, et al. A new generation of radiofluorinated pyrimidine-2,4,6-triones as MMP-targeted radiotracers for positron emission tomography. *J Med Chem.* 2012;55(1):223–232.

[251]. Wang J, Radomski MW, Medina C, et al. MMP inhibition by barbiturate homodimers. *Bioorg Med Chem Lett.* 2013;23(2):444–447.

[252]. Erdeljac N, Thiehoff C, Jumde RP, et al. Validating the 1,2-difluoro motif as a hybrid bioisostere of CF_3 and et using matrix metalloproteinases as structural probes. *J Med Chem.* 2020;63(11):6225–6237.

[253]. Reiter LA, Martinelli GJ, Reeves LA, et al. Difluoroketones as inhibitors of matrix metalloprotease-13. *Bioorg Med Chem Lett.* 2000;10(14):1581–1584.

[254]. Li JJ, Nahra J, Johnson AR, et al. Quinazolinones and pyrido[3,4-d]pyrimidin-4-ones as orally active and specific matrix metalloproteinase-13 inhibitors for the treatment of osteoarthritis. *J Med Chem.* 2008;51(4):835–841.

[255]. Schnute ME, O'Brien PM, Nahra J, et al. Discovery of (pyridin-4-yl)-2H-tetrazole as a novel scaffold to identify highly selective matrix metalloproteinase-13 inhibitors for the treatment of osteoarthritis. *Bioorg Med Chem Lett.* 2010;20(2):576–580.

[256]. Ruminski PG, Massa M, Strohbach J, et al. Discovery of N-(4-fluoro-3-methoxybenz yl)-6-(2-(((2S,5R)-5-(hydroxymethyl)-1,4-dioxan-2-yl)methyl)-2H-tetrazol-5-yl)-2 -methylpyrimidine-4-carboxamide. A highly selective and orally bioavailable matrix metalloproteinase-13 inhibitor for the potential treatment of osteoarthritis. *J Med Chem.* 2016;59(1):313–327.

[257]. Heim-Riether A, Taylor SJ, Liang S, et al. Improving potency and selectivity of a new class of non-Zn-chelating MMP-13 inhibitors. *Bioorg Med Chem Lett.* 2009;19(18):5321–5324.

[258]. Gao DA, Xiong Z, Heim-Riether A, et al. SAR studies of non-zinc-chelating MMP-13 inhibitors: Improving selectivity and metabolic stability. *Bioorg Med Chem Lett.* 2010;20(17):5039–5043.

[259]. De Savi C, Morley AD, Ting A, et al. Selective non zinc binding inhibitors of MMP-13. *Bioorg Med Chem Lett.* 2011;21(14):4215–4219.

[260]. De Savi C, Morley AD, Nash I, et al. Lead optimisation of selective non-zinc binding inhibitors of MMP-13. Part 2. *Bioorg Med Chem Lett.* 2012;22(1):271–277.

[261]. Nara H, Sato K, Naito T, et al. Thieno[2,3-d]pyrimidine-2-carboxamides bearing a carboxybenzene group at 5-position: Highly potent, selective, and orally avail-able MMP-13 inhibitors interacting with the S1' binding site. *Bioorg Med Chem.* 2014;22(19):5487–5505.

[262]. Nara H, Sato K, Naito T, et al. Discovery of novel, highly potent, and selective quin-azoline-2-carboxamide-based matrix metalloproteinase (MMP)-13 inhibitors with-out a zinc binding group using a structure-based design approach. *J Med Chem.* 2014;57(21):8886–8902.

[263]. Nara H, Sato K, Kaieda A, et al. Design, synthesis, and biological activity of novel, potent, and highly selective fused pyrimidine-2-carboxamide-4-one-based matrix metalloproteinase (MMP)-13 zinc-binding inhibitors. *Bioorg Med Chem.* 2016;24(23):6149–6165.

[264]. Nara H, Kaieda A, Sato K, et al. Discovery of novel, highly potent, and selective matrix metalloproteinase (MMP)-13 inhibitors with a 1,2,4-triazol-3-yl moiety as a zinc binding group using a structure-based design approach. *J Med Chem.* 2017;60(2):608–626.

[265]. Zhang YM, Fan X, Yang SM, et al. Syntheses and in vitro evaluation of arylsulfone-based MMP inhibitors with heterocycle-derived zinc-binding groups (ZBGs). *Bioorg Med Chem Lett.* 2008;18(1):405–408.

[266]. Zhang YM, Fan X, Chakaravarty D, et al. 1-Hydroxy-2-pyridinone-based MMP inhibitors: Synthesis and biological evaluation for the treatment of ischemic stroke. *Bioorg Med Chem Lett.* 2008;18(1):409–413.

[267]. Wilson LJ, Wang B, Yang SM, et al. Discovery of novel cobactin-T based matrix metalloproteinase inhibitors via a ring closing metathesis strategy. *Bioorg Med Chem Lett.* 2011;21(21):6485–6490.

[268]. Gege C, Bao B, Bluhm H, et al. Discovery and evaluation of a non-Zn chelating, selective matrix metalloproteinase 13 (MMP-13) inhibitor for potential intra-articu-lar treatment of osteoarthritis. *J Med Chem.* 2012;55(2):709–716.

[269]. Deng H, O'Keefe H, Davie CP, et al. Discovery of highly potent and selective small molecule ADAMTS-5 inhibitors that inhibit human cartilage degradation via encoded library technology (ELT). *J Med Chem.* 2012;55(16):7061–7079.

[270]. Johnson AR, Pavlovsky AG, Ortwine DF, et al. Discovery and characterization of a novel inhibitor of matrix metalloprotease-13 that reduces cartilage damage in vivo without joint fibroplasia side effects. *J Biol Chem.* 2007;282(38):27781–27791.

[271]. Engel CK, Pirard B, Schimanski S, et al. Structural basis for the highly selective inhibition of MMP-13. *Chem Biol.* 2005;12(2):181–189.

[272]. Pochetti G, Montanari R, Gege C, et al. Extra binding region induced by non-zinc chelating inhibitors into the S1' subsite of matrix metalloproteinase 8 (MMP-8). *J Med Chem.* 2009;52(4):1040–1049.

[273]. Dublanchet AC, Ducrot P, Andrianjara C, et al. Structure-based design and synthesis of novel non-zinc chelating MMP-12 inhibitors. *Bioorg Med Chem Lett.* 2005;15(16):3787–3790.

[274]. Vidal A, Sabatini M, Rolland-Valognes G, et al. Synthesis and in vitro evaluation of targeted tetracycline derivatives: Effects on inhibition of matrix metalloproteinases. *Bioorg Med Chem.* 2007;15(6):2368–2374.

[275]. Lauer-Fields JL, Minond D, Chase PS, et al. High throughput screening of potentially selective MMP-13 exosite inhibitors utilizing a triple-helical FRET substrate. *Bioorg Med Chem.* 2009;17(3):990–1005.

[276]. Vicini P, Crascì L, Incerti M, et al. Benzisothiazolyliminothiazolidin-4-ones with chondroprotective properties: Searching for potent and selective inhibitors of MMP-13. *ChemMedChem.* 2011;6(7):1199–1202.

[277]. Roth J, Minond D, Darout E, et al. Identification of novel, exosite-binding matrix metalloproteinase-13 inhibitor scaffolds. *Bioorg Med Chem Lett.* 2011;21(23):7180–7184.

[278]. Marques SM, Tuccinardi T, Nuti E, et al. Novel 1-hydroxypiperazine-2,6-diones as new leads in the inhibition of metalloproteinases. *J Med Chem.* 2011;54(24):8289–8298.

[279]. Panico AM, Vicini P, Geronikaki A, et al. Heteroarylimino-4-thiazolidinones as inhibitors of cartilage degradation. *Bioorg Chem.* 2011;39(1):48–52.

[280]. Shengule SR, Loa-Kum-Cheung WL, Parish CR, et al. A one-pot synthesis and biological activity of ageladine A and analogues. *J Med Chem.* 2011;54(7):2492–2503.

[281]. Wang L, Li X, Zhang S, et al. Natural products as a gold mine for selective matrix metalloproteinases inhibitors. *Bioorg Med Chem.* 2012;20(13):4164–4171.

[282]. Casalini F, Fugazza L, Esposito G, et al. Synthesis and preliminary evaluation in tumor bearing mice of new (18)F-labeled arylsulfone matrix metalloproteinase inhibitors as tracers for positron emission tomography. *J Med Chem.* 2013;56(6):2676–2689.

[283]. Lu HB, Wang SH, Li QM, et al. Design, synthesis and evaluation of 6-oxo-1, 6-dihydropyrimidine-2, 5-dicarboxamide derivatives as MMP 13 inhibitors. *Chem Res Chin Univ.* 2013;29(1):67–70.

[284]. Fischer T, Riedl R. Strategic targeting of multiple water-mediated interactions: A concise and rational structure-based design approach to potent and selective MMP-13 inhibitors. *ChemMedChem.* 2013;8(9):1457–1572.

[285]. Crascì L, Vicini P, Incerti M, et al. 2-Benzisothiazolylimino-5-benzylidene-4-thiazolidinones as protective agents against cartilage destruction. *Bioorg Med Chem.* 2015;23(7):1551–1556.

[286]. Lanz J, Riedl R. Merging allosteric and active site binding motifs: De novo generation of target selectivity and potency via natural-product-derived fragments. *ChemMedChem.* 2015;10(3):451–454.

[287]. Agamennone M, Belov DS, Laghezza A, et al. Fragment-based discovery of 5-arylisatin-based inhibitors of matrix metalloproteinases 2 and 13. *ChemMedChem.* 2016;11(17):1892–1898.

[288]. Hugenberg V, Wagner S, Kopka K, et al. Radiolabeled selective matrix metalloproteinase 13 (MMP-13) inhibitors: (Radio)syntheses and in vitro and first in vivo evaluation. *J Med Chem.* 2017;60(1):307–321.

[289]. Choi JY, Fuerst R, Knapinska AM, et al. Structure-based design and synthesis of potent and selective matrix metalloproteinase 13 inhibitors. *J Med Chem.* 2017;60(13):5816–5825.

[290]. Senn N, Ott M, Lanz J, et al. Targeted polypharmacology: Discovery of a highly potent non-hydroxamate dual matrix metalloproteinase (MMP)-10/-13 inhibitor. *J Med Chem.* 2017;60(23):9585–9598.

[291]. Fuerst R, Choi JY, Knapinska AM, et al. Development of matrix metalloproteinase-13 inhibitors - A structure-activity/structure-property relationship study. *Bioorg Med Chem.* 2018;26(18):4984–4995.

[292]. El Ashry ESH, Awad LF, Teleb M, et al. Structure-based design and optimization of pyrimidine- and 1,2,4-triazolo[4,3-a]pyrimidine-based matrix metalloproteinase-10/13 inhibitors via Dimroth rearrangement towards targeted polypharmacology. *Bioorg Chem.* 2020;96:103616.

[293]. Bendele AM, Neelagiri M, Neelagiri V, et al. Development of a selective matrix metalloproteinase 13 (MMP-13) inhibitor for the treatment of osteoarthritis. *Eur J Med Chem.* 2021;224:113666.

[294]. Knapinska AM, Singh C, Drotleff G, et al. Matrix metalloproteinase 13 inhibitors for modulation of osteoclastogenesis: Enhancement of solubility and stability. *ChemMedChem.* 2021;16(7):1133–1142.

5 Gelatinases and Their Inhibitors

Sk. Abdul Amin, Sanjib Das,
Shovanlal Gayen, and Tarun Jha

CONTENTS

ABSTRACT

Gelatinases, also called matrix metalloproteinase-2 (MMP-2) and matrix metallo-proteinase-9 (MMP-9), have been targets of choice for drug development for many years. Therefore, their inhibitors may serve as an important weapon against cancer, neurological conditions, and lung diseases, as well as cardiovascular disease prevention and treatment. In this chapter, the structure, as well as the function of

DOI: 10.1201/9781003303282-7

gelatinases, are discussed. Various gelatinase inhibitors with different zinc-binding groups (ZBGs) and non-zinc binding characters are illustrated. This chapter summarizes potent gelatinase-selective inhibitors. The prime objective is to give an overview and detailed insight into these gelatinase inhibitors to the scientific community to allow further development. This is a part of the continuous efforts toward the identification of potent gelatinase-selective inhibitors. This chapter provides crucial insights to explore inhibitors for future endeavors to speed up drug discovery efforts.

Keywords: Gelatinase; MMP-2; MMP-9; Gelatinase inhibitors

5.1 INTRODUCTION

Matrix metalloproteinase-2 (MMP-2) and matrix metalloproteinase-9 (MMP-9) are two important members of the MMP family. They are collectively called gelatinases: MMP-2 is known as gelatinase-A, and MMP-9 is gelatinase-B. Again, the structures of MMP-2 and MMP-9 are mostly similar to other members of the MMP family. However, regarding the N-terminus of the catalytic domain, gelatinases comprise a unique collagen-binding domain made up of three fibronectin type II tandem repeats [1, 2]. Gelatinases are predominantly liberated by leukocytes, vascular smooth muscle cells, and fibroblasts. In particular, gelatinase-A is released by leukocytes, platelets, monocytes, chondrocytes, endothelial cells, osteoblasts, dermal fibroblasts, and keratinocytes. On the other hand, MMP-9 is secreted by fibroblasts, osteoblasts, polymorphonuclear leucocytes, granulocytes, neutrophils, macrophages, T-cells, keratinocytes, epithelial cells, and dendritic cells [3]. Both are secreted as zymogens, which do not perform any catalytic activity. These zymogens or latent forms of gelatinases are then activated and directed preferentially into inter-spaces of cells and tissues. Active forms of these enzymes digest extracellular matrix (ECM) proteins and modulate cell surface proteins in several physiological and disease conditions [1]. Gelatinase-A is mostly responsible for the digestion of gelatin and type-IV collagen but may also digest other collagens such as type-V collagen, type-VIII collagen, type-X collagen, type-XI collagen, and type-XIV collagens [3]. The collagen degrading ability of MMP-2 is less than that of collagenases. Gelatinase-A degrades collagen in two phases: at first, triple helix collagens are denatured at a particular collagen cleavage sequence, and then, with the help of the fibronectin-like domain degraded collagen or gelatin is digested [1, 3]. Gelatinase-B is also responsible for the digestion of type-IV collagen as well as gelatin. Non-collagenous ECM proteins like elastin, fibronectin, aggrecan, proteoglycan core proteins, laminin, and versican are also substrates of gelatinases [2]. Additionally, several non-matrix proteins, for example, tumor necrosis factor-α (TNF-α), fibroblast growth factor receptor 1 (FGFR1), interleukin-1β (IL-1β), insulin-like growth factor-binding protein-3 and -5 (IGF-BP-3 and -5), and transforming growth factor-β (TGF-β) are found to be activated by gelatinases [1].

MMP-2 and MMP-9 have been highly correlated with tumor invasion, angiogenesis, and metastasis [4–7], particularly in cases of solid tumors such as melanoma [8], gastric cancer [9–11], colorectal cancer [12–14], breast cancer [15–17], lung cancer [18–22], hepatic cancer [23, 24], ovarian cancer [25, 26], prostate cancer [27, 28], and head and neck cancer [29]. Gelatinases are strongly related to solid tumors. However, the association between gelatinases and hematological malignancies has not yet been well studied [30, 31]. Over the last three decades, thousands of matrix metalloproteinase inhibitors (MMPIs) have been synthesized, but unfortunately, only doxycycline hydrate or Periostat® has received approval from the United States Food and Drug Administration (USFDA) for the treatment of periodontal disease [32]. Lack of selectivity as well as off-target adverse effects related to broad spectrum MMPIs, poor pharmacokinetic characters, metabolic instability, and dose-related toxicities such as musculoskeletal syndrome (MSS) are the prime reasons for the failure of MMPIs as anticancer agents in different phases of clinical trials [33]. In the post-era of consecutive failures of more than 50 MMPIs in clinical trial investigations, several pieces of evidence showed that selective gelatinase inhibition is not related to MSS [4, 33, 34]. The major objective of this chapter is to highlight the structure and function of gelatinases and discuss important inhibitors of gelatinases.

5.2 GENERAL STRUCTURE OF GELATINASES

Gelatinases consist of five major domains: (a) signal peptide domain, (b) pro-domain, (c) catalytic domain, (d) fibronectin domain, and (e) hemopexin domain (Figure 5.1).

5.2.1 SIGNAL PEPTIDE DOMAIN

The signal peptide domain (Figure 5.1) is made up of about 17–29 amino acids. These domains are responsible for the secretion of gelatinases outside the cell [35]. Except for MT-MMPs, most of these MMPs are attached to the cell surface by means of a transmembrane domain.

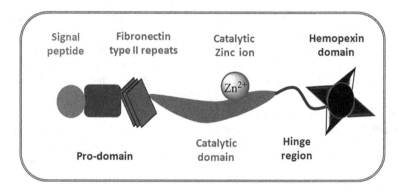

FIGURE 5.1 The domain structure of gelatinases.

5.2.2 PRO-DOMAIN

The pro-domains or pro-peptide domain (Figure 5.1) is made up of about 77–87 amino acids, and the amino acid sequence of the pro-domain of gelatinases is known as PRCGXPD. The pro-peptide domains are responsible for the enzymatic activation of gelatinases as well as other MMPs (except MMP-23) and are also known as "cysteine switch" [35–37]. The cysteine amino acid residue of the pro-peptide domain contains a sulfhydryl group that coordinates with the catalytic Zn^{2+} ion and is involved in the process of enzymatic latency [36–38]. The activities of gelatinases are suppressed due to this zinc-cysteine coordination. This "cysteine switch mechanism" prevents water molecules from attaching to the Zn^{2+} ion, which is necessary for enzyme catalysis [39]. The pro-peptide domain consists of three α chains attached by a flexible loop [40].

5.2.3 CATALYTIC DOMAIN

The catalytic domain contains (Figure 5.1) approximately 170 amino acids. This domain is crucial for the proteolytic activity of the gelatinases [41, 42]. This domain acts through a Zn^{2+}-binding consensus sequence (HEXXHXXGXXH) for its proteolytic activity [43]. The catalytic domain of gelatinases, as well as other MMP subtypes, is crucial for substrate hydrolysis, and structurally this domain is spherical with a diameter of about 40 Å [40, 41]. The catalytic domain comprises two zinc ions. Among these two zinc ions, one is responsible for the catalytic activity, and the other one imparts structural integrity of the domain [39]. Five calcium ions are also responsible for enzyme stability and integrity [44, 45]. The catalytic domain is divided into two subdomains by a shallow catalytic cleft. One is the C-terminal subdomain and another is the N-terminal subdomain [45]. The C-terminal and the N-terminal subdomains are attached to the highly open Ω loop. In the catalytic cleft, Zn^{2+} is coordinated with three histidine residues (His218, His222, His228) as well as a water molecule [45]. The catalytic cleft possesses six binding pockets or binding subsites named S1, S2, S3, S1′, S2′, and S3′ sites. The S1, S2, and S3 subsites are located at the left side of the catalytic Zn^{2+} ion, whereas the S2 and S3 pockets are solvent expounded. On the other hand, S1′, S2′, and S3′ pockets are located on the right side of this Zn^{2+} ion. Importantly, the depth and amino acid sequence of the S1′ pocket alter among various MMP subtypes [46]. Among various MMPs, there are shallow S1′ pocket-containing MMPs (MMP-1 and MMP-7); intermediate S1′ pocket-containing MMPs (MMP-2, MMP-8, MMP-9, MMP-12 and MMP-14); and deep S1′ pocket-containing MMPs (MMP-3, MMP-10 and MMP-13) [47, 48]. Considering the depth and volume of the S1′ pocket matrix, various MMPIs may be designed [49, 50]. The S1′ pocket of both these gelatinases is quite similar in size, and both are also exposed to the solvent. In the case of MMP-9, the residues 425–431 produce a loop that is absent in the case of MMP-2 [46].

5.2.4 FIBRONECTIN DOMAIN

The fibronectin domain (Figure 5.1) comprises three fibronectin type II repeats that is the modulator for collagen recognition. This domain is only specific for gelatinases, and in the case of other MMP subtypes, fibronectin type II repeats are absent. The fibronectin type-II motif may have the ability to bind collagen type-I, collagen type-IV gelatin, and laminin [39, 40, 46].

5.2.5 HEMOPEXIN DOMAIN

The hemopexin domain (Figure 5.1) comprises about 210 amino acids [42]. This domain contains four blades of β-propellers where each blade of the β-propeller consists of an α-helix and four antiparallel β-strands [39, 42]. Usually, chloride and calcium ions are located at the center of the propeller, and four blades of β-propellers are attached through a disulfide bond between the first and fourth blades [39]. The hemopexin domain is not present in MMP-7 (matrilysin 1), MMP-26 (matrilysin 2), and MMP-23. In the case of MMP-9, it plays a valuable role in binding the tissue inhibitor of metalloproteinases (TIMPs) and can interact with substrates like collagen and gelatin. Structurally, MMP-9 is one of the most complex MMPs, which comprises the linker peptide of variable length known as the hinge region [39, 42, 51].

5.3 ROLE OF GELATINASES IN DIFFERENT DISEASES

Much scientific literature has been published about how gelatinases are linked to various pathological events or diseases like cancer, neurodegenerative disorders, cardiovascular disorders, destructive lung diseases, arthritic diseases, and diabetes mellitus (DM) [2, 52, 53].

5.3.1 GELATINASES IN CANCER

Cancer research is currently focused on investigating the underlying functional mechanisms of cell transformation, tumor progression, and metastasis [6]. Cancer metastasis, which involves the migration of cancer cells from the primary tumor to nearby tissues and distant organs, is mediated by complex molecular changes in cell cycle regulation [6]. Emerging evidence suggests that epithelial-mesenchymal transition (EMT) is one of the key underlying functional mechanisms of cancer progression [6]. EMT allows a polarized epithelial cell to undergo multiple biochemical changes that enable it to assume a mesenchymal cell phenotype with the capability of enhanced migration, invasiveness, and elevated resistance to apoptosis [54]. Gelatinases are involved in the biochemical processes that trigger invasion and migration related to cancer cells [6, 55, 56]. Besides this, gelatinases have long been related to angiogenesis, which is another important pathological event in cancer progression [2, 52, 53]. Angiogenesis is the formation of new vasculature from pre-existing blood vessels. The initiation of tumor angiogenesis is required for tumor progression because malignant cells require oxygen and nutrients to survive, proliferate, and reside in close proximity to blood vessels [57]. Gelatinolytic activity develops tumor invasion and metastasis, notably in the case of solid tumors such as cancers of the breast, lung, gastric, hepatic, colorectal, prostate, ovarian, esophageal squamous cell carcinomas, melanoma, thyroid, and head and neck. The evidence available in the literature suggests that gelatinases are strongly associated with solid tumor malignancies. The association between gelatinases and hematological cancers has not been well investigated [2]. Although over 5,000 gelatinase inhibitors have been reported in the ChEMBL database, only a small fraction have been evaluated against leukemia or hematological malignancies [58].

5.3.2 GELATINASES IN NEUROLOGICAL DISORDERS

Neurological disorders are characterized by the functional deterioration of the nervous system due to the death of neurons. In normal physiological conditions, MMP-2 and MMP-9 play vital functions in the central nervous system (CNS), especially in growth and development. Gelatinases take part in important roles in the repairing process of degenerated neurons. In the CNS, they are expressed by neurons, microglia, and astrocytes. Through the activation of microglia, MMP-2 and MMP-9 disrupt the blood-brain barrier (BBB) and play physiopathological roles [59]. Gelatinases function significantly in various neurodegenerative diseases like Alzheimer's disease (AD) and Parkinson's disease (PD) by means of the remodeling of the ECM, disruption of the BBB, and activation of microglia [60]. In the early stages of AD-related pathology, expression of active MMP-2 increases markedly in the entorhinal cortex [61]. Some reports showed that the cerebrospinal fluid (CSF) of patients with AD possess a high MMP-9:TIMP-1 ratio as well as a lower level of TIMP-1 concerning cognitively healthy individuals. This higher ratio of MMP-9:TIMP-1 in AD patients correlates with the T-tau present in the CSF, a biomarker of neuronal degeneration [59, 62]. PD is characterized by the degeneration of dopaminergic neurons and lowered striatal dopamine and intraneuronal protein inclusions in the substantia nigra pars compacta. Several factors have been implicated in the pathogenesis of PD, such as inflammation, oxidative stress, excitotoxicity, mitochondrial dysfunction, the accumulation of misfolded proteins, apoptosis, necrosis, and autophagic degeneration [59]. The overexpression of MMP-2 causes neuronal damage in PD patients [63]. It was observed that activation of MMP-9 triggers cortical neuronal apoptosis during cerebral ischemia [64]. Gelatinases are also associated with the pathogenesis of epilepsy, psychiatric disorders (bipolar disorder, schizophrenia), multiple sclerosis, inflammatory diseases, and addiction [65].

5.3.3 GELATINASES IN CARDIOVASCULAR DISEASES

Gelatinases are associated with the pathogenesis of myocardial infarction, coronary thrombosis, atherosclerosis, and heart failure [66]. MMP-2 is widely distributed in subcellular parts of cardiac myocytes, including the nucleus, and has the ability to cleave the components of contractile apparatus like myosin 1 or troponin I [66]. Some studies reported that MMP-2 is abundantly retained within the cytoplasm [67–69]. MMP-2 takes part in cardiac injury and repair as well as directly impairs ventricular function in the absence of superimposed injury [70]. In the case of ischemia-reperfusion injury (IRI), a lowering in the Ca^{2+} ion sensitivity of myofilaments, as well as subsequent contractile dysfunction, occurs due to the degradation of a set of contractility-related myofilament proteins by MMP-2 [71]. MMP-9 has several potential substrates in cardiovascular disorders, including chemokines, cytokines, fibronectin, elastin, collagen fibers, and several other matricellular proteins. MMP-9 gene polymorphism increases aortic stiffness and the risk for the development of hypertension and the intensity of coronary atherosclerosis [72, 73]. In patients with essential hypertension, increased levels of MMP-9 and TIMP-1 are correlated to increased arterial stiffness [74]. In the preliminary stage, MMP-9 degrades collagen and actively participates in arterial debilitation, which can lead to hypertension [75]. In the case of atherosclerosis, MMP-9 activity is associated with the cleaving of an atherosclerotic plaque, which is formed by type-I, type-III, type-IV, type-V, type-XI, and type-XVI collagens [76]. MMP-9 may be linked to the lowering in the pathogenesis of atherosclerosis by inhibiting fibrin deposition, consequently reducing thrombus size [72]. Serum MMP-9 level is also strongly associated with biomarkers for predicting the risk of myocardial infarction (MI) like fibrinogen, the activity of C-reactive protein, and IL-6 [77]. Through active participation in the process of tissue remodeling and impaired angiogenesis, MMP-9 has been reported to take part in post-MI ventricular remodeling [78]. MMP-2 is produced by smooth muscle cells, whereas MMP-9 is produced by inflammatory cells like macrophages and neutrophils [79, 80]. MMP-2 acts as the primary factor in aneurysm etiology [79]. Increased levels of gelatinases take part in the breakdown of elastin and are crucial reasons for forming aneurysms [81].

5.3.4 GELATINASES IN LUNG DISEASES

Various lung cells like macrophages, epithelium, fibroblasts, and myofibroblasts can express gelatinases. Overexpression of gelatinases causes abnormal remodeling and excessive degradation of ECM present in lung tissue, which results from many respiratory disorders like bronchial asthma, chronic obstructive pulmonary diseases (COPD), and tuberculosis (TB) [82]. COPD is a group of growing inflammatory lung diseases, most frequently seen in the development of emphysema and chronic bronchitis due to the imbalance of protease and anti-protease in the lungs [83]. A significant increment of serum MMP-2 level has been reported in patients with COPD with respect to control groups [84]. In COPD, MMP-9 degrades ECM to enlarge the air space of the lungs [85]. In patients with emphysema, the elevated level of MMP-9 and a higher ratio of MMP-9/TIMP-1 were observed in comparison with other phenotypes [83]. Increased plasma levels of MMP-9, TIMP-1, and TIMP-2 are associated with disease intensity and are the best predictors of emphysema in COPD patients [83]. Gelatinases have been implicated in both acute and chronic asthma. In the case of acute asthma, elevated levels of MMP-9 have been reported in both sputum and bronchoalveolar lavage (BAL) fluid [86]. Increased levels of MMP concentrations, especially MMP-1, MMP -2, MMP -8, and MMP-9, are consistently reported in the sputum, BAL, and pleural fluid of TB patients compared with healthy controls [87]. These increased expressions of MMPs (most significantly MMP-1) are associated with various markers of pulmonary TB disease severity like sputum smear status, radiographic disease extent, and cavitation number [87].

5.3.5 GELATINASES IN ARTHRITIC DISEASES

The irrevocable digestion of the bone, tendon, and cartilage present in synovial joints is a characteristic of rheumatoid arthritis (RA) as well as osteoarthritis (OA) [88]. RA is an autoimmune and chronic inflammatory joint disease. RA is distinguished by hyperplasia of the cartilage and synovium, as well as bone erosion [89]. RA affects several joints throughout the body [88]. The pathogenesis of OA is primarily signaled by extensive degeneration of articular cartilage. OA is the most common type of arthritis that results in the loss of joint function, usually accompanied by severe pain [90]. OA develops from chronic overuse or injury and is prevalent in a small number of joints in comparison with RA [88]. Although MMP-1 and MMP-13 have leading roles in RA and OA, MMP-2 and MMP-9 have also been found to be elevated in RA and OA [88, 90]. The elevated expression of MMP-2 and MMP-9 results in the digestion of non-collagen matrix components of joints in the case of OA [88, 90]. In the case of RA, endogenous MMP-2 or MMP-9 contribute to the survival, proliferation, invasion, and migration of synovial fibroblasts. MMP-9 contributes predominantly by stimulating synovial fibroblast-mediated inflammation and degradation of cartilage. In contrast with MMP-9, MMP-2 inhibits these parameters of RA [89].

5.3.6 GELATINASES IN DIABETES MELLITUS

Hyperglycemia is one of the key features of DM, and its consequences damage the vascular system, nervous system, kidneys, eyes, and cardiovascular system [91]. It is considered a risk factor for cardiovascular diseases (CVD) [92]. Persistent hyperglycemia induces the synthesis of MMP-9 as well as generating oxidative stress (OS) in patients with DM. As a consequence of the generated OS, the expression and activity of MMP-9 are enhanced [93]. In the urine samples of type-1 DM and type-2 DM patients, the concentrations and activity of gelatinases are increased, especially in the case of patients having albuminuria and established renal injury [94]. By increasing extracellular collagen content, MMP-2 significantly involves the pathogenesis of diabetic cardiomyopathy [95]. In diabetes-induced retinal neuropathy and vasculopathy, MMP-9 has a role as an important mediator [96]. MMP-9 is also related to the severity of diabetic retinopathy [97]. In type-1 DM patients, the abnormal expression of MMP-2 and MMP-9 confers microangiopathic and macroangiopathic difficulties where MMP-2 is a prime indicator in the severity of microangiopathy, and MMP-9 is a potential biomarker of macroangiopathy [98].

5.4 INHIBITORS OF GELATINASES

Among different subtypes of MMPs, MMP-2 belongs to the gelatinase subfamily and has been identified as one of the most crucial targets for cancer, while MMP-9 is implicated as an anti-target in the advanced stages of cancer [45, 99–102].

5.4.1 HYDROXAMATE-BASED INHIBITORS

Curtin et al. [103] reported some Cα gem disubstituted succinimide hydroxamates as potential broad-spectrum MMPIs. Many molecules exhibited potent and MMP-2-selective inhibition over MMP-1 and -3. Compound **5.1** (Figure 5.2) was a potent MMP-2 inhibitor (IC_{50} = 2.3 nM), exhibiting high selectivity over MMP-1 and -3. Steinman et al. [104] designed some macrocyclic rings containing succinimide hydroxamates. Compound **5.2** (Figure 5.2) displayed potent MMP-2 inhibition (IC_{50} = 0.1 nM) with at least a 15-fold selectivity over MMP-1, -3, and -7.

Sheppard et al. [105] reported some nonselective broad-spectrum succinyl hydroxamate-based MMPIs. Compound **5.3** (Figure 5.2) was highly potent, but a nonselective MMP inhibitor (IC_{50}: MMP-1 = 0.26 nM, MMP-2 = 0.38 nM, MMP-3 = 1.20 nM and MMP-7 = 0.30 nM). At a 10 mg/kg/oral dose, Compound **5.3** displayed excellent oral bioavailability better than marimastat, the first compound tested in

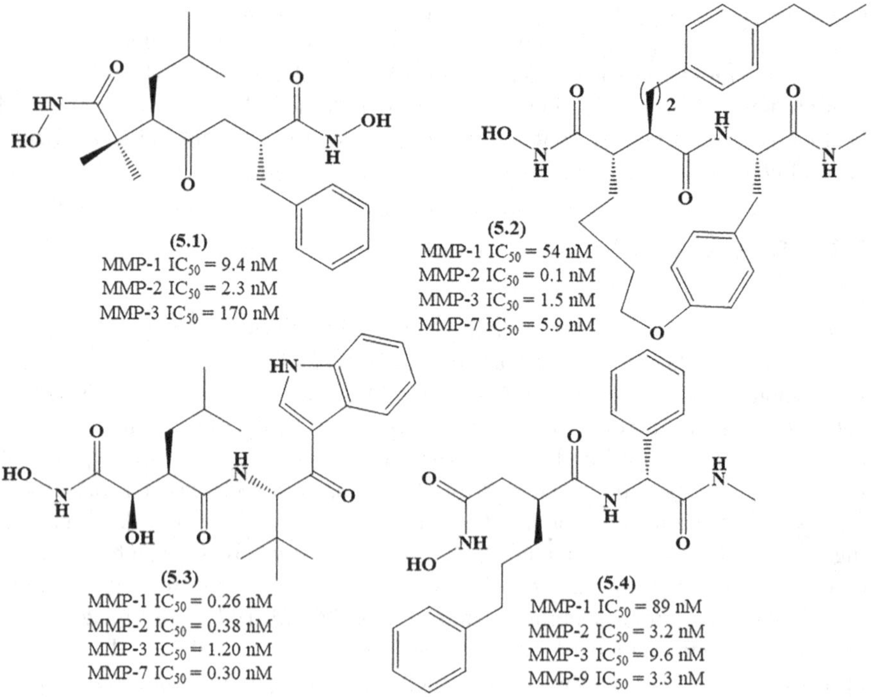

(5.1)
MMP-1 IC_{50} = 9.4 nM
MMP-2 IC_{50} = 2.3 nM
MMP-3 IC_{50} = 170 nM

(5.2)
MMP-1 IC_{50} = 54 nM
MMP-2 IC_{50} = 0.1 nM
MMP-3 IC_{50} = 1.5 nM
MMP-7 IC_{50} = 5.9 nM

(5.3)
MMP-1 IC_{50} = 0.26 nM
MMP-2 IC_{50} = 0.38 nM
MMP-3 IC_{50} = 1.20 nM
MMP-7 IC_{50} = 0.30 nM

(5.4)
MMP-1 IC_{50} = 89 nM
MMP-2 IC_{50} = 3.2 nM
MMP-3 IC_{50} = 9.6 nM
MMP-9 IC_{50} = 3.3 nM

FIGURE 5.2   Hydroxamate-based gelatinase inhibitors (compounds **5.1–5.4**).

the clinical trial. Yamamoto et al. [106] disclosed a set of hydroxamates as potent MMPIs. Compound **5.4** (Figure 5.2) was a potent but nonselective gelatinase inhibitor (IC_{50}: MMP-2 = 3.2 nM, MMP-9 = 3.3 nM) with at least a 2.5-fold selectivity over MMP-1 and -3.

Hanessian et al. [107] synthesized several acyclic sulfonamide-containing hydroxamates showing MMP-9-selective inhibition over MMP-1, -2, -3, and -13. However, Compound **5.5** (Figure 5.3) was a potent MMP-2 inhibitor (IC_{50} = 0.70 nM) bearing higher selectivity over MMP-9 and -13. Almstead et al. [108] reported some arylsulfonamido thiazine and thiazepine-containing hydroxamates as potent and broad-spectrum MMPIs. Compound **5.6** (Figure 5.3) yielded potent MMP-2 inhibition (IC_{50} = 1 nM) with at least a 2.3-fold selectivity over MMP-1, -2, -3, and -13. Cheng et al. [109] designed several arylsulfonamido proline-based hydroxamate derivatives as potent broad-spectrum MMPIs. All these molecules had a higher affinity toward MMP-2 and -13, maintaining greater selectivity over MMP-1, -3, and -7. Compound **5.7** (Figure 5.3) showed potent and nonselective inhibition for MMP-2 and -13 (IC_{50} = 0.2 nM for both) with at least a 25-fold selectivity over other MMPs.

Barta et al. [110] disclosed some arylhydroxamate sulfonamides as effective MMPIs. Most of them showed selective and potent MMP-2 inhibition over MMP-13 sparing MMP-1. Compound **5.8** (Figure 5.3) explored the most efficacious MMP-2 inhibition (IC_{50} = 1.3 nM), having 21-fold selectivity over MMP-13. Natchus et al. [111] reported a set of arylsulfonamido hydroxamates with functionalized 4-amino proline moiety. Compound **5.9** (Figure 5.4) exhibited effective MMP-13 inhibition

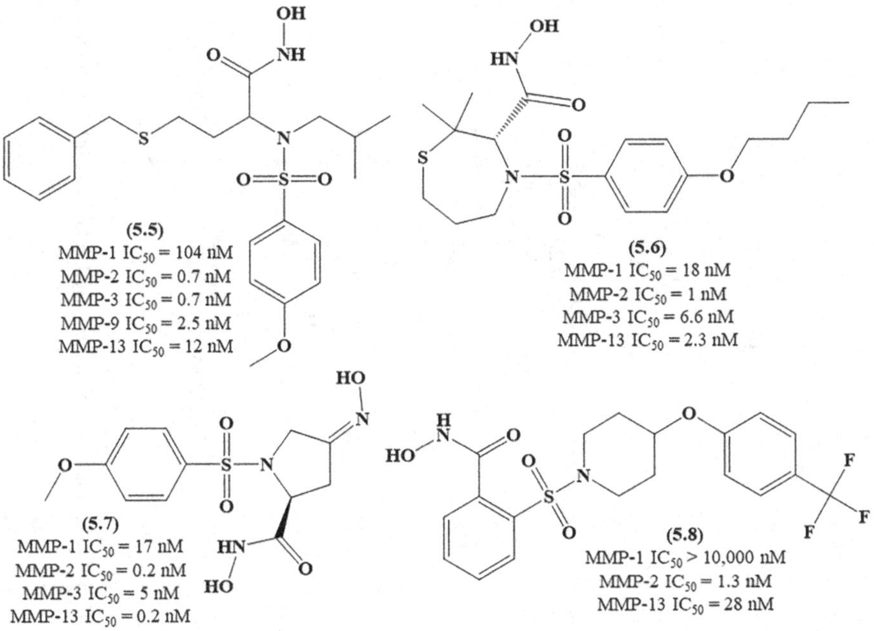

(5.5)
MMP-1 IC_{50} = 104 nM
MMP-2 IC_{50} = 0.7 nM
MMP-3 IC_{50} = 0.7 nM
MMP-9 IC_{50} = 2.5 nM
MMP-13 IC_{50} = 12 nM

(5.6)
MMP-1 IC_{50} = 18 nM
MMP-2 IC_{50} = 1 nM
MMP-3 IC_{50} = 6.6 nM
MMP-13 IC_{50} = 2.3 nM

(5.7)
MMP-1 IC_{50} = 17 nM
MMP-2 IC_{50} = 0.2 nM
MMP-3 IC_{50} = 5 nM
MMP-13 IC_{50} = 0.2 nM

(5.8)
MMP-1 IC_{50} > 10,000 nM
MMP-2 IC_{50} = 1.3 nM
MMP-13 IC_{50} = 28 nM

FIGURE 5.3 Another set of hydroxamate-based gelatinase inhibitors (compounds **5.5–5.8**).

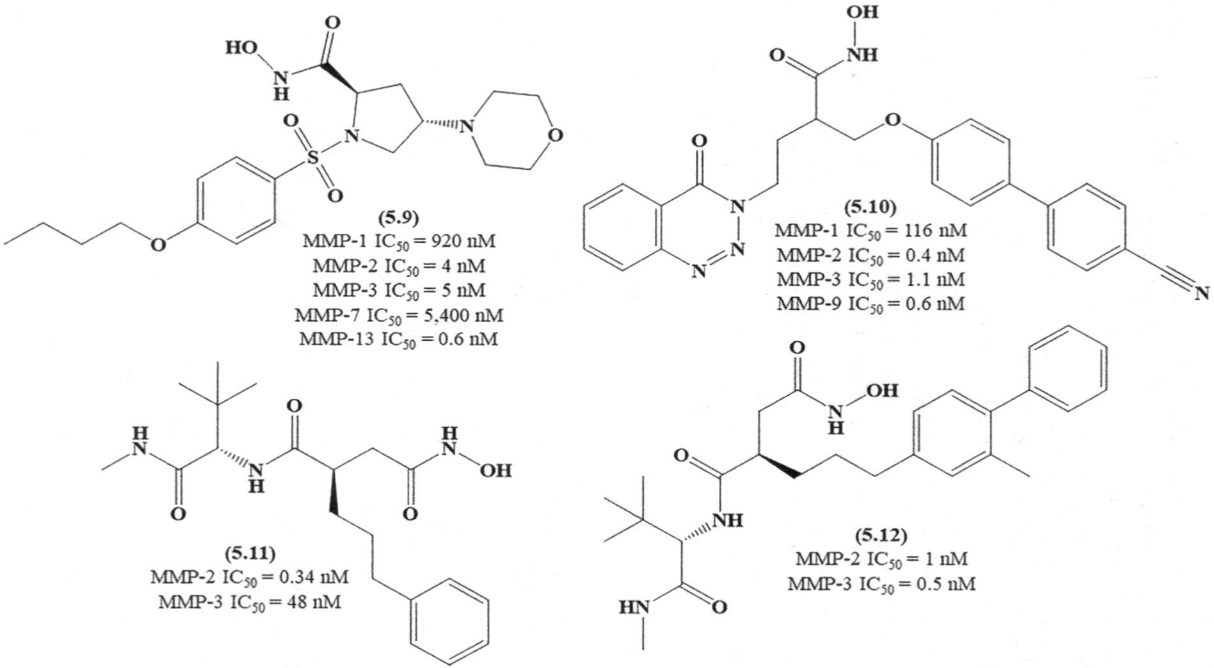

(5.9)
MMP-1 IC$_{50}$ = 920 nM
MMP-2 IC$_{50}$ = 4 nM
MMP-3 IC$_{50}$ = 5 nM
MMP-7 IC$_{50}$ = 5,400 nM
MMP-13 IC$_{50}$ = 0.6 nM

(5.10)
MMP-1 IC$_{50}$ = 116 nM
MMP-2 IC$_{50}$ = 0.4 nM
MMP-3 IC$_{50}$ = 1.1 nM
MMP-9 IC$_{50}$ = 0.6 nM

(5.11)
MMP-2 IC$_{50}$ = 0.34 nM
MMP-3 IC$_{50}$ = 48 nM

(5.12)
MMP-2 IC$_{50}$ = 1 nM
MMP-3 IC$_{50}$ = 0.5 nM

FIGURE 5.4 Various hydroxamate-based gelatinase inhibitors (compounds **5.9–5.12**).

$(IC_{50} = 0.6$ nM) with about seven-fold selectivity over MMP-2 $(IC_{50} = 4$ nM). Some 3-aryloxy propionic acid hydroxamates were found to be potent MMP-2-selective inhibitors [112]. Compound **5.10** (Figure 5.4) showed a higher affinity toward MMP-2 $(IC_{50} = 0.4$ nM) than MMP-3, -9, and -13. Despite the good pharmacokinetic profile, it also displayed a 40% reduction of tumors in the B16F10 melanoma model in mice at 100 mg/kg i.p. dose. Fray et al. [113] reported succinyl hydroxamate potent and MMP-2-selective inhibitors over MMP-3. Compound **5.11** (Figure 5.4) was the most potent MMP-2 inhibitor $(IC_{50} = 0.34$ nM), showing 141-fold selectivity over MMP-3. Fray and Dickinson [114] further disclosed several succinyl hydroxamates as highly effective MMPIs. Compound **5.12** (Figure 5.4) showed maximum MMP-2 inhibitory activity $(IC_{50} = 1$ nM) among these molecules.

Pikul et al. [115] disclosed several aryl sulfonamide-based hydroxamates having 6-oxohexahydropyridine and [1,4] diazepine moieties as potent MMPIs. Compound **5.13** (Figure 5.5) resulted in promising MMP-2 inhibition $(IC_{50} = 1$ nM) and selectivity compared with other MMPs.

Baxter et al. [116] synthesized a set of arylsulfonyl hydroxamates as effective MMPIs. Compound **5.14** (Figure 5.5) provided promising but nonselective MMP-2 inhibition with respect to MMP-8 $(IC_{50} = 3$ nM for both), maintaining greater selectivity over MMP-3 and -9. Apart from marked plasma level concentration at a 3 mg/kg dose, compound **5.14** produced 80% inhibition of B16F10 melanoma in a mouse model better than marimastat.

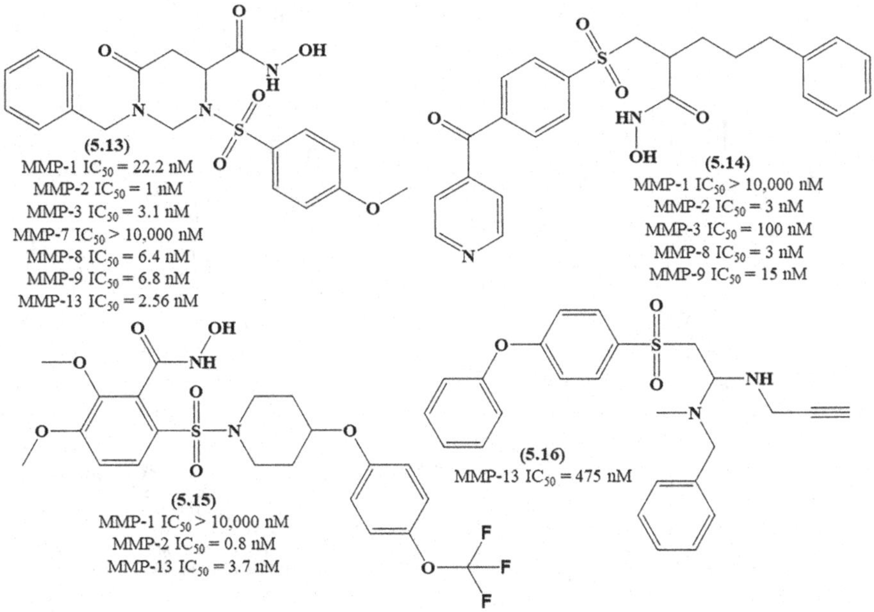

FIGURE 5.5   A set of hydroxamate-based gelatinase inhibitors (compounds **5.13–5.16**).

Some arylhydroxamate sulfonamides were designed as potent and MMP-2-selective inhibitors over MMP-13 [117]. Compound **5.15** (Figure 5.5) displayed promising MMP-2 inhibition ($IC_{50} = 0.8$ nM) with at least a five-fold selectivity over MMP-13 and good pharmacokinetic profiles in rats (Cmax = 5.16 μg/ml, t1/2 = 1.5 hour). A set of α-alkyl-α-amino-β-sulfone hydroxamate derivatives was disclosed as potent inhibitors of MMP-2 and -13 [118]. Compound **5.16** (Figure 5.5) resulted in the maximum MMP-2 inhibition ($IC_{50} = 0.2$ nM) and three-fold selectivity over MMP-13.

Holms et al. [119] explored a set of macrocyclic amide and ketone-based hydroxamates as potent inhibitors of TACE and MMP-1 and -2. Compound **5.17** (Figure 5.6) yielded potent MMP-2 inhibition ($IC_{50} = 0.23$ nM) with greater than 26-fold selectivity over TACE. Hanessian et al. [120] synthesized several arylsulfonyl homocysteine hydroxamates as highly efficacious MMPIs. Most of them exhibited potent and MMP-9-selective inhibition over other MMPs. Compound **5.18** (Figure 5.6) resulted in promising MMP-2 inhibition ($IC_{50} = 0.3$ nM), showing at least a 30-fold better affinity toward MMP-9 ($IC_{50} = 0.01$ nM). A further study conducted by Hanessian et al. [107] resulted in some arylsulfonamido hydroxamates as potential MMPIs. Compound **5.19** (Figure 5.6) yielded maximum MMP-2 inhibition ($IC_{50} = 1.64$ nM) but only a two-fold greater affinity toward MMP-9 ($IC_{50} = 0.9$ nM). Chollet et al. [121] reported some α-substituted 3-bis-arylthio N-hydroxy propionamides as potent MMP-2 inhibitors. Compound **5.20** (Figure 5.6) showed the highest MMP-2 inhibition ($IC_{50} = 0.06$ nM) with at least an eight-fold selectivity over other MMPs.

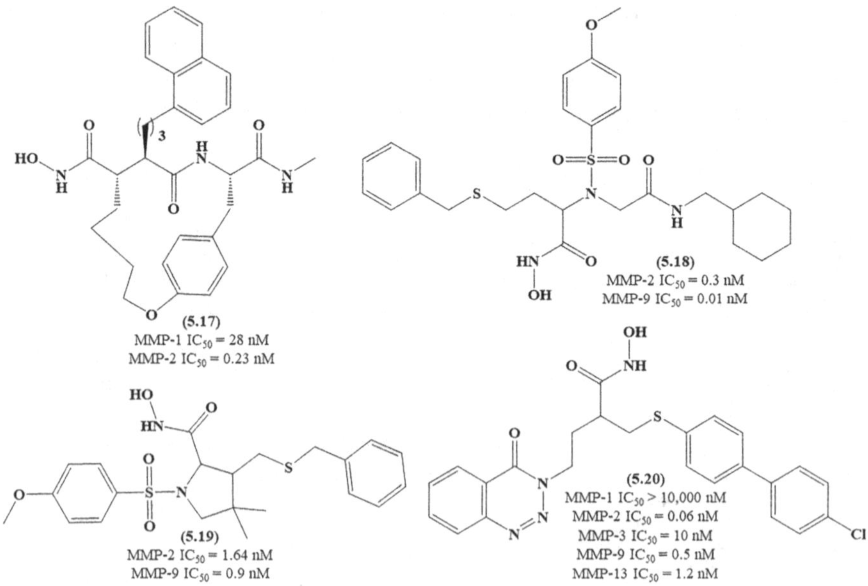

FIGURE 5.6 Another set of hydroxamate-based gelatinase inhibitors (compounds **5.17–5.20**).

Moreover, Compound **5.20** also displayed a 55% tumor reduction at 200 mg/kg i.p. dose in the B16F10 mice melanoma model and a significant reduction in the metastatic stage. It also showed moderate metabolic stability (20%) in human hepatic microsomes and excellent absorption (92%) in the caco-2 cell line monolayer permeability study.

Rossello et al. [122] developed some N-i-propoxy-N-biphenylsulphonyl-aminob utylhydroxamic acid derivatives as potent and MMP-2-selective inhibitors over other MMPs. Among these compounds, Compound **5.21** (Figure 5.7) displayed promising MMP-2 inhibition (IC_{50} = 0.09 nM) with a higher selectivity over other MMPs. Compound **5.21** also reduced the chemoinvasion of HUVEC cells while crossing the matrigel barrier, suggesting its antiangiogenic property. Another study by Rossello et al. [123] further produced several arylsulfonamido hydroxamic acids as MMP-2-selective inhibitors over other MMPs. Compound **5.22** (Figure 5.7) exhibited higher MMP-2 inhibition (IC_{50} = 0.41 nM) with at least a 19-fold selectivity over other MMPs. Becker et al. [124] reported a set of β- and α-piperidine-sulfone hydroxamic acids as potent MMPIs. Compound **5.23** (Figure 5.7) exhibited potent but nonselective MMP inhibition (IC_{50}: MMP-2 =0.33 nM, MMP-13 = 0.40 nM) but higher selectivity compared with other MMPs. At a dose of 50 mpk in the corneal neovascularization mouse model, compound **5.23** reduced 50% of neovascularization, which suggested its promising antiangiogenic activity.

Ikura et al. [125] developed some N-benzyl γ-aminobutyric acid hydroxamates as potent and MMP-2-selective inhibitors. Compound **5.24** (Figure 5.7) displayed maximum MMP-2 inhibition (IC_{50} = 2.9 nM) with 620-fold selectivity over MMP-3. Nakatani et al. [126] again developed a set of N-benzoyl γ-aminobutyric acid hydroxamates as promising MMP-2 inhibitors. Compound **5.25** (Figure 5.7) showed

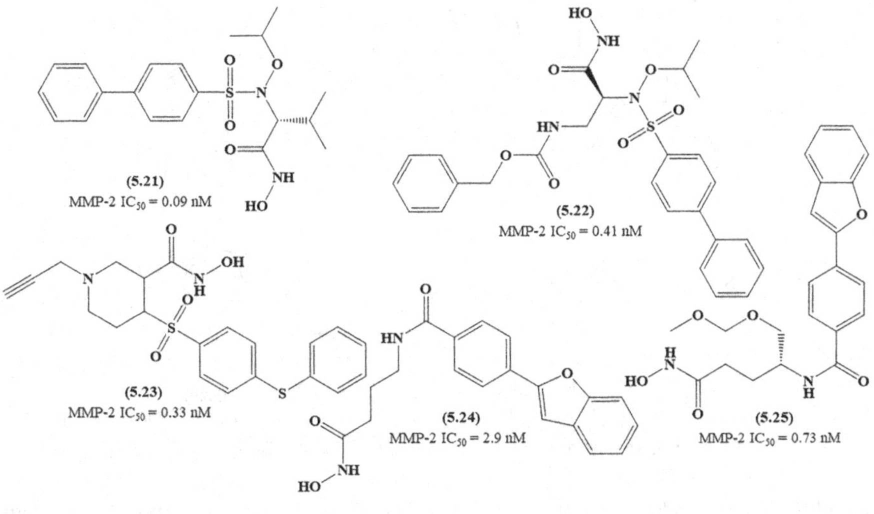

FIGURE 5.7 Hydroxamate-based gelatinase inhibitors (compounds **5.21–5.25**).

maximum MMP-2 inhibition (IC_{50} = 0.73 nM) and higher selectivity over other MMPs.

Yamamoto et al. [127] developed a set of N-phenoxy benzyl γ-aminobutyric acid hydroxamate derivatives. Compound **5.26** (Figure 5.8) displayed efficacious MMP-2 inhibition (IC_{50} = 0.5 nM) with two-fold selectivity over MMP-9. Condon et al. [128] reported some selective TACE inhibitors over MMP-2 and MMP-13. Among them, compound **5.27** (Figure 5.8) displayed effective MMP-2 inhibition (IC_{50} = 4 nM) with more than six-fold selectivity over MMP-13 (IC_{50} = 24.4 nM). Wagner et al. [129] disclosed several arylsulfonamido hydroxamates as potential broad-spectrum MMPIs. Compound **5.28** (Figure 5.8) displayed promising MMP-2 inhibition (IC_{50} = 2 nM) with at least a two-fold selectivity over other MMPs. Yang et al. [130] developed several β-N biaryl ether sulfonamido hydroxamate derivatives as potent and MMP-9-selective inhibitors over MMP-2. Compound **5.29** (Figure 5.8) exhibited effective MMP-9 inhibitory activity (IC_{50} = 2.9 nM) with 3.2-fold selectivity over MMP-2 (IC_{50} = 9.3 nM).

Some N-O-isopropyl sulfonamide-containing hydroxamates were reported by Nuti et al. [131] as highly efficacious MMPIs. Compound **5.30** (Figure 5.9) displayed potent MMP-13 inhibitory activity (IC_{50} = 3 nM) having 3.2-fold selectivity over MMP-2 (IC_{50} = 9.6 nM). Further investigations by Nuti et al. [132] led to the identification of arylsulfone-based hydroxamates as potential MMPIs. Although Compound **5.31** (Figure 5.9) resulted in promising MMP-2 inhibition (IC_{50} = 3.5 nM), it was more selective toward MMP-12 (IC_{50} = 0.20 nM). Some α-sulfone-α-piperidine and α-tetrahydropyranyl hydroxamate derivatives as potential MMPIs were developed

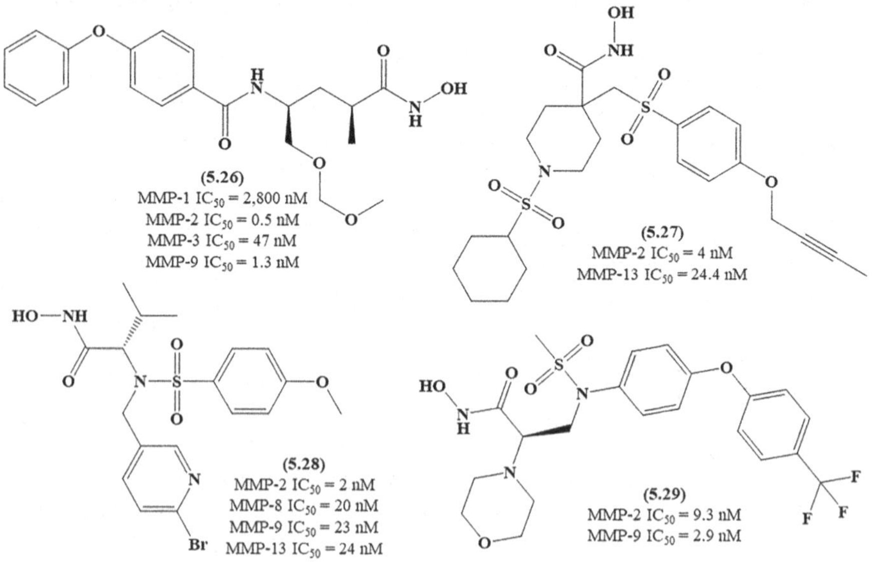

(5.26)
MMP-1 IC_{50} = 2,800 nM
MMP-2 IC_{50} = 0.5 nM
MMP-3 IC_{50} = 47 nM
MMP-9 IC_{50} = 1.3 nM

(5.27)
MMP-2 IC_{50} = 4 nM
MMP-13 IC_{50} = 24.4 nM

(5.28)
MMP-2 IC_{50} = 2 nM
MMP-8 IC_{50} = 20 nM
MMP-9 IC_{50} = 23 nM
MMP-13 IC_{50} = 24 nM

(5.29)
MMP-2 IC_{50} = 9.3 nM
MMP-9 IC_{50} = 2.9 nM

FIGURE 5.8 Another set of hydroxamate-based gelatinase inhibitors (compounds **5.26–5.29**).

by Becker et al. [133]. Compound **5.32** (Figure 5.9) showed potent but nonselective MMP inhibitory activity (IC_{50}: MMP-2 < 0.1 nM, MMP-13 < 0.1 nM). Further investigations by Fobian and co-workers [134] led to the development of α-sulfone hydroxamates as potent MMPIs. Compound **5.33** (Figure 5.9) disclosed promising MMP-2 inhibition (IC_{50} = 0.18 nM), but it was nonselective over MMP-8 and -13. Some (ethyl thiophene) sulfonamide-based hydroxamates were developed as potent MMPIs [135].

Compound **5.34** (Figure 5.10) displayed potent MMP-2 inhibitory activity (IC_{50} = 2.3 nM) with at least a 16.5-fold selectivity over other MMPs. In a dose-dependent manner, Compound **5.34** exhibited 12% cell viability and reduced 42.6% cellular invasion in U87MG glioblastoma cells.

Several α-tetrahydropyranyl-based arylsulfonyl hydroxamate derivatives were disclosed as potent and MMP-2-selective inhibitors over MMP-9 [136]. Compound **5.35** (Figure 5.10) yielded the maximum MMP-2 inhibitory activity (IC_{50} = 0.03 nM), maintaining at least a four-fold selectivity over other MMPs. Hugenberg et al. [137] synthesized several triazole-substituted hydroxamates as efficacious MMPIs. Compound **5.36** (Figure 5.10) displayed highly effective MMP-2 inhibition (IC_{50} = 0.13 nM) but exhibited 21-fold greater selectivity toward MMP-13 (IC_{50} = 0.006 nM). The *in vivo* study suggested that compound **5.36** was a promising MMP-targeted radiotracer for noninvasive positron emission tomography (PET)-imaging for activated MMPs. Fabre et al. [100] designed several triazolyl-containing arylsulfonyl hydroxamate derivatives as potent and gelatinase-selective inhibitors. Compound **5.37** (Figure 5.10) exhibited potent MMP-2 inhibition (IC_{50} = 1.7 nM) and 25.8-fold selectivity over MMP-9. It was also found to exhibit anti-invasive properties in the HT1080 cell line *in vitro* (37% inhibition at 10 μM) and showed effective water solubility and effective caco-2 cellular permeability. A set of γ-fluorinated α-aminocarboxylic and α-aminohydroxamic acid derivatives was synthesized by Behrends et al. [138] as effective gelatinase inhibitors. Compound **5.38** (Figure 5.11) showed promising MMP-2 inhibition (IC_{50} = 2 nM), maintaining 2.3-fold selectivity over MMP-9.

Nuti et al. [139] further disclosed a set of N-isopropoxy-aryl sulfonamide hydroxamates as promising and MMP-2-selective inhibitors. Although compound **5.39** (Figure 5.11) exhibited efficacious MMP-2 inhibition (IC_{50} = 0.67 nM), it had better MMP-9 and MMP-13 inhibitory properties. The *in vitro* study revealed that compound **5.39** also markedly reduced the migration and invasion of HUVEC at lower concentrations (1 nM). Nevertheless, it also interfered with the FBS-induced morphogenesis of HUVEC cells, suggesting its potential antiangiogenic activity dose dependently. Again, the western blot study and gelatin zymography analysis revealed that compound **5.39** was able to inhibit gelatinase. It also exerted effective cytotoxicity and apoptotic ability in endothelial cells. Nevertheless, it also responded well while assessed for the antiangiogenic efficacy *in vivo*, as suggested by the matrigel sponge assay model in mice. Zapico et al. [140] disclosed a set of synthesized arylsulfonamido hydroxamate derivatives as highly efficacious gelatinase inhibitors. Compound **5.40** (Figure 5.11) yielded promising MMP-2 inhibition (IC_{50} = 1.3 nM) and 95-fold selectivity over MMP-9. Sjoli et al. [141] developed several

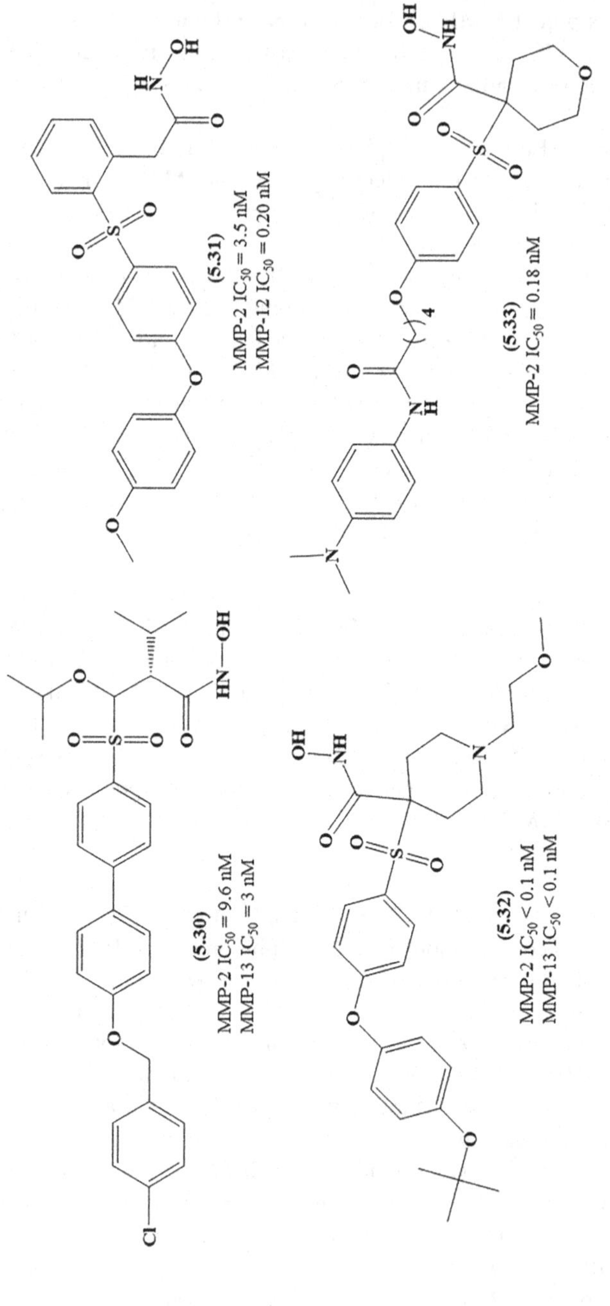

FIGURE 5.9 Various hydroxamate-based gelatinase inhibitors (compounds **5.30**–**5.33**).

(5.31)
MMP-2 IC$_{50}$ = 3.5 nM
MMP-12 IC$_{50}$ = 0.20 nM

(5.33)
MMP-2 IC$_{50}$ = 0.18 nM

(5.30)
MMP-2 IC$_{50}$ = 9.6 nM
MMP-13 IC$_{50}$ = 3 nM

(5.32)
MMP-2 IC$_{50}$ < 0.1 nM
MMP-13 IC$_{50}$ < 0.1 nM

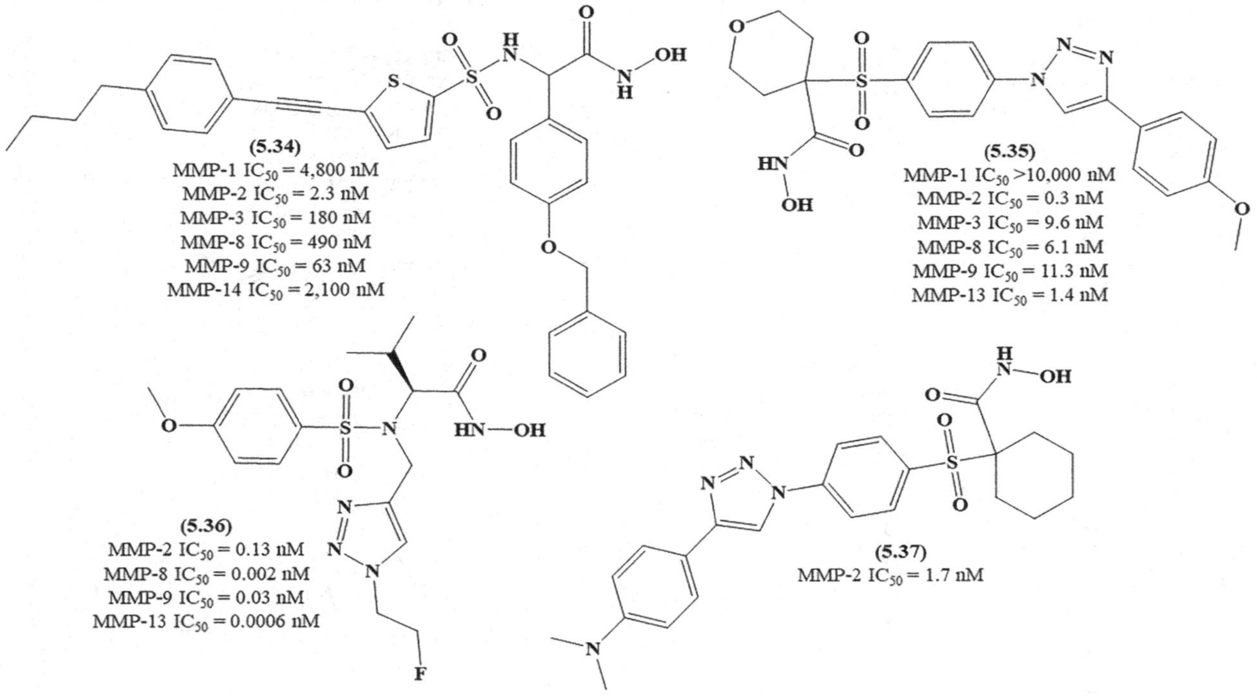

(5.35)
MMP-1 IC$_{50}$ >10,000 nM
MMP-2 IC$_{50}$ = 0.3 nM
MMP-3 IC$_{50}$ = 9.6 nM
MMP-8 IC$_{50}$ = 6.1 nM
MMP-9 IC$_{50}$ = 11.3 nM
MMP-13 IC$_{50}$ = 1.4 nM

(5.37)
MMP-2 IC$_{50}$ = 1.7 nM

(5.34)
MMP-1 IC$_{50}$ = 4,800 nM
MMP-2 IC$_{50}$ = 2.3 nM
MMP-3 IC$_{50}$ = 180 nM
MMP-8 IC$_{50}$ = 490 nM
MMP-9 IC$_{50}$ = 63 nM
MMP-14 IC$_{50}$ = 2,100 nM

(5.36)
MMP-2 IC$_{50}$ = 0.13 nM
MMP-8 IC$_{50}$ = 0.002 nM
MMP-9 IC$_{50}$ = 0.03 nM
MMP-13 IC$_{50}$ = 0.0006 nM

FIGURE 5.10 A set of hydroxamate-based gelatinase inhibitors (compounds **5.34–5.37**).

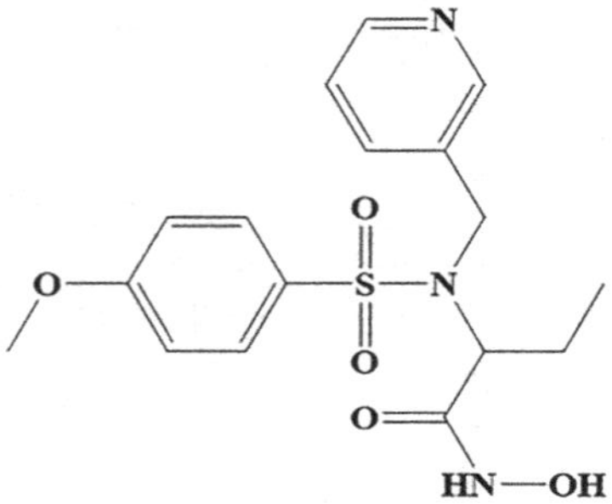

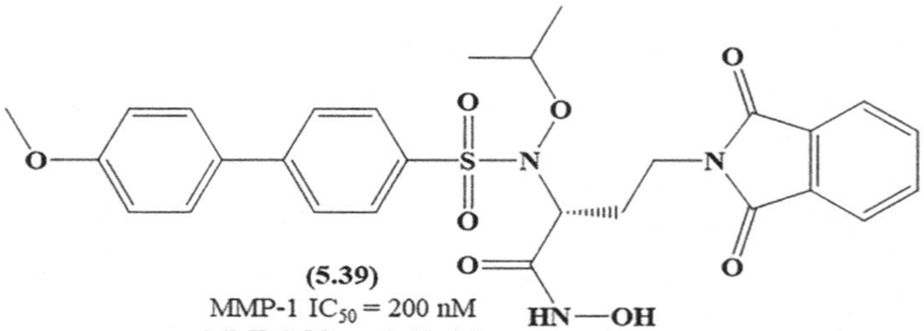

(5.39)

MMP-1 IC$_{50}$ = 200 nM
MMP-2 IC$_{50}$ = 0.67 nM
MMP-3 IC$_{50}$ = 105 nM
MMP-9 IC$_{50}$ = 0.43 nM
MMP-13 IC$_{50}$ = 0.19 nM
MMP-14 IC$_{50}$ = 3.9 nM

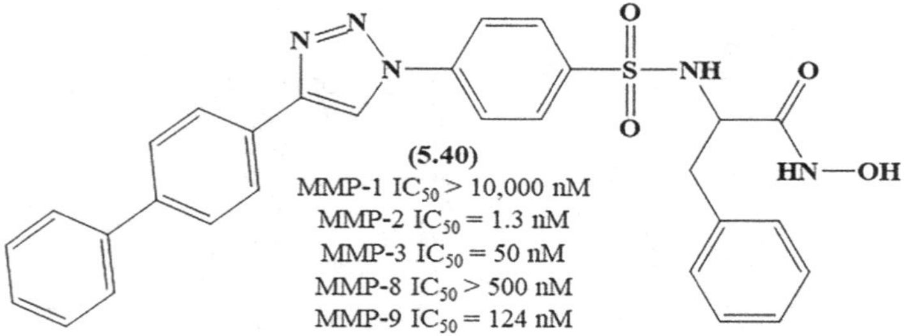

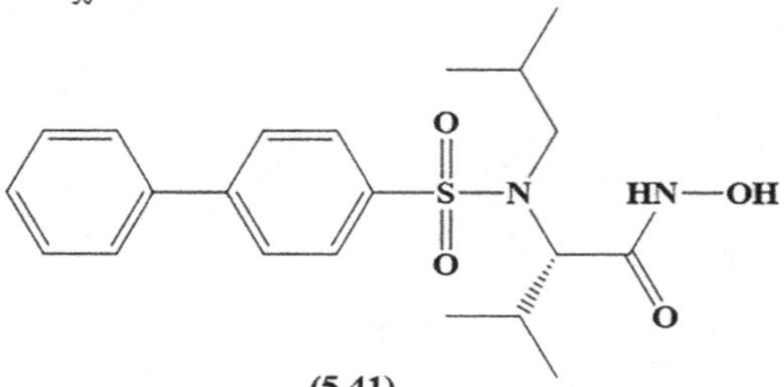

(5.41)

MMP-2 IC$_{50}$ = 0.003 nM
MMP-9 IC$_{50}$ = 0.0053 nM

(5.38)

MMP-2 IC$_{50}$ = 2 nM
MMP-9 IC$_{50}$ = 4.6 nM

(5.40)

MMP-1 IC$_{50}$ > 10,000 nM
MMP-2 IC$_{50}$ = 1.3 nM
MMP-3 IC$_{50}$ = 50 nM
MMP-8 IC$_{50}$ > 500 nM
MMP-9 IC$_{50}$ = 124 nM
MMP-12 IC$_{50}$ = 3.8 nM
MMP-14 IC$_{50}$ = 555.7 nM

FIGURE 5.11 Another set of hydroxamate-based MMP-2 inhibitors (compounds **5.38–5.41**).

hydroxamates as potential gelatinase and ADAM-17 inhibitors. Compound **5.41** (Figure 5.11) yielded potent MMP-2 inhibition (IC_{50} = 0.003 nM), having more than 17.6-fold selectivity over MMP-9.

5.4.2 NON-HYDROXAMATE-BASED INHIBITORS

5.4.2.1 Carboxylic Acid-Based Inhibitors

Kiyama et al. [142] produced several aryl sulfonamide-containing carboxylic acid derivatives as potential and MMP-2-selective inhibitors over MMP-9. Compound **5.42** (Figure 5.12) showed maximum MMP-2 inhibition (IC_{50} = 0.65 nM) among these molecules with selectivity over MMP-9.

Some biphenyl sulfonamide-based carboxylic acids as effective MMPIs were designed and synthesized by O'Brien and co-workers [143]. Compound **5.43** (Figure 5.12) resulted in promising MMP-2 inhibition (IC_{50} = 4 nM), having at least a two-fold selectivity over other MMPs sparing ACE, TACE, and endothelin converting enzyme (ECE). Pikul et al. [144] explored another series of aryl sulfonamide carboxylic acids with piperidine moiety as potent MMPIs. Compound **5.44** (Figure 5.12) produced efficacious MMP-2 inhibition (IC_{50} = 1 nM), bearing a three-fold selectivity over other MMPs. A pharmacokinetics study revealed that compound **5.44** showed good solubility (11.09 mg/ml at pH 7.0) and higher plasma protein binding ability (90.7%). Wu et al. [145] disclosed several biphenylsulfonamido carboxylic acid derivatives containing carboxamide function as highly efficacious MMP-13-selective inhibitors over MMP-2 and -14. Compound **5.45** (Figure 5.12) exhibited potent MMP-13 inhibitory activity (IC_{50} = 1.3 nM) with at least a four-fold selectivity over MMP-2 (IC_{50} = 5 nM). Zhang et al. [146] developed a set of biphenyl-sulfonamido carboxylic acid derivatives as promising gelatinase inhibitors. Most molecules of this set provided potent and MMP-2-selective inhibition over MMP-9. Compound **5.46** (Figure 5.13) yielded promising MMP-2 inhibition (IC_{50} = 1.8 nM) and 7.8-fold selectivity over MMP-9. It also exhibited a good pharmacokinetic profile in rats ($t_{1/2}$ = 1.4 hr, AUC= 18.23 μg h/ml, Vss= 0.4 L/kg, clearance rate = 0.6 ml/min/kg) and good metabolic stability in human liver microsomes (HLM). Li et al. [147] disclosed several biphenylsulfonamido carboxylic acids comprising a 3,4-disubstituted benzofuran scaffold as potent and highly MMP-13-selective inhibitors over MMP-2. Compound **5.47** (Figure 5.13) yielded promising MMP-13 inhibition (IC_{50} = 4 nM) with 145-fold selectivity over MMP-2 (IC_{50} = 581 nM). Selivanova et al. [148] reported some aryl sulfonamide carboxylic acid derivatives comprising indole moiety as effective gelatinase inhibitors. Compound **5.48** (Figure 5.13) displayed efficacious MMP-2 inhibition (IC_{50} = 1.8 nM) comprising four-fold selectivity over MMP-9. The ^{18}F-radiolabeled compound **5.48** was stable metabolically in human plasma as well as in C57BL mice, as suggested by *in vitro* and *in vivo* studies, respectively.

Halder et al. [149] designed and synthesized several L(+)-isoglutamine compounds possessing dual MMP-2 and histone deacetylase 8 (HDAC8) inhibitory properties. Compound **5.49** (Figure 5.13) was the maximum active MMP-2 inhibitor

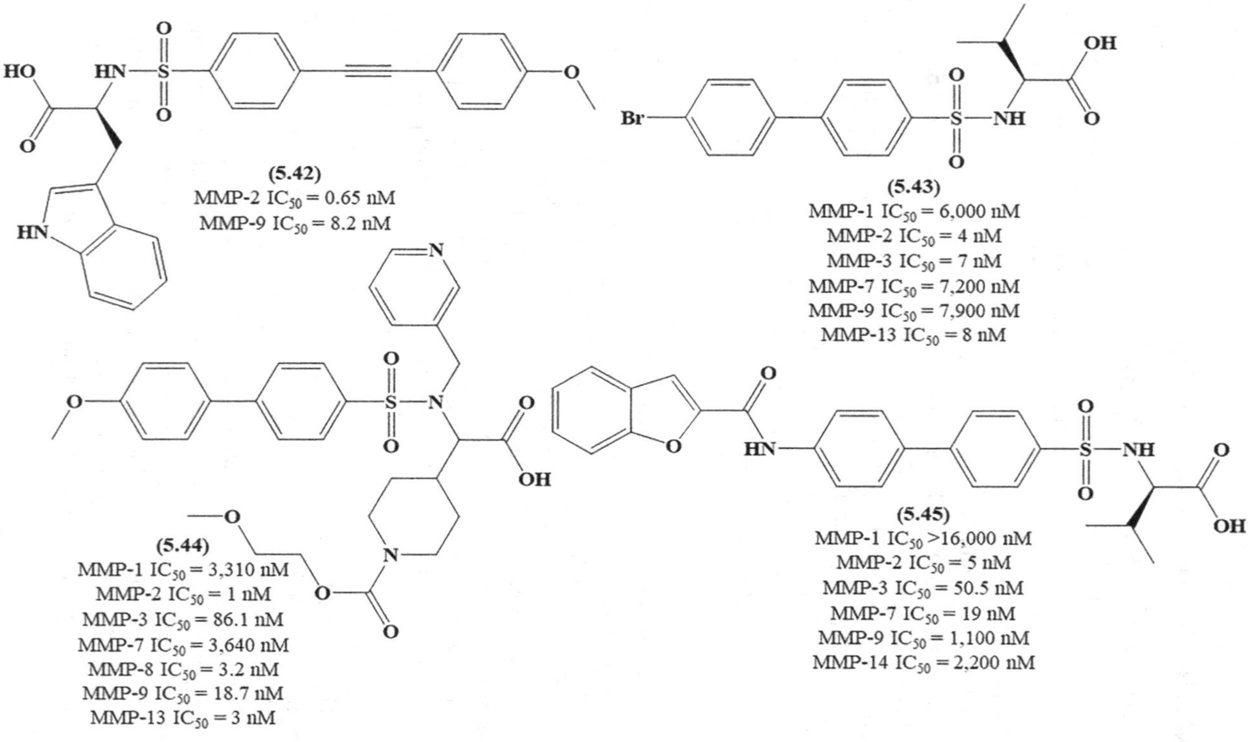

(5.42)
MMP-2 IC_{50} = 0.65 nM
MMP-9 IC_{50} = 8.2 nM

(5.43)
MMP-1 IC_{50} = 6,000 nM
MMP-2 IC_{50} = 4 nM
MMP-3 IC_{50} = 7 nM
MMP-7 IC_{50} = 7,200 nM
MMP-9 IC_{50} = 7,900 nM
MMP-13 IC_{50} = 8 nM

(5.44)
MMP-1 IC_{50} = 3,310 nM
MMP-2 IC_{50} = 1 nM
MMP-3 IC_{50} = 86.1 nM
MMP-7 IC_{50} = 3,640 nM
MMP-8 IC_{50} = 3.2 nM
MMP-9 IC_{50} = 18.7 nM
MMP-13 IC_{50} = 3 nM

(5.45)
MMP-1 IC_{50} >16,000 nM
MMP-2 IC_{50} = 5 nM
MMP-3 IC_{50} = 50.5 nM
MMP-7 IC_{50} = 19 nM
MMP-9 IC_{50} = 1,100 nM
MMP-14 IC_{50} = 2,200 nM

FIGURE 5.12 Carboxylic acid-based MMP-2 inhibitors (compounds **5.42–5.45**).

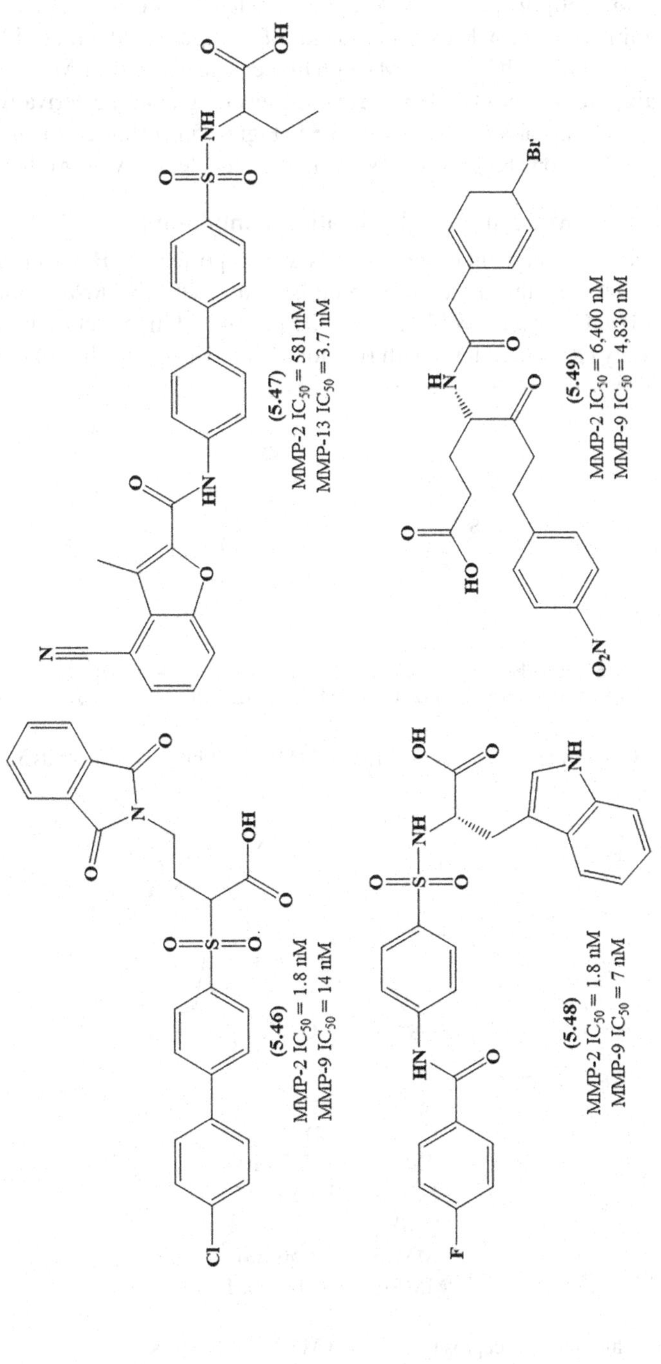

FIGURE 5.13 Several carboxylic acid-based MMP-2 inhibitors (compounds **5.46–5.49**).

(5.46)
MMP-2 IC$_{50}$ = 1.8 nM
MMP-9 IC$_{50}$ = 14 nM

(5.47)
MMP-2 IC$_{50}$ = 581 nM
MMP-13 IC$_{50}$ = 3.7 nM

(5.48)
MMP-2 IC$_{50}$ = 1.8 nM
MMP-9 IC$_{50}$ = 7 nM

(5.49)
MMP-2 IC$_{50}$ = 6,400 nM
MMP-9 IC$_{50}$ = 4,830 nM

(IC_{50} = 6.40 μM) among these compounds, but it exerted better affinity toward MMP-9 (IC_{50} = 4.83 μM).

Adhikari et al. [150] further developed a set of glutamine derivatives and initially screened for inhibitions of MMPs. Compound **5.50** (Figure 5.14) showed the most potent MMP-2 inhibition (IC_{50} = 24 nM) with higher selectivity over MMP-9 (IC_{50} = 492 nM). Again, Mukherjee et al. [151] disclosed several glutamine derivatives comprising good MMP inhibition. Compound **5.51** (Figure 5.14) showed the maximum active MMP-2 inhibition (IC_{50} = 0.21 μM) with higher selectivity over other MMPs.

5.4.2.2 Thiols and Mercaptosulfide Gelatinase Inhibitors

A set of mercaptosulfide-containing MMPIs was reported by Hurst et al. [152]. Maximum inhibitors of this series were promising and selective MMP-2 inhibitors over other MMPs. Compound **5.52** (Figure 5.15) exhibited highly effective MMP-2 inhibitory activity (Ki = 0.28 nM) with two-fold selectivity over other MMPs.

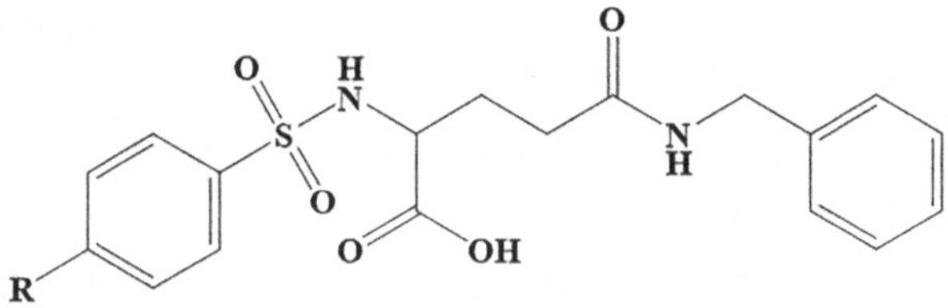

(**5.50**) R = Phenyl, MMP-2 IC_{50} = 24 nM; MMP-9 IC_{50} = 492.60 nM
(**5.51**) R = Nitro, MMP-2 IC_{50} = 210 nM; MMP-9 IC_{50} = 6,370 nM

FIGURE 5.14   Glutamine derivatives as potential MMP-2 inhibitors (compounds **5.50–5.51**).

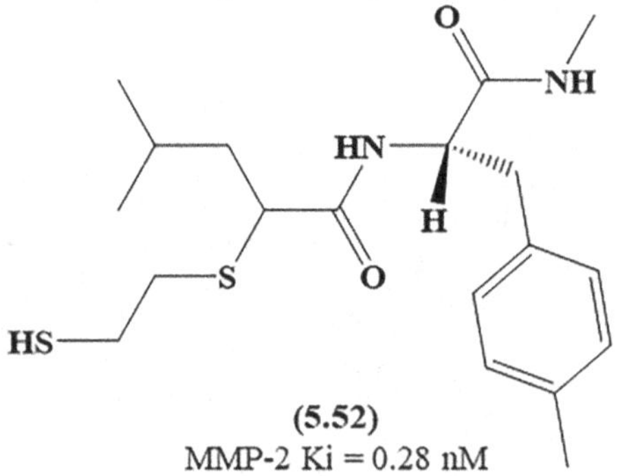

(**5.52**)
MMP-2 Ki = 0.28 nM
MMP-1 Ki = 52 nM
MMP-3 Ki = 250 nM
MMP-7 Ki = 56 nM
MMP-9 Ki = 0.43 nM

FIGURE 5.15   Thiol and mercaptosulfide-based MMP-2 inhibitors.

5.4.2.3 Phosphonate-Based Inhibitors

Caldwell et al. [153] reported some phosphinic acid-derived potential MMPIs. Compound **5.53** (Figure 5.16) resulted in promising but nonselective MMP-2 inhibition (Ki = 2.1 nM) compared with MMP-3 (Ki = 2.5 nM).

A series of α-biphenylsulfonylamido 2-methylpropyl phosphonate derivatives were reported as promising MMP-8-selective inhibitors compared with other MMPs by Biasone et al. [154]. Although compound **5.54** (Figure 5.16) exhibited maximum MMP-2 inhibition (IC_{50} = 0.39 nM), it was found to be nonselective toward MMP-8 (IC_{50} = 0.37 nM) but maintained the higher selectivity over other MMPs.

5.4.2.4 N-Hydroxyformamides-Based Inhibitors

Curtin et al. [155] further explored some biphenyl-ether retro hydroxamates as highly efficacious MMP-2 inhibitors selective over MMP-1. Compound **5.55** (Figure 5.17) resulted in promising MMP-2 inhibition (IC_{50} = 4 nM) with a minimum of ten-fold selectivity over other MMPs.

Compound **5.55** (Figure 5.17) also exhibited good pharmacokinetic properties in rats, dogs, and monkeys. At a 100 mg/kg b.i.d. dose for 21 days, compound **5.55** was found to effectively inhibit tumor growth in a B16 murine melanoma model with a 46% increased lifespan. In combination with paclitaxel, it also showed effective solid tumor inhibition without any major adverse effects. Wada et al. [156] developed a

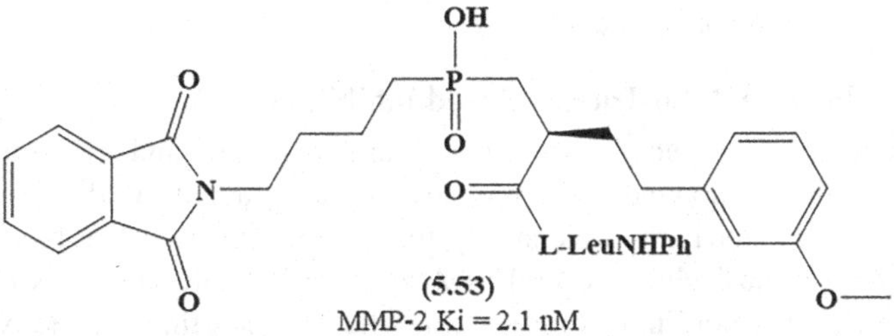

(5.53)
MMP-2 Ki = 2.1 nM
MMP-3 Ki = 2.5 nM

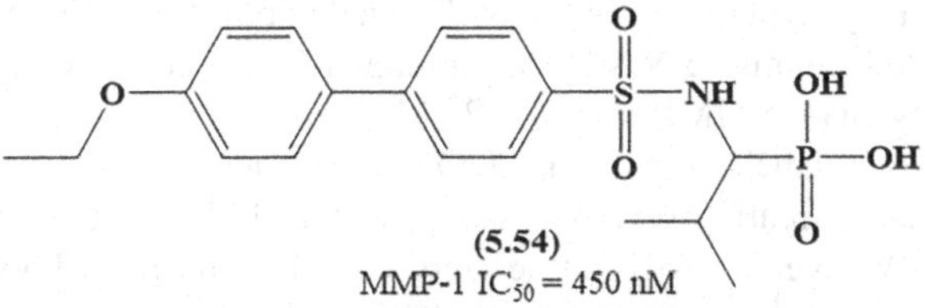

(5.54)
MMP-1 IC_{50} = 450 nM
MMP-2 IC_{50} = 0.39 nM
MMP-3 IC_{50} = 12 nM
MMP-7 IC_{50} = 450 nM
MMP-8 IC_{50} = 0.37 nM
MMP-9 IC_{50} = 0.56 nM
MMP-13 IC_{50} = 1.1 nM

FIGURE 5.16 Phosphonate and carbamoyl phosphonate as potential MMP-2 inhibitors (compounds **5.53–5.54**).

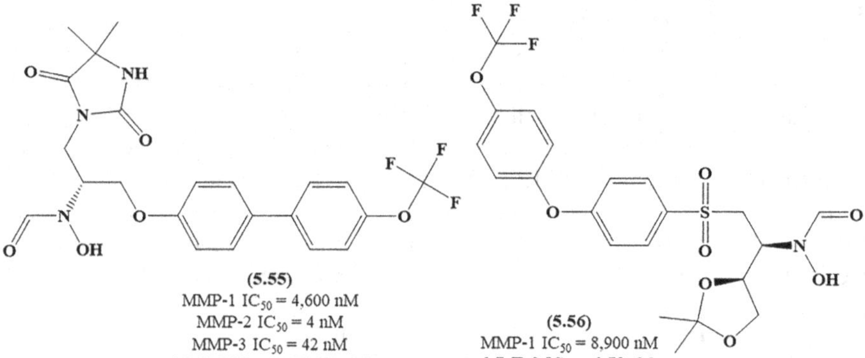

(5.55)
MMP-1 IC_{50} = 4,600 nM
MMP-2 IC_{50} = 4 nM
MMP-3 IC_{50} = 42 nM
MMP-7 IC_{50} = >10,000 nM
MMP-9 IC_{50} = 120 nM

(5.56)
MMP-1 IC_{50} = 8,900 nM
MMP-2 IC_{50} = 0.78 nM
MMP-9 IC_{50} = 0.50 nM

FIGURE 5.17 N-hydroxyformamides as potential MMP-2 inhibitors (compounds **5.55–5.56**).

set of phenoxyphenyl sulfone N-formylhydroxylamines as potential and orally bioavailable MMPIs. Compound **5.56** (Figure 5.17) was found to be a promising but nonselective MMP-2 inhibitor (IC_{50} = 0.78 nM) over MMP-9 (IC_{50} = 0.50 nM). At 3 mg/kg dose, it exhibited a good pharmacokinetic profile in cynomolgus monkeys ($t_{1/2}$ = 16.8 hr, AUC = 53 μM h/L). It also inhibited 48% of tumor growth in the murine synergistic B16 melanoma model.

5.4.2.5 Pyrimidine-2,4,6-Triones-Based Inhibitors

Among the nitrogen-based ZBGs, pyrimidine-2,4,6-trione and pyrimidine dione-thione-containing compounds were most extensively studied. As this class of compounds belonged to the barbiturate family, the metabolism, as well as bioavailability, were analyzed extensively in several FDA-approved barbiturate drugs [157]. Such types of inhibitors coordinate with the catalytic Zn^{2+} ion through the N3 atom of the barbiturate scaffold [158–159]. Several C-5 disubstituted barbiturates were disclosed as efficacious gelatinase inhibitors by Breyholz et al. [160]. Compound **5.57** (Figure 5.18) exerted promising MMP-2 inhibition (IC_{50} = 7 nM), comprising 3.5-fold greater activity against MMP-9 (IC_{50} = 2 nM).

Again, the ^{125}I-radiolabeled compound **5.57** was an effective radio-imaging tool that was efficacious in treating several diseases such as inflammation, atherosclerosis, and cancer. Wang et al. [161] synthesized several N-substituted homopiperazine barbiturate derivatives as promising gelatinase inhibitors. Compound **5.58** (Figure 5.18) produced promising MMP-2 inhibition (IC_{50} = 1.9 nM) with four-fold selectivity over MMP-9. It also effectively inhibited Caco-2 cellular invasion.

5.5 SUMMARY

Gelatinases exert crucial implications in tumorigenesis, angiogenesis, and apoptosis in various cancer conditions. It can be assumed that gelatinases may possess an

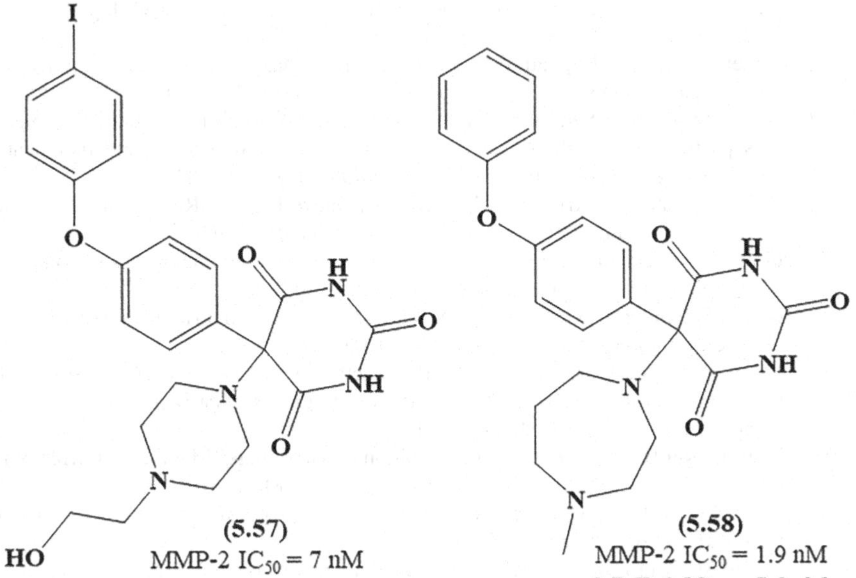

(5.57)
MMP-2 IC_{50} = 7 nM
MMP-9 IC_{50} = 2 nM

(5.58)
MMP-2 IC_{50} = 1.9 nM
MMP-9 IC_{50} = 7.5 nM

FIGURE 5.18 Pyrimidinetriones as potential MMP-2 inhibitors (compounds **5.57–5.58**).

indirect function in tumor progression. Thus, gelatinase inhibitors may be considered for targeting to be an efficacious remedy for the management of cancer as well as other related diseases. This chapter dealt with the structure of gelatinases and the potent gelatinase-selective inhibitors reported over past decades; these include hydroxamates and non-hydroxamates. The prime objective was to provide an outline of the gelatinase inhibitors to the scientific community to aid in further development processes. Identification of zinc-binding characters is a regulating factor to achieve gelatinase inhibitory efficacy. Hydrophobic and electrostatic properties of the S1′ pocket should also be considered to enhance gelatinase selectivity. Since the S1′ pocket shares vivid variability among various MMPs, the design of gelatinases inhibitors approaching this S1′ pocket may lead to excellent outcomes. This chapter may help in the development of potent gelatinase-selective inhibitors and ideas for designing target-specific gelatinase inhibitors. The gelatinase inhibitors discussed in this chapter may be utilized further in different rational drug-design strategies for newer effective and selective gelatinase inhibitors.

REFERENCES

[1]. Cui N, Hu M, Khalil RA. Biochemical and biological attributes of matrix metalloproteinases. *Prog Mol Biol Transl Sci.* 2017;147:1–73.

[2]. Das S, Amin SA, Jha T. Inhibitors of gelatinases (MMP-2 and MMP-9) for the management of hematological malignancies. *Eur J Med Chem.* 2021;223:113623.

[3]. Laronha H, Caldeira J. Structure and function of human matrix metalloproteinases. *Cells.* 2020;9(5):1076.

[4]. Winer A, Adams S, Mignatti P. Matrix metalloproteinase inhibitors in cancer therapy: Turning past failures into future successes. *Mol Cancer Ther.* 2018;17:1147–1155.

[5]. Gonzalez-Avila G, Sommer B, Mendoza-Posada DA, et al. Matrix metalloproteinases participation in the metastatic process and their diagnostic and therapeutic applications in cancer. *Crit Rev Oncol Hematol.* 2019;137:57–83.

[6]. Quintero-Fabián S, Arreola R, Becerril-Villanueva E, et al. Role of matrix metalloproteinases in angiogenesis and cancer. *Front Oncol.* 2019;9:1370.

[7]. Fields GB. Mechanisms of action of novel drugs targeting angiogenesis-promoting matrix metalloproteinases. *Front Immunol.* 2019;10:1278.

[8]. Napoli S, Scuderi C, Gattuso G, et al. Functional roles of matrix metalloproteinases and their inhibitors in melanoma. *Cells.* 2020;9:1151.

[9]. Yao Z, Yuan T, Wang H, et al. MMP-2 together with MMP-9 overexpression correlated with lymph node metastasis and poor prognosis in early gastric carcinoma. *Tumour Biol.* 2017;39:1010428317700411.

[10]. Zhao L, Niu H, Liu Y, et al. LOX inhibition downregulates MMP-2 and MMP-9 in gastric cancer tissues and cells. *J Cancer.* 2019;10:6481–6490.

[11]. Li J, Ma JM. Research progress in matrix metalloproteinase-2,9 in gastric cancer. *Chin Cancer.* 2015;24:403–407.

[12]. Heslin MJ, Yan J, Johnson MR, et al. Role of matrix metalloproteinases in colorectal carcinogenesis. *Ann Surg.* 2001;233:786–792.

[13]. Zucker S, Vacirca J. Role of matrix metalloproteinases (MMPs) in colorectal cancer. *Cancer Metastasis Rev.* 2004;23:101–117.

[14]. Langers AMJ, Verspaget HW, Hawinkels LJAC, et al. MMP-2 and MMP-9 in normal mucosa are independently associated with outcome of colorectal cancer patients. *Br J Cancer.* 2012;106:1495–1498.

[15]. Majumder A, Ray S, Banerji A. Epidermal growth factor receptor-mediated regulation of matrix metalloproteinase-2 and matrix metalloproteinase-9 in MCF-7 breast cancer cells. *Mol Cell Biochem.* 2019;452:111–121.

[16]. Pelekanou V, Villarroel-Espindola F, Schalper KA, et al. CD68, CD163, and matrix metalloproteinase 9 (MMP-9) co-localization in breast tumour microenvironment predicts survival differently in ER-positive and negative cancers. *Breast Cancer Res.* 2018;20:154.

[17]. Jung O, Lee J, Lee YJ, et al. Timosaponin AIII inhibits migration and invasion of A549 human non-small-cell lung cancer cells via attenuations of MMP-2 and MMP-9 by inhibitions of ERK1/2, Src/FAK and β-catenin signaling pathways. *Bioorg Med Chem Lett.* 2016;26:3963–3967.

[18]. Li Y, Yang F, Zheng W, et al. Punica granatum (pomegranate) leaves extract induces apoptosis through mitochondrial intrinsic pathway and inhibits migration and invasion in non-small cell lung cancer in vitro. *Biomed Pharmacother.* 2016;80:227–235.

[19]. Poudel B, Ki HH, Luyen BT, et al. Triticumoside induces apoptosis via caspase-dependent mitochondrial pathway and inhibits migration through downregulation of MMP-2/9 in human lung cancer cells. *Acta Biochim Biophys Sin (Shanghai).* 2016;48:153–160.

[20]. Zhao HJ, Liu T, Mao X, et al. Fructus phyllanthi tannin fraction induces apoptosis and inhibits migration and invasion of human lung squamous carcinoma cells in vitro via MAPK/MMP pathways. *Acta Pharmacol Sin.* 2015;36:758–768.

[21]. Adhikari N, Halder AK, Mallick S, et al. Robust design of some selective matrix metalloproteinase-2 inhibitors over matrix metalloproteinase-9 through in silico/fragment-based lead identification and de novo lead modification: Syntheses and biological assays. *Bioorg Med Chem.* 2016;24:4291–4309.

[22]. Shih YW, Chien ST, Chen PS, et al. Alpha-mangostin suppresses phorbol 12-myristate 13-acetate-induced MMP-2/MMP-9 expressions via alphavbeta3 integrin/FAK/ERK and NF-kappaB signaling pathway in human lung adenocarcinoma A549 cells. *Cell Biochem Biophys*. 2010;58:31–44.

[23]. Chen G, Qin GH, Dang YW, et al. The prospective role of matrix metalloproteinase-2/9 and transforming growth factor beta 1 in accelerating the progression of hepatocellular carcinoma. *Cancer Res*. 2017;6:S229–S231.

[24]. Daniele A, Abbate I, Oakley C, et al. Clinical and prognostic role of matrix metalloproteinase-2, -9 and their inhibitors in breast cancer and liver diseases: A review. *Int J Biochem Cell Biol*. 2016;77:91–101.

[25]. Sakata K, Shigemasa K, Nagai N, et al. Expression of matrix metalloproteinases (MMP-2, MMP-9, MT1-MMP) and their inhibitors (TIMP-1, TIMP-2) in common epithelial tumours of the ovary. *Int J Oncol*. 2000;17:673–681.

[26]. Hu X, Li L, Li DR, et al. Expression of matrix metalloproteinases-9,2,7,and tissue inhibitor of metalloproteinases-1,2,3 mRNA in ovarian tumours and their clinical significance. *Ai Zheng*. 2004;23:1194–1198.

[27]. Brehmer B, Biesterfeld S, Jakse G. Expression of matrix metalloproteinases (MMP-2 and -9) and their inhibitors (TIMP-1 and -2) in prostate cancer tissue. *Prostate Cancer Prostatic Dis*. 2003;6:217–222.

[28]. Gong Y, Chippada-Venkata UD, Oh WK. Roles of matrix metalloproteinases and their natural inhibitors in prostate cancer progression. *Cancers (Basel)* 2014;6: 1298–1327.

[29]. Pietruszewska W, Bojanowska-Poźniak K, Kobos J. Matrix metalloproteinases MMP-1, MMP-2, MMP-9 and their tissue inhibitors TIMP1, TIMP2, TIMP3 in head and neck cancer: An immunohistochemical study. *Otolaryngol Pol*. 2016;70:32–43.

[30]. Chaudhary AK, Pandya S, Ghosh K, et al. Matrix metalloproteinase and its drug targets therapy in solid and hematological malignancies: An overview. *Mutat Res*. 2013;753:7–23.

[31]. Amin SA, Adhikari N, Jha T. Is dual inhibition of metalloenzymes HDAC-8 and MMP-2 a potential pharmacological target to combat hematological malignancies? *Pharmacol Res*. 2017;122:8–19.

[32]. Li K, Tay FR, Yiu CKY. The past, present and future perspectives of matrix metalloproteinase inhibitors. *Pharmacol Ther*. 2020;207:107465.

[33]. Fields GB. The rebirth of matrix metalloproteinase inhibitors: Moving beyond the dogma. *Cells*. 2019;8:984.

[34]. Razai AS, Eckelman BP, Salvesen GS. Selective inhibition of matrix metalloproteinase 10 (MMP-10) with a single-domain antibody. *J Biol Chem*. 2020;295:2464–2472.

[35]. Travascio F (Ed.). (2017). *The Role of Matrix Metalloproteinase in Human Body Pathologies*. IntechOpen. https://doi.org/10.5772/66560.

[36]. Sela-Passwell N, Rosenblum G, Shoham T, et al. Structural and functional bases for allosteric control of MMP activities: Can it pave the path for selective inhibition? *Biochim Biophys Acta*. 2010;1803:29–38.

[37]. Van Wart HE, Birkedal-Hansen H. The cysteine switch: A principle of regulation of metalloproteinase activity with potential applicability to the entire matrix metalloproteinase gene family. *Proc Natl Acad Sci USA*. 1990;87:5578–5582.

[38]. Fischer T, Senn N, Riedl R. Design and structural evolution of matrix metalloproteinase inhibitors. *Chemistry*. 2019;25(34):7960–7980.

[39]. Nagase H, Visse R, Murphy G. Structure and function of matrix metalloproteinases and TIMPs. *Cardiovas Res*. 2006;69:562–573.

[40]. Cathcart J, Pulkoski-Gross A, Cao J. Targeting matrix metalloproteinases in cancer: Bringing new life to old disease. *Genes Dis*. 2015;2:26–34.

[41]. Klein G, Vellenge E, Fraaije MW, et al. The possible role of matrix metalloproteinase (MMP)-2 and MMP-9 in cancer, e.g. acute leukemia. *Crit Rev Oncol Hematol.* 2004;50:87–100.

[42]. Nagase H, Woessner F. Matrix metalloproteinases. *J Biol Chem.* 1999;274:21491–21494.

[43]. Itoh Y. Membrane-type matrix metalloproteinases: Their functions and regulations. *Matrix Biol.* 2015;46:207–223. https://www.intechopen.com/books/the-role-of-matrix-metalloproteinase-in-human-body-pathologies/overview-of-mmp-biology-and-gene-associations-in-human-diseases (Accessed 15 November 2022).

[44]. Travascio F. *The Role of Matrix Metalloproteinase in Human Body Pathologies.* 2017. IntechOpen. Available at: https://www.intechopen.com/books/5986.

[45]. Adhikari N, Mukherjee A, Saha A, et al. Arylsulfonamide and selectivity of matrix metalloproteinase-2: An overview. *Eur J Med Chem.* 2017;129:72–109.

[46]. Jacobsen JA, Jourden JLM, Miller MT, et al. Cohen To bind zinc or not to bind zinc: An examination of innovative approaches to improved metalloproteinase inhibition. *Biochim Byophys Acta.* 2010;1803:72–94.

[47]. Adhikari N, Amin SA, Jha T. Collagenases and gelatinases and their inhibitors as anticancer agents. In: SP Gupta (Ed.), *Cancer Leading Proteases.* Elsevier, 2020, 265–294.

[48]. Gimeno A, Beltrán-Debón R, Mulero M, et al. Garcia-Vallvé Understanding the variability of the S1' pocket to improve matrix metalloproteinase inhibitor selectivity profiles. *Drug Discov Today.* 2020;25:38–57.

[49]. Rao BG. Recent developments in the design of specific matrix metalloproteinase inhibitors aided by structural and computational studies. *Curr Pharma Des.* 2005;11:295–322.

[50]. Zhang C, Kim SK. Matrix metalloproteinase inhibitors (MMPIs) from marine natural products: The current situation and future prospects. *Mar Drugs.* 2009;7:71–84.

[51]. Huang H. Matrix metalloproteinase-9 (MMP-9) as a cancer biomarker and MMP-9 biosensors: Recent advances. *Sensors.* 2018;18:3249.

[52]. Das S, Amin SA, Jha T. Insight into the structural requirement of aryl sulphonamide based gelatinases (MMP-2 and MMP-9) inhibitors - Part I: 2D-QSAR, 3D-QSAR topomer CoMFA and Naïve Bayes studies - First report of 3D-QSAR Topomer CoMFA analysis for MMP-9 inhibitors and jointly inhibitors of gelatinases together. *SAR QSAR Environ Res.* 2021;32(8):655–687.

[53]. Das S, Amin SA, Gayen S, et al. Insight into the structural requirements of gelatinases (MMP-2 and MMP-9) inhibitors by multiple validated molecular modelling approaches: Part II. *SAR QSAR Environ Res.* 2022;33(3):167–192.

[54]. Kalluri R, Weinberg RA. The basics of epithelial-mesenchymal transition [published correction appears in J Clin Invest. 2010 May 3;120(5):1786]. *J Clin Invest.* 2009;119(6):1420–1428.

[55]. Li Y, He J, Wang F, et al. Role of MMP-9 in epithelial-mesenchymal transition of thyroid cancer. *World J Surg Oncol.* 2020;18(1):181.

[56]. Li S, Luo W. Matrix metalloproteinase 2 contributes to aggressive phenotype, epithelial-mesenchymal transition and poor outcome in nasopharyngeal carcinoma. *Onco Targets Ther.* 2019;12:5701–5711.

[57]. Lugano R, Ramachandran M, Dimberg A. Tumour angiogenesis: Causes, consequences, challenges and opportunities. *Cell Mol Life Sci.* 2020;77(9):1745–1770. https://www.ebi.ac.uk/chembl (Accessed 24 November 2022).

[59]. Cabral-Pacheco GA, Garza-Veloz I, Castruita-De la Rosa C, et al. The roles of matrix metalloproteinases and their inhibitors in human diseases. *Int J Mol Sci.* 2020;21(24):9739.

[60]. Tokito A, Jougasaki M. Matrix metalloproteinases in non-neoplastic disorders. *Int J Mol Sci.* 2016;17(7):1178.

[61]. Terni B, Ferrer I. Abnormal expression and distribution of MMP-2 at initial stages of alzheimer's disease-related pathology. *J Alzheimers Dis.* 2015;46:461–469.

[62]. Stomrud E, Bjorkqvist M, Janciauskiene S, et al. Alterations of matrix metalloproteinases in the healthy elderly with increased risk of prodromal Alzheimer's disease. *Alzheimers Res.* 2010;2:20.

[63]. Lorenzl S, Albers DS, Narr S, et al. Expression of MMP-2, MMP-9, and MMP-1 and their endogenous counterregulators TIMP-1 and TIMP-2 in postmortem brain tissue of Parkinson's disease. *Exp Neurol.* 2002;178(1):13–20.

[64]. Gu Z, Cui J, Brown S, et al. A highly specific inhibitor of matrixmetalloproteinase-9 rescues laminin from proteolysis and neurons from apoptosis in transient focal cerebral ischemia. *J Neurosci.* 2005;25:6401–6408.

[65]. Bronisz E, Kurkowska-Jastrzebska I. Matrix metalloproteinase 9 in epilepsy: The role of neuroinflammation in seizure development. *Mediators Inflamm.* 2016;2:1–14.

[66]. Kobusiak-Prokopowicz M, Krzysztofik J, Kaaz K, et al. MMP-2 and TIMP-2 in patients with heart failure and chronic kidney disease. *Open Med (Wars).* 2018;13:237–246.

[67]. Baghirova S, Hughes BG, Poirier M, et al. Nuclear matrix metalloproteinase-2 in the cardiomyocyte and the ischemic-reperfused heart. *J Mol Cell Cardiol.* 2016;94:153–161.

[68]. Fallata AM, Wyatt RA, Levesque JM, et al. Intracellular localization in zebrafish muscle and conserved sequence features suggest roles for gelatinase a moonlighting in sarcomere maintenance. *Biomedicines.* 2019;7(4):93.

[69]. Ali MA, Chow AK, Kandasamy AD, et al. Mechanisms of cytosolic targeting of matrix metalloproteinase-2. *J Cell Physiol.* 2012;227(10):3397–3404.

[70]. Wang GY, Bergman MR, Nguyen AP, et al. Cardiac transgenic matrix metalloproteinase-2 expression directly induces impaired contractility. *Cardiovasc Res.* 2006;69(3):688–696.

[71]. Gao L, Zheng YJ, Gu SS, et al. Degradation of cardiac myosin light chain kinase by matrix metalloproteinase-2 contributes to myocardial contractile dysfunction during ischemia/reperfusion. *J Mol Cell Cardiol.* 2014;77:102–112.

[72]. Yabluchanskiy A, Ma Y, Iyer RP, et al. Matrix metalloproteinase-9: Many shades of function in cardiovascular disease. *Physiology (Bethesda).* 2013;28(6):391–403.

[73]. Li T, Li X, Feng Y, et al. The role of matrix metalloproteinase-9 in atherosclerotic plaque instability. *Mediators Inflamm.* 2020;2020:3872367.

[74]. Tan J, Hua Q, Xing X, et al. Impact of the metalloproteinase-9/tissue inhibitor of metalloproteinase-1 system on large arterial stiffness in patients with essential hypertension. *Hypertens Res.* 2007;30(10):959–963.

[75]. Goh VJ, Le TT, Bryant J, et al. Novel index of maladaptive myocardial remodeling in hypertension. *Circ Cardiovasc Imaging.* 2017;10(9):e006840.

[76]. Lopes J, Adiguzel E, Gu S, et al. Type VIII collagen mediates vessel wall remodeling after arterial injury and fibrous cap formation in atherosclerosis. *Am J Pathol.* 2013;182(6):2241–2253.

[77]. Ferroni P, Basili S, Martini F, et al. Serum metalloproteinase 9 levels in patients with coronary artery disease: A novel marker of inflammation. *J Investig Med.* 2003;51(5):295–300.

[78]. Page-McCaw A, Ewald AJ, Werb Z. Matrix metalloproteinases and the regulation of tissue remodeling. *Nat Rev Mol Cell Biol.* 2007;8(3):221–233.

[79]. Goodall S, Crowther M, Hemingway DM, et al. Ubiquitous elevation of matrix metalloproteinase-2 expression in the vasculature of patients with abdominal aneurysms. *Circulation.* 2001;104(3):304–309.

[80]. Jones JA, Barbour JR, Lowry AS, et al. Spatiotemporal expression and localization of matrix metalloproteinas-9 in a murine model of thoracic aortic aneurysm. *J Vasc Surg.* 2006;44(6):1314–1321.

[81]. Dale MA, Suh MK, Zhao S, et al. Background differences in baseline and stimulated MMP levels influence abdominal aortic aneurysm susceptibility. *Atherosclerosis.* 2015;243(2):621–629.

[82]. Mohan V, Talmi-Frank D, Arkadash V, et al. Matrix metalloproteinase protein inhibitors: Highlighting a new beginning for metalloproteinases in medicine. *Metalloprotein Med.* 2016;3:31–47.

[83]. Uysal P, Uzun H. Relationship between circulating serpina3g, matrix metalloproteinase-9, and tissue inhibitor of metalloproteinase-1 and -2 with chronic obstructive pulmonary disease severity. *Biomolecules.* 2019;9(2):62.

[84]. Mahor D, Kumari V, Vashisht K, et al. Elevated serum matrix metalloprotease (MMP-2) as a candidate biomarker for stable COPD. *BMC Pulm Med.* 2020;20(1):302.

[85]. Churg A, Wang R, Wang X, et al. Wright, effect of an MMP-9/MMP-12 inhibitor on smoke-induced emphysema and airway remodeling in guinea pigs. *Thorax.* 2007;62:706–713.

[86]. Tonnel AB, Gosset P, Tillie-Leblond I. Characteristics of the inflammatory response in bronchial lavage fluids from patients with status asthmaticus. *Int Arch Allergy Immunol.* 2001;124(1–3):267–271.

[87]. Walker NF, Clark SO, Oni T, et al. Doxycycline and HIV infection suppress tuberculosis-induced matrix metalloproteinases. *Am J Respir Crit Care Med.* 2012;185(9):989–997.

[88]. Burrage PS, Mix KS, Brinckerhoff CE. Matrix metalloproteinases: Role in arthritis. *Front Biosci.* 2006;11:529–543.

[89]. Xue M, McKelvey K, Shen K, et al. Endogenous MMP-9 and not MMP-2 promotes rheumatoid synovial fibroblast survival, inflammation and cartilage degradation. *Rheumatology (Oxford).* 2014;53(12):2270–2279.

[90]. Mehana EE, Khafaga AF, El-Blehi SS. The role of matrix metalloproteinases in osteoarthritis pathogenesis: An updated review. *Life Sci.* 2019;234:116786.

[91]. Peeters SA, Engelen L, Buijs J, et al. Circulating matrix metalloproteinases are associated with arterial stiffness in patients with type 1 diabetes: Pooled analysis of three cohort studies. *Cardiovasc Diabetol.* 2017;16(1):139.

[92]. Wild S, Roglic G, Green A, et al. Global prevalence of diabetes: Estimates for the year 2000 and projections for 2030. *Diabetes Care.* 2004;27(5):1047–1053.

[93]. Uemura S, Matsushita H, Li W, et al. Diabetes mellitus enhances vascular matrix metalloproteinase activity: Role of oxidative stress. *Circ Res.* 2001;88(12):1291–1298.

[94]. Garcia-Fernandez N, Jacobs-Cachá C, Mora-Gutiérrez JM, et al. Matrix metalloproteinases in diabetic kidney disease. *J Clin Med.* 2020;9(2):472.

[95]. Lee HW, Lee SJ, Lee MY, et al. Enhanced cardiac expression of two isoforms of matrix metalloproteinase-2 in experimental diabetes mellitus. *PLoS One.* 2019;14(8):e0221798.

[96]. Opdenakker G, Abu El-Asrar A. Metalloproteinases mediate diabetes-induced retinal neuropathy and vasculopathy. *Cell Mol Life Sci.* 2019;76(16):3157–3166.

[97]. Jayashree K, Yasir M, Senthilkumar GP, et al. Circulating matrix modulators (MMP-9 and TIMP-1) and their association with severity of diabetic retinopathy. *Diabetes Metab Syndr.* 2018;12(6):869–873.

[98]. Derosa G, Avanzini MA, Geroldi D, et al. Matrix metalloproteinase 2 may be a marker of microangiopathy in children and adolescents with type 1 diabetes mellitus. *Diabetes Res Clin Pract.* 2005;70(2):119–125.

[99]. Adhikari N, Baidya S, Saha A, et al. Design and development of matrix metalloproteinase inhibitors containing zinc-binding groups, without zinc-binding groups, and mechanism-based. In: Gupta SP (Ed.), *Advances in Studies on Enzyme Inhibitors as Drugs: Miscellaneous Drugs*, Nova Science Publishers, 2017, 135–208.

[100]. Fabre B, Filipiak K, Zapico JM, et al. Progress towards water-soluble triazole-based selective MMP-2 inhibitors. *Org Biomol Chem.* 2013;11:6623–6641.

[101]. Overall CM, Kleifeld O. Validating matrix metalloproteinases as drug targets and anti-targets for cancer therapy. *Nature Rev.* 2006;6:227–239.

[102]. Zapico JM, Puckowska A, Filipiak K, et al. Design and synthesis of potent hydroxamate inhibitors with increased selectivity within the gelatinase family. *Org Biomol Chem.* 2015;13:142–156.

[103]. Curtin ML, Garland RB, Davidsen SK, et al. Broad spectrum matrix metalloproteinase inhibitors: An examination of succinamide hydroxamate inhibitors with P1 C alpha gem-disubstitution. *Bioorg Med Chem Lett.* 1998;8:1443–1448.

[104]. Steinman DH, Curtin ML, Garland RB, et al. The design, synthesis, and structure-activity relationships of a series of macrocyclic MMP inhibitors. *Bioorg Med Chem Lett.* 1998;8:2087–2092.

[105]. Sheppard GS, Florjancic AS, Giesler JR, et al. Aryl ketones as novel replacements for the C-terminal amide bond of succinyl hydroxamate MMP inhibitors. *Bioorg Med Chem Lett.* 1998;8:3261–3256.

[106]. Yamamoto M, Tsujishita H, Hori N, et al. Inhibition of membrane-type 1 matrix metalloproteinase by hydroxamate inhibitors: An examination of the subsite pocket. *J Med Chem.* 1998;41:1209–1217.

[107]. Hanessian S, Bouzbouz S, Boudon A, et al. Picking the S1, S1' and S2' pockets of matrix metalloproteinases: A niche for potent acyclic sulfonamide inhibitors. *Bioorg Med Chem Lett.* 1999;9:1691–1696.

[108]. Almstead NG, Bradley RS, Pikul S, et al. Design, synthesis, and biological evaluation of potent thiazine- and thiazepine-based matrix metalloproteinase inhibitors. *J Med Chem.* 1999;42:4547–4562.

[109]. Cheng M, De B, Almstead NG, et al. Design, synthesis, and biological evaluation of matrix metalloproteinase inhibitors derived from a modified proline scaffold. *J Med Chem.* 1999;42:5426–5436.

[110]. Barta TE, Becker DP, Bedell LJ, et al. Synthesis and activity of selective MMP inhibitors with an aryl backbone. *Bioorg Med Chem Lett.* 2000;10:2815–2817.

[111]. Natchus MG, Bookland RG, De B, et al. Development of new hydroxamate matrix metalloproteinase inhibitors derived from functionalized 4-aminoprolines. *J Med Chem.* 2000;43:4948–4963.

[112]. Chollet AM, Le Diguarher T, Murray L, et al. General synthesis of alpha-substituted 3-bisaryloxy propionic acid derivatives as specific MMP inhibitors. *Bioorg Med Chem Lett.* 2001;11:295–299.

[113]. Fray MJ, Burslem MF, Dickinson RP, et al. Selectivity of inhibition of matrix metalloproteases MMP-3 and MMP-2 by succinyl hydroxamates and their carboxylic acid analogues is dependent on P3' group chirality. *Bioorg Med Chem Lett.* 2001;11:567–570.

[114]. Fray MJ, Dickinson RP. Discovery of potent and selective succinyl hydroxamate inhibitors of matrix metalloprotease-3 (stromelysin-1). *Bioorg Med Chem Lett.* 2001;11:571–574.

[115]. Pikul S, Dunham KM, Almstead NG, et al. Heterocycle-based MMP inhibitors with P2' substituents. *Bioorg Med Chem Lett.* 2001;11:1009–1013.

[116]. Baxter AD, Bhogal R, Bird J, et al. Arylsulphonyl hydroxamic acids: Potent and selective matrix metalloproteinase inhibitors. *Bioorg Med Chem Lett.* 2001;11:1465–1468.

[117]. Barta TE, Becker DP, Bedell LJ, et al. Selective, orally active MMP inhibitors with an aryl backbone. *Bioorg Med Chem Lett.* 2001;11:2481–2483.

[118]. Becker DP, Barta TE, Bedell L, et al. Alpha-amino-beta-sulphone hydroxamates as potent MMP-13 inhibitors that spareMMP-1. *Bioorg Med Chem Lett.* 2001;11:2719–2722.

[119]. Holms J, Mast K, Marcotte P, et al. Discovery of selective hydroxamic acid inhibitors of tumour necrosis factor-alpha converting enzyme. *Bioorg Med Chem Lett.* 2001;11:2907–2910.

[120]. Hanessian S, Moitessier N, Gauchet C, et al. N-Aryl sulfonyl homocysteine hydroxamate inhibitors of matrix metalloproteinases: Further probing of the S(1), S(1)', and S(2)' pockets. *J Med Chem.* 2001;44:3066–3073.

[121]. Chollet AM, Le Diguarher T, Kucharczyk N, et al. Solid-phase synthesis of alpha-substituted 3-bisarylthio N-hydroxy propionamides as specific MMP inhibitors. *Bioorg Med Chem Lett.* 2002;10:531–544.

[122]. Rossello A, Nuti E, Carelli P, et al. N-i-propoxy-N-biphenylsulfonylaminobutylhydro xamic acids as potent and selective inhibitors of MMP-2 and MT1-MMP. *Bioorg Med Chem Lett.* 2005;15:1321–1326.

[123]. Rossello A, Nuti E, Catalani MP, et al. A new development of matrix metalloproteinase inhibitors: Twin hydroxamic acids as potent inhibitors of MMPs. *Bioorg Med Chem Lett.* 2005;15:2311–2314.

[124]. Becker DP, Villamil CI, Barta TE, et al. Synthesis and structure-activity relationships of beta- and alpha-piperidine sulfone hydroxamic acid matrix metalloproteinase inhibitors with oral antitumour efficacy. *J Med Chem.* 2005;48:6713–6730.

[125]. Ikura M, Nakatani S, Yamamoto S, et al. Discovery of a new chemical lead for a matrix metalloproteinase inhibitor. *Bioorg Med Chem.* 2006;14:4241–4252.

[126]. Nakatani S, Ikura M, Yamamoto S, et al. Design and synthesis of novel metalloproteinase inhibitors. *Bioorg Med Chem.* 2006;14:5402–5422.

[127]. Yamamoto S, Nakatani S, Ikura M, et al. Design and synthesis of an orally active matrix metalloproteinase inhibitor. *Bioorg Med Chem.* 2006;14:6383–6403.

[128]. Condon JS, Joseph-McCarthy D, Levin JI, et al. Identification of potent and selective TACE inhibitors via the S1 pocket. *Bioorg Med Chem Lett.* 2007;17:34–39.

[129]. Wagner S, Breyholz HJ, Law MP, et al. Novel fluorinated derivatives of the broad-spectrum MMP inhibitors N-hydroxy-2(R)-[[(4-methoxyphenyl)sulfonyl](benzyl)- and (3-picolyl)-amino]-3-methyl-butanamide as potential tools for the molecular imaging of activated MMPs with PET. *J Med Chem.* 2007;50:5752–5764.

[130]. Yang SM, Scannevin RH, Wang B, et al. beta-N-Biaryl ether sulfonamide hydroxamates as potent gelatinase inhibitors: Part 2. Optimization of alpha-amino substituents. *Bioorg Med Chem Lett.* 2008;18:1140–1145.

[131]. Nuti E, Casalini F, Avramova SI, et al. N-O-isopropyl sulfonamido-based hydroxamates: Design, synthesis and biological evaluation of selective matrix metalloproteinase-13 inhibitors as potential therapeutic agents for osteoarthritis. *J Med Chem.* 2009;52:4757–4773.

[132]. Nuti E, Panelli L, Casalini F, et al. Design, synthesis, biological evaluation, and NMR studies of a new series of arylsulfones as selective and potent matrix metalloproteinase-12 inhibitors. *J Med Chem.* 2009;52:6347–6361.

[133]. Becker DP, Barta TE, Bedell LJ, et al. Orally active MMP-1 sparing α-tetrahydropyranyl and α-piperidinyl sulfone matrix metalloproteinase (MMP) inhibitors with efficacy in cancer, arthritis, and cardiovascular disease. *J Med Chem.* 2010;53:6653–6680.

[134]. Fobian YM, Freskos JN, Barta TE, et al. MMP-13 selective alpha-sulfone hydroxamates: Identification of selective P1' amides. *Bioorg Med Chem Lett.* 2011;21:2823–2825.

[135]. Nuti E, Casalini F, Santamaria S, et al. Synthesis and biological evaluation in U87MG glioma cells of (ethynylthiophene)sulfonamido-based hydroxamates as matrix metalloproteinase inhibitors. *Eur J Med Chem.* 2011;46:2617–2629.

[136]. Zapico JM, Serra P, García-Sanmartín J, et al. Potent "clicked" MMP-2 inhibitors: Synthesis, molecular modeling and biological exploration. *Org Biomol Chem.* 2011;9:4587–4599.

[137]. Hugenberg V, Breyholz HJ, Riemann B, et al. A new class of highly potent matrix metalloproteinase inhibitors based on triazole-substituted hydroxamates: (radio)synthesis and in vitro and first in vivo evaluation. *J Med Chem.* 2012;55:4714–4727.

[138]. Behrends M, Wagner S, Kopka K, et al. New matrix metalloproteinase inhibitors based on γ-fluorinated α-aminocarboxylic and α-aminohydroxamic acids. *Bioorg Med Chem.* 2015;23:3809–3818.

[139]. Nuti E, Cantelmo AR, Gallo C, et al. N-O-isopropyl sulfonamido-based hydroxamates as matrix metalloproteinase inhibitors: Hit selection and in vivo antiangiogenic activity. *J Med Chem.* 2015;58:7224–7240.

[140]. Zapico JM, Puckowska A, Filipiak K, et al. Design and synthesis of potent hydroxamate inhibitors with increased selectivity within the gelatinase family. *Org. Biomol. Chem.* 2015;13:142–156.

[141]. Sjøli S, Nuti E, Camodeca C, et al. Synthesis, experimental evaluation and molecular modelling of hydroxamate derivatives as zinc metalloproteinase inhibitors. *Eur J Med Chem.* 2016;108:141–153.

[142]. Kiyama R, Tamura Y, Watanabe F, et al. Homology modeling of gelatinase catalytic domains and docking simulations of novel sulfonamide inhibitors. *J Med Chem.* 1999;42:1723–1728.

[143]. O'Brien PM, Ortwine DF, Pavlovsky AG, et al. Structure-activity relationships and pharmacokinetic analysis for a series of potent, systemically available biphenylsulfonamide matrix metalloproteinase inhibitors. *J Med Chem.* 2000;43:156–166.

[144]. Pikul S, Ohler NE, Ciszewski G, et al. Potent and selective carboxylic acid-based inhibitors of matrix metalloproteinases. *J Med Chem.* 2001;44:2499–2502.

[145]. Wu J, Rush TS. Hotchandani R, et al. Identification of potent and selective MMP-13 inhibitors. *Bioorg Med Chem Lett.* 2005;15:4105–4109.

[146]. Zhang YM, Fan X, Xiang B, et al. Synthesis and SAR of alpha-sulfonylcarboxylic acids as potent matrix metalloproteinase inhibitors. *Bioorg Med Chem Lett.* 2006;16:3096–3100.

[147]. Li W, Hu Y, Li J, et al. 3,4-Disubstituted benzofuran P1' MMP-13 inhibitors: Optimization of selectivity and reduction of protein binding. *Bioorg Med Chem Lett.* 2009;19:4546–4550.

[148]. Selivanova SV, Stellfeld T, Heinrich TK, et al. Design, synthesis, and initial evaluation of a high affinity positron emission tomography probe for imaging matrix metalloproteinases 2 and 9. *J Med Chem.* 2013;56:4912–4920.

[149]. Halder AK, Mallick S, Shikha D, et al. Design of dual MMP-2/HDAC8 inhibitors by pharmacophore mapping, molecular docking, synthesis and biological activity. *RSC Adv.* 2015;5:72373–72386.

[150]. Adhikari N, Halder AK, Mallick S, et al. Robust design of some selective matrix metalloproteinase-2 inhibitors over matrix metalloproteinase-9 through in silico/fragment-based lead identification and de novo lead modification: Syntheses and biological assays. *Bioorg Med Chem.* 2016;24:4291–4309.

[151]. Mukherjee A, Adhikari N, Jha T. A pentanoic acid derivative targeting matrix metalloproteinase-2 (MMP-2) induces apoptosis in a chronic myeloid leukemia cell line. *Eur J Med Chem.* 2017;141:37–50.

[152]. Hurst DR, Schwartz MA, Jin Y, et al. Inhibition of enzyme activity of and cell-mediated substrate cleavage by membrane type 1 matrix metalloproteinase by newly developed mercaptosulphide inhibitors. *Biochem J.* 2005;392:527–536.

[153]. Caldwell CG, Sahoo SP, Polo SA, et al. Phosphonic acid inhibitors of matrix metalloproteinases. *Bioorg Med Chem.* 1996;6:323–328.

[154]. Biasone A, Tortorella P, Campestre C, et al. alpha-Biphenylsulfonylamino 2-methyl-propyl phosphonates: Enantioselective synthesis and selective inhibition of MMPs. *Bioorg Med Chem.* 2007;15:791–799.

[155]. Curtin ML, Florjancic AS, Heyman HR, et al. Discovery and characterization of the potent, selective and orally bioavailable MMP inhibitor ABT-770. *Bioorg Med Chem Lett.* 2001;11:1557–1560.

[156]. Wada CK, Holms JH, Curtin ML, et al. Phenoxyphenyl sulfone N-formylhydroxylamines (retrohydroxamates) as potent, selective, orally bioavailable matrix metalloproteinase inhibitors. *J Med Chem.* 2002;45:219–232.

[157]. Grams F, Brandstetter H, D'Alò S, et al. Pyrimidine-2,4,6-triones: A new effective and selective class of matrix metalloproteinase inhibitors. *Biol Chem.* 2001;382:1277–1285.

[158]. Brandstetter H, Grams F, Glitz D, et al. The 1.8-A crystal structure of a matrix metalloproteinase 8-barbiturate inhibitor complex reveals a previously unobserved mechanism for collagenase substrate recognition. *J Biol Chem.* 2001;276:17405–17412.

[159]. Dunten P, Kammlott U, Crowther R, et al. X-ray structure of a novel matrix metalloproteinase inhibitor complexed to stromelysin. *Protein Sci.* 2001;10:923–926.

[160]. Breyholz HJ, Schäfers M, Wagner S, et al. C-5-disubstituted barbiturates as potential molecular probes for noninvasive matrix metalloproteinase imaging. *J Med Chem.* 2005;48:3400–3409.

[161]. Wang J, Medina C, Radomsk, MW, et al. N-substituted homopiperazine barbiturates as gelatinase inhibitors. *Bioorg Med Chem.* 2011;19:4985–4999.

6 Stromelysins and Their Inhibitors

Sandip Kumar Baidya, Suvankar Banerjee,
Nilanjan Adhikari, and Tarun Jha

CONTENTS

ABSTRACT

Stromelysins are a matrix metalloproteinase (MMP) family member—a zinc-dependent endopeptidase responsible for the breakdown of the extracellular matrix (ECM). However, many pathological and normal conditions, including the embryonic stage, osteogenesis, epithelium growth, morphogenesis, inflammation, tumor proliferation, and tissue inflammation, are associated with the widespread expression of stromelysin. Thus, it may be assumed that creating promising and selective stromelysin inhibitors will become a top priority in the near future for drug research and development. In this chapter, a broad description of different types of stromelysin inhibitors like hydroxamate, carboxylic acid, thiol and mercaptosulfide, phosphonates, N-hydroxyurea, hydrazide, N-hydroxyformamide, and pyrimidine-2,4,6-trione based molecules are shown, along with other miscellaneous stromelysins inhibitors. Additionally, the biological activity of these existing stromelysin inhibitors and crystallographic data are taken into account for the discovery of promising and selective stromelysin inhibitors using a variety of different drug-designing methodologies.

Keywords: Stromelysin; Hydroxamate; Carboxylic acid; Thiol and mercaptosulfide; Phosphonate; Other stromelysin inhibitors

DOI: 10.1201/9781003303282-8

6.1 INTRODUCTION

Stromelysins, namely stromelysin-1 (MMP-3), stromelysin-2 (MMP-10), and stromelysin-3 (MMP-11), are categorized as a special class of matrix metalloproteinases (MMPs). These stromelysins are mainly responsible for the proteolysis of the extracellular matrix (ECM). Being the family member MMPs, these are zinc-dependent endopeptidases associated with the breakdown of the ECM and remodeling of tissues [1–3]. Regarding the structure and substrate specificity, stromelysin-1 and -2 are closely associated, whereas stromelysin-3 is related distantly [4]. Stromelysin-1 (MMP-3) comprises 475-478 amino acids in mammals. The amino acid sequence of MMP-3 is highly conserved among various species, which indicates its efficacy for cross-species applications [5, 6]. MMP-3 consists of four major parts, including a propeptide domain (comprising 80 amino acids), a catalytic domain (comprising 170 amino acids), a ligating peptide of variable size, and a heme protein domain (200 amino acids). MMP-3 is a crucial part of modulating several cellular processes, including cellular differentiation and proliferation, as well as several disease progressions [5]. Stromelysin-2 (MMP-10) is liberated as a 53 kDa proenzyme and finally activated to a mature protease of 47 kDa [4]. It is important to note that MMP-10 possesses 82% structural homology with MMP-3 [7]. Importantly, MMP-10 is found to degrade several proteins like proteoglycans, type IV and IX collagens, laminin-I, fibronectin, the globular domains of collagens I and III, elastin, gelatin, and casein [8, 9]. On the other hand, stromelysin-3 (MMP-11) is widely expressed in both normal and pathological conditions, such as in the embryonic stage, osteogenesis, epithelium growth, morphogenesis, inflammation, tumor proliferation, and tissue inflammation) [1]. The structure of these stromelysins is depicted in Figure 6.1.

6.2 PATHOPHYSIOLOGY OF STROMELYSINS

Being a member of the MMP family, the stromelysins (MMP-3, MMP-10, and MMP-11), besides their normal functionalities inside the normal physiological condition, are also connected with various diseases and abnormal physiological conditions (Figure 6.2).

In the case of stromelysin-1 (MMP-3), it is noticed that MMP-3 is functionally associated with cardiovascular disorders [10, 11], gastric ulcer [12, 13], rheumatoid arthritis [14, 15], periodontitis [16], intervertebral disc disease [17], acute respiratory distress syndrome [18], carotid artery-related complications related to arthritis [19], virus-induced inflammation [20], neuronal inflammation [21], and mental disorders such as schizophrenia [22]. Besides the association with these physical and mental disorders, MMP-3 also contributes to a group of different neoplastic conditions such as bladder cancer [23], nasopharyngeal carcinoma [24], breast cancer [25, 26], lung adenocarcinoma [27], esophageal cancer [28], idiopathic pulmonary fibrosis [27], and tumors in the mammary gland [28].

Unlike MMP-3, the other members of the stromelysin family (stromelysin-2/MMP-10 and stromelysin-3/MMP-11) comparatively have less significance in pathophysiological conditions. However, both MMP-3 and MMP-10 are correlated with

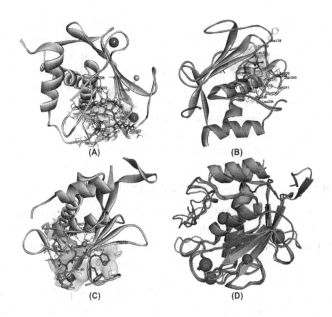

FIGURE 6.1 (A) General cartoon representation of stromelysins; ligand-bound crystal structure of (B) MMP-3 (PDB ID: 1SLN); (C) MMP-10 (PDB ID: 1Q3A); (D) MMP-11 (PDB ID: 1HV5); (E) superimposed structure of collagenases (MMP-3: light gray, MMP-10: gray, and MMP-11: dark gray).

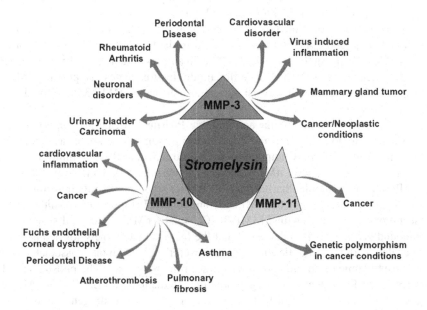

FIGURE 6.2 Role of stromelysins in various disease conditions.

human urinary bladder carcinoma [29, 30]. Also, studies have shown the potential of MMP-10 as a prognostic biomarker in breast cancer conditions as well as for idiopathic pulmonary fibrosis [30]. Abnormal MMP-10 expression can be associated with cardiovascular inflammation and atherothrombosis [31]. Additionally, MMP-10 is also associated with Fuchs endothelial corneal dystrophy (FECD) [32] and asthma [33]. Stromelysin-3 (MMP-11) is also associated with several pathophysiological conditions, including breast, prostate, gastric, colorectal, cervical, pancreatic cancer, hepatocellular carcinoma, head, and neck cancer, while being a contributor to genetic polymorphism in cancer conditions [34, 35].

6.3 HYDROXAMATE-BASED STROMELYSIN INHIBITORS

Several hydroxamate-based MMPIs have been identified to date as having potential efficacy against a variety of MMPs, including stromelysins. Researchers of Abbott Laboratory [36] disclosed a series of C_α gem disubstituted succinimide hydroxamates as effective broad-spectrum MMPIs. Compound **6.1** (Figure 6.3) was the most effective MMP-3 inhibitor (IC_{50} = 12 nM) in this series.

In the next study, the researcher of Abbott Laboratory [37] produced potential broad-spectrum MMPIs having macrocyclic ring-containing succinimide hydroxamates. Compound **6.2** (Figure 6.3) was the maximum effective MMP-3 inhibitor (IC_{50} = 1.5 nM) among these molecules.

Further study by Sheppard and co-workers from Abbott Laboratories [38] led to the identification of a set of succinyl hydroxamate-bearing potent broad-spectrum MMPIs by incorporating an aryl aminoketone moiety substituting the C-terminal amino acid amides. Among these compounds, compound **6.3** (Figure 6.3) exhibited the most potent MMP-3 inhibition (IC_{50} = 1.2 nM).

The researchers of Kanebo [39] reported some hydroxamate-based potential MMPIs. Compound **6.4** (Figure 6.3) resulted in the most potent MMP-3 inhibition (IC_{50} = 0.6 nM) among these molecules. Martin and co-workers from British Biotech [40] reported some nonpeptidic sulfonamido hydroxamates as potent MMPIs. Compound **6.5** (Figure 6.3) was the maximum efficacious MMP-3 inhibitor (IC_{50} = 7 nM) in this series.

Almstead et al. from Procter and Gamble Pharmaceuticals [41] reported a set of arylsulfonamido thiazepine and thiazine-containing hydroxamates as potent and broad-spectrum MMPIs. Compound **6.6** (Figure 6.3) was the maximum effective MMP-3 inhibitor (IC_{50} = 0.7 nM) among these molecules. Pikul and co-workers [42] from Procter and Gamble Pharmaceuticals further reported several phosphinamide-based hydroxamates as potent MMPIs. Compound **6.7** (Figure 6.3) resulted in the best inhibitory efficacy against MMP-3 (IC_{50} = 24.4 nM). The crystal structure of compound **6.7** and MMP-3 disclosed that the hydroxamate moiety formed a bidentate chelate with the catalytic Zn^{2+} ion. However, the phenyl moiety associated with the phosphinamide scaffold was moved toward the S1' pocket. The phosphinamide oxygen formed an effective hydrogen bonding interaction with Leu164 and Ala165. Again, the hydroxyl group of hydroxamate moiety formed hydrogen bonding with Glu202. The isobutyl group and N-benzyl moiety showed effective van der Waals

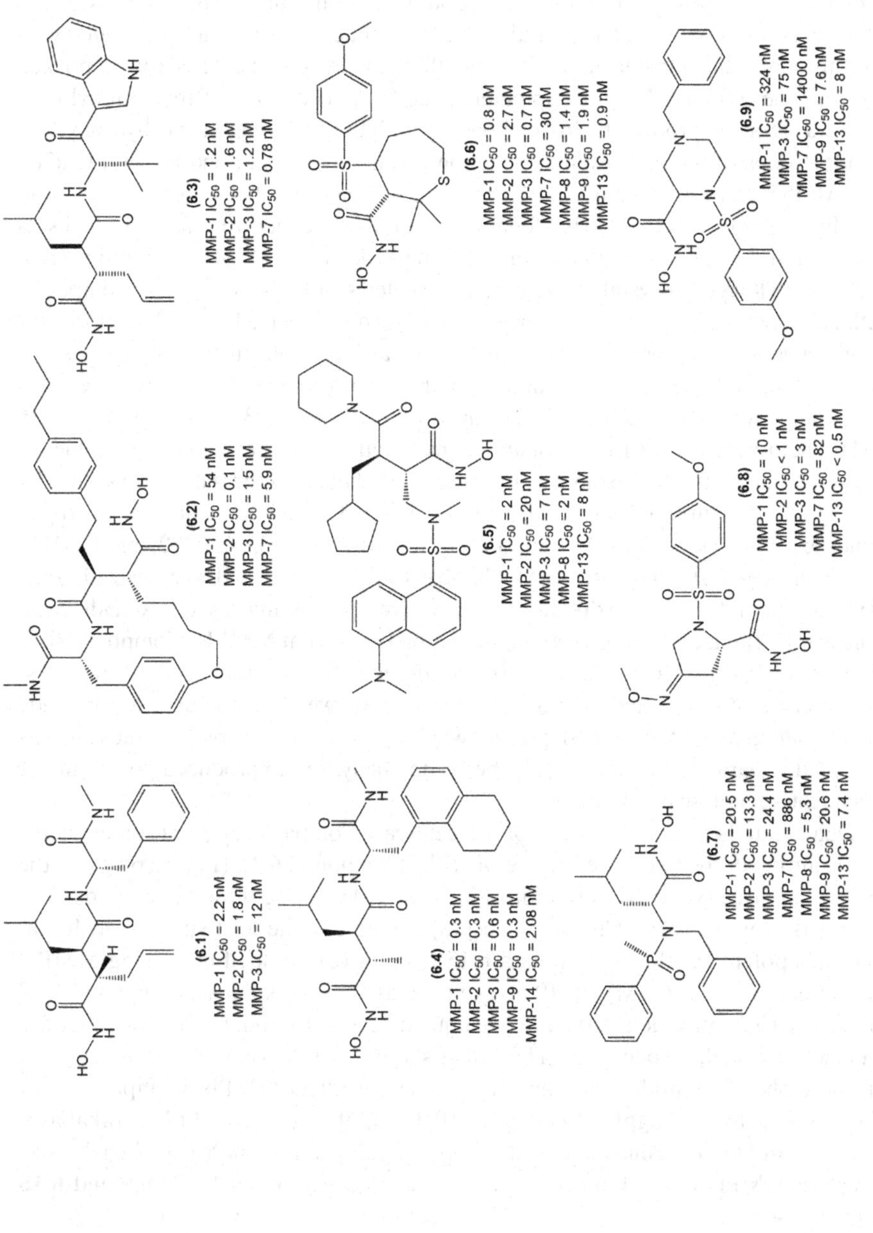

FIGURE 6.3 Hydroxamate-based potential MMP-3 inhibitors (compounds **6.1–6.9**).

(6.1)

MMP-1 IC$_{50}$ = 2.2 nM
MMP-2 IC$_{50}$ = 1.8 nM
MMP-3 IC$_{50}$ = 12 nM

(6.2)

MMP-1 IC$_{50}$ = 54 nM
MMP-2 IC$_{50}$ = 0.1 nM
MMP-3 IC$_{50}$ = 1.5 nM
MMP-7 IC$_{50}$ = 5.9 nM

(6.3)

MMP-1 IC$_{50}$ = 1.2 nM
MMP-2 IC$_{50}$ = 1.6 nM
MMP-3 IC$_{50}$ = 1.2 nM
MMP-7 IC$_{50}$ = 0.78 nM

(6.4)

MMP-1 IC$_{50}$ = 0.3 nM
MMP-2 IC$_{50}$ = 0.3 nM
MMP-3 IC$_{50}$ = 0.6 nM
MMP-9 IC$_{50}$ = 0.3 nM
MMP-14 IC$_{50}$ = 2.08 nM

(6.5)

MMP-1 IC$_{50}$ = 2 nM
MMP-2 IC$_{50}$ = 20 nM
MMP-3 IC$_{50}$ = 7 nM
MMP-8 IC$_{50}$ = 2 nM
MMP-13 IC$_{50}$ = 8 nM

(6.6)

MMP-1 IC$_{50}$ = 0.8 nM
MMP-2 IC$_{50}$ = 2.7 nM
MMP-3 IC$_{50}$ = 0.7 nM
MMP-7 IC$_{50}$ = 30 nM
MMP-8 IC$_{50}$ = 1.4 nM
MMP-9 IC$_{50}$ = 1.9 nM
MMP-13 IC$_{50}$ = 0.9 nM

(6.7)

MMP-1 IC$_{50}$ = 20.5 nM
MMP-2 IC$_{50}$ = 13.3 nM
MMP-3 IC$_{50}$ = 24.4 nM
MMP-7 IC$_{50}$ = 886 nM
MMP-8 IC$_{50}$ = 5.3 nM
MMP-9 IC$_{50}$ = 20.6 nM
MMP-13 IC$_{50}$ = 7.4 nM

(6.8)

MMP-1 IC$_{50}$ = 10 nM
MMP-2 IC$_{50}$ < 1 nM
MMP-3 IC$_{50}$ = 3 nM
MMP-7 IC$_{50}$ = 82 nM
MMP-13 IC$_{50}$ < 0.5 nM

(6.9)

MMP-1 IC$_{50}$ = 324 nM
MMP-3 IC$_{50}$ = 75 nM
MMP-7 IC$_{50}$ = 14000 nM
MMP-9 IC$_{50}$ = 7.6 nM
MMP-13 IC$_{50}$ = 8 nM

interaction with the hydrophobic side chain amino acids (namely Val163, Leu164, and His166).

Again, Cheng et al. [43] from Procter and Gamble reported a series of arylsulfon-amido proline-based hydroxamates bearing the oxime, hydrazone, and exomethylene moieties as potent broad-spectrum MMPIs. Compound **6.8** (Figure 6.3) resulted in broad-spectrum MMP inhibition with good MMP-3 inhibition (IC_{50} = 3 nM). The X-ray crystallographic data explored the hydroxamate function that coordinated with Zn^{2+} through a bidentate fashion. The p-methoxyphenyl group entered the S1′ pocket, whereas the iminomethoxy group entered the S2′ pocket. One of the sulfonyl oxygens was found to produce hydrogen bonding with Leu164, whereas the hydroxyl and amide groups of the hydroxamate function formed hydrogen bonding with Glu202 and Ala165, respectively. Further study by the same group of researchers [44] led to the discovery of a set of arylsulfonamido piperazine-containing hydroxamates as potential MMPIs. Compound **6.9** (Figure 6.3) yielded potent MMP-3 inhibition (IC_{50} = 75 nM). The X-ray crystallographic data revealed similar interactions to compound **6.8**. However, the carboxybenzyl group was placed between S1 and S2′ pockets.

Natchus and co-workers [45] from Procter and Gamble further reported some aryl sulfonamide-based hydroxamates with functionalized 4-aminoproline moiety. Compound **6.10** (Figure 6.4) displayed potential MMP-3 inhibition (IC_{50} = 16 nM). The p-n-butoxyphenyl sulfonamide group fitted into the deep hydrophobic S1′ pocket, whereas the hydroxamate group formed chelate to the Zn^{2+} ion as seen by the crystal structure of compound **6.10** and MMP-3. In addition, several hydrogen bonds are observed with the key amino acids (Leu164, Ala165, Glu202, and His211).

Again, scientists at Procter and Gamble [46] designed and synthesized some aryl sulfonamide-based hydroxamate derivatives possessing 6-oxohexahydropyri-dine and [1,4]diazepine moieties as potent broad-spectrum MMPIs. Compound **6.11** (Figure 6.4) resulted in potential MMP-3 inhibition (IC_{50} = 3.1 nM). The X-ray crystal structure of compound **6.11** and stromelysin showed that the aryl sulfonamide moiety plunged into the deep S1′ pocket, whereas the hexahydro pyrimidine ring was extended toward the S2′ pocket. The benzylic phenyl group produced good van der Waals interaction with a Leu222.

Duan et al. [47] from DuPont Pharmaceuticals Company reported some macro-cyclic amine derivatives as effective MMPIs. Compound **6.12** (Figure 6.4) was the maximum effective MMP-3 inhibitor (K_i = 38 nM) among these compounds. The scientists from Celltech Chiroscience [48] reported some aryl sulfonyl hydroxa-mates as potent MMPIs. Compound **6.13** (Figure 6.4) yielded promising MMP-3 inhibition (IC_{50} = 100 nM). At 10 mg/kg dose and 30 mg/kg dose, compound **6.13** produced 40% inhibition in the *in vivo* adjuvant arthritis model and B16F10 mouse melanoma model, respectively. The scientists of LEO Pharma [49] designed a set of cyclic phosphinamides and phosphonamides as potent MMPIs. Compound **6.14** (Figure 6.4) showed highly effective MMP-3 inhibition (IC_{50} = 13 nM). Takahashi et al. [50] of Ono Pharmaceuticals developed some γ-aminobutyric acid analogs as effective MMPIs through an *in silico* fragment-based approach. Compound **6.15** (Figure 6.4) displayed effective MMP-3 inhibition (IC_{50} = 1000 nM) among these compounds.

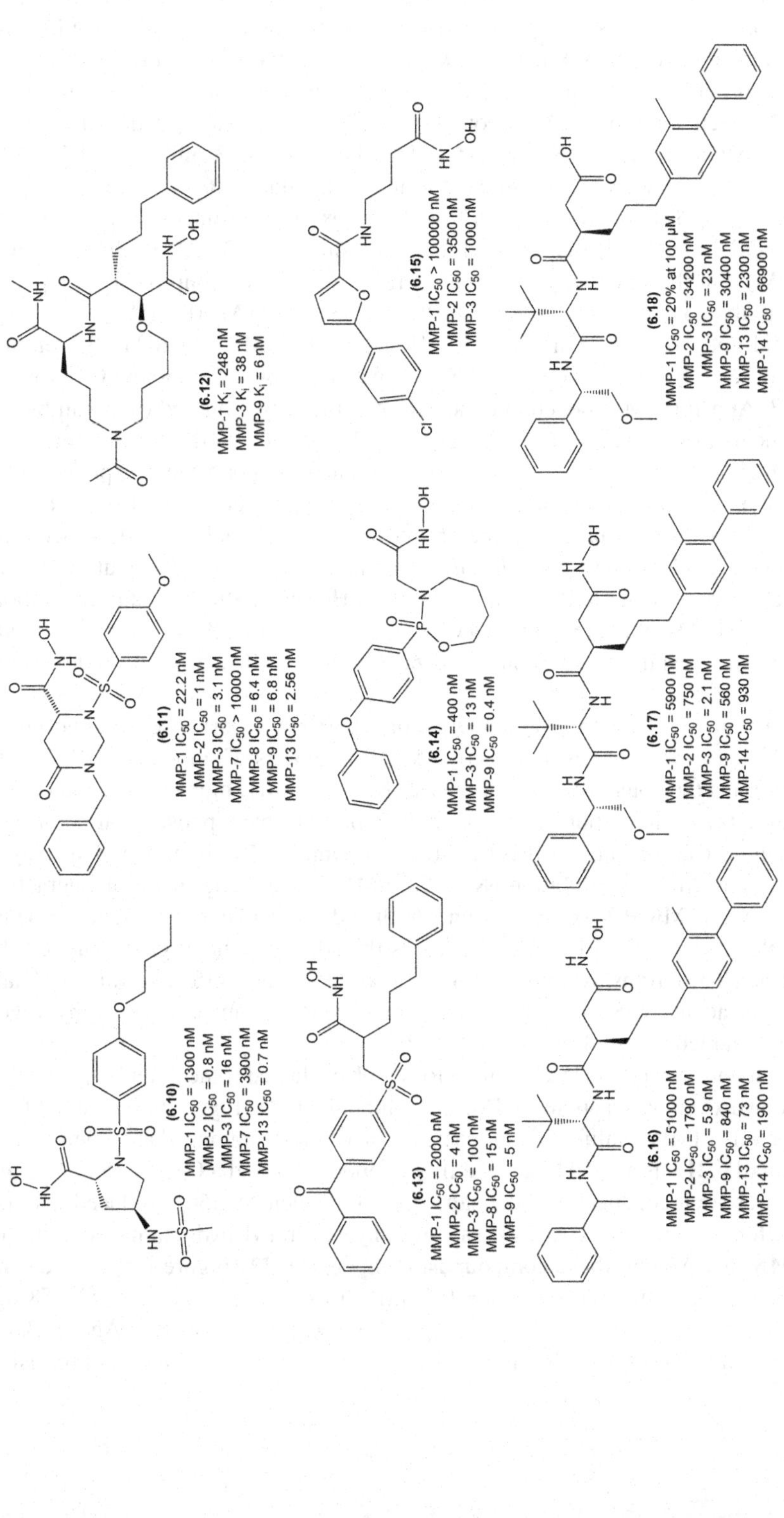

FIGURE 6.4 Some potential MMP-3 inhibitors (compounds **6.10–6.18**).

(6.10)
MMP-1 IC$_{50}$ = 1300 nM
MMP-2 IC$_{50}$ = 0.8 nM
MMP-3 IC$_{50}$ = 16 nM
MMP-7 IC$_{50}$ = 3900 nM
MMP-13 IC$_{50}$ = 0.7 nM

(6.11)
MMP-1 IC$_{50}$ = 22.2 nM
MMP-2 IC$_{50}$ = 1 nM
MMP-3 IC$_{50}$ = 3.1 nM
MMP-7 IC$_{50}$ > 10000 nM
MMP-8 IC$_{50}$ = 6.4 nM
MMP-9 IC$_{50}$ = 6.8 nM
MMP-13 IC$_{50}$ = 2.56 nM

(6.12)
MMP-1 K$_i$ = 248 nM
MMP-3 K$_i$ = 38 nM
MMP-9 K$_i$ = 6 nM

(6.13)
MMP-1 IC$_{50}$ = 2000 nM
MMP-2 IC$_{50}$ = 4 nM
MMP-3 IC$_{50}$ = 100 nM
MMP-8 IC$_{50}$ = 15 nM
MMP-9 IC$_{50}$ = 5 nM

(6.14)
MMP-1 IC$_{50}$ = 400 nM
MMP-3 IC$_{50}$ = 13 nM
MMP-9 IC$_{50}$ = 0.4 nM

(6.15)
MMP-1 IC$_{50}$ > 100000 nM
MMP-2 IC$_{50}$ = 3500 nM
MMP-3 IC$_{50}$ = 1000 nM

(6.16)
MMP-1 IC$_{50}$ = 51000 nM
MMP-2 IC$_{50}$ = 1790 nM
MMP-3 IC$_{50}$ = 5.9 nM
MMP-9 IC$_{50}$ = 840 nM
MMP-13 IC$_{50}$ = 73 nM
MMP-14 IC$_{50}$ = 1900 nM

(6.17)
MMP-1 IC$_{50}$ = 5900 nM
MMP-2 IC$_{50}$ = 750 nM
MMP-3 IC$_{50}$ = 2.1 nM
MMP-9 IC$_{50}$ = 560 nM
MMP-14 IC$_{50}$ = 930 nM

(6.18)
MMP-1 IC$_{50}$ = 20% at 100 μM
MMP-2 IC$_{50}$ = 34200 nM
MMP-3 IC$_{50}$ = 23 nM
MMP-9 IC$_{50}$ = 30400 nM
MMP-13 IC$_{50}$ = 2300 nM
MMP-14 IC$_{50}$ = 66900 nM

The researchers of Pfizer Global Research and Development [51] reported some succinyl hydroxamates as MMP-3-selective inhibitors over MMP-2. Compound **6.16** (Figure 6.4) was the most efficacious MMP-3-selective inhibitor (IC_{50} = 5.9 nM) over other MMPs, including MMP-1, -2, -9, -13, and -14. A further study conducted by the same group of researchers [52] led to the development of several other promising MMP-3-selective inhibitors. Compound **6.17** (Figure 6.4) bearing a biphenyl propyl group directed toward the S1′ pocket yielded better MMP-3 inhibition (IC_{50} = 2.1 nM) and selectivity than the earlier reported compound **6.16**. Replacement of the hydroxamate moiety of compound **6.17** with carboxylic acid function produced compound **6.18** (Figure 6.4) that showed a slight reduction in MMP-3 inhibition (IC_{50} = 23 nM), but the selectivity over other MMPs was greatly improved. Compound **6.18** was able to inhibit the cleavage of [^{3}H]-fibronectin by MMP-3 (IC_{50} = 320 nM), but it did not show any inhibition of [^{3}H]-gelatin by MMP-2 or MMP-9 even at a higher dose (100 µM). It indicated the selective behavior of compound **6.18** toward MMP-3. At a 100 µM dose, compound **6.18** significantly inhibited (68% inhibition) keratinocyte migration over a collagen matrix. The *in vitro* study revealed that compound **6.18** did not show any cytotoxic features and did not affect the proliferation of fibroblast, keratinocytes, or endothelial cells at higher doses. It also exhibited a good pharmacokinetic profile in the animal model, such as higher clearance with respect to liver blood flow (88 ml/min/kg) and moderate volume distribution (3.1 lit/kg), including a shorter half-life ($t_{1/2}$ = 23 min). However, after oral administration, the bioavailability of compound **6.18** was extremely low (< 5%). In the *ex vivo* study in rabbit Adriamycin wounds, compound **6.18** inhibited MMP-3 in a dose-dependent manner.

Sawa et al. [53] from the Nippon Organon laboratory reported several phosphonamide-based hydroxamates as effective MMP inhibitors. Compound **6.19** (Figure 6.5) exhibited the potent MMP-3 inhibition (K_i = 3.33 nM) among these compounds.

Again, the same group of researchers reported some phosphonamide-based hydroxamates as potential MMPIs [54]. Compound **6.20** (Figure 6.5) displayed highly potent MMP-3 inhibition (K_i = 5.2 nM). The binding mode of interaction study between MMP-3 and compound **6.20** indicated that the *p*-methoxyphenyl group plunged into the S1′ pocket, whereas the adjacent ethoxy group entered the S2′ subsite. The tetrahydro isoquinoline ring produced some effective van der Waals interaction at the S1/S2 site. The phosphonyl oxygen atom produced a hydrogen bonding interaction with Leu164 and Ala165.

Becker and co-workers [55] at Pfizer Research evaluated some β- and α-piperidine sulfone hydroxamates as potent MMPIs. Compound **6.21** (Figure 6.5) exhibited the most potent MMP-3 inhibitory efficacy (K_i = 0.3 nM) among these compounds. Compound **6.21** has a good bioavailability of about 36% and a C_{max} of 15,720 ng/ml. Further research conducted by the same group of scientists [56] produced a series of α-sulfone-α-piperidine, as well as α-tetrahydropyranyl hydroxamates as promising MMPIs. Among these compounds, compound **6.22** (Figure 6.5) showed the maximum MMP-3 inhibition (IC_{50} = 0.2 nM). It exhibited a high C_{max} (27158 ng/ml), modest half-life ($t_{1/2}$ = 1.1 hr), and good bioavailability (36.9%). Again, Barta et al. [57] of Pfizer Research reported some α-sulfone hydroxamates as promising

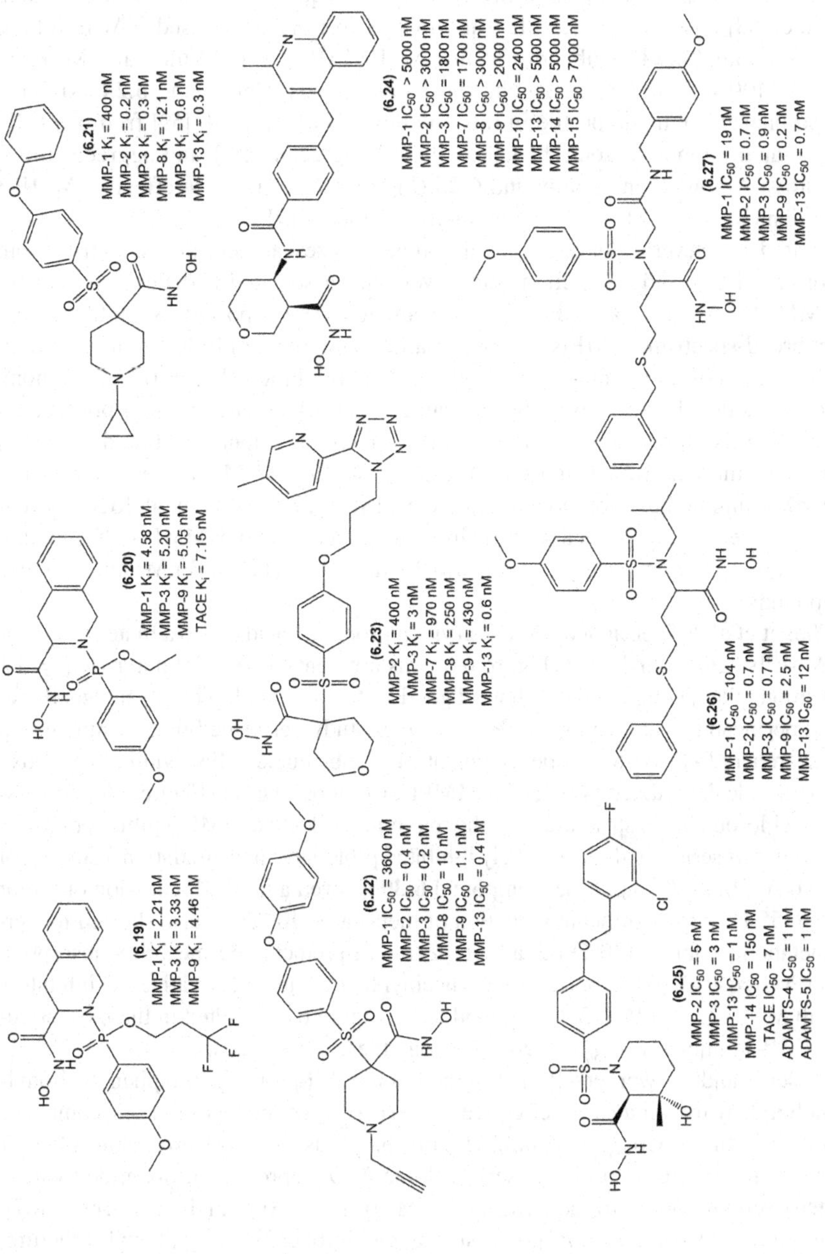

FIGURE 6.5 Another set of hydroxamate-based potential MMP-3 inhibitors (compounds **6.19–6.27**).

(6.19)
MMP-1 K_i = 2.21 nM
MMP-3 K_i = 3.33 nM
MMP-9 K_i = 4.46 nM

(6.20)
MMP-1 K_i = 4.58 nM
MMP-3 K_i = 5.20 nM
MMP-9 K_i = 5.05 nM
TACE K_i = 7.15 nM

(6.21)
MMP-1 K_i = 400 nM
MMP-2 K_i = 0.2 nM
MMP-3 K_i = 0.3 nM
MMP-8 K_i = 12.1 nM
MMP-9 K_i = 0.6 nM
MMP-13 K_i = 0.3 nM

(6.22)
MMP-1 IC_{50} = 3600 nM
MMP-2 IC_{50} = 0.4 nM
MMP-3 IC_{50} = 0.2 nM
MMP-8 IC_{50} = 10 nM
MMP-9 IC_{50} = 1.1 nM
MMP-13 IC_{50} = 0.4 nM

(6.23)
MMP-2 K_i = 400 nM
MMP-3 K_i = 3 nM
MMP-7 K_i = 970 nM
MMP-8 K_i = 250 nM
MMP-9 K_i = 430 nM
MMP-13 K_i = 0.6 nM

(6.24)
MMP-1 IC_{50} > 5000 nM
MMP-2 IC_{50} = 3000 nM
MMP-3 IC_{50} = 1800 nM
MMP-7 IC_{50} = 1700 nM
MMP-8 IC_{50} = 3000 nM
MMP-9 IC_{50} > 2000 nM
MMP-10 IC_{50} = 2400 nM
MMP-13 IC_{50} > 5000 nM
MMP-14 IC_{50} = 5000 nM
MMP-15 IC_{50} > 7000 nM

(6.25)
MMP-2 IC_{50} = 5 nM
MMP-3 IC_{50} = 3 nM
MMP-13 IC_{50} = 1 nM
MMP-14 IC_{50} = 150 nM
TACE IC_{50} = 7 nM
ADAMTS-4 IC_{50} = 1 nM
ADAMTS-5 IC_{50} = 1 nM

(6.26)
MMP-1 IC_{50} = 104 nM
MMP-2 IC_{50} = 0.7 nM
MMP-3 IC_{50} = 0.7 nM
MMP-9 IC_{50} = 2.5 nM
MMP-13 IC_{50} = 12 nM

(6.27)
MMP-1 IC_{50} = 19 nM
MMP-2 IC_{50} = 0.7 nM
MMP-3 IC_{50} = 0.9 nM
MMP-9 IC_{50} = 0.2 nM
MMP-13 IC_{50} = 0.7 nM

MMPIs. Among these compounds, compound **6.23** (Figure 6.5) resulted in the highest MMP-3 inhibition (K_i = 3 nM), having good selectivity over other MMPs except MMP-13.

Again, a group of scientists from Bristol Myers Squibb Pharmaceutical Research Institute [58] disclosed a set of β-amino hydroxamic acid-based TACE inhibitors. Compound **6.24** exhibited effective MMP-3 (IC_{50} = 1800 nM) and MMP-10 (IC_{50} = 2400 nM) inhibition among these compounds. Compound **6.24** exhibited a good pharmacokinetic profile in rats and dogs. Durham et al. [59] from Eli Lilly and Company reported some hydantoin-based aggrecanases-1 and aggrecanases-2 inhibitors. Among them, compound **6.25** (Figure 6.5) resulted in effective MMP-3 inhibition (IC_{50} = 3 nM) but non-specificity to other MMPs.

Apart from several pharmaceutical companies, researchers and scientists from various academic and research institutes were also associated with designing potential MMPIs. A set of arysulfonyl hydroxamates were reported as highly efficacious broad-spectrum MMPIs by Hanessian and co-workers [60]. Compound **6.26** (Figure 6.5) showed the most efficacious MMP-3 inhibition (IC_{50} = 0.7 nM) among these molecules. Further study by the same group of researchers [61] produced a series of arylsulfonyl homocysteine hydroxamates as potent and broad-spectrum MMPIs. Compound **6.27** (Figure 6.5) resulted in effective MMP-3 inhibition (IC_{50} = 0.9 nM) among these compounds. In the next study, Hanessian et al. [62] reported another series of arylsulfonamide hydroxamates as potential MMPIs. Compound **6.28** (Figure 6.6) displayed potential MMP-3 inhibition (IC_{50} = 3 nM) among these compounds.

Chollet et al. [63] designed some 3-aryloxy propionic acid hydroxamates as potential MMPIs. Compound **6.29** (Figure 6.6) was a potent MMP-3 inhibitor (IC_{50} = 1.1 nM) among these compounds. It showed good metabolic stability (42%) and good predicted permeability absorption (96%). A further study performed by the same group of researchers [64] led to the development of α-substituted 3-bisarylthio N-hydroxy propionamide derivatives as potential MMPIs. Compound **6.30** (Figure 6.6), possessing a *p*-chlorobiphenyl structure, was the maximum effective MMP-3 inhibitor (IC_{50} = 10 nM) in this series. It also effectively inhibited proteoglycan degradation at an IC_{50} of 1.1 µM. At 200mg/kg i.p. dose, compound **6.30** showed a marked reduction of tumor burden (55%) and a significant reduction of metastasis (100%). It also showed moderate metabolic stability (20%) but a high degree of predicted permeability absorption (92%). Marcq et al. [65] reported some succinyl hydroxamate derivatives as inhibitors of both MMP-2 and MMP-3. Compound **6.31** (Figure 6.6) resulted in the most effective MMP-3 inhibition (IC_{50} = 179 nM) among these compounds.

Rossello and co-workers [66] designed some *N-i*-propoxy-N-biphenylsulfonyl-aminobutyl hydroxamates as effective and MMP-2-selective inhibitors compared with other MMPs. Compound **6.32** (Figure 6.6) was the most promising MMP-3 inhibitor (IC_{50} = 1.6 nM) in this series. Some *N*-O-isopropyl sulfonamide hydroxamates were reported to be efficacious MMPIs by Nuti and co-workers [67]. Compound **6.33** (Figure 6.6), possessing a *p*-chlorobenzyloxy biphenyl structure, resulted in potent MMP-3 inhibition (IC_{50} = 180 nM). It also produced good results in a collagen degradation assay.

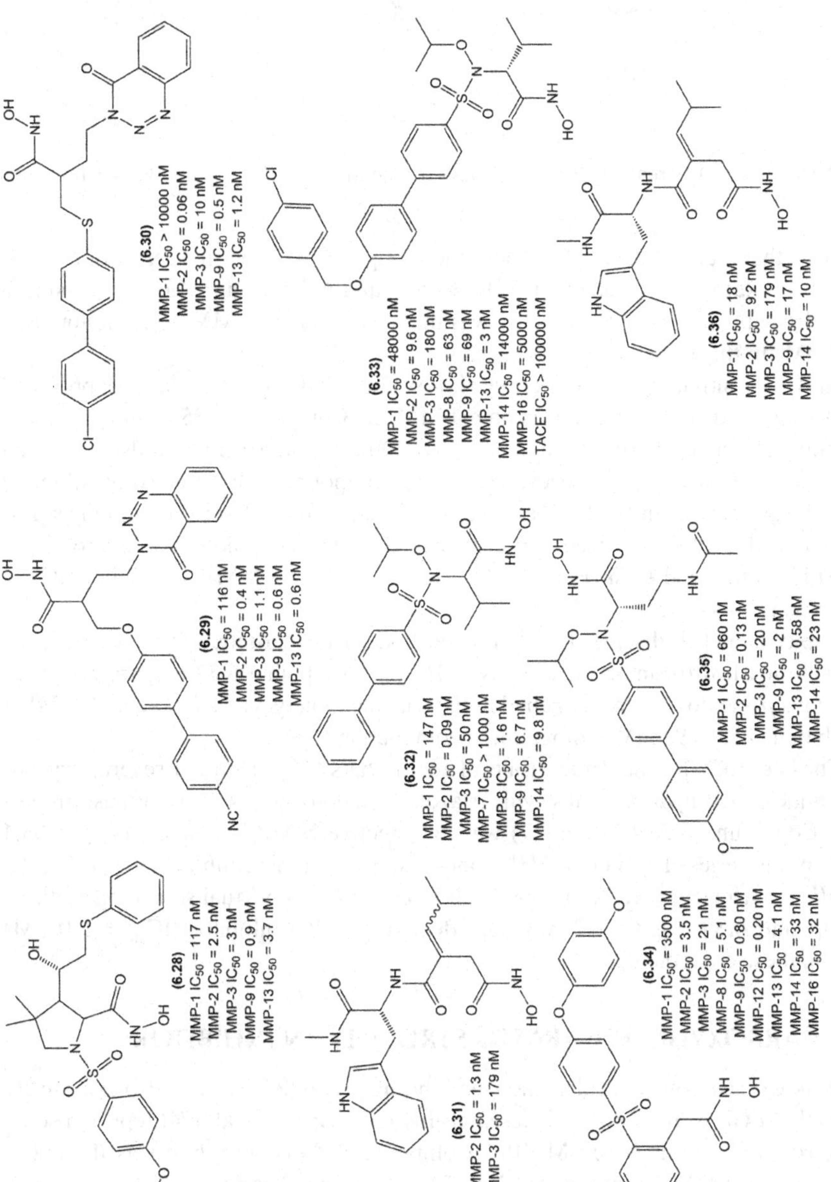

FIGURE 6.6 Another set of hydroxamate-based potential MMP-3 inhibitors (compounds **6.28–6.36**).

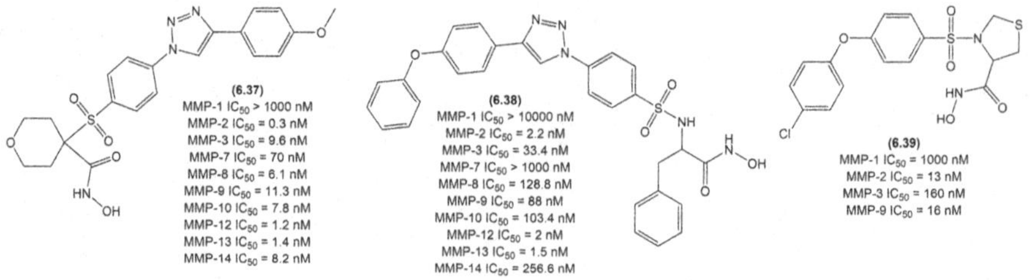

(6.37)
MMP-1 IC_{50} > 1000 nM
MMP-2 IC_{50} = 0.3 nM
MMP-3 IC_{50} = 9.6 nM
MMP-7 IC_{50} = 70 nM
MMP-8 IC_{50} = 6.1 nM
MMP-9 IC_{50} = 11.3 nM
MMP-10 IC_{50} = 7.8 nM
MMP-12 IC_{50} = 1.2 nM
MMP-13 IC_{50} = 1.4 nM
MMP-14 IC_{50} = 8.2 nM

(6.38)
MMP-1 IC_{50} > 10000 nM
MMP-2 IC_{50} = 2.2 nM
MMP-3 IC_{50} = 33.4 nM
MMP-7 IC_{50} = 1000 nM
MMP-8 IC_{50} = 128.8 nM
MMP-9 IC_{50} = 88 nM
MMP-10 IC_{50} = 103.4 nM
MMP-12 IC_{50} = 2 nM
MMP-13 IC_{50} = 1.5 nM
MMP-14 IC_{50} = 256.6 nM

(6.39)
MMP-1 IC_{50} = 1000 nM
MMP-2 IC_{50} = 13 nM
MMP-3 IC_{50} = 160 nM
MMP-9 IC_{50} = 16 nM

FIGURE 6.7 Different hydroxamate-based potential MMP-3 inhibitors (compounds 6.37–6.39).

A further study conducted by the same group [68] resulted in a series of arylsulfone hydroxamates as potent MMPIs. Compound **6.34** (Figure 6.6), possessing a *p*-methoxy phenyloxy phenyl group, was the most promising MMP-3 inhibitor (IC_{50} = 21 nM) in this set.

In their continuous effort, Nuti et al. [69] further designed some *N*-isopropoxy-arylsulfonamide hydroxamates as potent MMPIs. Compound **6.35** (Figure 6.6) was the most effective MMP-3 inhibitor (IC_{50} = 20 nM) in this series. It also displayed potential antiangiogenic efficacy. Moreover, compound **6.35** effectively inhibited both the gelatinases in HUVEC cells, as disclosed by the gelatin zymography study. Moroy et al. [70] synthesized and evaluated the analogs of ilomastat as promising MMPIs. Compound **6.36** (Figure 6.6) was the promising MMP-3 inhibitor (IC_{50} = 179 nM) in this series.

Zapico et al. [71] disclosed a set of potent and selective α-tetrahydropyranyl-based arylsulfonyl hydroxamates as effective MMPIs. Compound **6.37** (Figure 6.7), possessing a *p*-methoxy group attached to the triazole moiety, yielded potential MMP-3 inhibition (IC_{50} = 9.6 nM) among these compounds.

Further study by the same group of researchers [72] identified several arylsulfonamide-based hydroxamates with triazole functions as potent gelatinase inhibitors. Compound **6.38** (Figure 6.7) was an effective MMP-3 inhibitor (IC_{50} = 33.4 nM) in this series. Topai et al. [73] reported some gelatinase inhibitors by using the *in silico* pharmacophore-based approach followed by the virtual screening method. Compound **6.39** (Figure 6.7) was an effective MMP-3 inhibitor (IC_{50} = 160 nM) among these compounds.

6.4 CARBOXYLIC ACID-BASED STROMELYSIN INHIBITOR

MMPIs with carboxylic acid as the zinc-binding group (ZBG) were also extensively studied. At Glaxo Incorporated Research Institute, Brown et al. [74] reported some (carboxyalkyl) amino-based MMPIs. Compound **6.40** (Figure 6.8) was the maximum effective MMP-3 inhibitor (IC_{50} = 72 nM) among these molecules.

At Parke-Davis Pharmaceutical Research, O'Brien et al. [75] studied some biphenylsulfonamide-based carboxylic acids as potent MMPIs. Although compound **6.41** (Figure 6.8) was a potent MMP-3 inhibitor (IC_{50} = 3 nM), it also produced potent MMP-2 and MMP-13 inhibition.

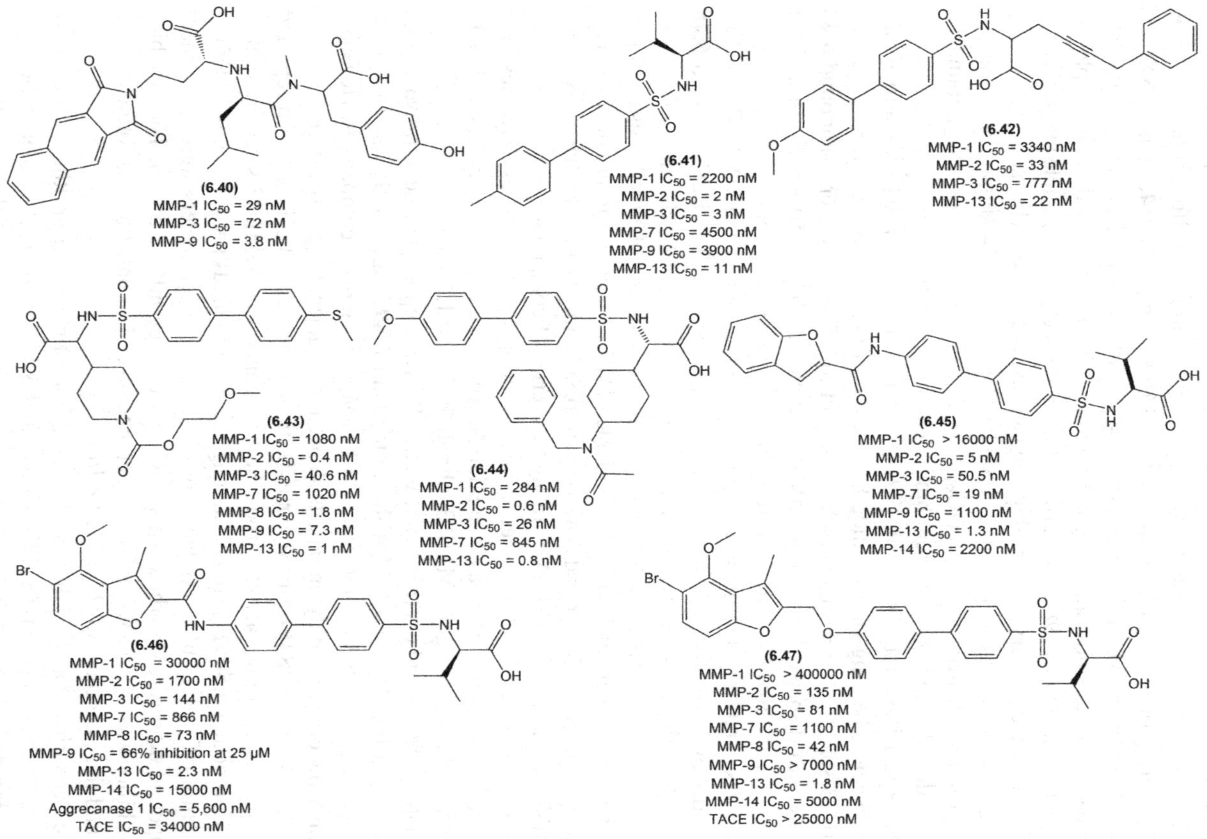

(6.40)
MMP-1 IC$_{50}$ = 29 nM
MMP-3 IC$_{50}$ = 72 nM
MMP-9 IC$_{50}$ = 3.8 nM

(6.41)
MMP-1 IC$_{50}$ = 2200 nM
MMP-2 IC$_{50}$ = 2 nM
MMP-3 IC$_{50}$ = 3 nM
MMP-7 IC$_{50}$ = 4500 nM
MMP-9 IC$_{50}$ = 3900 nM
MMP-13 IC$_{50}$ = 11 nM

(6.42)
MMP-1 IC$_{50}$ = 3340 nM
MMP-2 IC$_{50}$ = 33 nM
MMP-3 IC$_{50}$ = 777 nM
MMP-13 IC$_{50}$ = 22 nM

(6.43)
MMP-1 IC$_{50}$ = 1080 nM
MMP-2 IC$_{50}$ = 0.4 nM
MMP-3 IC$_{50}$ = 40.6 nM
MMP-7 IC$_{50}$ = 1020 nM
MMP-8 IC$_{50}$ = 1.8 nM
MMP-9 IC$_{50}$ = 7.3 nM
MMP-13 IC$_{50}$ = 1 nM

(6.44)
MMP-1 IC$_{50}$ = 284 nM
MMP-2 IC$_{50}$ = 0.6 nM
MMP-3 IC$_{50}$ = 26 nM
MMP-7 IC$_{50}$ = 845 nM
MMP-13 IC$_{50}$ = 0.8 nM

(6.45)
MMP-1 IC$_{50}$ > 16000 nM
MMP-2 IC$_{50}$ = 5 nM
MMP-3 IC$_{50}$ = 50.5 nM
MMP-7 IC$_{50}$ = 19 nM
MMP-9 IC$_{50}$ = 1100 nM
MMP-13 IC$_{50}$ = 1.3 nM
MMP-14 IC$_{50}$ = 2200 nM

(6.46)
MMP-1 IC$_{50}$ = 30000 nM
MMP-2 IC$_{50}$ = 1700 nM
MMP-3 IC$_{50}$ = 144 nM
MMP-7 IC$_{50}$ = 866 nM
MMP-8 IC$_{50}$ = 73 nM
MMP-9 IC$_{50}$ = 66% inhibition at 25 µM
MMP-13 IC$_{50}$ = 2.3 nM
MMP-14 IC$_{50}$ = 15000 nM
Aggrecanase 1 IC$_{50}$ = 5,600 nM
TACE IC$_{50}$ = 34000 nM

(6.47)
MMP-1 IC$_{50}$ > 400000 nM
MMP-2 IC$_{50}$ = 135 nM
MMP-3 IC$_{50}$ = 81 nM
MMP-7 IC$_{50}$ = 1100 nM
MMP-8 IC$_{50}$ = 42 nM
MMP-9 IC$_{50}$ > 7000 nM
MMP-13 IC$_{50}$ = 1.8 nM
MMP-14 IC$_{50}$ = 5000 nM
TACE IC$_{50}$ > 25000 nM

FIGURE 6.8 Carboxylic acid-based MMP-3 inhibitors (compounds **6.40–6.47**).

At Procter and Gamble Pharmaceuticals, Natchus et al. [76] designed a set of arylsulfonamido carboxylic acids with functionalized propargylglycines as potent MMPIs. Compound **6.42** (Figure 6.8) exhibited good MMP-3 inhibition ($IC_{50} = 777$ nM) but resulted in better affinity toward MMP-2 and MMP-13. In another study, Pikul et al. [77] of Procter and Gamble designed several arylsulfonamide carboxylic acids, bearing piperidine moiety, as potent MMPIs. Compound **6.43** (Figure 6.8) was the most promising MMP-3 inhibitor ($IC_{50} = 40.6$ nM) among these compounds. The pharmacokinetics study showed good solubility (3.50 mg/ml) with a higher plasma protein binding ability (98.2%). Further studies at Procter and Gamble by Tullis et al. [78] led to the discovery of some biphenylsulfonamide carboxylic acids with cyclohexylglycine scaffolds as potential MMPIs. Compound **6.44** (Figure 6.8) was the most promising MMP-3 inhibitor ($IC_{50} = 26$ nM) among this series of compounds. It also produced high plasma protein binding ability (98.5%).

At Wyeth Research, Wu et al. [79] reported a set of biphenylsulfonamide carboxylic acids, bearing carboxamide heterocyclic functions, as highly effective and MMP-13-selective inhibitors over MMP-2 and MMP-14. However, compound **6.45** (Figure 6.8) displayed promising MMP-3 inhibition ($IC_{50} = 50.5$ nM). In another study, Li et al. [80] at Wyeth Research reported another set of benzofuran 2-carboxamido-based biphenylsulfonamide carboxylic acids as potent and MMP-13-selective inhibitors over other MMPs as well as aggrecanase-1 and TACE. Compound **6.46** (Figure 6.8) showed effective MMP-3 inhibition ($IC_{50} = 144$ nM) among the series of compounds. A further study conducted by the scientists of Wyeth Research [81] reported some potent and orally bioavailable MMP-13-selective inhibitors for osteoarthritis treatment. Compound **6.47** (Figure 6.8) resulted in the highest efficacious MMP-3 inhibitor ($IC_{50} = 81$ nM) among this series of compounds.

Hudlicky et al. [82] reported some functionalized cyclohexylglycines and α-methylcyclohexylgycines as potential MMPIs. Among them, compound **6.48** (Figure 6.9) exhibited good MMP-3 inhibition ($IC_{50} = 1,220$ nM).

Matter and co-workers [83] from Aventis Pharma reported some tetrahydroisoquinoline-3-carboxylate-based MMPIs. Compound **6.49** (Figure 6.9) was the maximum effective MMP-3 inhibitor ($IC_{50} = 13$ nM) among these compounds. However, the pharmacokinetic study on rabbits showed insufficient C_{max} (1.6 μg/ml).

Monovich et al. [84] from Novartis Institutes for Biomedical Research reported some potent and orally active carboxylic acid-containing MMP-13-selective inhibitors. Compound **6.50** (Figure 6.9) among these compounds produced good MMP-3 inhibition ($IC_{50} = 18$ nM). As far as pharmacokinetic parameters were concerned, compound **6.50** was absorbed rapidly ($C_{max} = 0.58$ μg/ml at 0.56 hr). The oral bioavailability was 46.6%, which is quite appreciable. The half-life was found to be 7 hrs, and the clearance was high (112 ml/min/kg).

Le Diguarher et al. [85] disclosed a set of 5-substituted 2-bisarylthiocyclopentane carboxylic acids as potent MMPIs. Compound **6.51** (Figure 6.9) exhibited the most promising MMP-3-selective inhibition ($IC_{50} = 1.2$ nM) over other MMPs tested. Yuan et al. [86] reported some derivatives of methyl rosmarinate as potential MMP-1 inhibitors. Among these compounds, compound **6.52** (Figure 6.9) yielded effective MMP-3 inhibition ($IC_{50} = 3.4$ μM).

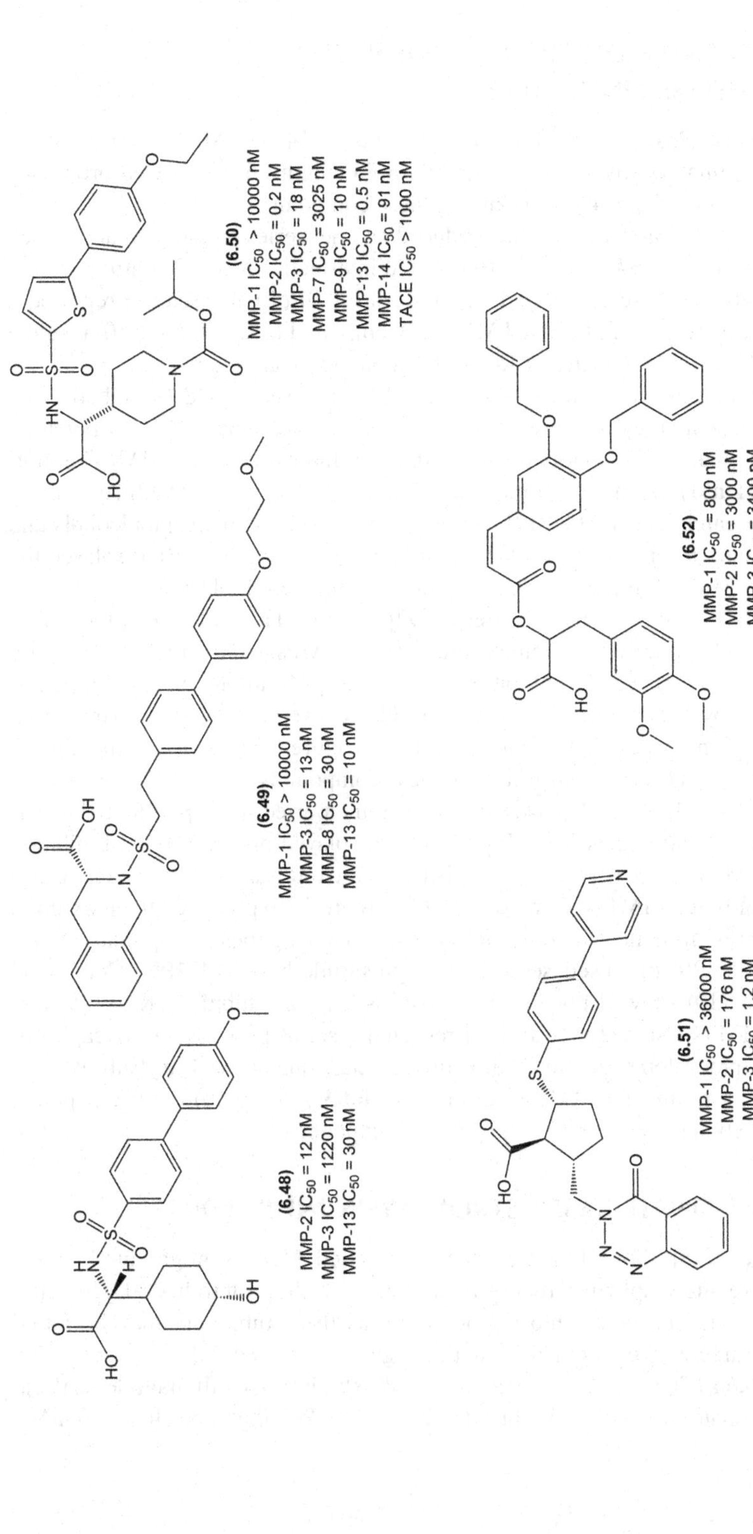

(6.50)
MMP-1 IC$_{50}$ > 10000 nM
MMP-2 IC$_{50}$ = 0.2 nM
MMP-3 IC$_{50}$ = 18 nM
MMP-7 IC$_{50}$ = 3025 nM
MMP-9 IC$_{50}$ = 10 nM
MMP-13 IC$_{50}$ = 0.5 nM
MMP-14 IC$_{50}$ = 91 nM
TACE IC$_{50}$ > 1000 nM

(6.49)
MMP-1 IC$_{50}$ > 10000 nM
MMP-3 IC$_{50}$ = 13 nM
MMP-8 IC$_{50}$ = 30 nM
MMP-13 IC$_{50}$ = 10 nM

(6.48)
MMP-2 IC$_{50}$ = 12 nM
MMP-3 IC$_{50}$ = 1220 nM
MMP-13 IC$_{50}$ = 30 nM

(6.52)
MMP-1 IC$_{50}$ = 800 nM
MMP-2 IC$_{50}$ = 3000 nM
MMP-3 IC$_{50}$ = 3400 nM
MMP-9 IC$_{50}$ = 6000 nM
MMP-12 IC$_{50}$ = 2300 nM
MMP-13 IC$_{50}$ = 5400 nM

(6.51)
MMP-1 IC$_{50}$ > 36000 nM
MMP-2 IC$_{50}$ = 176 nM
MMP-3 IC$_{50}$ = 1.2 nM
MMP-9 IC$_{50}$ = 341 nM
MMP-13 IC$_{50}$ = 275 nM

FIGURE 6.9 Various carboxylic acid-based MMP-3 inhibitors (compounds **6.48–6.52**).

6.5 THIOL- AND MERCAPTOSULFIDE-BASED STROMELYSIN INHIBITORS

At Chiroscience, Baxter et al. [87] reported some thiol-based MMPIs for the treatment of inflammatory disorders. Compound **6.53** (Figure 6.10) showed promising MMP-3 inhibition (IC_{50} = 430 nM) among these compounds.

Further study by Baxter et al. [88] produced another series of marcaptoacyl-based MMPIs. Compound **6.54** (Figure 6.10) resulted in effective MMP-3 inhibition (IC_{50} = 490 nM) among these compounds. Lynas et al. [89] of Chiroscience reported a series of N-α-mercaptoamide-based MMPIs. Compound **6.55** (Figure 6.10) resulted in good MMP-3 inhibition (IC_{50} = 1.47 µM) among these compounds.

The joint venture of Affimax and Wyeth-Ayrest Research led Campbell et al. [90] to discover malonyl α-mercaptoketones and α-mercaptoalcohols as potential MMPIs. Compound **6.56** (Figure 6.10) was the maximum efficacious MMP-3 inhibitor (IC_{50} = 11 nM) among these molecules. In another study at Wyeth-Ayrest and Affymax Research, Levin et al. [91] reported some succinyl mercaptoalcohols and mercaptoketones as promising MMPIs. Compound **6.57** (Figure 6.10) displayed the best effective MMP-3 inhibition (IC_{50} = 8 nM) among these molecules.

In Affimax Research, Szardenings et al. [92] developed a set of diketopiperazine-containing thiol derivatives as potent inhibitors of MMPs. Compound **6.58** (Figure 6.10) resulted in good MMP-3 inhibition (IC_{50} = 2.91 µM) among these compounds. Further study by Szardenings et al. [93] produced several diketopiperazine-based thiol analogs as potent MMPIs. Compound **6.59** (Figure 6.10) exhibited the highest MMP-3 inhibition (IC_{50} = 1.1 µM) among these compounds.

Freskos et al. [94] of Searle Discovery Research reported some γ-sulfone thiols as potent MMPIs. Compounds **6.60** (Figure 6.10) displayed potent MMP-3 inhibition (IC_{50} = 150 nM). Fink et al. [95] at Novartis Biomedical Research Institute reported a series of thiol-based MMPIs. Compound **6.61** (Figure 6.10) produced the maximum effective MMP-3 inhibitory activity (IC_{50} = 15 nM) among these compounds.

Hurst et al. [96] disclosed several mercaptosulfide-based MMPIs. Compound **6.62** (Figure 6.10) showed potent and MMP-3-selective inhibition (K_i = 1.5 nM) over other MMPs tested. Jin et al. [97] reported a set of pyrrolidine mercaptosulfide, 2-mercaptocyclopentane arylsulfonamide, and 3-mercapto-4-arylsulfonamide pyrrolidines as promising MMPIs. Compound **6.63** (Figure 10) exhibited potent MMP-3 inhibition (K_i = 37 nM) among these compounds.

6.6 PHOSPHONATE-BASED STROMELYSIN INHIBITORS

Pochetti et al. [98] showed that phosphonate-based MMPIs might bind to the MMP-8 active site employing two oxygen atoms forming a tetrahedral geometry. Phosphonates may be taken into consideration as these inhibitors may be found to exhibit characteristic interaction at the highly conserved MMP-8 active site. Compound **6.64** (Figure 6.11) bearing a *p*-methoxy biphenyl sulfonamido scaffold and a phosphonate ZBG group produced effective MMP-3 inhibition (IC_{50} = 40 nM).

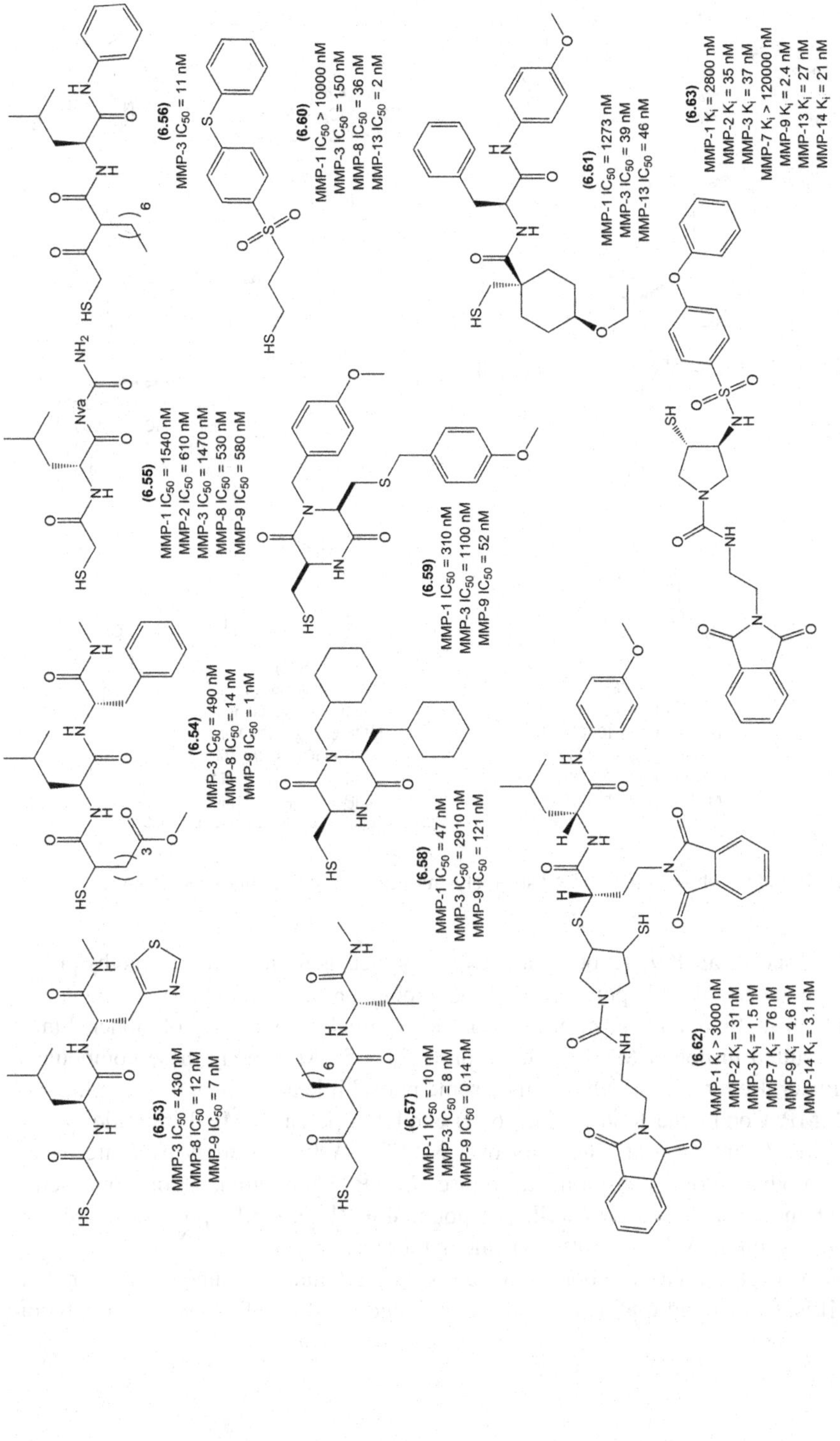

FIGURE 6.10 Thiol-based MMP-3 inhibitors (compounds 6.53–6.63).

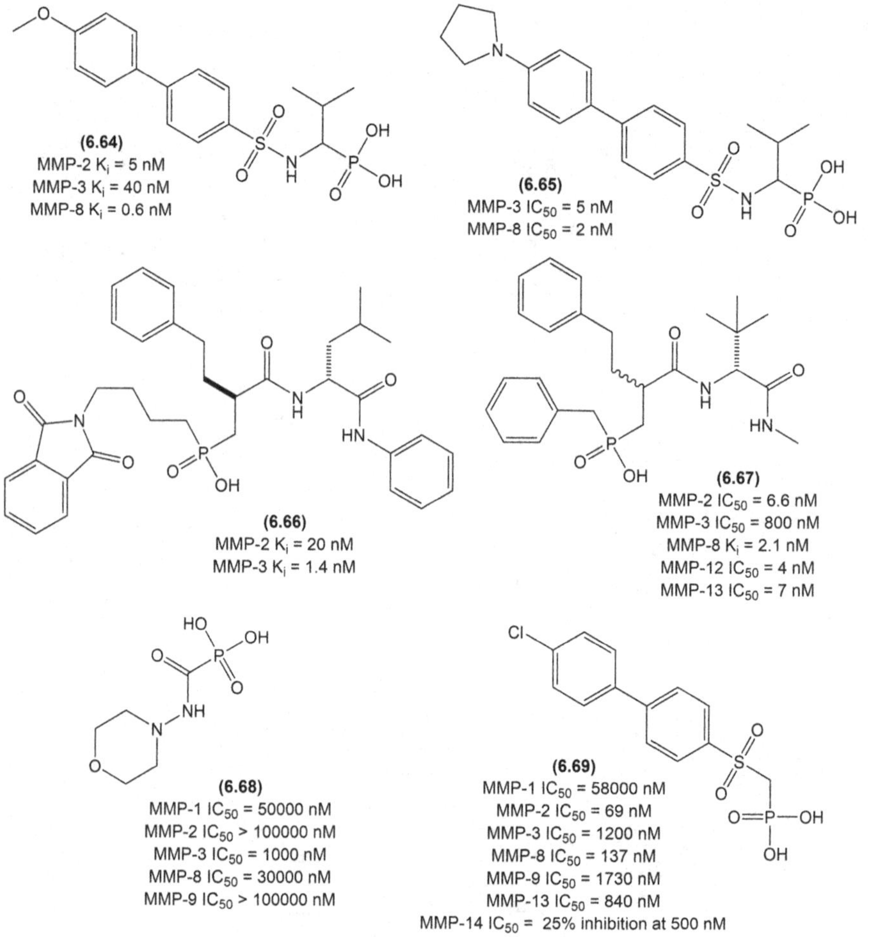

FIGURE 6.11   Phosphonate-based stromelysin inhibitors (compounds **6.64–6.69**).

Biasone et al. [99] reported a set of α-biphenylsulfonylamino 2-methylpropyl phosphonates as highly potent MMPIs. Compound **6.65** (Figure 6.11) bearing a pyrrolidinyl scaffold at the *para* position of the terminal phenyl group of biphenyl moiety resulted in potent MMP-3 inhibition (IC_{50} = 5 nM) among these compounds. At Pfizer, Reiter et al. [100] designed some phosphinic acids as potential inhibitors of MMP. Compound **6.66** (Figure 6.11) exhibited potent MMP-3 inhibition (K_i = 1.4 nM) having 14-fold selectivity over MMP-2. A further study by Reiter et al. [101] produced some phosphinic acid-based MMP-13 inhibitors, having some activity against MMP-1 and -3 as well. Compound **6.67** (Figure 6.11) possessed effective MMP-3 inhibition (IC_{50} = 800 nM) among these compounds.

Breuer et al. [102] reported a series of carbamoylphosphonates as potent MMPIs. Compound **6.68** (Figure 6.11) exhibited good MMP-3-selective inhibition

(IC_{50} = 1000 nM) over other MMPs tested. Rubino et al. [103] reported some α-sulfonylphosphonic acid-based promising MMPIs. Compound **6.69** (Figure 6.11) showed effective MMP-3 inhibition (IC_{50} = 1200 nM) among these compounds.

Matziari and co-workers [104] disclosed a set of phosphinic peptides as potent and MMP-11-selective inhibitors. Compound **6.70** (Table 6.1) bearing an *o*-bromo phenylthiomethyl group moved toward S1' pocket produced maximum MMP-11 inhibitory efficacy (K_i = 110 nM). It was also highly effective over other MMPs (MMP-2, -8, -9, -13, and -14). Slight modifications of the *o*-bromo group with ortho methoxy (compound **6.71**, Table 6.1) and ortho-trifluoro methoxy (compound **6.72**) also provided highly potent and MMP-11-selective inhibitors (**Table 6.1**). In another study, Matziari et al. [1] further modified the P1' substituents to derivatize these phosphinic-based peptides and reported a series of highly efficacious MMP-11-selective inhibitors (Compound **6.73–6.97**, Table 6.1).

6.7 N-HYDROXYUREA-BASED STROMELYSIN INHIBITORS

N-hydroxyurea function is an important ZBG due to its structural similarity with hydroxamates. As per the report of Campestre and co-workers [105], compound **6.98** (Figure 6.12) possessing a *p*-cyanobiphenyl group attached to the propionyloxy function yielded potent MMP-3 inhibition (IC_{50} = 200 μM). A slight modification of the aryl function with phenoxyphenyl moiety (compound **6.99,** Figure 6.12) also produced effective MMP-3 inhibitory (IC_{50} = 380 μM) efficacy.

6.8 HYDRAZIDE-BASED STROMELYSIN INHIBITORS

Hydrazides and sulfonylhydrazides were also found to be effective ZBGs. Being an isostere of hydroxamates, these ZBG also possess similar types of bidentate metal-chelating abilities. However, these hydrazides and sulfonylhydrazides were less effective MMPIs than the corresponding hydroxamates. LeDour and co-workers [106] reported some hydrazide-based analogs of Ilomastat as potent MMPIs. Compound **6.100** (Figure 6.13) possessing a *p*-bromo biphenylsulfonamido hydrazide group resulted in highly potent MMP-3 inhibition (IC_{50} = 53 nM).

6.9 N-HYDROXYFORMAMIDE-BASED STROMELYSIN INHIBITORS

N-hydroxyformamide was also found to be an effective ZBG for the development of potential MMPIs. Scientists of GlaxoSmithKline [107] reported some N-hydroxyformamide-based MMPIs. Compound **6.101** (Figure 6.14) was the most effective MMP-3 inhibitor (IC_{50} = 17 nM) in this series of compounds.

The researchers of Abbott laboratories [108] reported several retrohydroxamates as potent and orally bioavailable MMPIs. Compound **6.102** (**Figure 6.14**), possessing a *p*-trifluoromethoxy phenoxyphenyl sylfonylmethyl moiety attached to the retrohydroxamte scaffold, produced potent MMP-3 inhibition (IC_{50} = 12 nM). Compound **6.102** was highly bioavailable (>70%) when tested in rats, dogs, and monkeys. It had an AUC of 53μM.h and a half-life of 16.8 hrs when tested in cynomolgus monkeys.

TABLE 6.1
Phosphonate-Based Potential and Selective MMP-11 Inhibitors [K_i (nM)]

Cpd	R	MMP-1	MMP-2	MMP-7	MMP-8	MMP-9	MMP-11	MMP-13	MMP-14
6.70	$CH_2S(o\text{-}BrPh)$	—	4,650	—	18,400	3,910	110	8,700	30,100
6.71	$CH_2S(o\text{-}OMePh)$	—	30,000	—	38,900	35,600	230	15,700	160,000
6.72	$CH_2S(o\text{-}OCF_3Ph)$	—	200,000	—	200,000	148,000	410	200,000	30,000
6.73	CH_3	20% at 2 µM	0% at 2 µM	0% at 2 µM	9% at 2 µM	0% at 2 µM	2,700	—	0% at 2 µM
6.74	i-Pr	45% at 2 µM	202	210	40	65	22	—	192
6.75	Benzyl	10% at 2 µM	275	7% at 2 µM	45	110	9	—	660
6.76	CH_2Benzyl	23% at 2 µM	20	8% at 2 µM	2.5	10	5	—	105
6.77	β-naphthylmethyl	0% at 2 µM	330	1800	230	675	74	—	1,350
6.78	β-naphthyl$(CH_2)_2$	0% at 2 µM	30	2100	34	55	12	—	125
6.79	Benzyloxymethyl	9% at 2 µM	85	3% at 2 µM	20	55	16	—	545
6.80	Cyclohexyl thiomethyl	—	10,000	175,000	38,000	100,000	260	21,000	100,000

(Continued)

TABLE 6.1 (CONTINUED)
Phosphonate-Based Potential and Selective MMP-11 Inhibitors [K_i (nM)]

Cpd	R	MMP-1	MMP-2	MMP-7	MMP-8	MMP-9	MMP-11	MMP-13	MMP-14
6.81	Isobutylthiomethyl	—	6,500	450,000	1,250	10,000	165	1,850	21,000
6.82	Isopentylthiomethyl	—	4,500	450,000	660	10,000	165	850	21,000
6.83	CH_2SCH_2COOMe	—	6,300	300,000	2,000	10,000	300	1,350	15,000
6.84	CH_2SCH_2COOEt	—	6,300	>100,000	1,800	10,000	530	1,700	13,000
6.85	$CH_2S(CH_2)_2COOMe$	—	3,700	>100,000	900	2,000	380	1,400	16,000
6.86	$CH_2S(CH_2)_2COOEt$	—	2,500	>100,000	970	1,900	275	1,600	6,500
6.87	CH_2SPh	—	210	—	40	93	10	42	670
6.88	CH_2S(o-BrPh)	—	4,500	—	18,000	4,000	113	4,700	30,000
6.89	CH_2S(o-isopropylPh)	—	>100,000	—	11,000	29,000	300	10,000	24,000
6.90	CH_2S(o-EtPh)	—	>100,000	—	>100,000	>100,000	270	22,000	19,000
6.91	CH_2S(2, 4-di-t-ButPh)	—	765	—	3,400	6,700	77	1,700	13,000
6.92	CH_2S(o-OMePh)	—	30,000	—	40,000	35,600	230	16,000	160,000
6.93	CH_2S(2, 5-di-OMePh)	—	25,500	—	>100,000	85,000	430	31,000	25,000
6.94	CH_2S(o-OCF_3Ph)	—	>100,000	—	>100,000	—	413	>100,000	30,000
6.95	CH_2S(2-OCF_3, 4-BrPh)	—	14,000	—	>100,000	—	333	88,000	20,600
6.96	CH_2S(2-OCF_3, 4-PhPh)	—	15,800	—	100,000	20,000	615	9,000	23,700
6.97	CH_2S(m-OMePh)	—	2200	83,000	107	—	66	—	3,800

Cpd, compound.

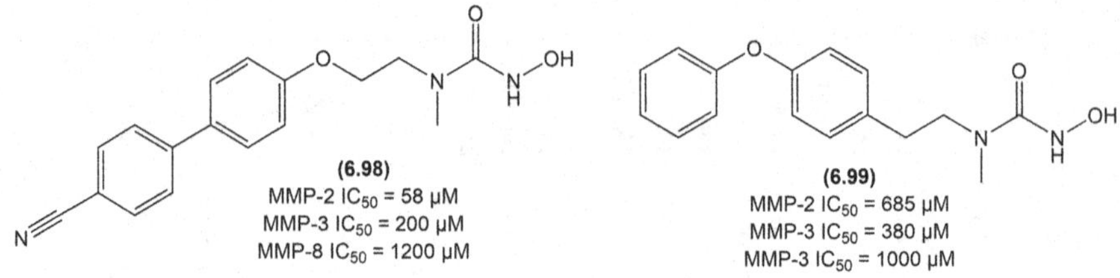

(6.98)
MMP-2 IC_{50} = 58 µM
MMP-3 IC_{50} = 200 µM
MMP-8 IC_{50} = 1200 µM

(6.99)
MMP-2 IC_{50} = 685 µM
MMP-3 IC_{50} = 380 µM
MMP-3 IC_{50} = 1000 µM

FIGURE 6.12   Hydroxyurea-based effective MMP-3 inhibitors (compounds **6.98–6.99**).

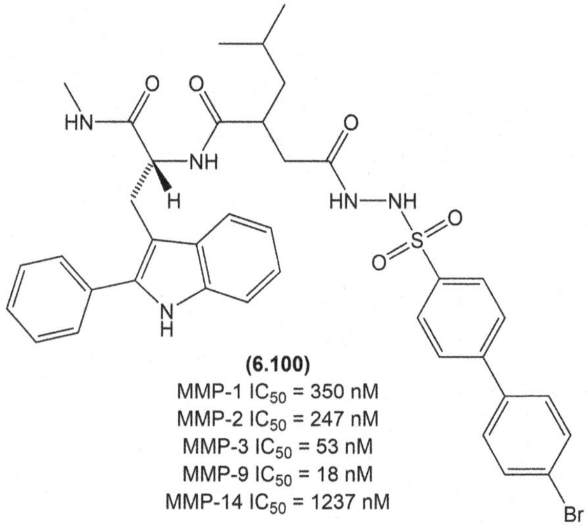

(6.100)
MMP-1 IC_{50} = 350 nM
MMP-2 IC_{50} = 247 nM
MMP-3 IC_{50} = 53 nM
MMP-9 IC_{50} = 18 nM
MMP-14 IC_{50} = 1237 nM

FIGURE 6.13   Hydrazide-based effective MMP-3 inhibitors (compound **6.100**).

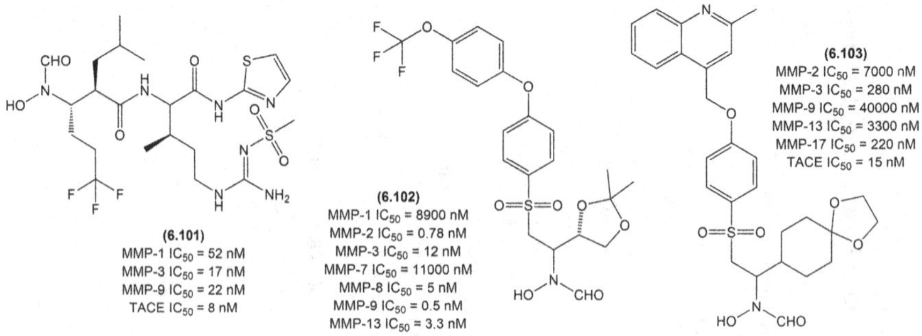

(6.101)
MMP-1 IC_{50} = 52 nM
MMP-3 IC_{50} = 17 nM
MMP-9 IC_{50} = 22 nM
TACE IC_{50} = 8 nM

(6.102)
MMP-1 IC_{50} = 8900 nM
MMP-2 IC_{50} = 0.78 nM
MMP-3 IC_{50} = 12 nM
MMP-7 IC_{50} = 11000 nM
MMP-8 IC_{50} = 5 nM
MMP-9 IC_{50} = 0.5 nM
MMP-13 IC_{50} = 3.3 nM

(6.103)
MMP-2 IC_{50} = 7000 nM
MMP-3 IC_{50} = 280 nM
MMP-9 IC_{50} = 40000 nM
MMP-13 IC_{50} = 3300 nM
MMP-17 IC_{50} = 220 nM
TACE IC_{50} = 15 nM

FIGURE 6.14   N-hydroxyformamide-based effective MMP-3 inhibitors (compounds **6.101–6.103**).

Again, it showed effective antitumor efficacy when administered orally in a murine B16 melanoma tumor growth model. Researchers of Kaken Pharmaceuticals [109] reported some reverse hydroxamates as selective TACE inhibitors. However, compound **6.103** (Figure 6.14) displayed potent MMP-3 inhibition (IC_{50} = 280 nM) among these compounds.

6.10 PYRIMIDINE-2,4,6-TRIONE-BASED STROMELYSIN INHIBITORS

Scientists at Hoffmann-La Roche [110] reported a series of 5,5-disubstituted pyrimidine-2,4,6-triones as effective MMP-3 inhibitors. Compound **6.104** (Figure 6.15) yielded effective inhibition against stromelysin (IC_{50} = 2 μM). The X-ray crystallographic structure of compound **6.104** with stromelysin shows the importance of C-5 substituents at the pyrimidine-2,4,6-trione scaffold. The N-1 amide groups formed chelation with the Zn^{2+} ion stabilized by three residues. The bulky aryl group entered the S1' pocket. Several hydrogen bonds are observed between the amide and carbonyl functions with Ala165, Leu164, and Glu202 amino acid residues.

A further study conducted by the researchers of Bristol Myers Squibb [111] led to the development of some pyrimidinetrione-based potent and MMP-13-selective inhibitors. Compound **6.105** (Figure 6.15), possessing a phenoxyphenyl group associated with the spiro ring structure, resulted in potent MMP-3 inhibition (K_i = 92 nM).

6.11 MISCELLANEOUS STROMELYSIN INHIBITORS

Zhang and co-workers [112] from Johnson and Johnson Pharmaceutical Research and Development reported some arylsulfone-based MMPIs containing heterocyclic ZBGs. Compound **6.106** (Figure 6.16), possessing a *p*-trifluoromethoxy

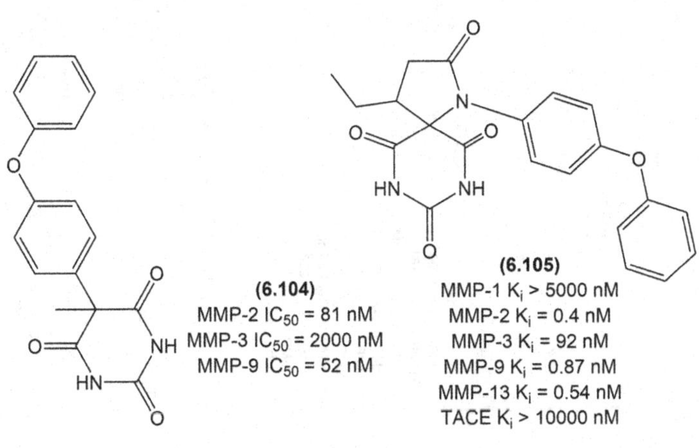

(6.104)
MMP-2 IC_{50} = 81 nM
MMP-3 IC_{50} = 2000 nM
MMP-9 IC_{50} = 52 nM

(6.105)
MMP-1 K_i > 5000 nM
MMP-2 K_i = 0.4 nM
MMP-3 K_i = 92 nM
MMP-9 K_i = 0.87 nM
MMP-13 K_i = 0.54 nM
TACE K_i > 10000 nM

FIGURE 6.15 Pyrimidine-2,4,6-trione-based effective MMP-3 inhibitors (compounds 6.104–6.105).

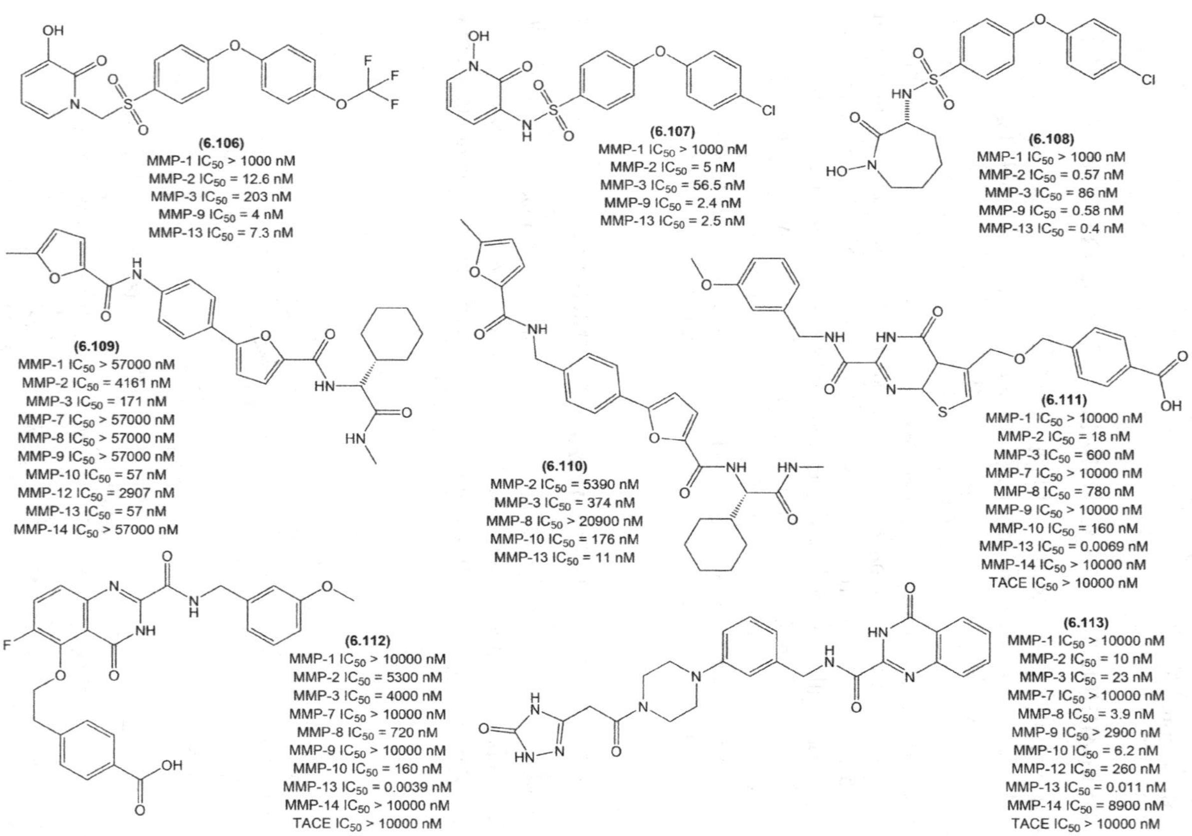

(6.106)
MMP-1 IC$_{50}$ > 1000 nM
MMP-2 IC$_{50}$ = 12.6 nM
MMP-3 IC$_{50}$ = 203 nM
MMP-9 IC$_{50}$ = 4 nM
MMP-13 IC$_{50}$ = 7.3 nM

(6.107)
MMP-1 IC$_{50}$ > 1000 nM
MMP-2 IC$_{50}$ = 5 nM
MMP-3 IC$_{50}$ = 56.5 nM
MMP-9 IC$_{50}$ = 2.4 nM
MMP-13 IC$_{50}$ = 2.5 nM

(6.108)
MMP-1 IC$_{50}$ > 1000 nM
MMP-2 IC$_{50}$ = 0.57 nM
MMP-3 IC$_{50}$ = 86 nM
MMP-9 IC$_{50}$ = 0.58 nM
MMP-13 IC$_{50}$ = 0.4 nM

(6.109)
MMP-1 IC$_{50}$ > 57000 nM
MMP-2 IC$_{50}$ = 4161 nM
MMP-3 IC$_{50}$ = 171 nM
MMP-7 IC$_{50}$ > 57000 nM
MMP-8 IC$_{50}$ > 57000 nM
MMP-9 IC$_{50}$ > 57000 nM
MMP-10 IC$_{50}$ = 57 nM
MMP-12 IC$_{50}$ = 2907 nM
MMP-13 IC$_{50}$ = 57 nM
MMP-14 IC$_{50}$ > 57000 nM

(6.110)
MMP-2 IC$_{50}$ = 5390 nM
MMP-3 IC$_{50}$ = 374 nM
MMP-8 IC$_{50}$ > 20900 nM
MMP-10 IC$_{50}$ = 176 nM
MMP-13 IC$_{50}$ = 11 nM

(6.111)
MMP-1 IC$_{50}$ > 10000 nM
MMP-2 IC$_{50}$ = 18 nM
MMP-3 IC$_{50}$ = 600 nM
MMP-7 IC$_{50}$ > 10000 nM
MMP-8 IC$_{50}$ = 780 nM
MMP-9 IC$_{50}$ > 10000 nM
MMP-10 IC$_{50}$ = 160 nM
MMP-13 IC$_{50}$ = 0.0069 nM
MMP-14 IC$_{50}$ > 10000 nM
TACE IC$_{50}$ > 10000 nM

(6.112)
MMP-1 IC$_{50}$ > 10000 nM
MMP-2 IC$_{50}$ = 5300 nM
MMP-3 IC$_{50}$ = 4000 nM
MMP-7 IC$_{50}$ > 10000 nM
MMP-8 IC$_{50}$ = 720 nM
MMP-9 IC$_{50}$ > 10000 nM
MMP-10 IC$_{50}$ = 160 nM
MMP-13 IC$_{50}$ = 0.0039 nM
MMP-14 IC$_{50}$ > 10000 nM
TACE IC$_{50}$ > 10000 nM

(6.113)
MMP-1 IC$_{50}$ > 10000 nM
MMP-2 IC$_{50}$ = 10 nM
MMP-3 IC$_{50}$ = 23 nM
MMP-7 IC$_{50}$ > 10000 nM
MMP-8 IC$_{50}$ = 3.9 nM
MMP-9 IC$_{50}$ = 2900 nM
MMP-10 IC$_{50}$ = 6.2 nM
MMP-12 IC$_{50}$ = 260 nM
MMP-13 IC$_{50}$ = 0.011 nM
MMP-14 IC$_{50}$ = 8900 nM
TACE IC$_{50}$ > 10000 nM

FIGURE 6.16   Miscellaneous stromelysin inhibitors (compounds 6.106–6.113).

phenoxyphenyl sylfonylmethyl moiety attached to the heterocyclic hydroxypyridinone ZBG, resulted in effective MMP-3 inhibition (IC_{50} = 203 nM).

In the next study, Zhang et al. [113] reported some 1-hydroxy-2-pyridinone-based MMPIs. Compound **6.107** (Figure 6.16), having a p-chlorophenoxyphenyl sulfonamido moiety attached to the hydroxypyridinone ZBG, produced effective MMP-3 inhibition (IC_{50} = 56.5 nM). Compound **6.107** showed effective pharmacokinetic parameters in rats at an oral dose of 10 mg/kg ($t_{1/2}$ = 47 hrs; AUC = 179 µg.h/ml; volume distribution = 1.75 L/kg; clearance = 0.5 ml/min/kg). Compound **6.107** also produced promising results in focal cerebral ischemia in the tMCAO mice model.

Wilson and co-workers from Johnson Pharmaceutical Research and Development [114] discovered some cobactin-T-based MMPIs through a ring-closing metathesis method. Compound **6.108** (Figure 6.16), having p-chlorophenoxyphenyl sulfonamido moiety attached to the N-hydroxyoxoazepan ring, produced potent MMP-3 inhibition (IC_{50} = 86 nM). Compound **6.108** at 0.5 mg/kg i.v. provided good pharmacokinetic properties (C_{max} = 4.6 µM; $t_{1/2}$ = 14 hrs; AUC = 1226 ng h/ml; volume distribution = 3.3 L/kg; clearance = 7 ml/min/kg) in the rat model.

Heim-Riether et al. [115] at Boehringer Ingelheim Pharmaceuticals reported a series of non-zinc chelating MMP-13 inhibitors. Compound **6.109** (Figure 6.16) yielded both effective MMP-3 and MMP-10 inhibition (IC_{50} of 171 nM and 57 nM, respectively). A further study conducted by the researchers of Boehringer Ingelheim Pharmaceuticals [116] produced a series of non-zinc chelating MMP-13 inhibitors. Compound **6.110** (Figure 6.16), having similarity with compound **6.109**, produced good MMP-3 and MMP-10 inhibition (IC_{50} of 374 nM and 176 nM, respectively).

Nara et al. [117] from Takeda Pharmaceutical company reported some thieno[2,3-d]pyrimidine-2-carboxamide derivatives as potent and MMP-13-selective inhibitors. However, compound **6.111** (Figure 6.16) showed effective MMP-3 and MMP-10 inhibition (IC_{50} of 600 nM and 160 nM, respectively). It significantly inhibited the breakdown of collagenase (87.4% inhibition at 0.1 µM). Compound **6.111** produced good pharmacokinetic properties in guinea pigs (AUC = 8357 ng h/ml; C_{max} = 1445 ng/ml). Further research conducted by the same group of researchers [118] guided the discovery of some potent quinazoline-2-carboxamides-based MMP-13-selective inhibitors by the structure-based drug design approach. However, compound **6.112** (Figure 6.16) showed good MMP-10 inhibition (IC_{50} = 160 nM) with moderate efficacy against MMP-3 (IC_{50} = 4000 nM). Compound **6.112** displayed moderate metabolic stability in rat microsomes, providing high total body clearance and low plasma AUC. In the monoiodoacetate (MIA)-induced rat arthritis model, compound **6.112**, when administered orally, was found to decrease cartilage degradation with no higher toxicity. Again, Nara et al. [119] reported some fused pyrimidine-2-ca rboxamide-4-one-containing non-zinc binding MMP-13 inhibitors. However, compound **6.113** (Figure 6.16) displayed both potent MMP-3 and MMP-10 inhibition (IC_{50} of 23 nM and 6.20 nM, respectively).

Nara et al. [120] developed some highly potent and MMP-13-selective inhibitors containing 1,2,4-triazol-3-yl ZBG moiety through a structure-based drug design (SBDD) approach. Compound **6.114** (Figure 6.17) exhibited potent MMP-10 inhibition (IC_{50} = 55 nM) with a lower affinity toward MMP-3 (IC_{50} = 1100 nM).

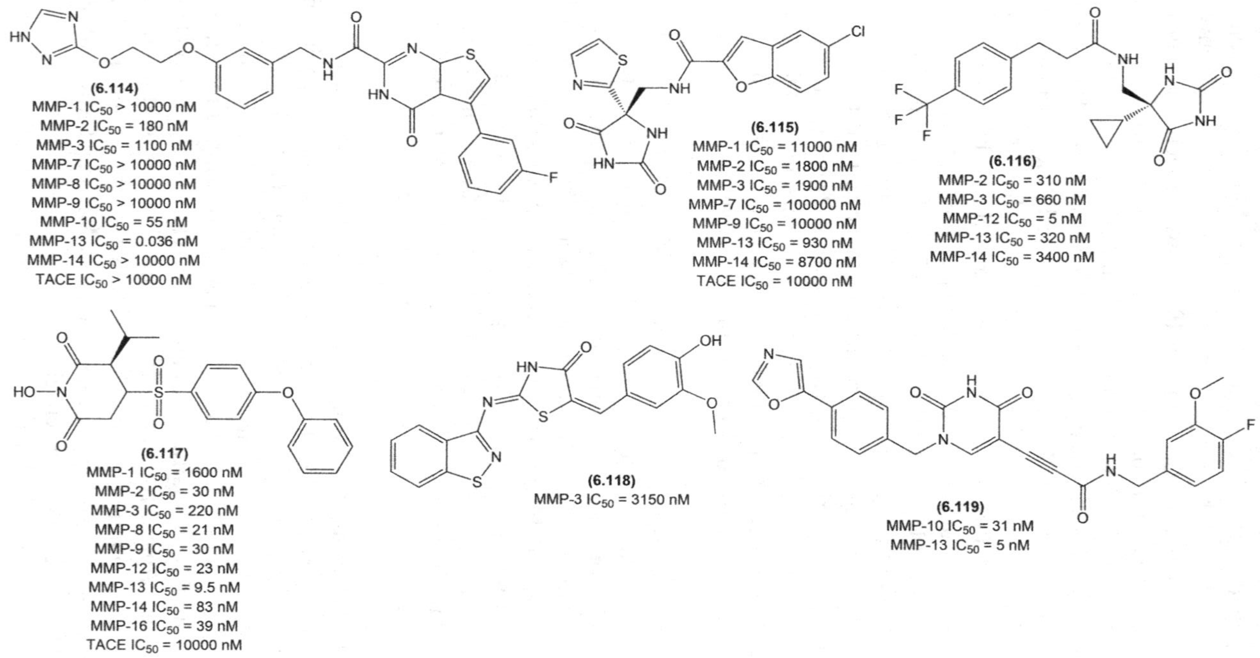

(6.114)

MMP-1 IC$_{50}$ > 10000 nM
MMP-2 IC$_{50}$ = 180 nM
MMP-3 IC$_{50}$ = 1100 nM
MMP-7 IC$_{50}$ > 10000 nM
MMP-8 IC$_{50}$ > 10000 nM
MMP-9 IC$_{50}$ > 10000 nM
MMP-10 IC$_{50}$ = 55 nM
MMP-13 IC$_{50}$ = 0.036 nM
MMP-14 IC$_{50}$ > 10000 nM
TACE IC$_{50}$ > 10000 nM

(6.115)

MMP-1 IC$_{50}$ = 11000 nM
MMP-2 IC$_{50}$ = 1800 nM
MMP-3 IC$_{50}$ = 1900 nM
MMP-7 IC$_{50}$ = 100000 nM
MMP-9 IC$_{50}$ > 10000 nM
MMP-13 IC$_{50}$ = 930 nM
MMP-14 IC$_{50}$ = 8700 nM
TACE IC$_{50}$ = 10000 nM

(6.116)

MMP-2 IC$_{50}$ = 310 nM
MMP-3 IC$_{50}$ = 660 nM
MMP-12 IC$_{50}$ = 5 nM
MMP-13 IC$_{50}$ = 320 nM
MMP-14 IC$_{50}$ = 3400 nM

(6.117)

MMP-1 IC$_{50}$ = 1600 nM
MMP-2 IC$_{50}$ = 30 nM
MMP-3 IC$_{50}$ = 220 nM
MMP-8 IC$_{50}$ = 21 nM
MMP-9 IC$_{50}$ = 30 nM
MMP-12 IC$_{50}$ = 23 nM
MMP-13 IC$_{50}$ = 9.5 nM
MMP-14 IC$_{50}$ = 83 nM
MMP-16 IC$_{50}$ = 39 nM
TACE IC$_{50}$ = 10000 nM

(6.118)

MMP-3 IC$_{50}$ = 3150 nM

(6.119)

MMP-10 IC$_{50}$ = 31 nM
MMP-13 IC$_{50}$ = 5 nM

FIGURE 6.17 Some other miscellaneous stromelysin inhibitors (compounds 6.114–6.119).

Compound **6.114** was found to inhibit the curtilage degradation in a dose-dependent manner (70.8% inhibition at 1 μM).

Wiley et al. [121] reported some hydantoin-containing aggrecanase inhibitors. Compound **6.115** (Figure 6.17), possessing a benzofuryl carboxamide moiety attached to the hydantoin scaffold, resulted in effective MMP-3 inhibition (IC_{50} = 1,900 nM).

Durham et al. [122] further reported some aggrecanase inhibitors. Among these compounds, compound **6.116** (Figure 6.17), possessing a p-trifluromethyl phenylethyl carboxamide moiety attached to the hydantoin scaffold, produced good MMP-3 inhibition (IC_{50} = 660 nM).

Marques and co-workers [123] reported some 1-hydroxypiperazine-2,6-diones as potent MMPIs. Compound **6.117** (Figure 6.17), possessing a phenoxyphenyl sulfonyl group attached to the hydroxypiperazine-2,6-dione scaffold, exhibited potent MMP-3 inhibition (IC_{50} = 220 nM) among these compounds.

Crascì et al. [124] reported some 2-benzisothiazolylimino-5-benzylidene-4-thiaz olidinones as effective MMPIs. Compound **6.118** (Figure 6.17) resulted in the highest MMP-3 inhibition (IC_{50} = 3,150 nM). Compound **6.118** also effectively reduced the cytokine-induced NO production (66%) associated with osteoarthritis. Compound **6.118** also decreased NF-κB levels and MMP-3 production in IL-1β mediated human chondrocytes, as evidenced by the western blot analysis study. It indicated the crucial role of compound **6.118** as a chondroprotective MMP-3 inhibitor for reducing the inflammatory process related to osteoarthritis. Senn and co-workers [125] disclosed some non-hydroxamate-based dual MMP-10/-13 inhibitors. Among these compounds, compound **6.119** (Figure 6.17) exhibited the most potent inhibitory efficacy against both MMP-10 (IC_{50} = 31 nM) and MMP-13 (IC_{50} = 5 nM). Compound **6.119** was inactive against other MMPs (MMP-1, -2, -3, -7, -8, -9, -12, and -14) at a dose of 10 μM.

6.12 SUMMARY

Although the proper mechanisms of stromelysins (MMP-3, -10, and -11) have not yet been well explored, several experimental pieces of evidence revealed their crucial roles in various disease conditions. Based on this evidence, designing potent and selective inhibitors of stromelysins can be considered, which may be a task for future drug development and discovery. As stromelysins have some structural and functional similarities with other classes of MMPs like collagenase, gelatinases, and so on, the crucial mechanisms of stromelysins in various pathophysiology and disease conditions should be investigated properly. This may be an added advantage and alternative strategy for essential aspects of stromelysins related to well-known disease conditions, as well as to reduce the off-target effects of commonly used drug candidates. This chapter illustrated different stromelysins (MMP-3, -10, and -11); their mechanisms in disease conditions have been described. In this context, some potential MMP-3 inhibitors have also been mentioned. Researchers are not trying to design promising and selective inhibitors of stromelysins because the mechanisms of stromelysins have not been well-explored. However, based on some preliminary reports, potent and selective stromelysin inhibitors may be tried to manage such disease conditions. This chapter mentions potential stromelysin inhibitors based on which selective and more potent stromelysin inhibitors may be designed. In addition, the available crystallographic data and the biological activity of such available stromelysin inhibitors may be taken into consideration for designing more potent and selective stromelysin inhibitors through several ligand- and structure-based drug design (LBDD and SBDD) methodologies. This chapter, therefore, may provide helpful information to the researchers for future endeavors related to the discovery of promising stromelysins inhibitors.

REFERENCES

[1]. Matziari M, Dive V, Yiotakis A. Matrix metalloproteinase 11 (MMP-11; stromelysin-3) and synthetic inhibitors. *Med Res Rev.* 2007;27(4):528–552.

[2]. Nagase H, Visse R, Murphy G. Structure and function of matrix metalloproteinases and TIMPs. *Cardiovasc Res.* 2006;69(3):562–573.

[3]. Laronha H, Caldeira J. Structure and function of human matrix metalloproteinases. *Cells.* 2020;9(5):1076.

[4]. Piskór BM, Przylipiak A, Dąbrowska E, Niczyporuk M, Ławicki S. Matrilysins and stromelysins in pathogenesis and diagnostics of cancers. *Cancer Manag Res.* 2020;12:10949–10964.

[5]. Wan J, Zhang G, Li X, et al. Matrix metalloproteinase 3: A promoting and destabilizing factor in the pathogenesis of disease and cell differentiation. *Front Physiol.* 2021;12:663978.

[6]. Adamcova M, Šimko F. Multiplex biomarker approach to cardiovascular diseases. *Acta Pharmacol Sin.* 2018;39(7):1068–1072.

[7]. Klein T, Bischoff R. Physiology and pathophysiology of matrix metalloproteases. *Amino Acids.* 2011;41(2):271–290.

[8]. Krampert M, Bloch W, Sasaki T, et al. Activities of the matrix metalloproteinase stromelysin-2 (MMP-10) in matrix degradation and keratinocyte organization in wounded skin. *Mol Biol Cell.* 2004;15(12):5242–5254.

[9]. Madlener M, Mauch C, Conca W, et al. Regulation of the expression of stromelysin-2 by growth factors in keratinocytes: Implications for normal and impaired wound healing. *Biochem J.* 1996;320:659–664.

[10]. Eyyupkoca F, Sabanoglu C, Altintas MS, et al. Higher levels of TWEAK and matrix metalloproteinase-3 during the acute phase of myocardial infarction are associated with adverse left ventricular remodeling. *Postepy Kardiol Interwencyjnej.* 2021;17(4):356–365. doi: 10.5114/aic.2021.111967.

[11]. Wang X, Han W, Han L, et al. Levels of Serum sST2, MMP-3, and Gal-3 in patients with essential hypertension and their correlation with left ventricular hypertrophy. *Evid Based Complement Alternat Med.* 2021;2021:7262776.

[12]. Choudhary P, Roy T, Chatterjee A, et al. Melatonin rescues swim stress induced gastric ulceration by inhibiting matrix metalloproteinase-3 via down-regulation of inflammatory signaling cascade. *Life Sci.* 2022;297:120426.

[13]. Ming S, Yin H, Li X, et al. GITR promotes the polarization of TFH-like cells in *Helicobacter pylori*-positive gastritis. *Front Immunol.* 2021;12:736269.

[14]. Kvacskay P, Yao N, Schnotz JH, et al. Increase of aerobic glycolysis mediated by activated T helper cells drives synovial fibroblasts towards an inflammatory phenotype: New targets for therapy? *Arthritis Res Ther.* 2021;23(1):56.

[15]. Mirtaheri E, Khabbazi A, Nazemiyeh H, et al. Stachys schtschegleevii tea, matrix metalloproteinase, and disease severity in female rheumatoid arthritis patients: A randomized controlled clinical trial. *Clin Rheumatol.* 2022;41(4):1033–1044.

[16]. Hashimoto H, Hashimoto S, Shimazaki Y. Functional impairment and periodontitis in rheumatoid arthritis. *Int Dent J.* 2022;72:641–647.

[17]. Ravichandran D, Pillai J, Krishnamurthy K. Genetics of intervertebral disc disease: A review. *Clin Anat.* 2022;35(1):116–120. doi: 10.1002/ca.23803.

[18]. Artham S, Verma A, Newsome AS, et al. Patients with acute respiratory distress syndrome exhibit increased stromelysin1 activity in the blood samples. *Cytokine.* 2020;131:155086. doi: 10.1016/j.cyto.2020.155086.

[19]. Klimontov VV, Koroleva EA, Khapaev RS, et al. Carotid artery disease in subjects with type 2 diabetes: Risk factors and biomarkers. *J Clin Med.* 2021;11(1):72.

[20]. Sengupta S, Addya S, Biswas D, et al. Matrix metalloproteinases and tissue inhibitors of metalloproteinases in murine β-coronavirus-induced neuroinflammation. *Virology.* 2022;566:122–135.

[21]. Lefevere E, Salinas-Navarro M, Andries L, et al. Tightening the retinal glia limitans attenuates neuroinflammation after optic nerve injury. *Glia.* 2020;68(12):2643–2660.

[22]. Ordak M, Libman-Sokolowska M, Nasierowski T, et al. Matrix metalloproteinase-3 serum levels in schizophrenic patients. *Int J Psychiatry Clin Pract.* 2022;27:1–7.

[23]. Ay A, Alkanli N, Cevik G. Investigation of the relationship between MMP-1 (−1607 1G/2G), MMP-3 (−1171 5A/6A) gene variations and development of bladder cancer. *Mol Biol Rep.* 2021;48(12):7689–7695.

[24]. Allen DZ, Aljabban J, Silverman D, et al. Meta-analysis illustrates possible role of lipopolysaccharide (LPS)-induced tissue injury in nasopharyngeal carcinoma (NPC) pathogenesis. *PLoS One.* 2021;16(10):e0258187.

[25]. Argote Camacho AX, González Ramírez AR, Pérez Alonso AJ, et al. Metalloproteinases 1 and 3 as potential biomarkers in breast cancer development. *Int J Mol Sci.* 2021;22(16):9012.

[26]. Suhaimi SA, Chan SC, Rosli R. Matrix metallopeptidase 3 polymorphisms: Emerging genetic markers in human breast cancer metastasis. *J Breast Cancer.* 2020;23(1):1–9.

[27]. Kreus M, Lehtonen S, Skarp S, et al. Extracellular matrix proteins produced by stromal cells in idiopathic pulmonary fibrosis and lung adenocarcinoma. *PLoS One.* 2021;16(4):e0250109.

[28]. Sharma R, Chattopadhyay TK, Mathur M, Ralhan R. Prognostic significance of stromelysin-3 and tissue inhibitor of matrix metalloproteinase-2 in esophageal cancer. *Oncology.* 2004;67(3–4):300–309.

[29]. Kudelski J, Młynarczyk G, Gudowska-Sawczuk M, et al. Enhanced expression but decreased specific activity of matrix metalloproteinase 10 (MMP-10) in comparison with matrix metalloproteinase 3 (MMP-3) in human urinary bladder carcinoma. *J Clin Med.* 2021;10(16):3683.

[30]. Sokai A, Handa T, Tanizawa K, et al. Matrix metalloproteinase-10: A novel biomarker for idiopathic pulmonary fibrosis. *Respir Res.* 2015;16:120.

[31]. Rodriguez JA, Orbe J, Martinez de Lizarrondo S, et al. Metalloproteinases and atherothrombosis: MMP-10 mediates vascular remodeling promoted by inflammatory stimuli. *Front Biosci.* 2008;13:2916–2921.

[32]. Xu I, Thériault M, Brunette I, et al. Matrix metalloproteinases and their inhibitors in Fuchs endothelial corneal dystrophy. *Exp Eye Res.* 2021;205:108500.

[33]. Kuo CS, Pavlidis S, Zhu J, et al. Contribution of airway eosinophils in airway wall remodeling in asthma: Role of MMP-10 and MET. *Allergy.* 2019;74(6):1102–1112.

[34]. Ma B, Ran R, Liao HY, Zhang HH. The paradoxical role of matrix metalloproteinase-11 in cancer. *Biomed Pharmacother.* 2021;141:111899.

[35]. Matziari M, Dive V, Yiotakis A. Matrix metalloproteinase 11 (MMP-11; stromelysin-3) and synthetic inhibitors. *Med Res Rev.* 2007;27(4):528–552.

[36]. Curtin ML, Garland RB, Davidsen SK, et al. Broad spectrum matrix metalloproteinase inhibitors: An examination of succinamide hydroxamate inhibitors with P1 C alpha gem-disubstitution. *Bioorg Med Chem Lett.* 1998;8(12):1443–1448.

[37]. Steinman DH, Curtin ML, Garland RB, et al. The design, synthesis, and structure-activity relationships of a series of macrocyclic MMP inhibitors. *Bioorg Med Chem Lett.* 1998;8(16):2087–2092.

[38]. Sheppard GS, Florjancic AS, Giesler JR, et al. Aryl ketones as novel replacements for the C-terminal amide bond of succinyl hydroxamate MMP inhibitors. *Bioorg Med Chem Lett.* 1998;8(22):3251–3256.

[39]. Yamamoto M, Tsujishita H, Hori N, et al. Inhibition of membrane-type 1 matrix metalloproteinase by hydroxamate inhibitors: An examination of the subsite pocket. *J Med Chem.* 1998;41(8):1209–1217.

[40]. Martin FM, Beckett RP, Bellamy CL, et al. The synthesis and biological evaluation of non-peptidic matrix metalloproteinase inhibitors. *Bioorg Med Chem Lett.* 1999;9(19):2887–2892.

[41]. Almstead NG, Bradley RS, Pikul S, et al. Design, synthesis, and biological evaluation of potent thiazine- and thiazepine-based matrix metalloproteinase inhibitors. *J Med Chem.* 1999;42(22):4547–4562.

[42]. Pikul S, McDow Dunham KL, Almstead NG, et al. Design and synthesis of phosphinamide-based hydroxamic acids as inhibitors of matrix metalloproteinases. *J Med Chem.* 1999;42(1):87–94.

[43]. Cheng M, De B, Almstead NG, et al. Design, synthesis, and biological evaluation of matrix metalloproteinase inhibitors derived from a modified proline scaffold. *J Med Chem.* 1999;42(26):5426–5436.

[44]. Cheng M, De B, Pikul S, et al. Design and synthesis of piperazine-based matrix metalloproteinase inhibitors. *J Med Chem.* 2000;43(3):369–380.

[45]. Natchus MG, Bookland RG, De B, et al. Development of new hydroxolate matrix metalloproteinase inhibitors derived from functionalized 4-aminoprolines. *J Med Chem.* 2000;43(26):4948–4963.

[46]. Pikul S, Dunham KM, Almstead NG, et al. Heterocycle-based MMP inhibitors with P2' substituents. *Bioorg Med Chem Lett.* 2001;11(8):1009–1013.

[47]. Duan JJ, Chen L, Xue CB, et al. P1, P2'-linked macrocyclic amine derivatives as matrix metalloproteinase inhibitors. *Bioorg Med Chem Lett.* 1999;9(10):1453–1458.

[48]. Baxter AD, Bhogal R, Bird J, et al. Arylsulphonyl hydroxamic acids: Potent and selective matrix metalloproteinase inhibitors. *Bioorg Med Chem Lett.* 2001;11(11): 1465–1468.

[49]. Sørensen MD, Blaehr LK, Christensen MK, et al. Cyclic phosphinamides and phosphonamides, novel series of potent matrix metalloproteinase inhibitors with antitumour activity. *Bioorg Med Chem.* 2003;11(24):5461–5484.

[50]. Takahashi K, Ikura M, Habashita H, et al. Novel matrix metalloproteinase inhibitors: Generation of lead compounds by the in silico fragment-based approach. *Bioorg Med Chem.* 2005;13(14):4527–4543.

[51]. Fray MJ, Dickinson RP. Discovery of potent and selective succinyl hydroxamate inhibitors of matrix metalloprotease-3 (stromelysin-1). *Bioorg Med Chem Lett.* 2001;11(4):571–574.

[52]. Fray MJ, Dickinson RP, Huggins JP, et al. A potent, selective inhibitor of matrix metalloproteinase-3 for the topical treatment of chronic dermal ulcers. *J Med Chem.* 2003;46(16):3514–3525.

[53]. Sawa M, Kondo H, Nishimura S. Encounter with unexpected collagenase-1 selective inhibitor: Switchover of inhibitor binding pocket induced by fluorine atom. *Bioorg Med Chem Lett.* 2002;12(4):581–584.

[54]. Sawa M, Kiyoi T, Kurokawa K, et al. New type of metalloproteinase inhibitor: Design and synthesis of new phosphonamide-based hydroxamic acids. *J Med Chem.* 2002;45(4):919–929.

[55]. Becker DP, Villamil CI, Barta TE, et al. Synthesis and structure-activity relationships of beta- and alpha-piperidine sulfone hydroxamic acid matrix metalloproteinase inhibitors with oral antitumour efficacy. *J Med Chem.* 2005;48(21):6713–6730.

[56]. Becker DP, Barta TE, Bedell LJ, et al. Orally active MMP-1 sparing α-tetrahydropyranyl and α-piperidinyl sulfone matrix metalloproteinase (MMP) inhibitors with efficacy in cancer, arthritis, and cardiovascular disease. *J Med Chem.* 2010;53(18):6653–6680.

[57]. Barta TE, Becker DP, Bedell LJ, et al. MMP-13 selective α-sulfone hydroxamates: A survey of P1' heterocyclic amide isosteres. *Bioorg Med Chem Lett.* 2011;21(10):2820–2822.

[58]. Chen XT, Ghavimi B, Corbett RL, et al. A new 4-(2-methylquinolin-4-ylmethyl)phenyl P1' group for the beta-amino hydroxamic acid derived TACE inhibitors. *Bioorg Med Chem Lett.* 2007;17(7):1865–1870.

[59]. Durham TB, Klimkowski VJ, Rito CJ, et al. Identification of potent and selective hydantoin inhibitors of aggrecanase-1 and aggrecanase-2 that are efficacious in both chemical and surgical models of osteoarthritis. *J Med Chem.* 2014;57(24):10476–10485.

[60]. Hanessian S, Bouzbouz S, Boudon A, et al. Picking the S1, S1' and S2' pockets of matrix metalloproteinases. A niche for potent acyclic sulfonamide inhibitors. *Bioorg Med Chem Lett.* 1999;9(12):1691–1696.

[61]. Hanessian S, Moitessier N, Gauchet C, et al. N-Aryl sulfonyl homocysteine hydroxamate inhibitors of matrix metalloproteinases: Further probing of the S(1), S(1)', and S(2)' pockets. *J Med Chem.* 2001;44(19):3066–3073.

[62]. Hanessian S, MacKay DB, Moitessier N. Design and synthesis of matrix metalloproteinase inhibitors guided by molecular modeling. Picking the S(1) pocket using conformationally constrained inhibitors. *J Med Chem.* 2001;44(19):3074–3082.

[63]. Chollet AM, Le Diguarher T, Murray L, et al. General synthesis of alpha-substituted 3-bisaryloxy propionic acid derivatives as specific MMP inhibitors. *Bioorg Med Chem Lett.* 2001;11(3):295–299.

[64]. Chollet AM, Le Diguarher T, Kucharczyk N, et al. Solid-phase synthesis of alpha-substituted 3-bisarylthio N-hydroxy propionamides as specific MMP inhibitors. *Bioorg Med Chem.* 2002;10(3):531–544.

[65]. Marcq V, Mirand C, Decarme M, et al. MMPs inhibitors: New succinylhydroxamates with selective inhibition of MMP-2 over MMP-3. *Bioorg Med Chem Lett.* 2003;13(17):2843–2846.

[66]. Rossello A, Nuti E, Carelli P, et al. N-i-propoxy-N-biphenylsulfonylaminobutylhydroxamic acids as potent and selective inhibitors of MMP-2 and MT1-MMP. *Bioorg Med Chem Lett.* 2005;15(5):1321–1326.

[67]. Nuti E, Casalini F, Avramova SI, et al. N-O-isopropyl sulfonamido-based hydroxamates: Design, synthesis and biological evaluation of selective matrix metalloproteinase-13 inhibitors as potential therapeutic agents for osteoarthritis. *J Med Chem.* 2009;52(15):4757–4773.

[68]. Nuti E, Panelli L, Casalini F, et al. Design, synthesis, biological evaluation, and NMR studies of a new series of arylsulfones as selective and potent matrix metalloproteinase-12 inhibitors. *J Med Chem.* 2009;52(20):6347–6361.

[69]. Nuti E, Cantelmo AR, Gallo C, et al. N-O-isopropyl sulfonamido-based hydroxamates as matrix metalloproteinase inhibitors: Hit selection and in vivo antiangiogenic activity. *J Med Chem.* 2015;58(18):7224–7240.

[70]. Moroy G, Denhez C, El Mourabit H, et al. Simultaneous presence of unsaturation and long alkyl chain at P'1 of Ilomastat confers selectivity for gelatinase A (MMP-2) over gelatinase B (MMP-9) inhibition as shown by molecular modelling studies. *Bioorg Med Chem.* 2007;15(14):4753–4766.

[71]. Zapico JM, Serra P, García-Sanmartín J, et al. Potent "clicked" MMP-2 inhibitors: Synthesis, molecular modeling and biological exploration. *Org Biomol Chem.* 2011;9(12):4587–4599.

[72]. Zapico JM, Puckowska A, Filipiak K, et al. Design and synthesis of potent hydroxamate inhibitors with increased selectivity within the gelatinase family. *Org Biomol Chem.* 2015;13(1):142–156.

[73]. Topai A, Breccia P, Minissi F, et al. In silico scaffold evaluation and solid phase approach to identify new gelatinase inhibitors. *Bioorg Med Chem.* 2012;20(7):2323–2337.

[74]. Brown FK, Brown PJ, Bickett DM, et al. Matrix metalloproteinase inhibitors containing a (carboxyalkyl)amino zinc ligand: Modification of the P1 and P2' residues. *J Med Chem.* 1994;37(5):674–688.

[75]. O'Brien PM, Ortwine DF, Pavlovsky AG, et al. Structure-activity relationships and pharmacokinetic analysis for a series of potent, systemically available biphenylsulfonamide matrix metalloproteinase inhibitors. *J Med Chem.* 2000;43(2):156–166.

[76]. Natchus MG, Bookland RG, Laufersweiler MJ, et al. Development of new carboxylic acid-based MMP inhibitors derived from functionalized propargylglycines. *J Med Chem.* 2001;44(7):1060–1071.

[77]. Pikul S, Ohler NE, Ciszewski G, et al. Potent and selective carboxylic acid-based inhibitors of matrix metalloproteinases. *J Med Chem.* 2001;44(16):2499–2502.

[78]. Tullis JS, Laufersweiler MJ, VanRens JC, et al. The development of new carboxylic acid-based MMP inhibitors derived from a cyclohexylglycine scaffold. *Bioorg Med Chem Lett.* 2001;11(15):1975–1979.

[79]. Wu J, Rush TS 3rd, Hotchandani R, et al. Identification of potent and selective MMP-13 inhibitors. *Bioorg Med Chem Lett.* 2005;15(18):4105–4109.

[80]. Li J, Rush TS 3rd, Li W, et al. Synthesis and SAR of highly selective MMP-13 inhibitors. *Bioorg Med Chem Lett.* 2005;15(22):4961–4966.

[81]. Hu Y, Xiang JS, DiGrandi MJ, et al. Potent, selective, and orally bioavailable matrix metalloproteinase-13 inhibitors for the treatment of osteoarthritis. *Bioorg Med Chem.* 2005;13(24):6629–6644.

[82]. Hudlicky T, Oppong K, Duan C, et al. Chemoenzymatic synthesis of functionalized cyclohexylglycines and alpha-methylcyclohexylglycines via Kazmaier-Claisen rearrangement. *Bioorg Med Chem Lett.* 2001;11(5):627–629.

[83]. Matter H, Schudok M, Schwab W, et al. Tetrahydroisoquinoline-3-carboxylate based matrix-metalloproteinase inhibitors: Design, synthesis and structure-activity relationship. Bioorg Med Chem. 2002;10(11):3529–3544.

[84]. Monovich LG, Tommasi RA, Fujimoto RA, et al. Discovery of potent, selective, and orally active carboxylic acid based inhibitors of matrix metalloproteinase-13. *J Med Chem.* 2009;52(11):3523–3538.

[85]. Le Diguarher T, Chollet AM, Bertrand M, et al. Stereospecific synthesis of 5-substituted 2-bisarylthiocyclopentane carboxylic acids as specific matrix metalloproteinase inhibitors. *J Med Chem.* 2003;46(18):3840–3852.

[86]. Yuan H, Lu W, Wang L, et al. Synthesis of derivatives of methyl rosmarinate and their inhibitory activities against matrix metalloproteinase-1 (MMP-1). *Eur J Med Chem.* 2013;62:148–157.

[87]. Baxter AD, Bird J, Bhogal R, et al. A novel series of matrix metalloproteinase inhibitors for the treatment of inflammatory disorders. *Bioorg Med Chem Lett.* 1997;7(7):897–902.

[88]. Baxter AD, Bhogal R, Bird JB, et al. Mercaptoacyl matrix metalloproteinase inhibitors: The effect of substitution at the mercaptoacyl moiety. *Bioorg Med Chem Lett.* 1997;7(21):2765–2770.

[89]. Lynas JF, Martin SL, Walker B, et al. Solid-phase synthesis and biological screening of N-alpha-mercaptoamide template-based matrix metalloprotease inhibitors. *Comb Chem High Throughput Screen.* 2000;3(1):37–41.

[90]. Campbell DA, Xiao XY, Harris D, et al. Malonyl alpha-mercaptoketones and alpha-mercaptoalcohols, a new class of matrix metalloproteinase inhibitors. *Bioorg Med Chem Lett.* 1998;8(10):1157–1162.

[91]. Levin JI, DiJoseph JF, Killar LM, et al. The asymmetric synthesis and in vitro characterization of succinyl mercaptoalcohol and mercaptoketone inhibitors of matrix metalloproteinases. *Bioorg Med Chem Lett.* 1998;8(10):1163–1168.

[92]. Szardenings AK, Harris D, Lam S, et al. Rational design and combinatorial evaluation of enzyme inhibitor scaffolds: Identification of novel inhibitors of matrix metalloproteinases. *J Med Chem.* 1998;41(13):2194–2200.

[93]. Szardenings AK, Antonenko V, Campbell DA, et al. Identification of highly selective inhibitors of collagenase-1 from combinatorial libraries of diketopiperazines. *J Med Chem.* 1999;42(8):1348–1357.

[94]. Freskos JN, Mischke BV, DeCrescenzo GA, et al. Discovery of a novel series of selective MMP inhibitors: Identification of the gamma-sulfone-thiols. *Bioorg Med Chem Lett.* 1999;9(7):943–948.

[95]. Fink CA, Carlson JE, Boehm C, et al. Design and synthesis of thiol containing inhibitors of matrix metalloproteinases. *Bioorg Med Chem Lett.* 1999;9(2):195–200.

[96]. Hurst DR, Schwartz MA, Jin Y, et al. Inhibition of enzyme activity of and cell-mediated substrate cleavage by membrane type 1 matrix metalloproteinase by newly developed mercaptosulphide inhibitors. *Biochem J.* 2005;392(Pt 3):527–536.

[97]. Jin Y, Roycik MD, Bosco DB, et al. Matrix metalloproteinase inhibitors based on the 3-mercaptopyrrolidine core. *J Med Chem.* 2013;56(11):4357–4373.

[98]. Pochetti G, Gavuzzo E, Campestre C, et al. Structural insight into the stereoselective inhibition of MMP-8 by enantiomeric sulfonamide phosphonates. *J Med Chem.* 2006;49(3):923–931.

[99]. Biasone A, Tortorella P, Campestre C, et al. alpha-Biphenylsulfonylamino 2-methylpropyl phosphonates: Enantioselective synthesis and selective inhibition of MMPs. *Bioorg Med Chem.* 2007;15(2):791–799.

[100]. Reiter LA, Rizzi JP, Pandit J, et al. Inhibition of MMP-1 and MMP-13 with phosphinic acids that exploit binding in the S2 pocket. *Bioorg Med Chem Lett.* 1999;9(2):127–132.

[101]. Reiter LA, Mitchell PG, Martinelli GJ, et al. Phosphinic acid-based MMP-13 inhibitors that spare MMP-1 and MMP-3. *Bioorg Med Chem Lett.* 2003;13(14):2331–2336.

[102]. Breuer E, Salomon CJ, Katz Y, et al. Carbamoylphosphonates, a new class of in vivo active matrix metalloproteinase inhibitors. 1. Alkyl- and cycloalkylcarbamoylphosphonic acids. *J Med Chem.* 2004;47(11):2826–2832.

[103]. Rubino MT, Agamennone M, Campestre C, et al. Synthesis, SAR, and biological evaluation of alpha-sulfonylphosphonic acids as selective matrix metalloproteinase inhibitors. *ChemMedChem.* 2009;4(3):352–362.

[104]. Matziari M, Beau F, Cuniasse P, et al. Evaluation of P1'-diversified phosphinic peptides leads to the development of highly selective inhibitors of MMP-11. *J Med Chem.* 2004;47(2):325–336.

[105]. Campestre C, Agamennone M, Tortorella P, et al. N-hydroxyurea as zinc binding group in matrix metalloproteinase inhibition: Mode of binding in a complex with MMP-8. *Bioorg Med Chem Lett.* 2006;16(1):20–24.

[106]. Ledour G, Moroy G, Rouffet M, et al. Introduction of the 4-(4-bromophenyl)benzene-sulfonyl group to hydrazide analogs of Ilomastat leads to potent gelatinase B (MMP-9) inhibitors with improved selectivity. *Bioorg Med Chem.* 2008;16(18):8745–8759.

[107]. Rabinowitz MH, Andrews RC, Becherer JD, et al. Design of selective and soluble inhibitors of tumour necrosis factor-alpha converting enzyme (TACE). *J Med Chem.* 2001;44(24):4252–4267.

[108]. Wada CK, Holms JH, Curtin ML, et al. Phenoxyphenyl sulfone N-formylhydroxylamines (retrohydroxamates) as potent, selective, orally bioavailable matrix metalloproteinase inhibitors. *J Med Chem.* 2002;45(1):219–232.

[109]. Kamei N, Tanaka T, Kawai K, et al. Reverse hydroxamate-based selective TACE inhibitors. *Bioorg Med Chem Lett.* 2004;14(11):2897–2900.

[110]. Foley LH, Palermo R, Dunten P, et al. Novel 5,5-disubstitutedpyrimidine-2,4,6-triones as selective MMP inhibitors. *Bioorg Med Chem Lett.* 2001;11(8):969–972.

[111]. Kim SH, Pudzianowski AT, Leavitt KJ, et al. Structure-based design of potent and selective inhibitors of collagenase-3 (MMP-13). *Bioorg Med Chem Lett.* 2005;15(4):1101–1106.

[112]. Zhang YM, Fan X, Yang SM, et al. Syntheses and in vitro evaluation of arylsulfone-based MMP inhibitors with heterocycle-derived zinc-binding groups (ZBGs). *Bioorg Med Chem Lett.* 2008;18(1):405–408.

[113]. Zhang YM, Fan X, Chakaravarty D, et al. 1-Hydroxy-2-pyridinone-based MMP inhibitors: Synthesis and biological evaluation for the treatment of ischemic stroke. *Bioorg Med Chem Lett.* 2008;18(1):409–413.

[114]. Wilson LJ, Wang B, Yang SM, et al. Discovery of novel cobactin-T based matrix metalloproteinase inhibitors via a ring closing metathesis strategy. *Bioorg Med Chem Lett.* 2011;21(21):6485–6490.

[115]. Heim-Riether A, Taylor SJ, Liang S, et al. Improving potency and selectivity of a new class of non-Zn-chelating MMP-13 inhibitors. *Bioorg Med Chem Lett.* 2009;19(18):5321–5324.

[116]. Gao DA, Xiong Z, Heim-Riether A, et al. SAR studies of non-zinc-chelating MMP-13 inhibitors: Improving selectivity and metabolic stability. *Bioorg Med Chem Lett.* 2010;20(17):5039–5043.

[117]. Nara H, Sato K, Naito T, et al. Thieno[2,3-d]pyrimidine-2-carboxamides bearing a carboxybenzene group at 5-position: Highly potent, selective, and orally available MMP-13 inhibitors interacting with the S1″ binding site. *Bioorg Med Chem.* 2014;22(19):5487–5505.

[118]. Nara H, Sato K, Naito T, et al. Discovery of novel, highly potent, and selective quinazoline-2-carboxamide-based matrix metalloproteinase (MMP)-13 inhibitors without a zinc binding group using a structure-based design approach. *J Med Chem.* 2014;57(21):8886–8902.

[119]. Nara H, Sato K, Kaieda A, et al. Design, synthesis, and biological activity of novel, potent, and highly selective fused pyrimidine-2-carboxamide-4-one-based matrix metalloproteinase (MMP)-13 zinc-binding inhibitors. *Bioorg Med Chem.* 2016;24(23):6149–6165.

[120]. Nara H, Kaieda A, Sato K, et al. Discovery of novel, highly potent, and selective matrix metalloproteinase (MMP)-13 inhibitors with a 1,2,4-triazol-3-yl moiety as a zinc binding group using a structure-based design approach. *J Med Chem.* 2017;60(2):608–626.

[121]. Wiley MR, Durham TB, Adams LA, et al. Use of osmotic pumps to establish the pharmacokinetic-pharmacodynamic relationship and define desirable human performance characteristics for aggrecanase inhibitors. *J Med Chem.* 2016;59(12):5810–5822.

[122]. Durham TB, Marimuthu J, Toth JL, et al. A highly selective hydantoin inhibitor of aggrecanase-1 and aggrecanase-2 with a low projected human dose. *J Med Chem.* 2017;60(13):5933–5939.

[123]. Marques SM, Tuccinardi T, Nuti E, et al. Novel 1-hydroxypiperazine-2,6-diones as new leads in the inhibition of metalloproteinases. *J Med Chem.* 2011;54(24):8289–8298.

[124]. Crascì L, Vicini P, Incerti M, et al. 2-Benzisothiazolylimino-5-benzylidene-4-thiazolidinones as protective agents against cartilage destruction. *Bioorg Med Chem.* 2015;23(7):1551–1556.

[125]. Senn N, Ott M, Lanz J, et al. Targeted polypharmacology: Discovery of a highly potent non-hydroxamate dual matrix metalloproteinase (MMP)-10/-13 inhibitor. *J Med Chem.* 2017;60(23):9585–9598.

7 Matrilysin and Their Inhibitors

Sandip Kumar Baidya, Suvankar Banerjee,
Nilanjan Adhikari, and Tarun Jha

CONTENTS

ABSTRACT

The design and discovery of matrilysin inhibitors are being disregarded because the roles and activities of matrilysin in numerous disease conditions have not been well-explored. However, matrilysin inhibitors (particularly MMP-7) presented in this chapter are assessed to judge the selective pattern of other specific MMP isoforms (usually collagenases or gelatinases) over MMP-7. Newer, more promising MMP-7 inhibitors may be made in accordance with their structures and activities. The research of matrilysin in many biological contexts and subsequent construction of selective inhibitors of such class might be anticipated to be targeted in this context. Selective matrilysin inhibitors are thus further examined in light of the potential roles and functions of matrilysin in many pathophysiological circumstances. This might reveal additional facets of matrilysin and associated inhibitors in the future.

Keywords: Matrilysin; Cancer; Hydroxamate; Thiazine and thiazepine; Diverse matrilysin inhibitors

7.1 INTRODUCTION

Matrix metalloproteinases (MMPs) are proteolytic enzymes that are responsible for the degradation of the extracellular matrix (ECM). The general structure of MMPs consists of the propeptide, catalytic domain (CD), a linker peptide having a variable length, and a hemopexin-like domain (HPx) [1, 2]. MMPs include matrilysin such as matrilysin-1 (MMP-7) and matrilysin-2 (MMP-26), which lack a hemopexin domain and a linker peptide. Therefore, matrilysins are considered the smallest subset of

DOI: 10.1201/9781003303282-9

MMPs in the MMP family [3]. Matrilysins consist of a single peptide, a catalytic domain, and a propeptide having a molecular mass of 28 kDa [4]. Interestingly, X-ray crystallographic data demonstrated the composition of the human matrilysin having a complex form with inhibitors. A five-stranded β-sheet, three α-helices, and a Zn^{2+} ion are essential for matrilysin enzyme activity. Moreover, one Zn^{2+} ion and two Ca^{2+} ions are essential for regulating enzyme stability [5]. These enzymes are found in several wounds of an organ like the brain, lung, breast, stomach, and colon. The matrilysins play crucial roles in tumor invasion and metastasis as they degrade ECM components along with gelatin I, III, IV, and V, as well as basement membrane type IV collagen, proteoglycan, fibronectin, laminin, vitronectin, and elastin [4]. From this point of view, matrilysin could be a promising target, and the development of matrilysin inhibitors is beneficial for therapeutic efficacy.

MMP-7 (also known as putative metalloproteinase, punctuated metalloproteinase; PUMP1) has been considered an important regulator of cell surface proteolysis and conjugates with different cell surface proteins like β-integrin, cadherin, TNF-α, heparin sulfate, and so on [6]. In fact, among all other MMPs, MMP-7 is overexpressed by carcinoma cells rather than stromal cells. Moreover, overexpression of MMP-7 is noticed in different malignancies, including breast cancer, lung cancer, stomach cancer, colorectal cancer, and squamous cell carcinoma of the head and neck [7]. Furthermore, some reports explored the expression of MMP-7 in epithelial ovarian carcinoma. Researchers have found that vascular epithelial growth factor (VEGF) and interleukin-8 (IL-8) significantly increased the secretion of MMP-7 in the DOV13 human ovarian carcinoma cell line [7]. MMP-7 itself may affect the structure of casein, laminin, fibronectin, collagen III/IV/V/IX/X/XI, type I/II/IV/V gelatins, elastin, and proteoglycan, thereby inducing their degradation [8]. Again, it helps to regulate different biochemical processes like activation, degradation, and shedding of non-ECM proteins. Heparin-binding epidermal growth factor (proHB-EGF) precursor, membrane-bound Fas ligand (FasL), TNF-α precursor, and E-cadherin are broken down by MMP-7 into mature HB-EGF, soluble FasL, TNF-α, and N-cadherin, which is responsible for promoting cellular proliferation and invasion [9].

Another matrilysin from the MMP family is matrilysin-2 (MMP-26), a small enzyme having an unclassical cysteine switch for latency preservation. Therefore, like no other MMPs, it can go through autocatalytic activation [10]. However, MMP-26 is responsible for the breakdown of ECM proteins (namely fibrinogen, vitronectin, and denatured collagen), blood plasma protein (such as fibrinogen and insulin-like growth factor-binding protein 1), and the inhibitor-like α1-antitrypsin and α2-macroglobulin and even integrin receptors (β4-integrin) [11]. Nonetheless, expression of MMP-26 in healthy tissue is decreased and may enhance cancerous tissue of the epithelial element [12]. In general, MMP-26 expression is found in the sclera of the human eye and T-cells; in the case of women, MMP-26 expression is found in ovarian theca granulosa cells and different endometrial cells, for example, surface and granular epithelial cells and vascular endothelial and endometrial stromal cells [13, 14].

A group of researchers confirmed increasing gene expression of MMP-26 in different tumor cell lines along with MCF-7 breast carcinoma cells [15]. Moreover, MMP-26 is involved in destroying the necrotic tissue of oxygen-deficient tumors and is engaged in neovascularization and angiogenesis [15]. In fact, some research demonstrated that matrilysin can activate gelatinases (i.e., MMP-2 and MMP-9) [16–18]. Moreover, it is active at the specific site of the pro-MMP-9 to generate a more stable active MMP-9 [10, 19]. It has been reported that regulation of both MMP-26 and TIMP-4 expression was found during the progression of various disease conditions [11]. Furthermore, MMP-7 also might enhance the proteolytic activity of MMP-9, and it has effects on a transient increase in the proteolytic activity of MMP-2 [17].

7.2 STRUCTURAL OVERVIEW OF MATRILYSIN

Matrilysin-1 is an enzyme, first discovered in 1980, that was found in the involuting uterus of the rat [20]. This enzyme was not fully purified until 1988 and was then characterized in more detail [21]. Matrilysin-1 is structurally different from other MMPs. In general, all MMP structures consist of major domains such as a single peptide, a pro-domain, one hemopexin domain, and one catalytic center. A few MMPs, like MMP-14, MMP-15, MMP-16, and MMP-24, comprise transmembrane domains, and MMP-23 consists of a cysteine array and Ig-like domain [1]. Despite these domains, furin cleavage, fibronectin repeat, and the hinge region are the various segments of different MMP structures. However, among these MMPs, matrilysin (MMP-7 and MMP-26) is the smallest among all MMPs in this metalloproteinase family. The structure of matrilysin consists of a single peptide, a pro-domain, and one catalytic center (Figure 7.1) [1]. A hemopexin domain is absent in matrilysin [22]. The gene encoding MMP-7 is located at 11q21-q22 and has 13 exons. The cDNA of the enzyme is 1,094 bp long and encodes 267 amino acids [23].

7.3 MATRILYSIN IN DIFFERENT DISEASE CONDITIONS

Matrilysins are overexpressed in invasive tumors of several organs, such as the stomach [24, 25], colon [26], esophagus [27], liver [28], and pancreas [29]. MMP-7

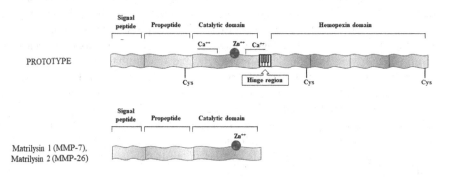

FIGURE 7.1   Prototype structure of MMPs and the domain structure of matrilysin.

expression is considered pro-cancerous, which is involved in the development of several digestive system tumors. Moreover, matrilysin overexpression is not only responsible for different digestive tumors but also responsible for intestinal lung disease [30, 31], fibrosing lung disease [32], renal tubular damage [33], kidney disease [34], and several other diseases like periodontal disease [35], Paget's disease [36], biliary atresia [37], myeloma growth and osteolytic bone disease [38], and coronary artery disease [39]. Moreover, combined overexpression of MMP-7, MMP-26, and MMP-8 might increase the risk of ischemic stroke [40]. Furthermore, MMP-7 also works as a biomarker in diseases like laryngopharyngeal reflux disease [41] and nonalcoholic fatty liver disease [42]. Most of the early research focused on the expression of matrilysin in gastrointestinal tumors. It was established that MMP-7 and MMP-26 are produced by tumor epithelium, and it is identified by using localization techniques like *in situ* hybridization and immunohistochemistry along with more quantitative methods, such as northern blotting. Interestingly, it was found that matrilysin expression is upregulated in tumors in comparison with adjacent normal tissue [43]. In the case of gastrointestinal tumors, the matrilysin mRNA was detected by about 80% in northern blot analysis, and about 90% of colorectal tumors were investigated by *in situ* hybridization [43]. In the case of chronic pancreatitis, the plasma concentration of MMP-7 could be a diagnostic marker in differentiating periampullary carcinoma. One group of researchers [44] used Luminex-100 technologies to identify MMP-7 expression in the serum of colorectal cancer patients and healthy controls. They found significantly higher expression of MMP-7 in the serum of patients than that of the control group. It concluded that the patient's survival rate is lower with higher MMP-7 concentration in serum than those with lower MMP-7 serum concentration levels.

Researchers found that higher MMP-7 expression is found in epithelial cells of Barrett esophagus and esophageal cancer, especially in terms of invasiveness. Therefore, MMP-7 may be a potential biomarker in the progression of esophageal cancer [23]. Again, Sharma and co-workers [45] found MMP-7 expression in the progression of gallbladder cancer. These findings express the carcinogenic effects of MMP-7, and the expression of MMP-7 might crucially take part in regulating and developing gallbladder and esophageal cancer.

Another study by Szarvas et al. [46] found that the expression of MMP-7 significantly increases plasma concentration in patients having bladder cancer in comparison with healthy controls. Therefore, increasing MMP-7 concentration is an independent risk factor for the higher stage of cancer metastasis and cancer-related death. Moreover, MMP-7 also plays a prime role in the invasion and migration of ovarian cancer. Overexpression of MMP-7 was found in high-grade ovarian cancer and low-grade ovarian tumors in a sample of 44 patients. At the same time, it is interesting to know that no such MMP-7 expression was found in healthy ovaries [47]. Therefore, matrilysin-1 could be a promising biomarker for ovarian carcinoma.

Another study found that MMP-7 was expressed in human breast tissue. Researchers found a common genetic variation in the MMP-7 gene related to breast cancer risk in a large population-dependent case-control study in Chinese women. It was found that MMP-7 has several functions that might contribute to the development and progression of breast cancer [48]. In addition, it was noticed that MMP-7 is elevated in idiopathic pulmonary fibrosis and can be considered a predictive biomarker during disease progression [49].

MMP-7 is expressed rarely in normal adult kidneys but is overexpressed in acute kidney injury (AKI) as well as chronic kidney disease (CKD). The function of MMP-7 in kidney diseases is complex, and by degrading ECM, MMP-7 breaks down several substrates like E-cadherin to control various cellular processes. Therefore, increased MMP-7 is observed in AKI patients and may be considered a promising biomarker of kidney diseases [50].

7.4 MATRILYSIN INHIBITORS

Xue et al. from DuPont Pharmaceuticals Company [51] reported some macrocyclic hydroxamic acids. Compounds **7.1** and **7.2** (Figure 7.2) were the potent but nonselective MMP-7 inhibitors (Ki of 0.8 and 1.5 nM, respectively). However, the pharmacokinetic study conducted on beagle dogs showed rapid absorption but short half-lives and lower oral bioavailability. Xue and co-workers from DuPont Pharmaceuticals Company [52] further reported a series of macrocyclic hydroxamate-based biphenyl derivatives. Compound **7.3** (Figure 7.2) was the maximum effective MMP-7 inhibitor (Ki = 177 nM) among these molecules.

Castelhano and co-workers from Syntex Discovery Research [53] reported some indolactam-based MMPIs. Compound **7.4** (Figure 7.2) was the most potent but nonselective inhibitor of matrilysin-1 (Ki = 3 nM). Vassiliou et al. [54] reported some phosphinic pseudo-tripeptides as potential MMPIs. Compound **7.5** (Figure 7.2) was the maximum effective MMP-7 inhibitor (Ki = 117 nM).

Ott and co-workers from Bristol-Myers Squibb Research and Development [55] reported some α,β-cyclic-β-benzamido hydroxamic acids as potential TACE inhibitors. Among these molecules, compound **7.6** (Figure 7.2) was the most potent MMP-7 inhibitor (Ki = 6 nM). Compound **7.6** yielded relatively low clearance (3.3 L/h/kg) with a lower half-life (2.9 h) and low oral bioavailability (25%).

Chen and co-workers from Bristol-Myers Squibb Pharmaceutical Research Institute [56] disclosed a set of β-amino hydroxamic acid-dependent TACE inhibitors. Among these molecules, compound **7.7** (Figure 7.3) was the most effective MMP-7 inhibitor (IC$_{50}$ = 1700 nM). At 8 mg/kg PO dose, compound **7.7** displayed good pharmacokinetic profiles tested in rats and dogs.

Gilmore et al. from Bristol-Myers Squibb Pharmaceutical Research Institute [57] reported some hydroxamate-based potent TACE inhibitors. Among these molecules, compound **7.8** (Figure 7.3) exerted the most effective MMP-7 inhibition (Ki = 635 nM). Ott and co-workers from Bristol-Myers Squibb Research and Development [58] obtained some orally bioavailable 2-substituted-1H-benzo[d]imidazol-1-yl)methyl)benzamide-based TACE inhibitors. Among these compounds, compound **7.9** (Figure 7.3) was the most effective MMP-7 inhibitor (IC$_{50}$ = 3,502 nM). Lu et al. from Bristol-Myers Squibb Pharmaceutical Research Institute [59] further reported some orally bioavailable TACE inhibitors. Among these molecules, compounds **7.10** and **7.11** (Figure 7.3) resulted in promising MMP-7 inhibitory efficacy (Ki of 852 and

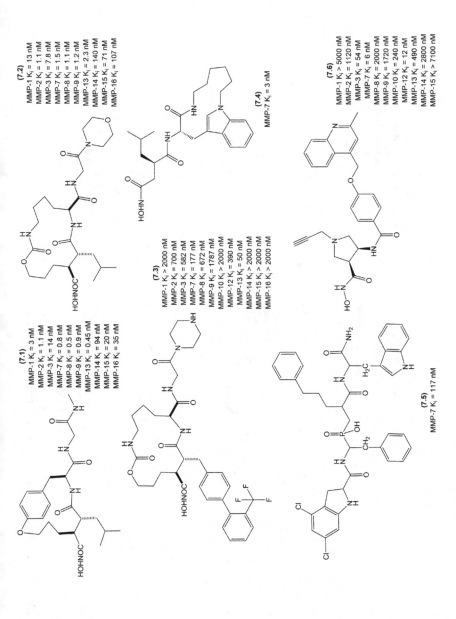

FIGURE 7.2 Some potential MMP-7 inhibitors (compounds 7.1–7.6).

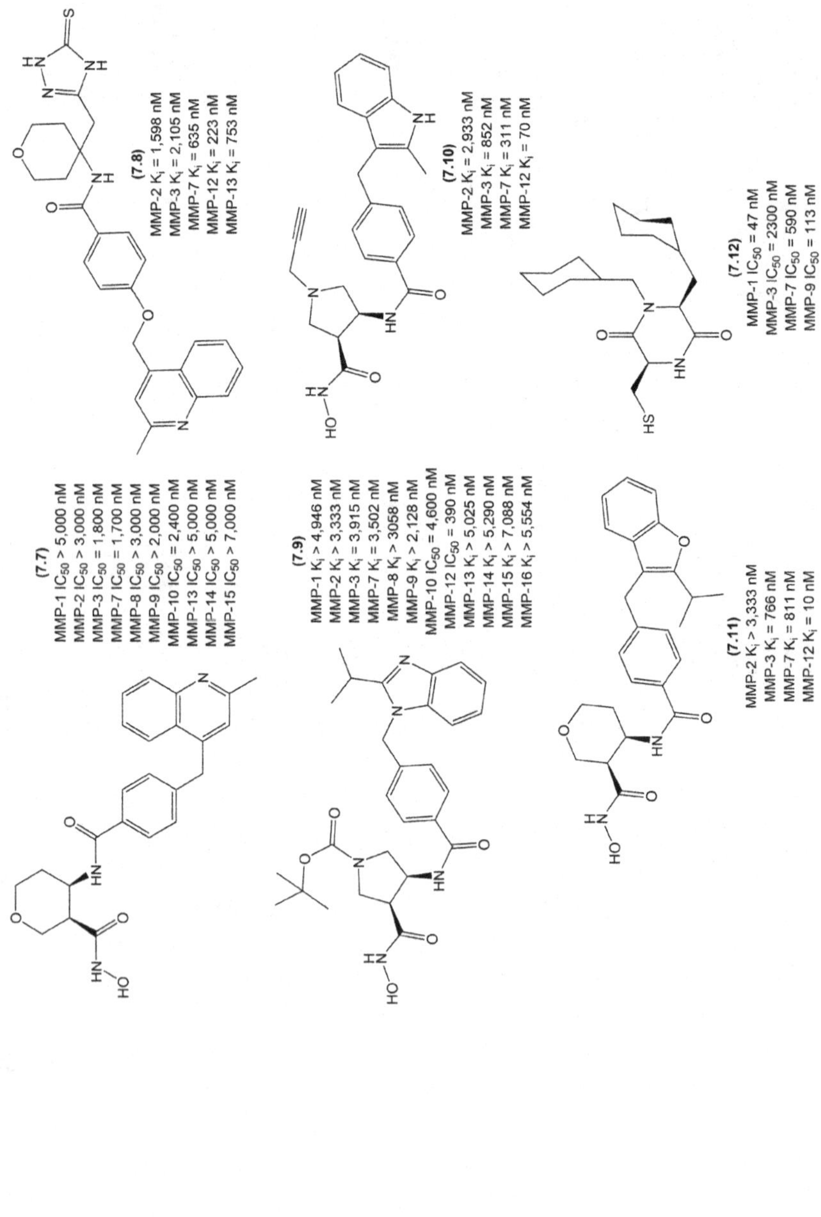

(7.7)

MMP-1 IC$_{50}$ > 5,000 nM
MMP-2 IC$_{50}$ > 3,000 nM
MMP-3 IC$_{50}$ = 1,800 nM
MMP-7 IC$_{50}$ = 1,700 nM
MMP-8 IC$_{50}$ > 3,000 nM
MMP-9 IC$_{50}$ > 2,000 nM
MMP-10 IC$_{50}$ = 2,400 nM
MMP-13 IC$_{50}$ > 5,000 nM
MMP-14 IC$_{50}$ > 5,000 nM
MMP-15 IC$_{50}$ > 7,000 nM

(7.8)

MMP-2 K$_i$ = 1,598 nM
MMP-3 K$_i$ = 2,105 nM
MMP-7 K$_i$ = 635 nM
MMP-12 K$_i$ = 223 nM
MMP-13 K$_i$ = 753 nM

(7.9)

MMP-1 K$_i$ > 4,946 nM
MMP-2 K$_i$ > 3,333 nM
MMP-3 K$_i$ = 3,915 nM
MMP-7 K$_i$ = 3,502 nM
MMP-8 K$_i$ = 3058 nM
MMP-9 K$_i$ > 2,128 nM
MMP-10 IC$_{50}$ = 4,600 nM
MMP-12 IC$_{50}$ = 390 nM
MMP-13 K$_i$ > 5,025 nM
MMP-14 K$_i$ = 5,290 nM
MMP-15 K$_i$ > 7,088 nM
MMP-16 K$_i$ = 5,554 nM

(7.10)

MMP-2 K$_i$ = 2,933 nM
MMP-3 K$_i$ = 852 nM
MMP-7 IC$_{50}$ = 311 nM
MMP-12 K$_i$ = 70 nM

(7.11)

MMP-2 K$_i$ > 3,333 nM
MMP-3 K$_i$ = 766 nM
MMP-7 K$_i$ = 811 nM
MMP-12 K$_i$ = 10 nM

(7.12)

MMP-1 IC$_{50}$ = 47 nM
MMP-3 IC$_{50}$ = 2300 nM
MMP-7 IC$_{50}$ = 590 nM
MMP-9 IC$_{50}$ = 113 nM

FIGURE 7.3   Various effective MMP-7 inhibitors (compounds **7.7–7.12**).

766 nM, respectively). Szardenings and co-workers from Affymax Research Institute [60] reported some thiol-based effective MMPIs. Compound **7.12** (Figure 7.3) was the most effective matrilysin inhibitor (IC_{50} = 590 nM) among these molecules.

Almstead and co-workers from Procter and Gamble Pharmaceuticals [61] reported some potent thiazine- and thiazepine-based MMPIs. Some of the molecules (compounds **7.13**–**7.20**) were found to be potent MMP-7 inhibitors (Table 7.1).

Pikul and co-workers from Procter and Gamble Pharmaceuticals [62] reported some achiral potent MMPIs. Compound **7.21** (Figure 7.4) was the most potent MMP-7 inhibitor (IC_{50} = 30 nM) among these molecules. Cheng and co-workers from Procter and Gamble Pharmaceuticals [63] reported a series of proline-based MMPIs. Compounds **7.22** and **7.23** (Figure 7.4) were effective MMP-7 inhibitors among these molecules.

Natchus and co-workers from Procter and Gamble Pharmaceuticals [64] reported some functionalized 4-aminoproline-based hydroxamates as potential MMPIs. Compounds **7.24** and **7.25** (Figure 7.4) were effective MMP-7 inhibitors (IC_{50} of 310 and 450 nM, respectively). Pikul et al. from Procter and Gamble Pharmaceuticals [65] reported some heterocycle-based MMPIs. Among these molecules, compound **7.26** (Figure 7.4) was the most effective MMP-7 inhibitor (IC_{50} = 88 nM).

A further study by Tullis and co-workers from Procter and Gamble Pharmaceuticals [66] resulted in some carboxylic acid-based MMPIs comprising cyclohexylglycine moiety. Among these molecules, compound **7.27** (Figure 7.5) was the most effective MMP-7 inhibitor (IC_{50} = 845 nM). Pikul et al. from Procter and Gamble Pharmaceuticals further reported some selective carboxylic acid-based selective MMPIs [67]. However, compound **7.28** (Figure 7.5), containing a hydroxamate moiety, was the most promising MMP-7 inhibitor among these molecules (IC_{50} = 20 nM).

A further study by Cheng et al. [68] produced some piperazine-based MMPIs. Compound **7.29** (Figure 7.5) was the most effective MMP-7 inhibitor among these molecules (IC_{50} = 232 nM). Compound **7.29** exhibited good pleural absorption and *ex vivo* results (absorption 59%, logP = 1.76, explant IC_{50} = 43 nM). Apfel et al. from Hoffmann-La Roche Ltd. reported [69] some hydroxamates as potential peptide deformylase inhibitors. Among these molecules, compound **7.30** (Figure 7.5) was the most effective matrilysin inhibitor (IC_{50} = 290 nM). Mazzola Jr et al. from Schering Plough Research Institute [70] reported some highly potent TACE inhibitors. Compounds **7.31** and **7.32** (Figure 7.5) were promising MMP-7 inhibitors (Ki of 110 and 128 nM, respectively) among these molecules. However, compound **7.32** failed to show detectable plasma levels in rat pharmacokinetics. Again, it displayed low oral bioavailability and, subsequently, poor absorption, as evidenced by the Caco-2 assay.

Steinman et al. from Abbott Laboratories [71] reported some macrocyclic MMPIs. Many of these molecules (compounds **7.33**–**7.41**) were found to be potential MMP-7 inhibitors (Table 7.2).

Sheppard et al. from Abbott Laboratories [72] reported some succinyl hydroxamate-based MMPIs. Some compounds (compounds **7.42**–**7.67**) exhibited potential MMP-7 inhibitory activity (Table 7.3).

TABLE 7.1

Thiazine- and Thiazepine-Based Potential MMP-7 Inhibitors (IC$_{50}$ in nM)

(7.13-7.16)   (7.17-7.19)   (7.20)

Cpd	R	n	Ar	MMP-1	MMP-2	MMP-3	MMP-7	MMP-8	MMP-9	MMP-13
7.13	S	0	-	0.4	1.4	0.7	23	0.7	0.9	1.0
7.14	S	1	-	0.8	2.7	0.7	30	1.4	1.9	0.9
7.15	CH$_2$	1	-	2.4	1.4	3.3	18	1.9	0.5	-
7.16	S	3	-	3.0	2.4	7.2	30	0.6	3.7	1.0
7.17	S	-	-p-Br-Ph	0.7	6.8	10	17	-	-	1.3
7.18	SO$_2$	-	-p-Br-Ph	19	1.2	2.7	27	-	-	0.4
7.19	S	-	-Ph-O-Ph	2.3	-	11	16	-	-	<0.4
7.20	-	-	-	1.0	1.8	1.0	38	-	-	1.4

Cpd, compound.

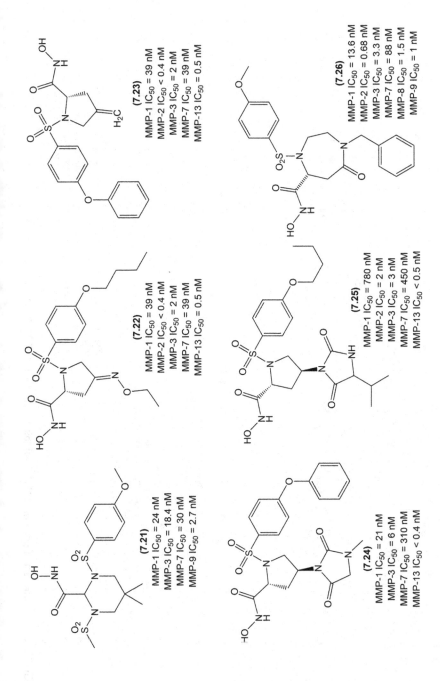

FIGURE 7.4 Several other potential MMP-7 inhibitors (compounds **7.21–7.26**).

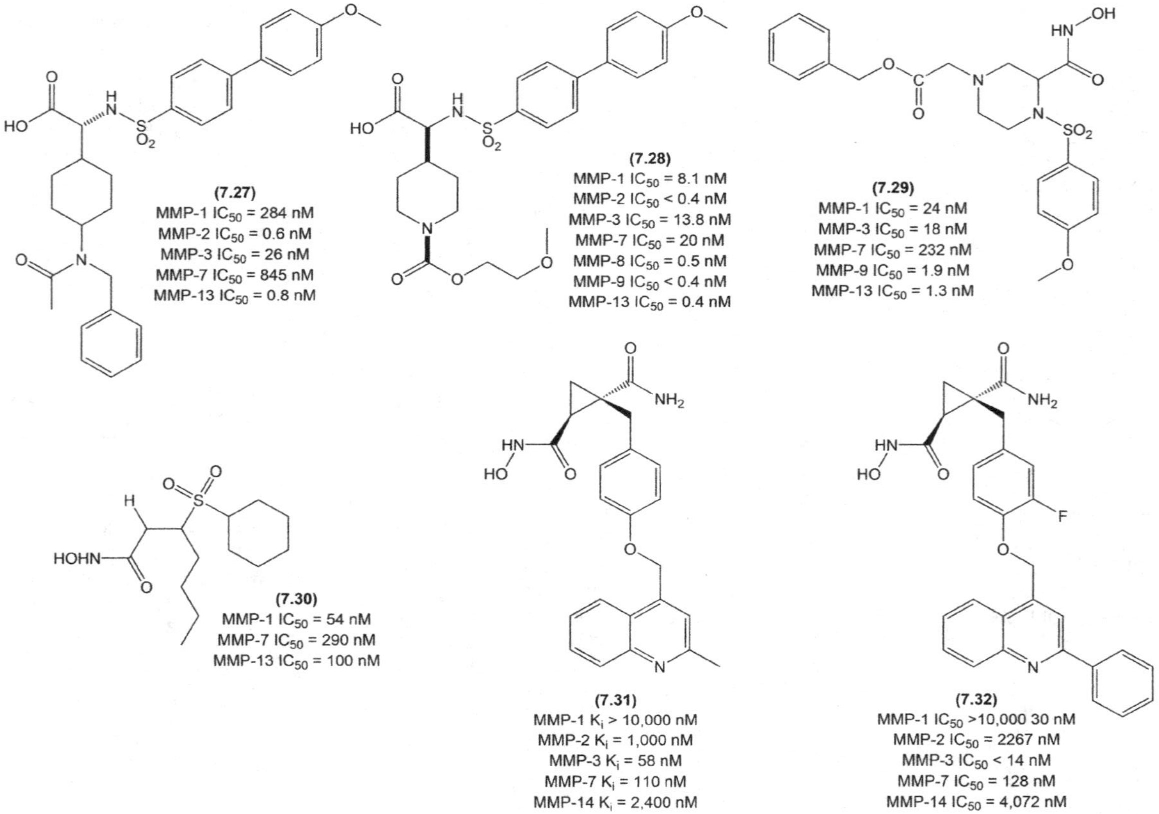

(7.29)

MMP-1 IC$_{50}$ = 24 nM
MMP-3 IC$_{50}$ = 18 nM
MMP-7 IC$_{50}$ = 232 nM
MMP-9 IC$_{50}$ = 1.9 nM
MMP-13 IC$_{50}$ = 1.3 nM

(7.28)

MMP-1 IC$_{50}$ = 8.1 nM
MMP-2 IC$_{50}$ < 0.4 nM
MMP-3 IC$_{50}$ = 13.8 nM
MMP-7 IC$_{50}$ = 20 nM
MMP-8 IC$_{50}$ = 0.5 nM
MMP-9 IC$_{50}$ < 0.4 nM
MMP-13 IC$_{50}$ = 0.4 nM

(7.27)

MMP-1 IC$_{50}$ = 284 nM
MMP-2 IC$_{50}$ = 0.6 nM
MMP-3 IC$_{50}$ = 26 nM
MMP-7 IC$_{50}$ = 845 nM
MMP-13 IC$_{50}$ = 0.8 nM

(7.32)

MMP-1 IC$_{50}$ >10,000 30 nM
MMP-2 IC$_{50}$ = 2267 nM
MMP-3 IC$_{50}$ < 14 nM
MMP-7 IC$_{50}$ = 128 nM
MMP-14 IC$_{50}$ = 4,072 nM

(7.31)

MMP-1 K$_i$ > 10,000 nM
MMP-2 K$_i$ = 1,000 nM
MMP-3 K$_i$ = 58 nM
MMP-7 K$_i$ = 110 nM
MMP-14 K$_i$ = 2,400 nM

(7.30)

MMP-1 IC$_{50}$ = 54 nM
MMP-7 IC$_{50}$ = 290 nM
MMP-13 IC$_{50}$ = 100 nM

FIGURE 7.5　Another set of potential MMP-7 inhibitors (compounds **7.27–7.32**).

TABLE 7.2

Some macrocyclic potential MMP-7 inhibitors (IC$_{50}$ in nM)

Cpd	R$_1$	R$_2$	n	MMP-1	MMP-2	MMP-3	MMP-7
7.33	i-butyl	Me	1	1.8	2.2	1.6	3.9
7.34	(CH$_2$)$_3$Ph(p-CH$_3$)	Me	1	6.1	0.8	2.8	9.1
7.35	(CH$_2$)$_2$Ph(CH$_2$)$_2$CH$_3$	Me	1	54	0.1	5.9	1.5
7.36	i-butyl	Me	0	3.0	2.6	3.0	7.8
7.37	i-butyl	Me	2	2.1	2.3	2.6	6.1
7.38	i-butyl	Me	3	2.2	5.9	5.7	12
7.39	i-butyl	2-pyridyl	1	4.6	2.1	1.6	2.6
7.40	i-butyl	CH$_2$CH$_2$SMe	1	2.7	3.8	2.5	4.2
7.41	i-butyl	CH$_2$CH$_2$N(CH$_3$)$_2$	1	6.6	6.5	4.2	12

Cpd, compound.

O'Brien et al. from Parke-Davis Pharmaceutical Research [73] reported a series of biphenyl sulfonamides as potent MMPIs. Some of these molecules (compounds **7.68–7.81**) resulted in highly potent MMP-7 inhibitory efficacy. Among these molecules, compound **7.74** showed an increase in potency against MMP-7 compared with the *in vitro* activity of MMP-2 and MMP-3 (Table 7.4).

Li and co-workers from Wyeth Research [74] reported a set of potent and highly MMP-13-selective inhibitors. Among these molecules, compounds **7.82** and **7.83** (Figure 7.6) were found to be promising MMP-7 inhibitors (IC$_{50}$ of 534 and 458 nM, respectively).

Barta and co-workers from Pfizer Research & Development [75] reported some α-sulfone hydroxamates as selective MMP-13 inhibitors. Among these molecules, compound **7.84** (Figure 7.6) displayed the most effective MMP-7 inhibitory efficacy (Ki = 970 nM). Nara and co-workers from Takeda Pharmaceutical Company Limited [76] reported fused pyrimidine-2-carboxamide-4-one-dependent selective MMP-13 inhibitors. Compounds **7.85** and **7.86** (Figure 7.6) were found to be the most effective

TABLE 7.3

Some Succinyl Hydroxamate-Based Potential MMP-7 Inhibitors (IC$_{50}$ in nM)

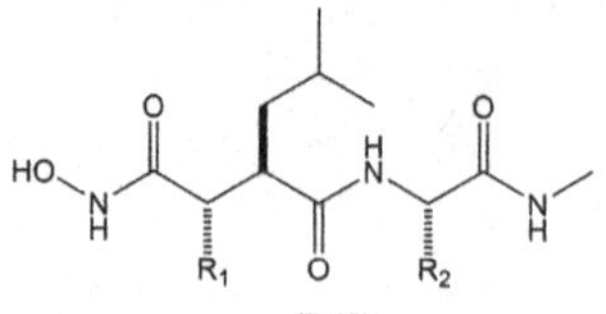

(7.42)

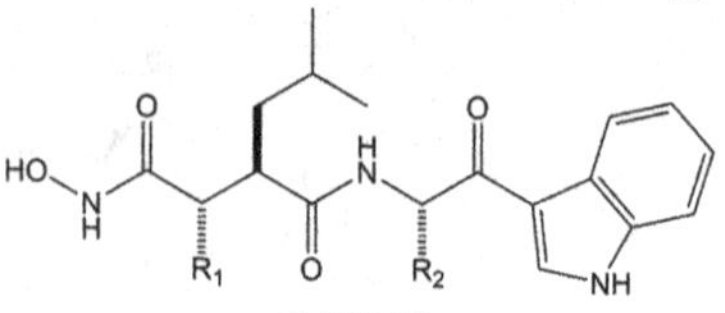

(7.43-7.47)

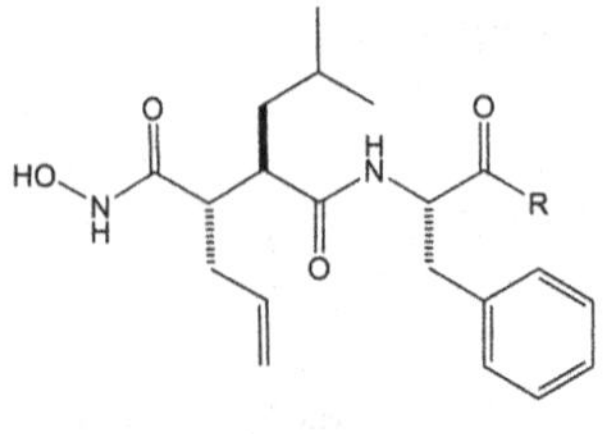

(7.48-7.58)

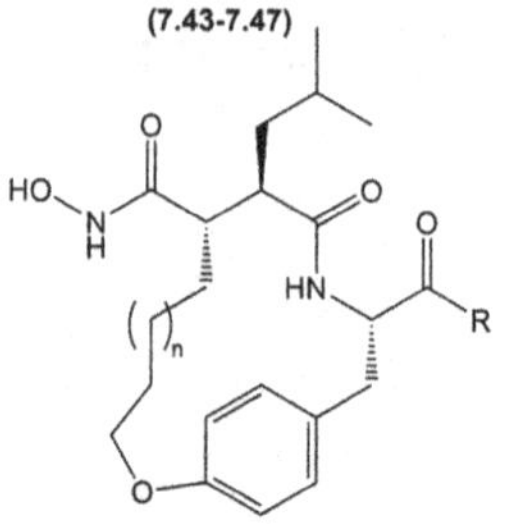

(7.59-7.67)

Cpd	R	R$_1$	R$_2$	n	MMP-1	MMP-2	MMP-3	MMP-7
7.42	-	allyl	CH$_2$Ph	-	2.2	1.8	12	11
7.43	-	allyl	CH$_2$Ph	-	1.1	1.1	2.3	2.2
7.44	-	allyl	t-Bu	-	1.2	1.6	1.2	0.78
7.45	-	OH	CH$_2$Ph	-	5.0	0.60	7.8	1.1
7.46	-	OH	t-Bu	-	0.26	0.38	1.2	0.30
7.47	-	H	CH$_2$Ph	-	5.1	1.0	5.6	4.3
7.48	3-(1-Me-indolyl)	-	-	-	4.7	23	36	29
7.49	3-pyrrolyl	-	-	-	6.2	2.7	6.6	8.0
7.50	2-pyrrolyl	-	-	-	2.6	1.1	1.7	1.2
7.51	2-thiazolyl	-	-	-	-	1100	360	220
7.52	2-oxazolyl	-	-	-	2.7	7.2	1.8	4.2
7.53	2-benzimidazolyl	-	-	-	180	110	54	68
7.54	3-pyridyl	-	-	-	14	8.6	10	8.6
7.55	phenyl	-	-	-	10	3.4	4.	3.6
7.56	2-thienyl	-	-	-	-	6.5	3.2	13
7.57	methyl	-	-	-	-	22	16	45
7.58	ethyl	-	-	-	40	33	82	39
7.59	NHMe	-	-	1	1.8	5.6	4.0	1.6
7.60	NHMe	-	-	2	2.1	2.3	2.6	6.1
7.61	3-indolyl	-	-	2	4.8	6.1	5.1	3.1
7.62	phenyl	-	-	2	9.1	3.9	2.7	2.2
7.63	phenyl	-	-	1	13	9.5	8.9	3.3
7.64	2-pyrrolyl	-	-	1	1.9	7.2	7.2	4.2
7.65	4-(t-Bu)-Ph	-	-	1	270	91	110	40
7.66	4-(SO$_2$Me)-Ph	-	-	1	60	8.5	9.8	5.7
7.67	4-(HOCH$_3$)Ph	-	-	1	5.0	5.1	3.4	1.5

Cpd, compound.

TABLE 7.4

Biphenylsulfonamide-Based Potential MMP-7 Inhibitors (IC$_{50}$ in nM)

Cpd	R	MMP-1	MMP-2	MMP-3	MMP-7	MMP-9	MMP-13
7.68	H	5,400	40	38	71,000	26,000	62
7.69	4-F	4,200	39	10	4,800	64,000	43
7.70	4-F	8,600	49	17	22,000	65,000	150
7.71	4-Br	6,000	4	7	7,200	7,900	8
7.72	3-Br	1,00,000	535	290	1,00,000	1,00,000	710
7.73	3-Cl	6,500	11	9	7,500	16,000	48
7.74	2-F, 4-Br	3,600	5	16	2,100	4,900	7
7.75	4-Me	2,200	2	3	4,500	3,900	11
7.76	4-OMe	1,500	3	8	7,200	2,200	6
7.77	4-NH$_2$	26,000	36	36	31,000	20,000	105
7.78	4-CF$_3$	4,200	13	9	7,900	20,000	23
7.79	4-CN	18,000	33	6	7,000	59,000	37
7.80	4-CHO	3,200	12	8	4,500	17,000	16
7.81	4-NO$_2$	12,000	61	15	5,600	38,000	102

Cpd, compound.

MMP-7 inhibitors (IC$_{50}$ = 7.3 and 30 nM, respectively). Miller and co-workers from British Biotech Pharmaceuticals Ltd. reported [77] some phenylalanine analogs as effective MMPIs. Compound **7.87** (Figure 7.6) was the most effective matrilysin inhibitor (IC$_{50}$ = 20 nM) among these molecules. Chen et al. from Roche Bioscience [78] reported some potent benzimidazole-based MMPIs. Many of these molecules (compounds **7.88–7.98**) were highly effective matrilysin inhibitors (Table 7.5).

Ma et al. [79] reported several tetrahydroisoquinoline-based sulfonamido hydroxamates as potent MMPIs. However, many of these molecules (compounds **7.99–7.107**) in this series exhibited potent MMP-26 inhibitory efficacy (Table 7.6). Among these molecules, compounds **7.105** and **7.107** were found to be better effective MMP-7 inhibitors (IC$_{50}$ of 2.424 and 3.192 µM).

Subramaniam et al. [80] disclosed some bis-(arylsulfonamido) hydroxamate-dependent MMPIs. Some molecules (compounds **7.108–7.113**) yielded potential MMP-7 inhibitory activity (Table 7.7).

Jin et al. [81] designed some 3-mercaptopyrrolidine-containing MMPIs. Among these compounds, compounds **7.114** and **7.115** (Figure 7.7) were found to be the most effective MMP-7 inhibitors (Ki = 12 and 11 nM, respectively). Campestre et al. [82] reported some peptidyl 3-substituted 1-hydroxyureas as potential MMPIs. Compounds **7.116** and **7.117** (Figure 7.7) were the most effective MMP-7 inhibitors

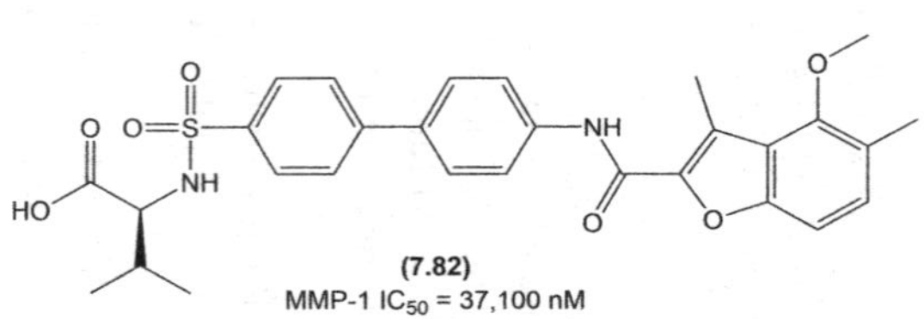

(7.82)
MMP-1 IC$_{50}$ = 37,100 nM
MMP-2 IC$_{50}$ = 1,610 nM
MMP-3 IC$_{50}$ = 442 nM
MMP-7 IC$_{50}$ = 534 nM
MMP-8 IC$_{50}$ = 52 nM
MMP-13 IC$_{50}$ = 4.9 nM
MMP-14 IC$_{50}$ = 15,000 nM

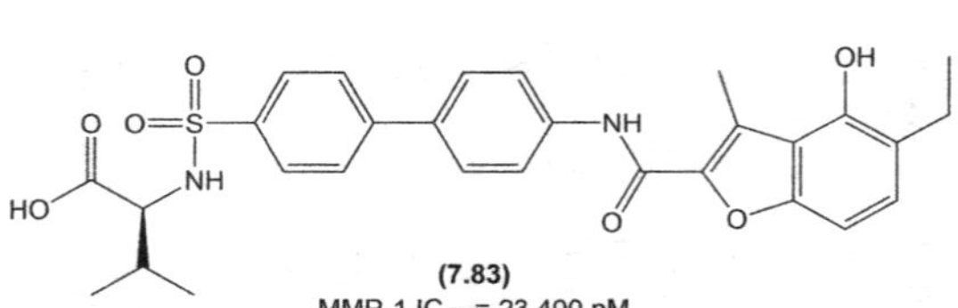

(7.83)
MMP-1 IC$_{50}$ = 23,400 nM
MMP-2 IC$_{50}$ = 1,760 nM
MMP-3 IC$_{50}$ = 492 nM
MMP-7 IC$_{50}$ = 458 nM
MMP-8 IC$_{50}$ = 94 nM
MMP-13 IC$_{50}$ = 7.1 nM
MMP-14 IC$_{50}$ = 15,800 nM

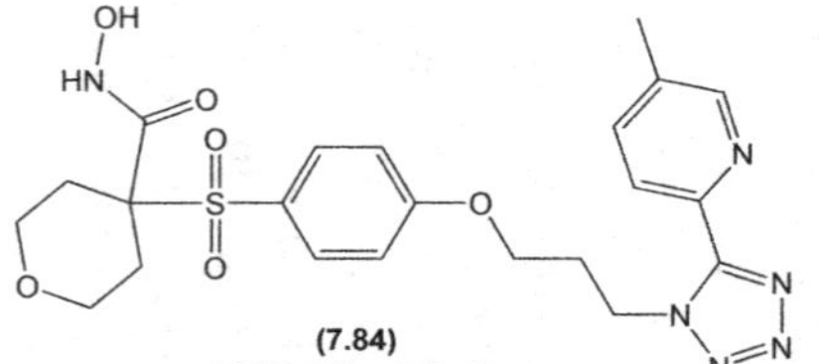

(7.84)
MMP-2 K$_i$ = 400 nM
MMP-3 K$_i$ = 3 nM
MMP-7 K$_i$ = 970 nM
MMP-8 K$_i$ = 250 nM
MMP-9 K$_i$ = 430 nM
MMP-13 K$_i$ = 0.60 nM

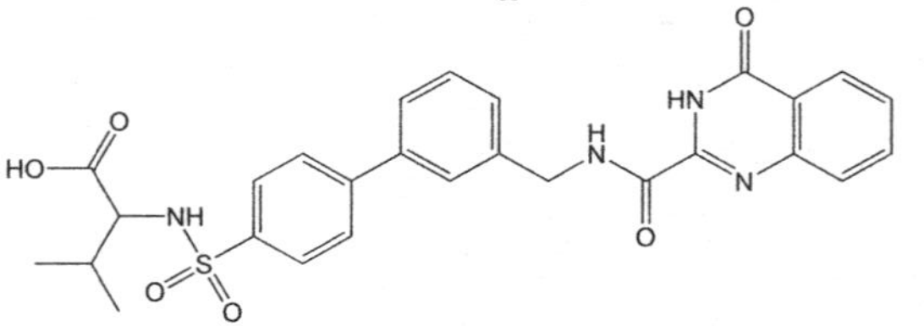

(7.85)
MMP-1 IC$_{50}$ = 11 nM
MMP-2 IC$_{50}$ = 1.9 nM
MMP-3 IC$_{50}$ = 1.5 nM
MMP-7 IC$_{50}$ = 7.3 nM
MMP-8 IC$_{50}$ = 0.82 nM
MMP-9 IC$_{50}$ = 4.7 nM
MMP-10 IC$_{50}$ = 0.30 nM
MMP-12 IC$_{50}$ = 8.1 nM
MMP-13 IC$_{50}$ = 0.0032 nM
MMP-14 IC$_{50}$ = 3.8 nM

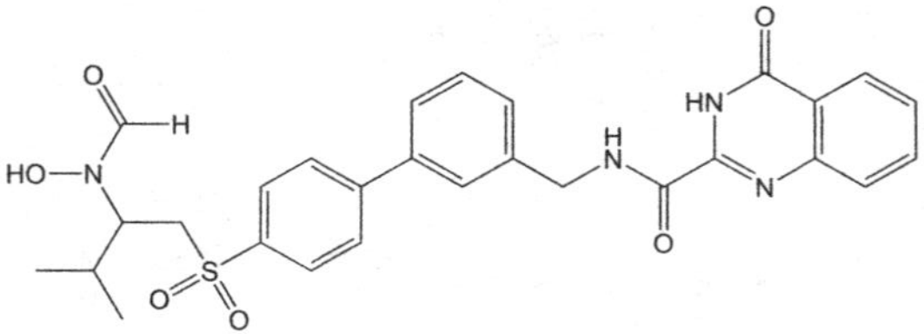

(7.86)
MMP-1 IC$_{50}$ = 18 nM
MMP-2 IC$_{50}$ = 3 nM
MMP-3 IC$_{50}$ = 2.5 nM
MMP-7 IC$_{50}$ = 30 nM
MMP-8 IC$_{50}$ = 1.3 nM
MMP-9 IC$_{50}$ = 5.3 nM
MMP-10 IC$_{50}$ = 0.35 nM
MMP-12 IC$_{50}$ = 8.5 nM
MMP-13 IC$_{50}$ = 0.051 nM
MMP-14 IC$_{50}$ = 5.4 nM

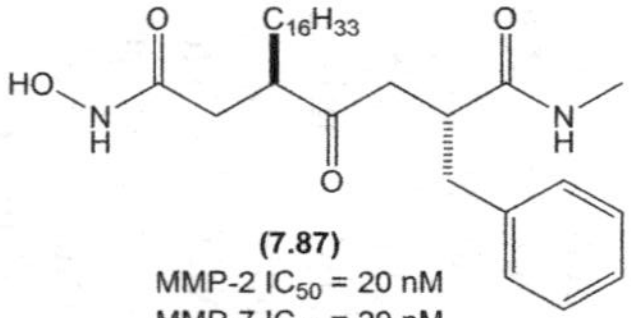

(7.87)
MMP-2 IC$_{50}$ = 20 nM
MMP-7 IC$_{50}$ = 20 nM

FIGURE 7.6 Different potential MMP-7 inhibitors (compounds **7.82–7.87**).

TABLE 7.5

Some Potential Benzimidazole-Based MMP-7 Inhibitors (IC$_{50}$ in nM)

(7.88-7.93)　　　　　　　　　(7.94-7.98)

Cpd	R$_1$	R$_2$	X	Y	MMP-7
7.88	-	CH$_2$CHMe$_2$	H	H	2
7.89	-	CH$_2$CHMe$_2$	H	CF$_3$	10
7.90	-	CH$_2$CHMe$_2$	H	OCF$_3$	10
7.91	-	CH$_2$CHMe$_2$	H	CO$_2$CH$_3$	1
7.92	-	CH$_2$CHMe$_2$	Cl	Cl	33
7.93	-	3-indolylmethyl	H	H	10
7.94	CH$_2$CHMe$_2$	CH$_2$CHMe$_2$	H	H	50
7.95	CH$_2$CHMe$_2$	CH$_2$CHMe$_2$	H	Ph	1
7.96	CH$_2$CHMe$_2$	CH$_2$CHMe$_2$	CO$_2$Me	Ph	70
7.97	c-C$_6$H$_{11}$	CH$_2$CHMe$_2$	H	Ph	3.1
7.98	CH$_2$CHMe$_2$	3-indolylmethyl	H	H	18

Cpd, compound.

(Ki = 0.0083 and 4.1 nM, respectively). Gona and co-workers [83] reported some potent and selective MMP-12 inhibitors. Among these molecules, compounds **7.118** and **7.119** (Figure 7.7) were the most promising MMP-7 inhibitors (Ki of 14.6 and 17.2 nM, respectively).

As per the report of Mahasenan et al. [84], compound **7.120** (Figure 7.8) was found to be a highly effective MMP-7 inhibitor (K$_i$ = 75 nM). Biasone et al. [85] reported a set of α-biphenylsulfonylamino 2-methylpropyl phosphonates as effective MMPIs. Among these molecules, compound **7.121** (Figure 7.8) was the maximum effective MMP-7 inhibitor (IC$_{50}$ = 150 nM). Attolino et al. [86] reported some N-arylsulfonyl-based water-soluble MMPIs. Compound **7.122** (Figure 7.8) among the molecules resulted in the most potent MMP-7 inhibition (Ki = 344 nM). Ledour and co-workers reported some hydrazide-based ilomastat derivatives [87] as effective MMPIs. Among these molecules, compounds **7.123** and **7.124** (Figure 7.8) exerted potent MMP-7 inhibitory efficacy (IC$_{50}$ of 110 and 475 nM, respectively).

Aihara et al. [88] reported some methylated epigallocatechin gallate derivatives as promising MMP inhibitors. Among these molecules, compounds **7.125–7.127** (Figure 7.9) resulted in effective MMP-7 inhibitory activity. Testero et al. [89] reported some thiiranes as potent and selective gelatinase inhibitors. Some of these

TABLE 7.6

Tetrahydroisoquinoline-Based Sulfonamide Hydroxamates as Potential MMP-7 Inhibitors (IC$_{50}$ in nM)

Cpd	R	R$_1$	Y	MMP-1	MMP-2	MMP-7	MMP-9	MMP-12	MMP-14	MMP-15	MMP-16	MMP-26
7.99	H	H	H	6.319	0.430	–	0.335	0.421	1.102	0.218	0.184	0.858
7.100	H	H	4-Me	152	18	10,500	40	29	52	19	21	97
7.101	H	H	4-NO$_2$	41	76	21,420	258	59	521	126	177	791
7.102	H	H	2-Cl, 5-Cl	–	853	21,380	1,882	170	4,613	1,798	1,834	7,903
7.103	H	Bn	H	452	24	7,136	35	57	39	17	35	1,453
7.104	H	Bn	4-Me	462	33	12,040	130	72	62	44	56	2,046
7.105	H	Bn	4-OMe	88	16	2,424	30	57	34	4	22	744
7.106	OMe	H	H	595	27	10,690	100	65	867	29	40	146
7.107	OMe	H	4-OMe	123	26	3,192	46	20	68	6	16	86

Cpd, compound.

TABLE 7.7

Bis-(arylsulfonamide) Hydroxamate-Based Potential MMP-7 Inhibitors (K_i in nM)

Cpd	Ar	MMP-7	MMP-9	MMP-10
7.108	p-OMe-Ph	605	39	335
7.109	p-F-Ph	625	2,750	4,570
7.110	p-Cl-Ph	237	230	ND
7.111	p-I-Ph	1,800	2.6	1600
7.112	m-CF$_3$-Ph	602	NI	NI
7.113	2,4-diOMe-Ph	289	1,24,000	3,72,000

Cpd, compound.

molecules (compounds **7.128–7.131**) (Figure 7.9) exhibited promising MMP-7 inhibition. All these molecules displayed good metabolic stability with good intrinsic clearance and solubility.

7.5 SUMMARY

The design and discovery of matrilysin inhibitors have been ignored because the roles and functions of matrilysins are not well-explored in several disease conditions. Researchers have primarily focused on the exploration of designing inhibitors of gelatinases and collagenases and, to some extent, on designing MMP-12 inhibitors, because the roles and functions of such types of MMPs in various disease conditions have been explored. However, because of the similarity, these matrilysins are likely to participate significantly in diverse disease conditions. Therefore, the area is an open and challenging field. It is important to note that the matrilysin inhibitors (especially MMP-7) discussed in this chapter are evaluated by the researchers to judge the selective pattern of other specific MMP isoforms (generally collagenases or gelatinases) over MMP-7. New promising MMP-7 inhibitors may be designed accordingly based on their structures and activity. In this context, it may be assumed that the exploration of matrilysins in diverse biological conditions and the subsequent designing of selective inhibitors is intended. Therefore, selective matrilysin inhibitors can be evaluated further by considering the promising roles and functions of matrilysins in different pathophysiological conditions. This may open new aspects of matrilysins and related inhibitors in the future.

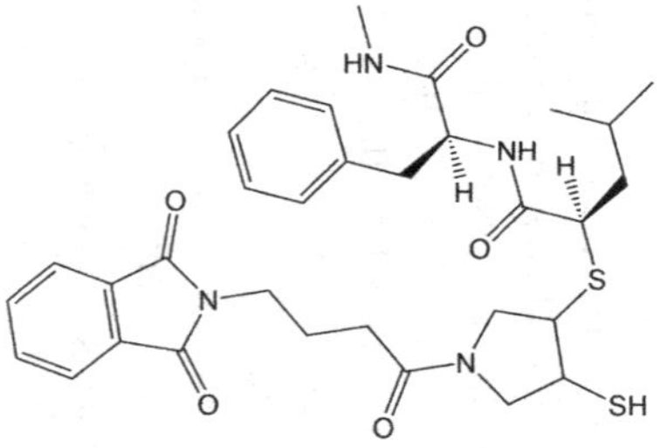

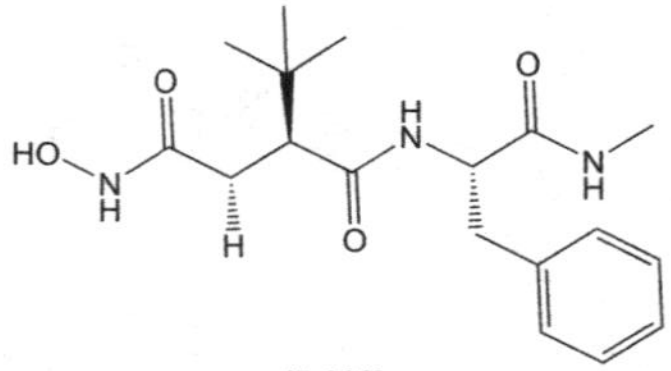

(7.116)
MMP-1 IC$_{50}$ = 25 nM
MMP-2 IC$_{50}$ = 0.7 nM
MMP-3 IC$_{50}$ = 43 nM
MMP-7 IC$_{50}$ = 8.3 nM
MMP-8 IC$_{50}$ = 0.046 nM
MMP-9 IC$_{50}$ = 0.38 nM

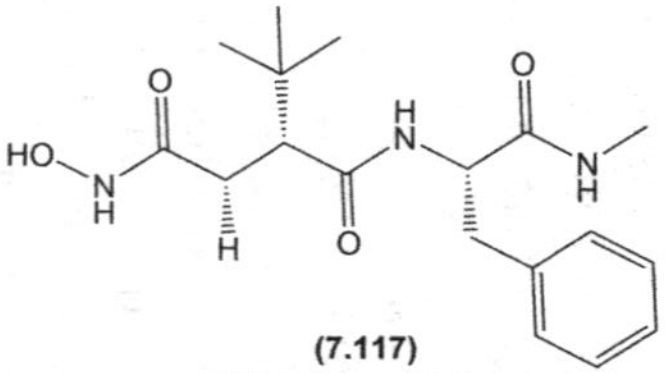

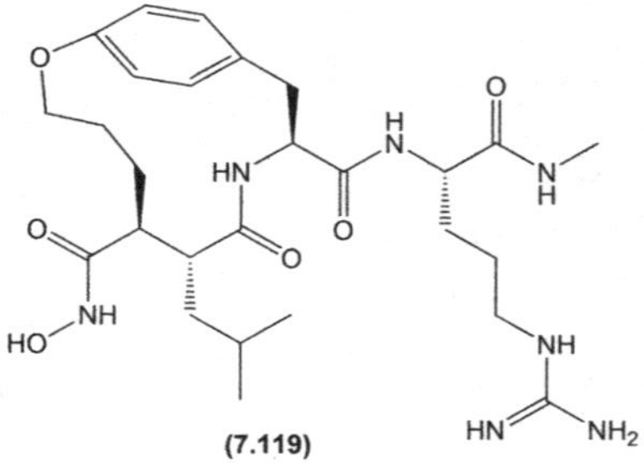

(7.119)
MMP-2 K$_i$ = 5.8 nM
MMP-7 K$_i$ = 17.2 nM
MMP-9 K$_i$ = 20.4 nM
MMP-12 K$_i$ = 1 nM
MMP-13 K$_i$ = 15.3 nM

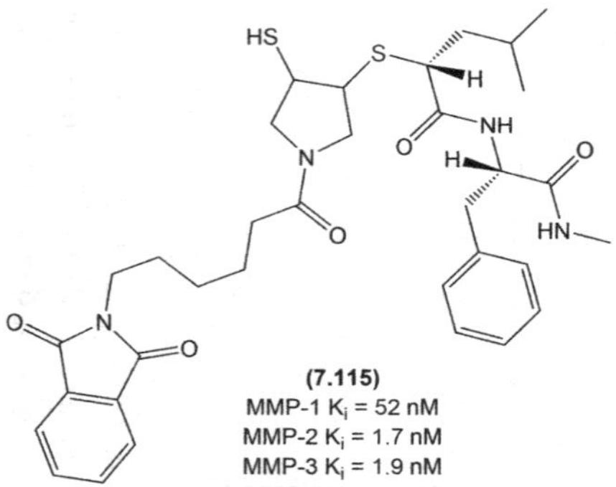

(7.115)
MMP-1 K$_i$ = 52 nM
MMP-2 K$_i$ = 1.7 nM
MMP-3 K$_i$ = 1.9 nM
MMP-7 K$_i$ = 11 nM
MMP-9 K$_i$ = 0.98 nM
MMP-14 K$_i$ = 7 nM

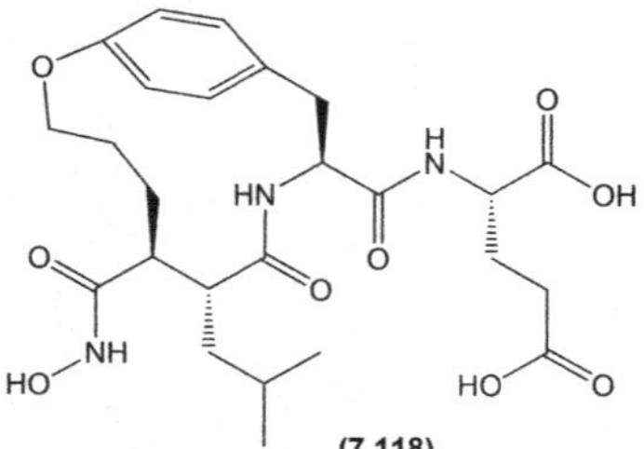

(7.118)
MMP-2 K$_i$ = 396 nM
MMP-7 K$_i$ = 14.6 nM
MMP-9 K$_i$ = 2107 nM
MMP-12 K$_i$ = 1.2 nM
MMP-13 K$_i$ = 89 nM

(7.114)
MMP-1 K$_i$ = 75 nM
MMP-2 K$_i$ = 8.5 nM
MMP-3 K$_i$ = 31 nM
MMP-7 K$_i$ = 12 nM
MMP-9 K$_i$ = 3.9 nM
MMP-14 K$_i$ = 6 nM

(7.117)
MMP-1 IC$_{50}$ = 640 nM
MMP-2 IC$_{50}$ = 170 nM
MMP-3 IC$_{50}$ = 20,000 nM
MMP-7 IC$_{50}$ = 4,100 nM
MMP-8 IC$_{50}$ = 48 nM
MMP-9 IC$_{50}$ = 150 nM

FIGURE 7.7   A set of effective MMP-7 inhibitors (compounds **7.114–7.119**).

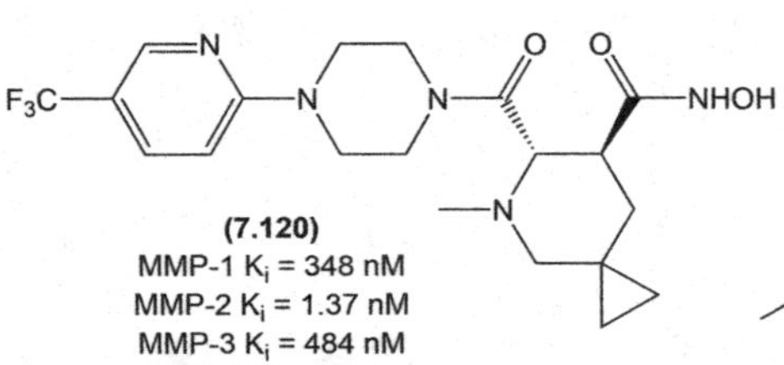

FIGURE 7.8 Another set of potential MMP-7 inhibitors (compounds 7.120–7.124).

(7.120)
MMP-1 K_i = 348 nM
MMP-2 K_i = 1.37 nM
MMP-3 K_i = 484 nM
MMP-7 K_i = 75 nM
MMP-8 K_i = 3.01 nM
MMP-9 K_i = 10.4 nM
MMP-12 K_i = 29.5 nM
MMP-14 K_i = 67.6 nM

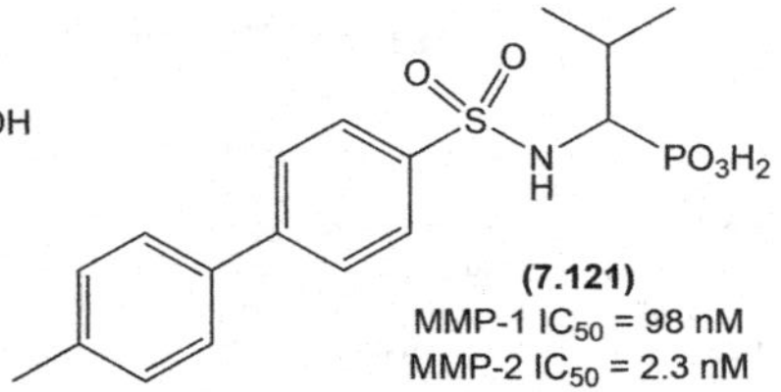

(7.121)
MMP-1 IC_{50} = 98 nM
MMP-2 IC_{50} = 2.3 nM
MMP-3 IC_{50} = 45 nM
MMP-7 IC_{50} = 150 nM
MMP-8 IC_{50} = 0.39 nM
MMP-9 IC_{50} = 4.1 nM
MMP-13 IC_{50} = 3.3 nM
MMP-14 IC_{50} = 11 nM

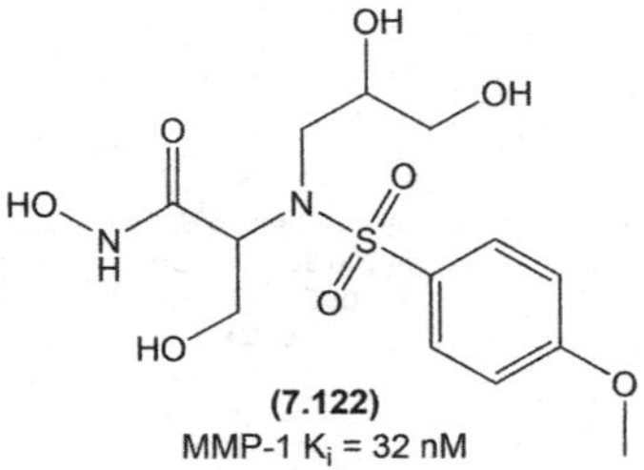

(7.122)
MMP-1 K_i = 32 nM
MMP-7 K_i = 344 nM
MMP-8 K_i = 8 nM
MMP-12 K_i = 7 nM
MMP-13 K_i = 1.7 nM

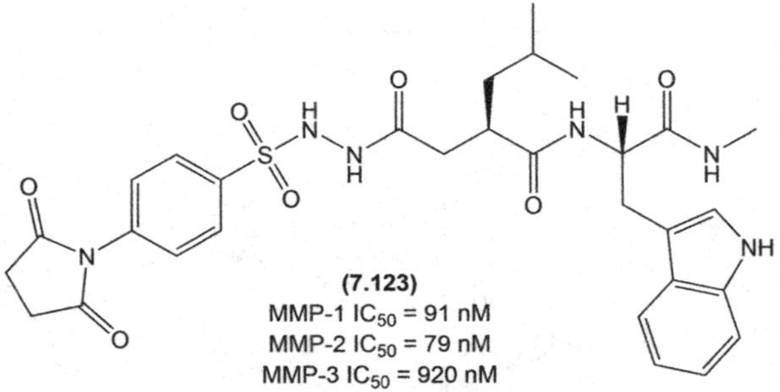

(7.123)
MMP-1 IC_{50} = 91 nM
MMP-2 IC_{50} = 79 nM
MMP-3 IC_{50} = 920 nM
MMP-7 IC_{50} = 110 nM
MMP-9 IC_{50} = 8.5 nM
MMP-14 IC_{50} = 720 nM

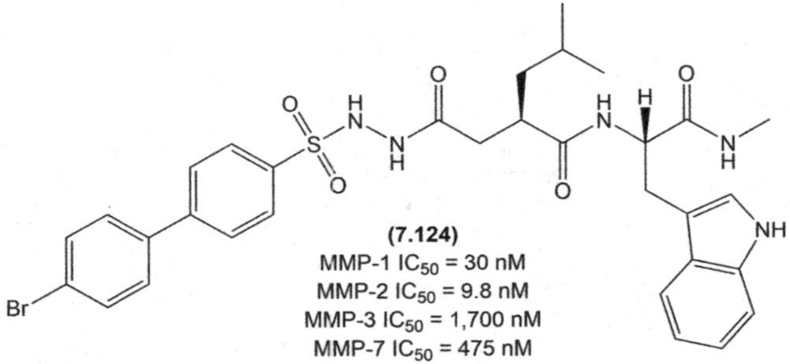

(7.124)
MMP-1 IC_{50} = 30 nM
MMP-2 IC_{50} = 9.8 nM
MMP-3 IC_{50} = 1,700 nM
MMP-7 IC_{50} = 475 nM
MMP-9 IC_{50} = 3 nM
MMP-14 IC_{50} = 17,000 nM

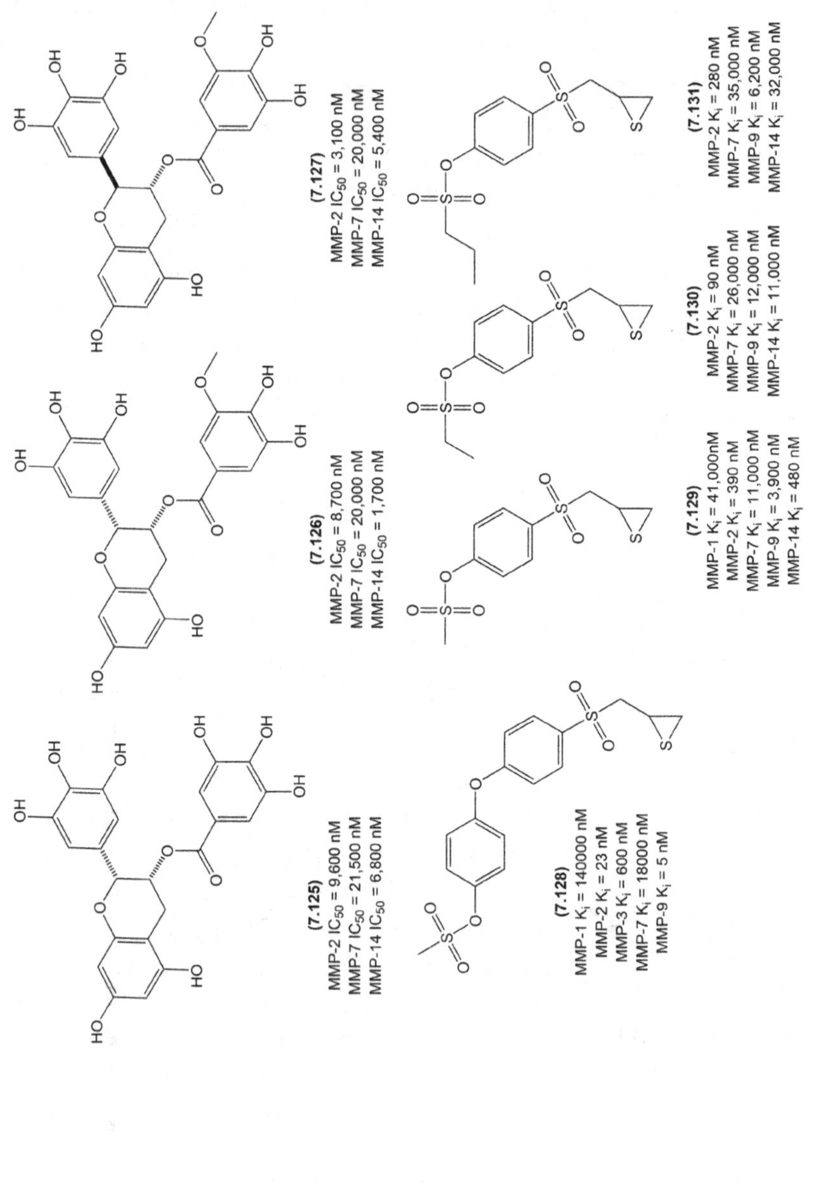

(7.125)

MMP-2 IC$_{50}$ = 9,600 nM
MMP-7 IC$_{50}$ = 21,500 nM
MMP-14 IC$_{50}$ = 6,800 nM

(7.126)

MMP-2 IC$_{50}$ = 8,700 nM
MMP-7 IC$_{50}$ = 20,000 nM
MMP-14 IC$_{50}$ = 1,700 nM

(7.127)

MMP-2 IC$_{50}$ = 3,100 nM
MMP-7 IC$_{50}$ = 20,000 nM
MMP-14 IC$_{50}$ = 5,400 nM

(7.128)

MMP-1 K$_i$ = 140000 nM
MMP-2 K$_i$ = 23 nM
MMP-3 K$_i$ = 600 nM
MMP-7 K$_i$ = 18000 nM
MMP-9 K$_i$ = 5 nM

(7.129)

MMP-1 K$_i$ = 41,000nM
MMP-2 K$_i$ = 390 nM
MMP-7 K$_i$ = 11,000 nM
MMP-9 K$_i$ = 3,900 nM
MMP-14 K$_i$ = 480 nM

(7.130)

MMP-2 K$_i$ = 90 nM
MMP-7 K$_i$ = 26,000 nM
MMP-9 K$_i$ = 12,000 nM
MMP-14 K$_i$ = 11,000 nM

(7.131)

MMP-2 K$_i$ = 280 nM
MMP-7 K$_i$ = 35,000 nM
MMP-9 K$_i$ = 6,200 nM
MMP-14 K$_i$ = 32,000 nM

FIGURE 7.9　Some other effective MMP-7 inhibitors (compounds **7.125–7.131**).

REFERENCES

[1]. Adhikari N, Mukherjee A, Saha A, et al. Arylsulfonamides and selectivity of matrix metalloproteinase-2: An overview. *Eur J Med Chem*. 2017;129:72–109.

[2]. Baidya SK, Banerjee S, Adhikari N, et al. Selective inhibitors of medium-size S1' pocket matrix metalloproteinases: A stepping stone of future drug discovery. *J Med Chem*. 2022;65(16):10709–10754.

[3]. Nagase H, Visse R, Murphy G. Structure and function of matrix metalloproteinases and TIMPs. *Cardiovasc Res*. 2006;69(3):562–573.

[4]. Oneda H, Shiihara M, Inouye K. Inhibitory effects of green tea catechins on the activity of human matrix metalloproteinase 7 (matrilysin). *J Biochem*. 2003;133(5):571–576.

[5]. Browner MF, Smith WW, Castelhano AL. Matrilysin-inhibitor complexes: Common themes among metalloproteases. *Biochemistry*. 1995;34(20):6602–6610.

[6]. Masaki T, Matsuoka H, Sugiyama M, et al. Matrilysin (MMP-7) as a significant determinant of malignant potential of early invasive colorectal carcinomas. *Br J Cancer*. 2001;84(10):1317–1321.

[7]. Wang FQ, So J, Reierstad S, Fishman DA. Matrilysin (MMP-7) promotes invasion of ovarian cancer cells by activation of progelatinase. *Int J Cancer*. 2005;114(1):19–31.

[8]. Piskór BM, Przylipiak A, Dąbrowska E, et al. Plasma concentrations of matrilysins MMP-7 and MMP-26 as diagnostic biomarkers in breast cancer. *J Clin Med*. 2021;10(7):1436.

[9]. Li M, Yamamoto H, Adachi Y, et al. Role of matrix metalloproteinase-7 (matrilysin) in human cancer invasion, apoptosis, growth, and angiogenesis. *Exp Biol Med (Maywood)*. 2006;231(1):20–27.

[10]. Amălinei C, Căruntu ID, Bălan RA. Biology of metalloproteinases. *Rom J Morphol Embryol*. 2007;48(4):323–334.

[11]. Romanowicz L, Gogiel T, Galewska Z, et al. Divergent changes in the content and activity of MMP-26 and TIMP-4 in human umbilical cord tissues associated with preeclampsia. *Eur J Obstet Gynecol Reprod Biol*. 2018;231:48–53.

[12]. Cui N, Hu M, Khalil RA. Biochemical and biological attributes of matrix metalloproteinases. *Prog Mol Biol Transl Sci*. 2017;147:1–73.

[13]. Ripley D, Tunuguntla R, Susi L, et al. Expression of matrix metalloproteinase-26 and tissue inhibitors of metalloproteinase-3 and -4 in normal ovary and ovarian carcinoma. *Int J Gynecol Cancer*. 2006;16(5):1794–1800.

[14]. Chegini N, Rhoton-Vlasak A, Williams RS. Expression of matrix metalloproteinase-26 and tissue inhibitor of matrix metalloproteinase-3 and -4 in endometrium throughout the normal menstrual cycle and alteration in users of levonorgestrel implants who experience irregular uterine bleeding. *Fertil Steril*. 2003;80(3):564–570.

[15]. Marchenko GN, Ratnikov BI, Rozanov DV, et al. Characterization of matrix metalloproteinase-26, a novel metalloproteinase widely expressed in cancer cells of epithelial origin. *Biochem J*. 2001;356(Pt 3):705–718.

[16]. Uría JA, López-Otín C. Matrilysin-2, a new matrix metalloproteinase expressed in human tumors and showing the minimal domain organization required for secretion, latency, and activity. *Cancer Res*. 2000;60(17):4745–4751.

[17]. von Bredow DC, Cress AE, Howard EW, et al. Activation of gelatinase-tissue-inhibitors-of-metalloproteinase complexes by matrilysin. *Biochem J*. 1998;331(Pt 3):965–972.

[18]. Christensen J, Shastri VP. Matrix-metalloproteinase-9 is cleaved and activated by cathepsin K. *BMC Res Notes*. 2015;8:322.

[19]. Löffek S, Schilling O, Franzke CW. Series "matrix metalloproteinases in lung health and disease": Biological role of matrix metalloproteinases: A critical balance. *Eur Respir J*. 2011;38(1):191–208.

[20]. Sellers A, Woessner JF Jr. The extraction of a neutral metalloproteinase from the involuting rat uterus, and its action on cartilage proteoglycan. *Biochem J.* 1980;189(3):521–531.

[21]. Woessner JF Jr, Taplin CJ. Purification and properties of a small latent matrix metalloproteinase of the rat uterus. *J Biol Chem.* 1988;263(32):16918–16925.

[22]. Woessner JF Jr. Matrix metalloproteinases and their inhibitors in connective tissue remodeling. *FASEB J.* 1991;5(8):2145–2154.

[23]. Liao HY, Da CM, Liao B, et al. Roles of matrix metalloproteinase-7 (MMP-7) in cancer. *Clin Biochem.* 2021;92:9–18.

[24]. Aihara R, Mochiki E, Nakabayashi T, et al. Clinical significance of mucin phenotype, beta-catenin and matrix metalloproteinase 7 in early undifferentiated gastric carcinoma. *Br J Surg.* 2005;92(4):454–462.

[25]. Huachuan Z, Xiaohan L, Jinmin S, et al. Expression of matrix metalloproteinase-7 involving in growth, invasion, metastasis and angiogenesis of gastric cancer. *Chin Med Sci J.* 2003;18(2):80–86.

[26]. Yamamoto H, Iku S, Adachi Y, et al. Association of trypsin expression with tumour progression and matrilysin expression in human colorectal cancer. *J Pathol.* 2003;199(2):176–184.

[27]. Yamamoto H, Adachi Y, Itoh F, et al. Association of matrilysin expression with recurrence and poor prognosis in human esophageal squamous cell carcinoma. *Cancer Res.* 1999;59(14):3313–3316.

[28]. Yamamoto H, Itoh F, Adachi Y, et al. Relation of enhanced secretion of active matrix metalloproteinases with tumor spread in human hepatocellular carcinoma. *Gastroenterology.* 1997;112(4):1290–1296.

[29]. Yamamoto H, Itoh F, Iku S, et al. Expression of matrix metalloproteinases and tissue inhibitors of metalloproteinases in human pancreatic adenocarcinomas: Clinicopathologic and prognostic significance of matrilysin expression. *J Clin Oncol.* 2001;19(4):1118–1127.

[30]. Xu Z, Chen W, Chen C. Matrix metalloproteinase 7 is a candidate biomarker in systemic sclerosis-associated interstitial lung disease. Matrix metalloproteinase 7 is a candidate biomarker in systemic sclerosis-associated interstitial lung disease. *Acta Reumatol Port.* 2020;45(3):191–200.

[31]. Matson SM, Lee SJ, Peterson RA, et al. The prognostic role of matrix metalloproteinase-7 in scleroderma-associated interstitial lung disease. *Eur Respir J.* 2021;58(6):2101560.

[32]. Cosgrove GP, du Bois RM. Matrix metalloproteinase-7 expression in fibrosing lung disease: Restoring the balance. *Chest.* 2008;133(5):1058–1060.

[33]. Surendran K, Simon TC, Liapis H, et al. Matrilysin (MMP-7) expression in renal tubular damage: Association with Wnt4. *Kidney Int.* 2004;65(6):2212–2222.

[34]. Liu Z, Tan RJ, Liu Y. The many faces of matrix metalloproteinase-7 in kidney diseases. *Biomolecules.* 2020;10(6):960.

[35]. de Oliveira Nóbrega FJ, de Oliveira DHIP, Vasconcelos RG, et al. Study of the participation of MMP-7, EMMPRIN and cyclophilin A in the pathogenesis of periodontal disease. *Arch Oral Biol.* 2016;72:172–178.

[36]. Kuivanen T, Tanskanen M, Jahkola T, et al. Matrilysin-1 (MMP-7) and MMP-19 are expressed by Paget's cells in extramammary Paget's disease. *J Cutan Pathol.* 2004;31(7):483–491.

[37]. Jiang J, Wang J, Shen Z, et al. Serum MMP-7 in the diagnosis of biliary atresia. *Pediatrics.* 2019;144(5):e20190902.

[38]. Lwin ST, Fowler JA, Drake MT, et al. A loss of host-derived MMP-7 promotes myeloma growth and osteolytic bone disease in vivo. *Mol Cancer.* 2017;16(1):49.

[39]. Nilsson L, Jonasson L, Nijm J, et al. Increased plasma concentration of matrix metalloproteinase-7 in patients with coronary artery disease. *Clin Chem.* 2006;52(8):1522–1527.

[40]. Hsieh FI, Chiou HY, Hu CJ, et al. Combined effects of MMP-7, MMP-8 and MMP-26 on the risk of ischemic stroke. *J Clin Med.* 2019;8(11):2011.

[41]. Im NR, Kim B, Jung KY, et al. Usefulness of matrix metalloproteinase-7 in saliva as a diagnostic biomarker for laryngopharyngeal reflux disease. *Sci Rep.* 2021;11(1):17071.

[42]. Irvine KM, Okano S, Patel PJ, et al. Serum matrix metalloproteinase 7 (MMP-7) is a biomarker of fibrosis in patients with non-alcoholic fatty liver disease. *Sci Rep.* 2021;11(1):2858.

[43]. Fingleton BM, Heppner Goss KJ, Crawford HC, et al. Matrilysin in early stage intestinal tumorigenesis. *APMIS.* 1999;107(1):102–110.

[44]. Klupp F, Neumann L, Kahlert C, et al. Serum MMP-7, MMP-10 and MMP-12 level as negative prognostic markers in colon cancer patients. *BMC Cancer.* 2016;16:494.

[45]. Sharma KL, Misra S, Kumar A, et al. Higher risk of matrix metalloproteinase (MMP-2, 7, 9) and tissue inhibitor of metalloproteinase (TIMP-2) genetic variants to gallbladder cancer. *Liver Int.* 2012;32(8):1278–1286.

[46]. Szarvas T, Jäger T, Becker M, et al. Validation of circulating MMP-7 level as an independent prognostic marker of poor survival in urinary bladder cancer. *Pathol Oncol Res.* 2011;17(2):325–332.

[47]. Tanimoto H, Underwood LJ, Shigemasa K, et al. The matrix metalloprotease pump-1 (MMP-7, Matrilysin): A candidate marker/target for ovarian cancer detection and treatment. *Tumour Biol.* 1999;20(2):88–98.

[48]. Beeghly-Fadiel A, Long JR, Gao YT, et al. Common MMP-7 polymorphisms and breast cancer susceptibility: A multistage study of association and functionality. *Cancer Res.* 2008;68(15):6453–6459.

[49]. Bauer Y, White ES, de Bernard S, et al. MMP-7 is a predictive biomarker of disease progression in patients with idiopathic pulmonary fibrosis. *ERJ Open Res.* 2017;3(1):00074-2016.

[50]. Liu Z, Tan RJ, Liu Y. The many faces of matrix metalloproteinase-7 in kidney diseases. *Biomolecules.* 2020;10(6):960.

[51]. Xue CB, Voss ME, Nelson DJ, et al. Design, synthesis, and structure-activity relationships of macrocyclic hydroxamic acids that inhibit tumor necrosis factor alpha release in vitro and in vivo. *J Med Chem.* 2001;44(16):2636–2660.

[52]. Xue CB, He X, Corbett RL, et al. Discovery of macrocyclic hydroxamic acids containing biphenylmethyl derivatives at P1', a series of selective TNF-alpha converting enzyme inhibitors with potent cellular activity in the inhibition of TNF-alpha release. *J Med Chem.* 2001;44(21):3351–3354.

[53]. Castelhano AL, Billedeau R, Dewdney N, et al. Novel indolactam-based inhibitors of matrix metalloproteinases. *Bioorg Med Chem Lett.* 1995;5(13):1415–1420.

[54]. Vassiliou S, Mucha A, Cuniasse P, et al. Phosphinic pseudo-tripeptides as potent inhibitors of matrix metalloproteinases: A structure-activity study. *J Med Chem.* 1999;42(14):2610–2620.

[55]. Ott GR, Asakawa N, Lu Z, et al. Alpha,beta-cyclic-beta-benzamido hydroxamic acids: Novel templates for the design, synthesis, and evaluation of selective inhibitors of TNF-alpha converting enzyme (TACE). *Bioorg Med Chem Lett.* 2008;18(2):694–699.

[56]. Chen XT, Ghavimi B, Corbett RL, et al. A new 4-(2-methylquinolin-4-ylmethyl)phenyl P1' group for the beta-amino hydroxamic acid derived TACE inhibitors. *Bioorg Med Chem Lett.* 2007;17(7):1865–1870.

[57]. Gilmore JL, King BW, Asakawa N, et al. Synthesis and structure-activity relationship of a novel, non-hydroxamate series of TNF-alpha converting enzyme inhibitors. *Bioorg Med Chem Lett.* 2007;17(16):4678–4682.

[58]. Ott GR, Asakawa N, Lu Z, et al. Potent, exceptionally selective, orally bioavailable inhibitors of TNF-alpha converting enzyme (TACE): Novel 2-substituted-1H-benzo[d]imidazol-1-yl)methyl)benzamide P1' substituents. *Bioorg Med Chem Lett.* 2008;18(5):1577–1582.

[59]. Lu Z, Ott GR, Anand R, et al. Potent, selective, orally bioavailable inhibitors of tumor necrosis factor-alpha converting enzyme (TACE): Discovery of indole, benzofuran, imidazopyridine and pyrazolopyridine P1' substituents. *Bioorg Med Chem Lett.* 2008;18(6):1958–1962.

[60]. Szardenings AK, Harris D, Lam S, et al. Rational design and combinatorial evaluation of enzyme inhibitor scaffolds: Identification of novel inhibitors of matrix metalloproteinases. *J Med Chem.* 1998;41(13):2194–2200.

[61]. Almstead NG, Bradley RS, Pikul S, et al. Design, synthesis, and biological evaluation of potent thiazine- and thiazepine-based matrix metalloproteinase inhibitors. *J Med Chem.* 1999;42(22):4547–4562.

[62]. Pikul S, McDow Dunham KL, Almstead NG, et al. Discovery of potent, achiral matrix metalloproteinase inhibitors. *J Med Chem.* 1998;41(19):3568–3571.

[63]. Cheng M, De B, Almstead NG, et al. Design, synthesis, and biological evaluation of matrix metalloproteinase inhibitors derived from a modified proline scaffold. *J Med Chem.* 1999;42(26):5426–5436.

[64]. Natchus MG, Bookland RG, De B, et al. Development of new hydroxamate matrix metalloproteinase inhibitors derived from functionalized 4-aminoprolines. *J Med Chem.* 2000;43(26):4948–4963.

[65]. Pikul S, Dunham KM, Almstead NG, et al. Heterocycle-based MMP inhibitors with P2' substituents. *Bioorg Med Chem Lett.* 2001;11(8):1009–1013.

[66]. Tullis JS, Laufersweiler MJ, VanRens JC, et al. The development of new carboxylic acid-based MMP inhibitors derived from a cyclohexylglycine scaffold. *Bioorg Med Chem Lett.* 2001;11(15):1975–1979.

[67]. Pikul S, Ohler NE, Ciszewski G, et al. Potent and selective carboxylic acid-based inhibitors of matrix metalloproteinases. *J Med Chem.* 2001;44(16):2499–2502.

[68]. Cheng M, De B, Pikul S, et al. Design and synthesis of piperazine-based matrix metalloproteinase inhibitors. *J Med Chem.* 2000;43(3):369–380.

[69]. Apfel C, Banner DW, Bur D, et al. Hydroxamic acid derivatives as potent peptide deformylase inhibitors and antibacterial agents. *J Med Chem.* 2000;43(12):2324–2331.

[70]. Mazzola RD Jr, Zhu Z, Sinning L, et al. Discovery of novel hydroxamates as highly potent tumor necrosis factor-alpha converting enzyme inhibitors. Part II: Optimization of the S3' pocket. *Bioorg Med Chem Lett.* 2008;18(21):5809–5814.

[71]. Steinman DH, Curtin ML, Garland RB, et al. The design, synthesis, and structure-activity relationships of a series of macrocyclic MMP inhibitors. *Bioorg Med Chem Lett.* 1998;8(16):2087–2092.

[72]. Sheppard GS, Florjancic AS, Giesler JR, et al. Aryl ketones as novel replacements for the C-terminal amide bond of succinyl hydroxamate MMP inhibitors. *Bioorg Med Chem Lett.* 1998;8(22):3251–3256.

[73]. O'Brien PM, Ortwine DF, Pavlovsky AG, et al. Structure-activity relationships and pharmacokinetic analysis for a series of potent, systemically available biphenylsulfonamide matrix metalloproteinase inhibitors. *J Med Chem.* 2000;43(2):156–166.

[74]. Li J, Rush TS 3rd, Li W, et al. Synthesis and SAR of highly selective MMP-13 inhibitors. *Bioorg Med Chem Lett.* 2005;15(22):4961–4966.

[75]. Barta TE, Becker DP, Bedell LJ, et al. MMP-13 selective α-sulfone hydroxamates: A survey of P1' heterocyclic amide isosteres. *Bioorg Med Chem Lett.* 2011;21(10):2820–2822.

[76]. Nara H, Sato K, Kaieda A, et al. Design, synthesis, and biological activity of novel, potent, and highly selective fused pyrimidine-2-carboxamide-4-one-based matrix metalloproteinase (MMP)-13 zinc-binding inhibitors. *Bioorg Med Chem.* 2016;24(23):6149–6165.

[77]. Miller A, Askew M, Beckett RP, et al. Inhibition of matrix metalloproteinases: An examination of the S1' pocket. *Bioorg Med Chem Lett.* 1997;7(2):193–198.

[78]. Chen JJ, Zhang Y, Hammond S, et al. Design, synthesis, activity, and structure of a novel class of matrix metalloproteinase inhibitors containing a heterocyclic P2′-P3′ amide bond isostere, *Bioorg Med Chem Lett*.1996;6(13):1601–1606.

[79]. Ma D, Wu W, Yang G, et al. Tetrahydroisoquinoline based sulfonamide hydroxamates as potent matrix metalloproteinase inhibitors. *Bioorg Med Chem Lett*. 2004;14(1):47–50.

[80]. Subramaniam R, Haldar MK, Tobwala S, et al. Novel bis-(arylsulfonamide) hydroxamate-based selective MMP inhibitors. *Bioorg Med Chem Lett*. 2008;18(11):3333–3337.

[81]. Jin Y, Roycik MD, Bosco DB, et al. Matrix metalloproteinase inhibitors based on the 3-mercaptopyrrolidine core. *J Med Chem*. 2013;56(11):4357–4373.

[82]. Campestre C, Tortorella P, Agamennone M, et al. Peptidyl 3-substituted 1-hydroxyureas as isosteric analogues of succinylhydroxamate MMP inhibitors. *Eur J Med Chem*. 2008;43(5):1008–1014.

[83]. Gona K, Toczek J, Ye Y, et al. Hydroxamate-based selective macrophage elastase (MMP-12) inhibitors and radiotracers for molecular imaging. *J Med Chem*. 2020;63(23):15037–15049.

[84]. Mahasenan KV, Ding D, Gao M, et al. In search of selectivity in inhibition of ADAM10. *ACS Med Chem Lett*. 2018;9(7):708–713.

[85]. Biasone A, Tortorella P, Campestre C, et al. Alpha-biphenylsulfonylamino 2-methylpropyl phosphonates: Enantioselective synthesis and selective inhibition of MMPs. *Bioorg Med Chem*. 2007;15(2):791–799.

[86]. Attolino E, Calderone V, Dragoni E, et al. Structure-based approach to nanomolar, water soluble matrix metalloproteinases inhibitors (MMPIs). *Eur J Med Chem*. 2010;45(12):5919–5925.

[87]. Ledour G, Moroy G, Rouffet M, et al. Introduction of the 4-(4-bromophenyl)benzenesulfonyl group to hydrazide analogs of Ilomastat leads to potent gelatinase B (MMP-9) inhibitors with improved selectivity. *Bioorg Med Chem*. 2008;16(18):8745–8759.

[88]. Aihara Y, Yoshida A, Furuta T, et al. Regioselective synthesis of methylated epigallocatechin gallate via nitrobenzenesulfonyl (Ns) protecting group. *Bioorg Med Chem Lett*. 2009;19(15):4171–4174.

[89]. Testero SA, Lee M, Staran RT, et al. Sulfonate-containing thiiranes as selective gelatinase inhibitors. *ACS Med Chem Lett*. 2010;2(2):177–181.

8 Membrane-Type MMPs and Their Inhibitors

*Suvankar Banerjee, Sandip Kumar Baidya,
Nilanjan Adhikari, and Tarun Jha*

CONTENTS

ABSTRACT

Membrane-type matrix metalloproteinases (MT-MMPs) affect several diseases, including cancer, cardiovascular diseases, and neurodegenerative diseases. These MMPs are expressed on the cell membrane. Instead of MT-MMPs, researchers are primarily working to develop alternative MMP inhibitors, such as collagenase and gelatinase inhibitors. As a result, there is much scope for developing MMP-14 inhibitors. Potential MMP-14 inhibitors can be designed using ligand- and structure-based molecular modeling techniques and X-ray crystallographic data. In this chapter, although not a lot of information is available on other membrane-type MMPs, the majority of molecules having potential roles of MMP-14 and their inhibitors will be discussed.

Keywords: Membrane-type MMP; Cancer; Cardiovascular disease; Neurodegenerative disorder; Arylsulfonamide; Hydroxamates

8.1 INTRODUCTION

Matrix metalloproteinases (MMPs) belong to zinc-dependent endopeptidases that take part in prime roles during the normal and pathological remodeling of the extracellular matrix (ECM), and they promote diverse biological events [1–3]. Among these MMPs, membrane type-matrix metalloproteinases (MT-MMPs) are a unique

DOI: 10.1201/9781003303282-10

class of MMPs associated with the cell membrane through a transmembrane domain or a glycosylphosphatidylinositol (GPI) anchor [3, 4]. After the first MT-MMP, i.e., MT1-MMP (also called MMP-14), was discovered, MT2-MMP (also called MMP-15), MT3-MMP (also called MMP-16), and MT4-MMP (also called MMP-17) were discovered in a short period, and later, MT5-MMP (MMP-24) and MT6-MMP (MMP-26) were further discovered. Among these MT-MMPs, MT1-MMP was identified first, and it plays a crucial role in cellular invasion and migration in tumors [3, 5, 6]. MT1-MMP is found to hydrolyze the ECM and subsequently trigger the activation of proMMP-2 effectively [3, 7, 8]. Finally, the activated MMP-2 is found to break the basement membrane type IV collagen [9, 10]. As MMP-14 is localized at the cancer cells, having to invade characters with effective proteolytic efficacy, it can be considered a potential target for inhibition [11]. MMP-14 is bound to the cell membrane with the help of the type 1 transmembrane region and is expressed in an active form on the cell surface by the activity of furin-like serine proteinases [2, 12]. Moreover, MMP-14 consists of a pro-peptide domain, a catalytic domain linker, and a hemopexin domain [2, 13]. The hemopexin domain may exert its function by the protein substrate recognition that is crucial for the breakdown of type I collagen [2, 14–16]. The hemopexin domain plays crucial roles in the modulation of enzyme and cellular localization [2, 17, 18]. Nevertheless, the linker region between the hemopexin and catalytic domains helps tether the collagen [2, 19].

8.2 STRUCTURAL ASPECTS OF MT-MMPs

The structure of MT-MMPs is quite similar to that of the other isoforms of the matrix metalloenzyme family, containing an N-terminal signal peptide sequence, a pro-peptide domain, a conserved catalytic domain with one structural and one catalytic Zn^{2+}, and two Ca^{2+} ions. Similarly, a hemopexin domain is also followed by the conserved catalytic domain, whereas the presence of a fibronectin domain followed by a cytoplasmic tail at the C-terminal end of these MT-MMP isoforms is unique to the rest of the MMP subclasses (Figure 8.1A) [20]. Additionally, unlike the other classes of MMPs, the MT-MMPs are the only isoform that contains a hydrophobic phenylalanine residue among its Ω-loop amino acids [21, 22]. The crystal structure of MT1-MMP (PDB ID: 1BQQ) and MT3-MMP (PDB ID: 1RM8) with the active sites, along with their superimposed structures, are given in Figure 8.1B, C, and D, respectively [21, 22].

8.3 MMP-14 PATHOPHYSIOLOGY IN DISEASE CONDITIONS

Among these MT-MMPs, MT1-MMP (MMP-14) plays major roles in diverse pathophysiological and disease conditions, including cancer, cardiovascular disease, and neurodegenerative diseases [23].

8.3.1 CANCER

The hemopexin domain of MMP-14 is found to modulate the molecular crosstalk that is found to initiate and trigger cancer cell migration and metastatic events [24].

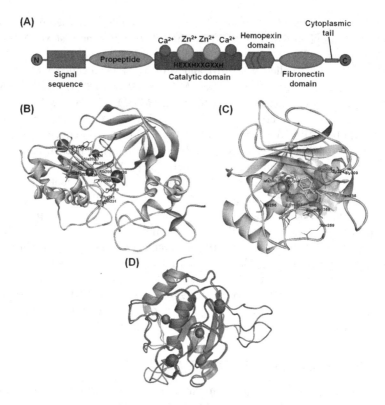

FIGURE 8.1 (A) General cartoon representation of membrane-type MMPs; ligand-bound crystal structure of (B) MT1-MMP (PDB ID: 1BQQ); (C) MT3-MMP (PDB ID: 1RM8); (D) superimposed structure of collagenases (MT1-MMP: gray, MT3-MMP: dark gray).

Nevertheless, it has also been found that MMP-14 is regulated by a novel mechanism through the involvement of interleukin-6 (IL-6) and p53, which is related to the tumor microenvironment and stimulation of molecular changes in cancer cells [25]. MMP-14 degrades the ECM for cell migration, shedding cell surface molecules for migratory signals, and activating extracellular signal-regulated protein kinase (ERK) for enhancing cell migration, as well as angiogenesis and invasion [26, 27]. MMP-14 is a crucial enzyme responsible for breaching basement membranes by cancer cells and invasion mediated by interstitial type I collagen tissues. MMP-14 is found to be accumulated in invadopodia, which are specialized ECM-degrading membrane protrusions of invasive cells [28]. MMP-14 has been found to take part crucial roles in the progression of several cancers, including ovarian cancer [29, 30], esophageal cancer [31], gastric cancer [32], breast cancer [33, 34], non-small cell lung cancer [35], digestive system carcinoma [36], urinary bladder carcinoma [37], nasopharyngeal carcinoma [38], glioma [39], prostate cancer [40], pancreatic cancer [41], laryngeal squamous cell carcinoma [42], synovial sarcoma [43], colorectal cancer [44], epithelial skin cancers [45], and melanoma [46]. Therefore, considering the crucial roles of MMP-14 in several cancers, it can be targeted to design effective and MMP-14-selective inhibitors for managing several cancers.

8.3.2 Cardiovascular Disease

It was noted that the MMP-14/MMP-2 ratio may modulate the degree of Pro-MMP-2 activation as a key regulator in the development of an aortic aneurysm [47]. MMP-14 has been found to cleave mature elastin of the skin to produce various bioactive peptides and, subsequently, may take part in the development of cardiovascular diseases [48]. MMP-14 expression is highly associated with the angiogenic efficacy of vascular endothelial growth factor (VEGF) and MMP-9 in the mechanisms of proliferative diabetic retinopathy (PDR) [49]. It was found that estrogenic loss or gain may alter MMP-13 and MMP-14 profiles and take part in crucial roles in postmenopausal hypertension [50]. MMP-14 is expressed in atherosclerotic plaques and plays a crucial role in the development of vulnerable carotid plaques. Nevertheless, MMP-14 gene polymorphisms may have an influence on the bioactivity or expression of MMP-14 [51]. MMP-14 from bone marrow-derived cells can trigger collagen accumulation in the formation of atherosclerotic plaques [52]. Again, deep venous thrombosis (DVT) is highly correlated with the enhanced transcriptional activity of MMP-2 and MMP-14 [53]. MMP-14 is found to be correlated with alterations in left ventricular mass (LVM) and body weight (BW) in chronic phases of hypertension [54]. The expression levels of C-reactive protein (CRP), MMP-14, and tissue inhibitor of MMP-2 (TIMP-2) have been established as inflammatory markers for the progression of periodontal inflammation related to type 2 diabetes mellitus [55]. Moreover, the MMP-14 level is found to be higher in the case of diabetic retinopathy [56].

8.3.3 Neurodegenerative Disorders

Apart from other MMPs, MMP-14 has been found to play crucial roles in neuroinflammation and cerebral ischemia [57]. In the case of familial amyloidotic polyneuropathy (FAP), MMP-14 is found to be highly expressed in FAP nerves, upregulated in sciatic nerves, and with an increased rate in the plasma of FAP patients, correlating with disease progression [58]. Nevertheless, it helps to shed cell surface neuronal-glial antigen 2 (NG2) proteoglycan on macrophages and, subsequently, it regulates peripheral nerve injury [59]. Macrophage MMP-14 expression is upregulated in other major neuroinflammatory and neurodegenerative diseases, namely Alzheimer's disease, multiple sclerosis, human amyotrophic lateral sclerosis (ALS), and acute brain trauma [60].

8.3.4 Other Diseases

In addition, MMP-14 has been found to have a good correlation with eye-related diseases. MMP-14 has a direct relation with Fuchs endothelial corneal dystrophy [61]. Moreover, enhanced expression of MMP-14 has been noticed in glaucoma patients [62]. Along with MMP-13, MMP-14 has been found in the peritoneal fluid of women with endometriosis [63]. Along with MMP-2, MMP-14 has been found to play a crucial role in Dupuytren's disease fibroblast-mediated contraction [64]. Fibroblast-derived MMP-14 is also found to control collagen homeostasis in adult skin [65]. MMP-14 also modulates collagen degradation and the migration of mononuclear cells during genotype VII Newcastle disease virus [66]. MMP-14 expression also has a good relationship with sepsis [67].

8.4 INHIBITORS OF MMP-14

Considering the roles of MMP-14 in such types of diverse disease conditions, potential and selective MMP-14 inhibitors can be designed to combat these diseases.

Yamamoto and co-workers from the New Drug Discovery Research Laboratory of Kanebo Ltd. [68] reported some hydroxamate-based MT1-MMP inhibitors. All these molecules (compounds **8.1–8.11**, Table 8.1), although nonselective, were found to be potent MT1-MMP inhibitors.

Xue and co-workers from DuPont Pharmaceuticals Company [69] reported some macrocyclic hydroxamic acids as effective tumor necrosis factor-α

TABLE 8.1

Hydroxamate-Based Analogs as Promising MMP-14 Inhibitors (IC$_{50}$ in nM)

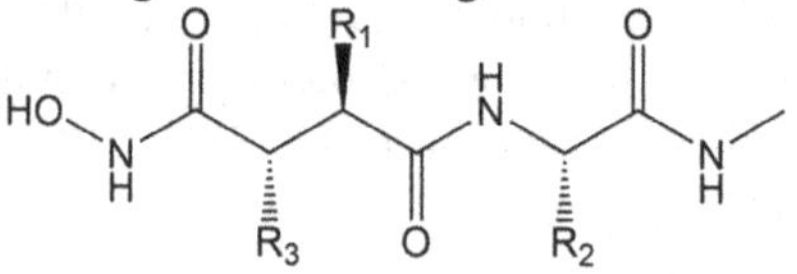

Cpd	R$_1$	R$_2$	R$_3$	MMP-1	MMP-2	MMP-3	MMP-9	MMP-14
8.1	i-But	Ph	H	15	42.5	4.4	14	19.3
8.2	-(CH$_2$)$_2$Ph	Ph	H	92	46.3	17	11	105
8.3	-(CH$_2$)$_3$Ph	Ph	H	89	3.2	9.6	3.3	8.5
8.4	-(CH$_2$)$_8$CH$_3$	Ph	H	90	1.6	100	0.2	17.6
8.5	i-But	c-Hex	H	5.4	8.4	2.3	5	2.3
8.6	i-But	Ph	CH$_3$	3	7.5	1.9	3.9	59
8.7	i-But	Ph	(4-morpholino)CH$_2$	3.5	-	61	45	72
8.8	i-But	(5,6,7,8-tetrahydro-1-napthyl)methyl	CH$_3$	03	0.3	0.3	0.3	2.08
8.9	-(CH$_2$)$_3$Ph	-C(CH$_3$)$_3$	H	21	-	-	1.3	1.9
8.10	-(CH$_2$)$_3$Ph	-CH(CH$_3$)$_2$	H	93	-	-	2.8	2.5
8.11	i-But	-C$_6$H$_{11}$	CH$_3$	2.9	-	-	0.9	13

Cpd, compound.

converting enzyme (TACE) inhibitors. Among these molecules, compound **8.12** (Figure 8.2) was the most effective MMP-14 inhibitor (K_i = 94 nM). It exhibited a good pharmacokinetic profile in beagle dogs.

Aranapakam and co-workers from Wyeth Research [70] reported a series of N-substituted 4-arylsulfonylpiperidine-4-hydroxamic acid derivatives as orally active MMPIs. Compound **8.13** (Figure 8.2) was the most effective MMP-14 inhibitor (IC_{50} = 1 nM) among these molecules. Compound **8.13** at a 25 mg/kg dose resulted in good oral bioavailability in rats (55%) and dogs (47%) with a good $T_{1/2}$ of 10.7 hr and 17.6 hr, respectively. Wu et al. from Wyeth Research [71] reported some selective MMP-13 inhibitors. Compound **8.14** (Figure 8.2) was the most effective MMP-14 inhibitor (IC_{50} = 1.5 nM) among these molecules. Park et al. from Wyeth Research [72] reported some butynyloxyphenyl β-sulfone piperidine hydroxamates as TACE inhibitors. Among these molecules, compound **8.15** (Figure 8.2) was the most promising MMP-14 inhibitor (IC_{50} = 12 nM), although it was nonselective. Condon and co-workers from Wyeth Research [73] reported some selective TACE inhibitors. Compound **8.16** (Figure 8.2) was the most promising MMP-14 inhibitor (IC_{50} = 583 nM) among these molecules. Further study by Lombart et al. from Wyeth Research [74] led to the identification of a set of 3,3-piperidine hydroxamate-based TACE inhibitors. Among these molecules, compound **8.17** (Figure 8.2) was the most effective MMP-14 inhibitor (IC_{50} = 1,020 nM). Huang and co-workers from Wyeth Research [75] reported some selective TACE inhibitors through structure-based drug design. Compound **8.18** (Figure 8.3) was the most effective MMP-14 inhibitor (IC_{50} = 1,000 nM) among these molecules.

Park and co-workers from Wyeth Research [76] reported some tryptophan sulfonamide derivatives as potent TACE inhibitors. Compound **8.19** (Figure 8.3) was the most efficacious MMP-14 inhibitor (IC_{50} = 6.82 μM) among these molecules. Hopper et al. from Wyeth Research [77] reported a series of ((4-keto)-phenoxy)methyl biphenyl-4-sulfonamides as aggrecanase inhibitors. Among these molecules, compound **8.20** (Figure 8.3) was the most effective MMP-14 inhibitor (IC_{50} = 220 nM).

Fray et al. from Pfizer Global Research and Development [78] reported some potent MMP-3 inhibitors. Among these molecules, compound **8.21** (Figure 8.3) was the most effective MMP-14 inhibitor (IC_{50} = 930 nM). Reiter and co-workers from Pfizer Global Research and Development [79] reported some pyran-containing sulfonamide hydroxamic acids as MMP-1-sparing potent MMPIs. Among these molecules, compound **8.22** (Figure 8.3) was the most effective MMP-14 inhibitor (IC_{50} = 7.4 nM). Further study by the scientists of Pfizer Global Research and Development [80] led to the development of 3-hydroxy-4-arylsulfonyltetrahydropyranyl-3-hydroxamic acids as potent inhibitors of TACE and aggrecanases. Among these molecules, compound **8.23** (Figure 8.3) was the most effective MMP-14 inhibitor (IC_{50} = 150 nM). Blagg and co-workers from Pfizer Global Research and Development [81] further reported some pyrimidinetrione-based MMP-13 inhibitors selective over MMP-14. Although these molecules were highly MMP-13-selective inhibitors, many of these compounds (compounds **8.24–8.33**, Table 8.2) exerted potent MMP-14 inhibitory efficacy.

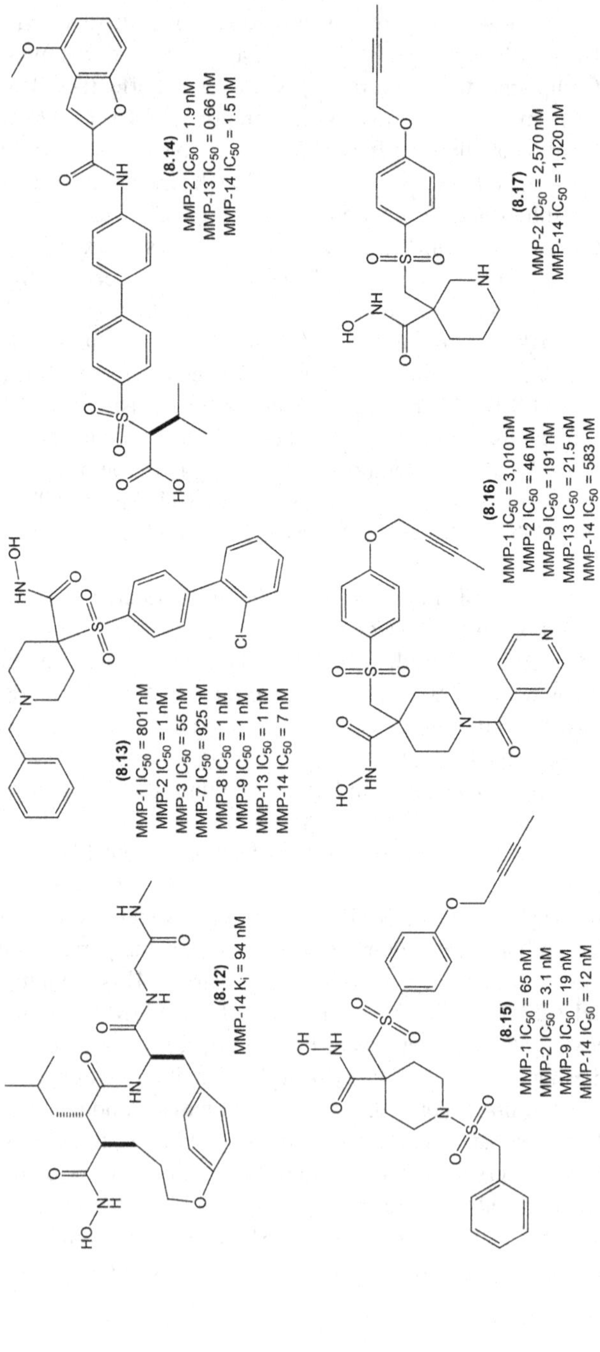

FIGURE 8.2 Some potential MMP-14 inhibitors (compounds **8.12–8.17**).

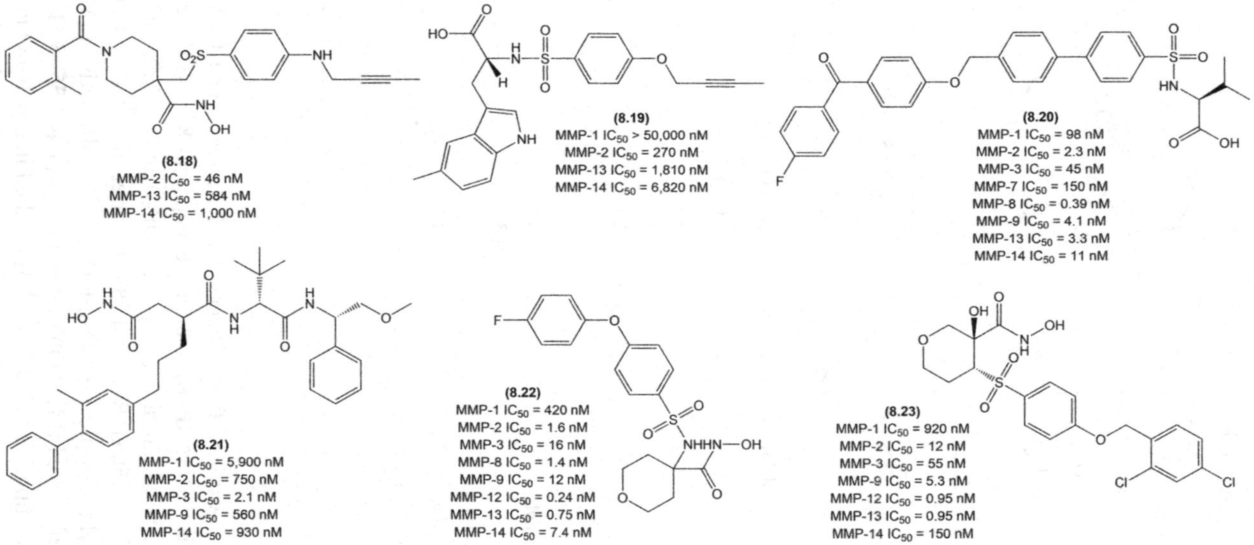

(8.18)

MMP-2 IC_{50} = 46 nM
MMP-13 IC_{50} = 584 nM
MMP-14 IC_{50} = 1,000 nM

(8.19)

MMP-1 IC_{50} > 50,000 nM
MMP-2 IC_{50} = 270 nM
MMP-13 IC_{50} = 1,810 nM
MMP-14 IC_{50} = 6,820 nM

(8.20)

MMP-1 IC_{50} = 98 nM
MMP-2 IC_{50} = 2.3 nM
MMP-3 IC_{50} = 45 nM
MMP-7 IC_{50} = 150 nM
MMP-8 IC_{50} = 0.39 nM
MMP-9 IC_{50} = 4.1 nM
MMP-13 IC_{50} = 3.3 nM
MMP-14 IC_{50} = 11 nM

(8.21)

MMP-1 IC_{50} = 5,900 nM
MMP-2 IC_{50} = 750 nM
MMP-3 IC_{50} = 2.1 nM
MMP-9 IC_{50} = 560 nM
MMP-14 IC_{50} = 930 nM

(8.22)

MMP-1 IC_{50} = 420 nM
MMP-2 IC_{50} = 1.6 nM
MMP-3 IC_{50} = 16 nM
MMP-8 IC_{50} = 1.4 nM
MMP-9 IC_{50} = 12 nM
MMP-12 IC_{50} = 0.24 nM
MMP-13 IC_{50} = 0.75 nM
MMP-14 IC_{50} = 7.4 nM

(8.23)

MMP-1 IC_{50} = 920 nM
MMP-2 IC_{50} = 12 nM
MMP-3 IC_{50} = 55 nM
MMP-9 IC_{50} = 5.3 nM
MMP-12 IC_{50} = 0.95 nM
MMP-13 IC_{50} = 0.95 nM
MMP-14 IC_{50} = 150 nM

FIGURE 8.3 Various effective MMP-14 inhibitors (compounds **8.18–8.23**).

TABLE 8.2

A Series of Pyrimidinetrione-Based Analogs as Potential MMPIs (IC_{50} in nM)

(8.24, 8.26-8.33)   (8.25)

Cpd	R	MMP-13	MMP-14
8.24	F	0.87	23
8.25	-	3.1	16
8.26	Cl	1.4	18
8.27	CH_3	2.1	23
8.28	Br	0.87	19
8.29	5-Oxazolyl	0.54	3.0
8.30	Pyrrolyl	3.1	22
8.31	Imidazolyl	0.95	18
8.32	5-Pyrazolyl	4.1	27
8.33	4-Pyrazolyl	0.61	11

Cpd, compound.

Whitlock and co-workers from Pfizer Global Research and Development [82] reported some selective MMP-3 inhibitors. Compound **8.34** (Figure 8.4) was the most promising MMP-14 inhibitor (IC_{50} = 1,710 nM) among these molecules.

Becker et al. from Pfizer Research [83] reported a series of MMP-1 sparing α-tetrahydropyranyl and α-piperidinyl sulfone-based orally active MMPIs. Many of them were highly effective MMP-14 inhibitors (compounds **8.35–8.61**, Table 8.3). At a 20 mg/kg dose, compound **8.53** (Table 8.3) resulted in excellent bioavailability in female mice (80%), female rats (82.2%), male dogs (64%), and female dogs (69.2%).

Thompson and co-workers from Bristol-Myers Squibb Pharmaceutical Research Institute [84] reported a set of succinyl-caprolactam γ-secretase inhibitors.

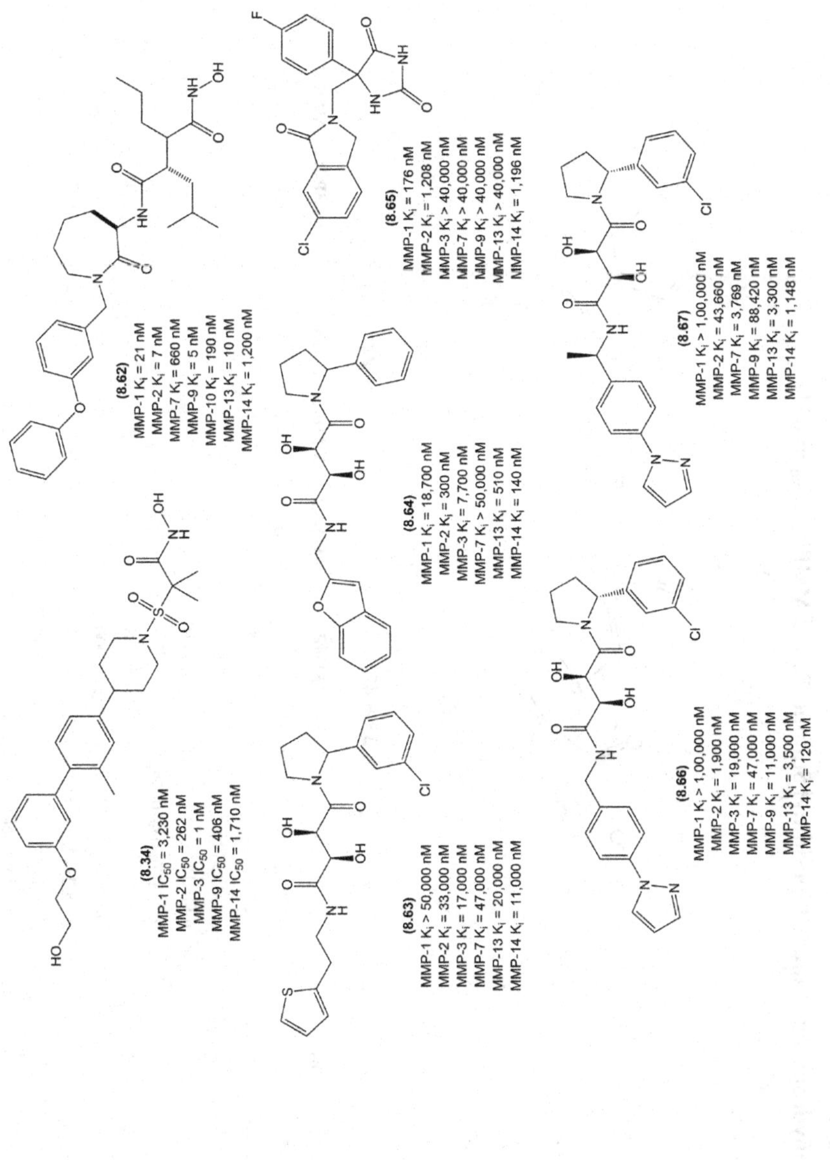

(8.34)
MMP-1 IC$_{50}$ = 3,230 nM
MMP-2 IC$_{50}$ = 262 nM
MMP-3 IC$_{50}$ = 1 nM
MMP-9 IC$_{50}$ = 406 nM
MMP-14 IC$_{50}$ = 1,710 nM

(8.62)
MMP-1 K$_i$ = 21 nM
MMP-2 K$_i$ = 7 nM
MMP-7 K$_i$ = 660 nM
MMP-9 K$_i$ = 5 nM
MMP-10 K$_i$ = 190 nM
MMP-13 K$_i$ = 10 nM
MMP-14 K$_i$ = 1,200 nM

(8.63)
MMP-1 K$_i$ > 50,000 nM
MMP-2 K$_i$ = 33,000 nM
MMP-3 K$_i$ = 17,000 nM
MMP-7 K$_i$ = 47,000 nM
MMP-13 K$_i$ = 20,000 nM
MMP-14 K$_i$ = 11,000 nM

(8.64)
MMP-1 K$_i$ = 18,700 nM
MMP-2 K$_i$ = 300 nM
MMP-3 K$_i$ = 7,700 nM
MMP-7 K$_i$ > 50,000 nM
MMP-13 K$_i$ = 510 nM
MMP-14 K$_i$ = 140 nM

(8.65)
MMP-1 K$_i$ = 176 nM
MMP-2 K$_i$ = 1,208 nM
MMP-3 K$_i$ > 40,000 nM
MMP-7 K$_i$ > 40,000 nM
MMP-9 K$_i$ > 40,000 nM
MMP-13 K$_i$ > 40,000 nM
MMP-14 K$_i$ = 1,196 nM

(8.66)
MMP-1 K$_i$ > 1,00,000 nM
MMP-2 K$_i$ = 1,900 nM
MMP-3 K$_i$ = 19,000 nM
MMP-7 K$_i$ = 47,000 nM
MMP-9 K$_i$ = 11,000 nM
MMP-13 K$_i$ = 3,500 nM
MMP-14 K$_i$ = 120 nM

(8.67)
MMP-1 K$_i$ > 1,00,000 nM
MMP-2 K$_i$ = 43,660 nM
MMP-7 K$_i$ = 3,769 nM
MMP-9 K$_i$ = 88,420 nM
MMP-13 K$_i$ = 3,300 nM
MMP-14 K$_i$ = 1,148 nM

FIGURE 8.4 A set of potential MMP-14 inhibitors (compounds **8.34, 8.62–8.67**).

TABLE 8.3

α-Tetrahydropyranyl and α-Piperidinyl Sulfone-Based MMPIs (IC$_{50}$ in nM)

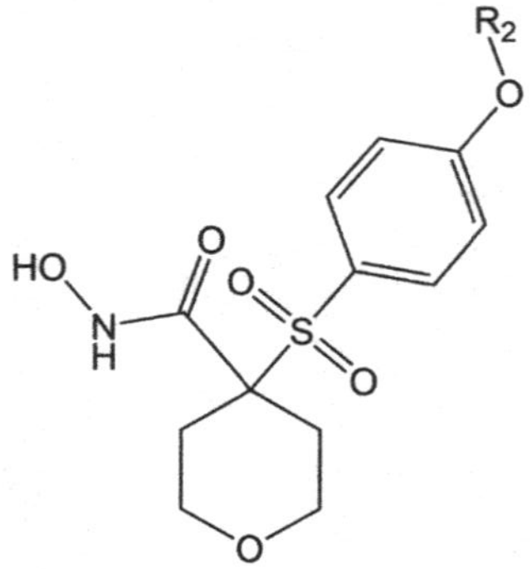

Cpd		R$_1$	R$_2$	MMP-1	MMP-2	MMP-3	MMP-7	MMP-8	MMP-9	MMP-13	MMP-14
				(8.35–8.43)					(8.44–8.61)		
8.35	–		m-ClPh	1,800	0.3	18.1	–	0.4	2.9	0.45	4.5
8.36	–		p-ClPh	435	<0.1	18.1	–	1.2	0.3	0.15	5.6
8.37	–		3,4-diClPh	3,600	0.35	35	–	4.0	5.4	0.8	47
8.38	–		p-OHPh	400	0.2	–	–	-	<0.1	0.3	1.71
8.39	–		p-isopropoxy phenyl	300	<0.1	-	–	-	<0.1	0.1	10.5
8.40	–		p-PhPh	1,400	0.1	50	–	2.4	1.7	0.25	20
8.41	–		m-CF$_3$Ph	>10,000	0.8	55.3	–	30	42.5	0.8	24
8.42	–		p-OCF$_3$Ph	1,140	<0.1	35	–	0.9	0.2	<0.1	10.6
8.43	–		p-SCH$_3$Ph	2,500	<0.1	-	–	-	<0.1	<0.1	3.63
8.44	–		2-pyridylmethyl	4,500	0.2	20.6	–	1.9	0.1	0.3	3.1

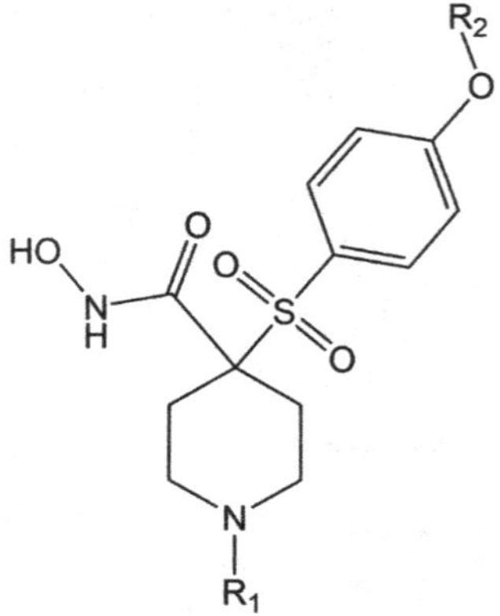

(Continued)

TABLE 8.3 (CONTINUED)
α-Tetrahydropyranyl and α-Piperidinyl Sulfone-Based MMPIs (IC$_{50}$ in nM)

Cpd	R$_1$	R$_2$	MMP-1	MMP-2	MMP-3	MMP-7	MMP-8	MMP-9	MMP-13	MMP-14
8.45	cyclopropyl	p-OEtPh	1,000	0.1	-	-	-	0.2	0.25	6.8
8.46	methoxyethyl	p-isopropoxy phenyl	2,000	0.3	-	-	-	-	0.5	25.8
8.47	cyclopropyl	p-isopropoxy phenyl	770	0.1	-	-	-	0.21	0.1	13.3
8.48	prppargyl	methylenedioxyphenyl-methyl	2,000	0.2	18.1	-	1.3	0.3	0.6	14.9
8.49	methoxyethyl	methylenedioxyphenyl-methyl	2400	0.25	20	-	1.2	0.27	0.2	4.0
8.50	cyclopropyl	cyclopropyl	1,000	0.5	-	-	-	<0.1	0.3	0.73

(Continued)

TABLE 8.3 (CONTINUED)
α-Tetrahydropyranyl and α-Piperidinyl Sulfone-Based MMPIs (IC$_{50}$ in nM)

Cpd	R$_1$	R$_2$	MMP-1	MMP-2	MMP-3	MMP-7	MMP-8	MMP-9	MMP-13	MMP-14
8.51	(cyclopropyl)	(benzodioxole)	6,000	0.2	21.5	-	1.5	1.9	0.5	49.4
8.52	N-morpholinyl-ethyl	p-CF$_3$Ph	>10,000	0.3	-	-	-	0.1	0.35	7.4
8.53	methoxyethyl	p-OCF$_3$Ph	>10,000	<0.1	28.7	7,000	1.7	0.18	<0.1	13
8.54		p-OCF$_3$Ph	4,000	<0.1	22	7,000	1.2	0.15	0.1	4.6
8.55	2-pyridylmethyl	p-OCF$_3$Ph	6,000	0.2	115	>10,000	0.6	0.2	<0.1	4.1
8.56	3-pyridylmethyl	p-OCF$_3$Ph	4,600	<0.1	42.5	>10,000	1.5	0.6	0.2	3.7
8.57	ethoxyethyl	p-OCF$_3$Ph	5,900	<0.1	-	-	-	0.1	<0.1	9.5
8.58	Acetyl	p-OCF$_3$Ph	3,600	0.1	18.1	-	1.6	0.1	0.2	9.0
8.59	Propargyl	p-OCF$_3$Ph	2,600	<0.1	-	-	-	<0.1	0.2	1.33
8.60	Methyl	p-OCF$_3$Ph	>10,000	<0.1	-	-	-	0.18	0.6	24.9
8.61	isopropyl	p-OCF$_3$Ph	>10,000	<0.1	-	-	0.4	<0.1	<0.1	7.1

Cpd, compound.

Compound **8.62** (Figure 8.4) was the most effective MMP-14 inhibitor (K_i = 1,200 nM) in this series. Rosner and co-workers from Schering-Plough Research Institute [85] reported some tartrate-based TACE inhibitors. Among these molecules, compounds **8.63** and **8.64** (Figure 8.4) displayed the most promising MMP-14 inhibitory efficacy (K_i = 11 nM and 0.14 nM, respectively). Yu and co-workers from Merck Research Laboratories [86] reported a series of hydantoin-based TACE inhibitors. Compound **8.65** (Figure 8.4) was the most promising MMP-14 inhibitor (Ki = 1,196 nM) among these molecules. A further study conducted by Merck scientists [87] led to the development of some tartrate-based TACE inhibitors. Among these molecules, compound **8.66** (Figure 8.4) was the most effective MMP-14 inhibitor (K_i = 120 nM). At a dose of 10 mg/kg, compound **8.66** also exhibited 20% bioavailability in rats. Again, some 2-(2-aminothiazol-4-yl)pyrrolidine-containing tartrate diamides were reported as potent, orally bioavailable, and selective TACE inhibitors by Dai et al. [88] of Merck Research Laboratories. Among these molecules, compound **8.67** (Figure 8.4) was the most effective MMP-14 inhibitor (K_i = 1,148 nM).

De Savi and co-workers of AstraZeneca [89] reported some N-hydroxyformamide-based aggrecanase 1 inhibitors. Several molecules exhibited potent MMP-14 inhibitory efficacy (compounds **8.68–8.70**, Figure 8.5).

Further study by the same group of researchers [90] reported some hydantoin-based MMP-13 inhibitors. Among these molecules, compound **8.71** (Figure 8.5) was the most effective MMP-14 inhibitor (IC_{50} = 62 nM).

Nara and co-workers from Takeda Pharmaceutical Company [91] reported a series of thieno[2,3-d]pyrimidine-2-carboxamides as highly potent, orally active, and MMP-13-selective inhibitors. Compound **8.72** (Figure 8.5) among these molecules was the most effective MMP-14 inhibitor (IC_{50} = 1.1 nM). Nara et al. [92] further reported some potent and highly selective fused pyrimidine-2-carboxamide-4-one-containing MMP-13 inhibitors. Among these molecules, compounds **8.73** and **8.74** (Figure 8.5) were the most effective MMP-14 inhibitors (IC_{50} of 3.8 nM and 5.4 nM, respectively).

Durham and co-workers from Eli Lilly and Company [93] reported some hydantoin-based aggrecanase inhibitors. Among these molecules, compound **8.75** (Figure 8.6) was the most effective MMP-14 inhibitor (IC_{50} = 150 nM).

Durham et al. from Eli Lilly and Company [94] reported some hydantoin-based potential aggrecanase inhibitors. Compound **8.76** (Figure 8.6) was the most effective MMP-14 inhibitor (IC_{50} = 150 nM). Boiteau et al. from Nestlé Skin Health R&D [95] reported some TACE inhibitors. Compounds **8.77** and **8.78** (Figure 8.6) were the most effective MMP-14 inhibitors in this series (IC_{50} = 6.5 μM and 4.4 μM, respectively).

Schro¨der et al. [96] reported some 6H-1,3,4-thiadiazine-based potent MMPIs. Two molecules (compounds **8.79–8.80**, Figure 8.6) resulted in potential MMP-14 inhibitors (Ki of 100 nM and 50 nM, respectively). Krumme and Tschesche [97] reported some oxal hydroxamic acid derivatives as effective MMPIs. Among them, compound **8.81** (Figure 8.7) was the most efficacious MMP-14 inhibitor (IC_{50} = 1.4 μM).

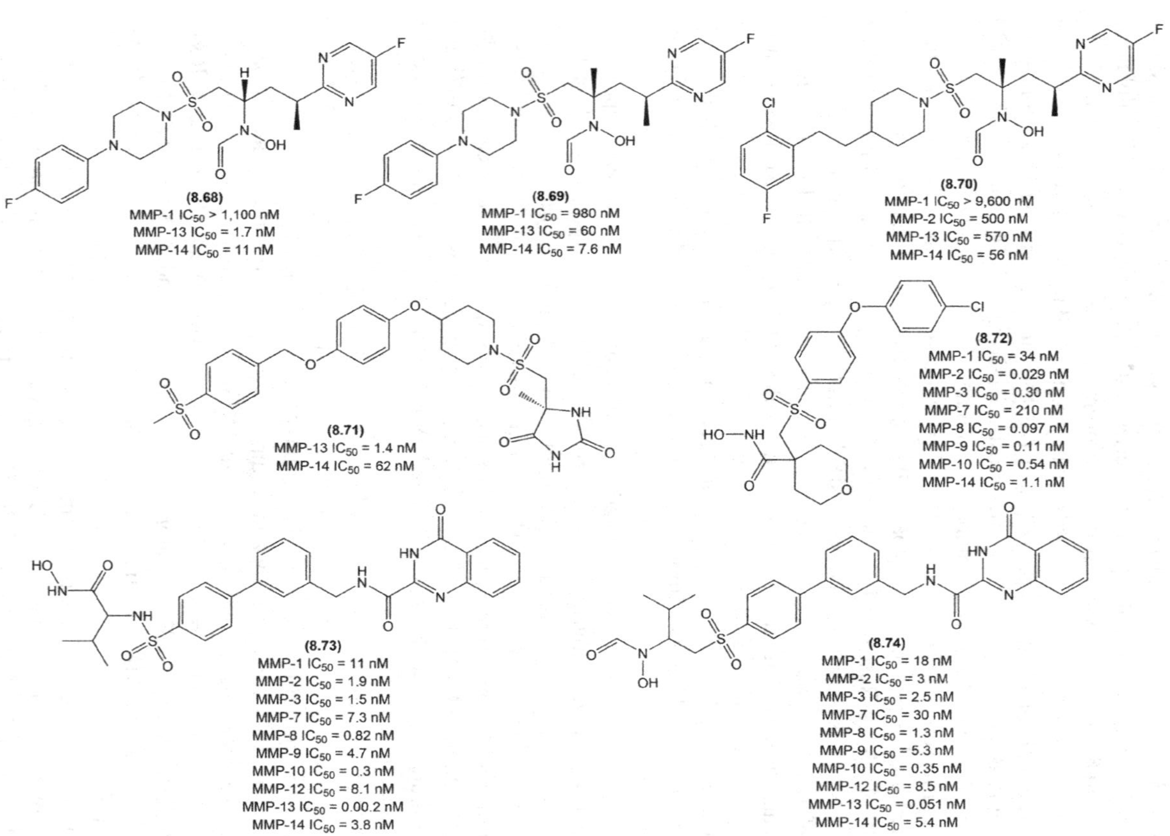

FIGURE 8.5 Another set of potential MMP-14 inhibitors (compounds **8.68**–**8.74**).

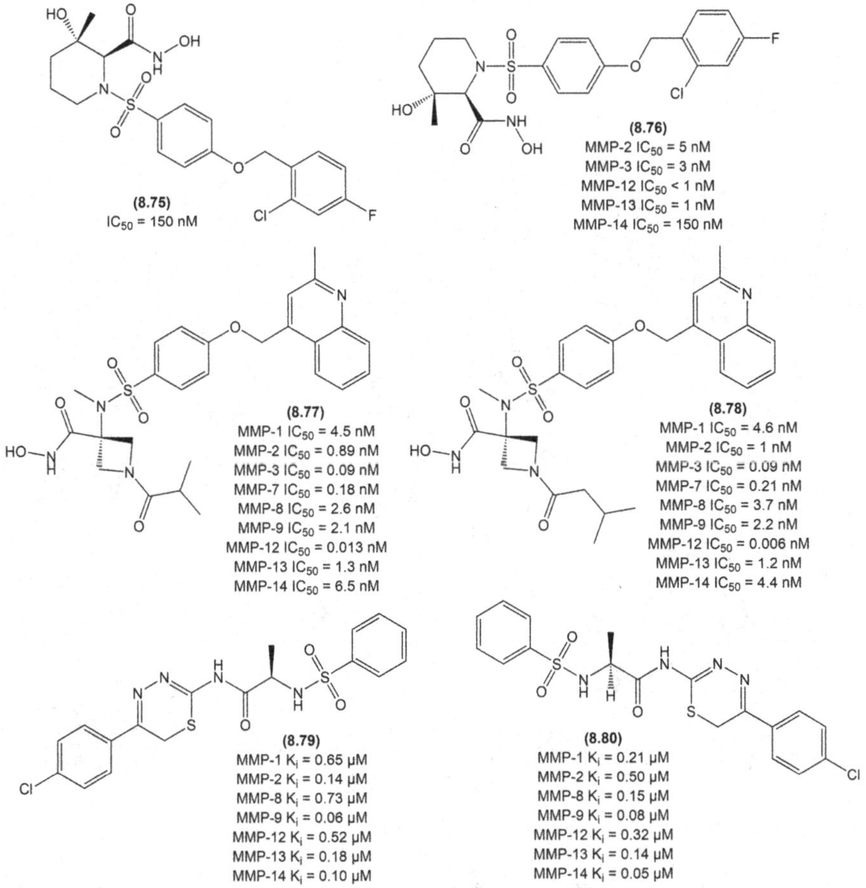

FIGURE 8.6 Different effective MMP-14 inhibitors (compounds **8.75–8.80**).

Ma et al. [98] reported some tetrahydroisoquinoline-based sulfonamide hydroxamates as potential MMPIs. Although all these molecules were nonselective MMPIs, most of these molecules exhibited promising inhibitory activity against MMP-14, MMP-15, and MMP-16 (compounds **8.82–8.90**, Table 8.4).

Biasone et al. [99] designed some α-biphenylsulfonylamino 2-methylpropyl phosphonates as potential MMPIs. Compounds **8.91** and **8.92** (Figure 8.7) were the most promising MMP-14 inhibitors among these molecules. Tauro et al. [100] reported some arylamino methylene bisphosphonate derivatives as bone-seeking MMPIs. Among these molecules, compound **8.93** (Figure 8.7) was nonselective but the most promising MMP-14 inhibitor (IC$_{50}$ = 3,900 nM). Moroy and co-workers [101] reported some ilomastat analogs as potential MMPIs. Compound **8.94** (Figure 8.7) was the most effective MMP-14 inhibitor (IC$_{50}$ = 10 nM) among these molecules.

LeDour et al. [102] reported some hydrazide analogs of ilomastat as potential MMPIs. Compounds **8.95** and **8.96** (Figure 8.7) were the most promising MMP-14

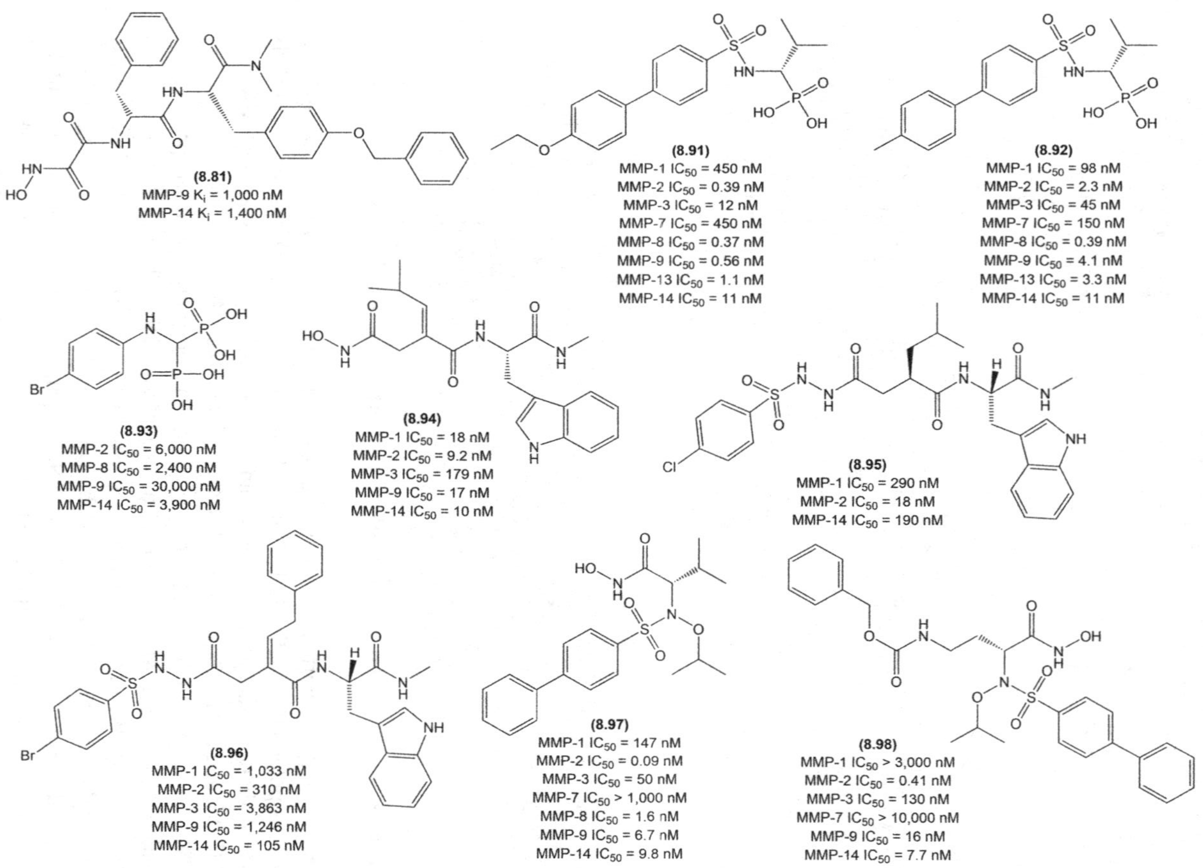

FIGURE 8.7 Another set of potential MMP-14 inhibitors (compounds **8.81, 8.91–8.98**).

TABLE 8.4
Tetrahydroisoquinoline-Based Sulfonamide Hydroxamates Analogs as Promising MMPIs (IC$_{50}$ in μM)

Cpd	R	R$_1$	Y	MMP-1	MMP-2	MMP-7	MMP-9	MMP-12	MMP-14	MMP-15	MMP-16	MMP-26
8.82	H	H	H	6.319	0.430	N.A.	0.335	0.421	1.102	0.218	0.184	0.858
8.83	H	H	4'-Me	0.0152	0.018	10.50	0.040	0.029	0.052	0.019	0.021	0.097
8.84	H	H	4'-NH$_2$	13.19	0.150	N.A.	0.248	0.191	0.835	0.385	0.202	0.492
8.85	H	H	4'-NO$_2$	0.041	0.076	21.42	0.258	0.059	0.521	0.126	0.177	0.791
8.86	H	Bn	H	0.452	0.024	7.136	0.035	0.057	0.039	0.017	0.035	1.453
8.87	H	Bn	4'-Me	0.462	0.033	12.04	0.130	0.072	0.062	0.044	0.056	2.046
8.88	H	Bn	4'-OMe	0.088	0.016	2.424	0.03	0.057	0.034	0.004	0.022	0.744
8.89	OMe	H	H	0.595	0.027	10.69	0.10	0.065	0.867	0.029	0.040	0.146
8.90	OMe	H	4'-OMe	0.123	0.026	3.192	0.046	0.020	0.068	0.006	0.016	0.086

Cpd, compound.

inhibitors in this series (IC$_{50}$ of 190 nM and 105 nM, respectively). Rossello and co-workers [103] reported some N-i-propoxy-N-biphenylsulfonylaminobutylhydroxam ic acid compounds as potential MMP-2 and MMP-14 inhibitors. Compounds **8.97** and **8.98** (Figure 8.7) resulted in excellent MMP-14 inhibitory efficacy (IC$_{50}$ of 9.8 nM and 7.7 nM, respectively). Both these compounds inhibited the chemoinvasion of HUVEC cells, suggesting these are potent antiangiogenic agents. At a 10 µM dose, compound **8.98** yielded 35% dead cells in the trypan blue test conducted on HT1080 cells [104]. Marques and co-workers [105] reported a set of iminodiacetyl-containing hydroxamate-benzenesulfonamide conjugates as dual inhibitors of carbonic anhydrase and MMPs. However, several molecules (compounds **8.99–8.104**, Table 8.5) displayed potential MMP-14 and MMP-16 inhibitory activity.

Nuti et al. [106] disclosed some N-O-isopropyl sulfonamido-containing hydroxamates as potential MMP-13 inhibitors. Many of these molecules (compounds **8.105–8.108**, Figure 8.8) were found to exert potential MMP-14 inhibitory efficacy.

Nuti et al. [107] developed further some arylsulfones as promising MMP-12 inhibitors. Several molecules (compounds **8.109–8.113**, Table 8.6) were found as potent MMP-14 inhibitors. Also, compound **8.110** (Table 8.6) exhibited potent MMP-16 inhibitory activity.

Again, Nuti et al. [108] disclosed some arylsulfonamide-based TACE inhibitors. Several compounds (compounds **8.114–8.126**, Table 8.7) were reported as effective MMP-14 inhibitors.

Nuti et al. [109] reported a set of (ethynylthiophene) sulfonamido-based hydroxamates as potential MMPIs. Among these molecules, compound **8.127** (Figure 8.8) was the most promising MMP-14 inhibitor (IC$_{50}$ = 112 nM). Marques et al. [110] reported some 1-hydroxypiperazine-2,6-diones as promising MMPIs. Compound **8.128** (Figure 8.8) was the most effective MMP-14 inhibitor in this series (IC$_{50}$ = 83 nM), which was also potent against MMP-16 (IC$_{50}$ = 39 nM). Nuti et al. [111] further proposed some arylsulfonamide-based aggrecanase inhibitors. Several molecules (compounds **8.129–8.133**, Table 8.8) were found to be highly potent MMP-14 inhibitors.

Nuti and co-workers [112] further produced several arylsulfonamides as potential ADAM-17 inhibitors. However, some of these molecules exhibited potent MMP-14 inhibitory activity (compounds **8.134–8.136**, Figure 8.9).

Nuti et al. [113] produced some N-O-isopropyl sulfonamido-based hydroxamates as potential MMPIs. Some compounds were found to be highly effective MMP-14 inhibitors (compounds **8.137–8.144**, Table 8.9).

Nuti et al. [114] further reported some bifunctional potential MMPIs. Among these compounds, compound **8.145** (Figure 8.9) was the most effective MMP-14 inhibitor (IC$_{50}$ = 23 nM). Nuti et al. [115] further reported some thioaryl-based potent MMP-12 inhibitors. However, compound **8.146** (Figure 8.9) was the most effective MMP-14 inhibitor (IC$_{50}$ = 710 nM) among these molecules.

Cuffaro and co-workers [116] reported some bifunctional MT1-MMP inhibitors. Compounds **8.147** and **8.148** (Figure 8.10) were potent MT1-MMP inhibitors in this series. Compound **8.147** decreased MT1-MMP-dependent proMMP-2 activation, collagen degradation, and collagen invasion in a dose-dependent manner. At a

TABLE 8.5

A Series of Iminodiacetyl-Based Hydroxamate-Benzenesulfonamide Analogs as Promising MMPIs (IC$_{50}$ in nM)

$$SPE = \text{---CH}_2\text{CH}_2\text{---Ph---SO}_2\text{NH}_2$$

Cpd	R	R$_1$	R$_2$	MMP-1	MMP-2	MMP-8	MMP-9	MMP-13	MMP-14	MMP-16
8.99	i-Pr	-SO$_2$PhOCH$_3$	OH	235	145	29.2	62.0	-	353	-
8.100	i-Pr	-SO$_2$PhPh	OH	236	24.7	4.3	27.7	-	306	-
8.101	i-Pr	-SO$_2$PhOPh	OH	59	0.50	0.40	0.77	0.33	3.9	1.56
8.102	H	-SO$_2$PhOPh	NH-SPE	532	25.3	59.0	53.7	-	89.8	44.0
8.103	H	-SO$_2$PhOPh	NH-SPE	143	1.57	0.74	0.51	-	2.1	1.00
8.104	H	-SO$_2$PhOPh	OH	1,530	1.2	3.7	3.2	1.6	14	11.4

Cpd, compound.

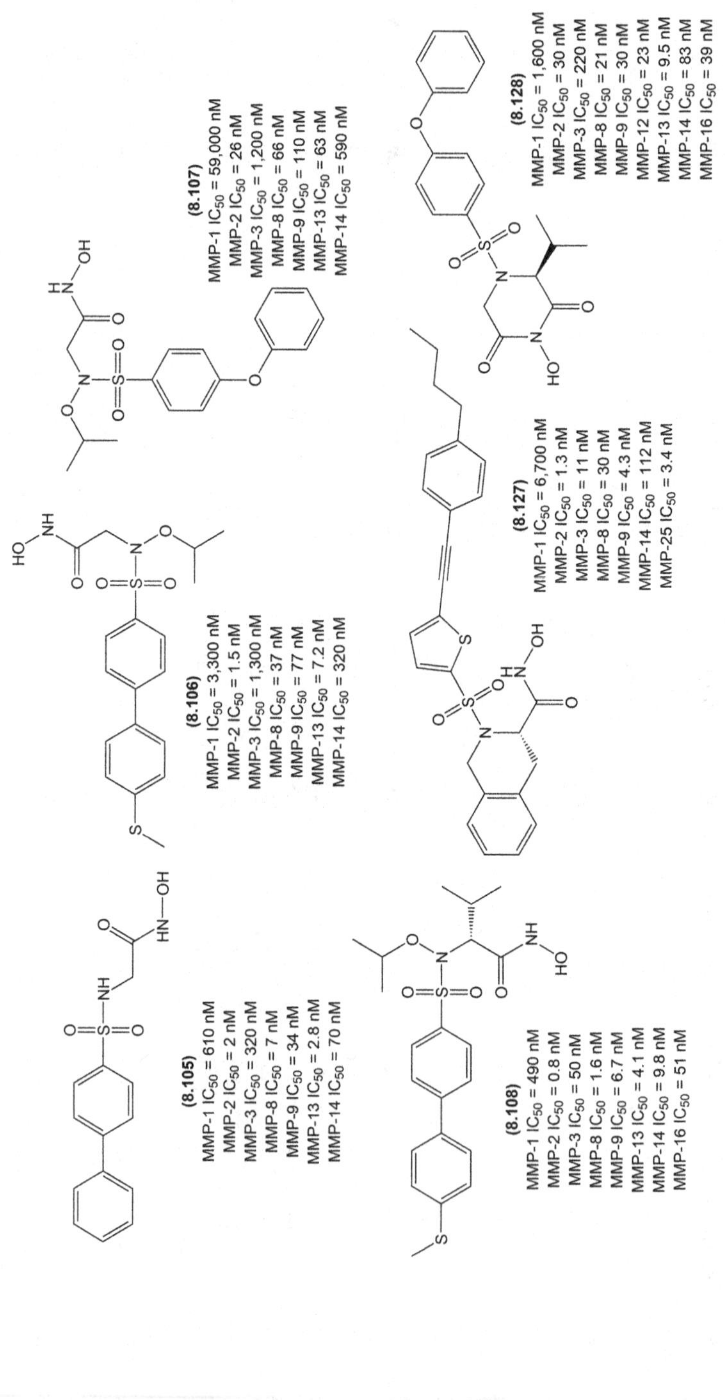

(8.107)
MMP-1 IC$_{50}$ = 59,000 nM
MMP-2 IC$_{50}$ = 26 nM
MMP-3 IC$_{50}$ = 1,200 nM
MMP-8 IC$_{50}$ = 66 nM
MMP-9 IC$_{50}$ = 110 nM
MMP-13 IC$_{50}$ = 63 nM
MMP-14 IC$_{50}$ = 590 nM

(8.128)
MMP-1 IC$_{50}$ = 1,600 nM
MMP-2 IC$_{50}$ = 30 nM
MMP-3 IC$_{50}$ = 220 nM
MMP-8 IC$_{50}$ = 21 nM
MMP-9 IC$_{50}$ = 30 nM
MMP-12 IC$_{50}$ = 23 nM
MMP-13 IC$_{50}$ = 9.5 nM
MMP-14 IC$_{50}$ = 83 nM
MMP-16 IC$_{50}$ = 39 nM

(8.106)
MMP-1 IC$_{50}$ = 3,300 nM
MMP-2 IC$_{50}$ = 1.5 nM
MMP-3 IC$_{50}$ = 1,300 nM
MMP-8 IC$_{50}$ = 37 nM
MMP-9 IC$_{50}$ = 77 nM
MMP-13 IC$_{50}$ = 7.2 nM
MMP-14 IC$_{50}$ = 320 nM

(8.127)
MMP-1 IC$_{50}$ = 6,700 nM
MMP-2 IC$_{50}$ = 1.3 nM
MMP-3 IC$_{50}$ = 11 nM
MMP-8 IC$_{50}$ = 30 nM
MMP-9 IC$_{50}$ = 4.3 nM
MMP-14 IC$_{50}$ = 112 nM
MMP-25 IC$_{50}$ = 3.4 nM

(8.105)
MMP-1 IC$_{50}$ = 610 nM
MMP-2 IC$_{50}$ = 2 nM
MMP-3 IC$_{50}$ = 320 nM
MMP-8 IC$_{50}$ = 7 nM
MMP-9 IC$_{50}$ = 34 nM
MMP-13 IC$_{50}$ = 2.8 nM
MMP-14 IC$_{50}$ = 70 nM

(8.108)
MMP-1 IC$_{50}$ = 490 nM
MMP-2 IC$_{50}$ = 0.8 nM
MMP-3 IC$_{50}$ = 50 nM
MMP-8 IC$_{50}$ = 1.6 nM
MMP-9 IC$_{50}$ = 6.7 nM
MMP-13 IC$_{50}$ = 4.1 nM
MMP-14 IC$_{50}$ = 9.8 nM
MMP-16 IC$_{50}$ = 51 nM

FIGURE 8.8   Several other effective MMP-14 inhibitors (compound **8.105–8.108, 8.127–8.128**).

TABLE 8.6
A Series of Arylsulfones as Promising MMP-14 and MMP-16 Inhibitors (IC$_{50}$ in nM)

Cpd	Ar	R	X	MMP-1	MMP-2	MMP-3	MMP-8	MMP-9	MMP-12	MMP-13	MMP-14	MMP-16
8.109	p-OMePh	H	NHOH	4,100	230	730	280	98	32	84	200	130
8.110	p-OMePhOPh	H	NHOH	3,500	3.5	21	5.1	0.8	0.2	4.1	33	32
8.111	p-OMeBiPh	H	NHOH	8,300	9.7	1,600	120	94	4.8	25	710	130
8.112	p-OMeBiPh	CH$_3$	NHOH	>10,000	7	1,400	54	69	2.7	12	360	150
8.113	p-OMeBiPh	H	OH	4,400	47	7,500	99	730	140	78	740	730

Cpd, compound.

TABLE 8.7

A Series of Arylsulfonamide-Based MMP-14 Inhibitors (IC_{50} in nM)

Cpd	R	R_1	R_2	MMP-1	MMP-2	MMP-9	MMP-14
8.114	i-Bu	H	Ph	4,800	12	34	530
8.115	H	H	Ph	610	2.0	34	70
8.116	i-Bu	H	OMe	300	13	4.8	13
8.117	H	H	OMe	3,000	32	130	210
8.118	H	H	Br	270	40	290	360
8.119	O-iPr	i-Pr	OMe	1,100	190	170	240
8.120	i-Bu	i-Pr	OMe	56	29	7.2	16
8.121	H	$(CH_2)_2NHCOCH_3$	Ph	196	0.70	8.6	34
8.122	H	$(CH_2)_2NHCOCH_3$	Br	1,500	190	190	300
8.123	H	$(CH_2)_2Pht$	Br	4.0	1.5	1.1	0.9
8.124	H	$(CH_2)_2NHCbz$	OCH_2CCCH_3	1,100	17	46	210
8.125	H	$(CH_2)_2Pht$	OCH_2CCCH_3	350	4.2	3.5	4.3
8.126	i-Bu	$(CH_2)_2Pht$	OCH_2CCCH_3	400	21	13	29

Cpd, compound.

10 μM concentration, compound **8.147** completely abolished collagen degradation and reduced MT1-MMP-dependent collagen invasion significantly.

Aihara et al. [117] reported some methylated epigallocatechin gallate derivatives. Some of these molecules (compounds **8.148–8.151**, Table 8.10) exhibited potential MMP-14 inhibitory efficacy.

Topai et al. [118] disclosed some gelatinase inhibitors designed by an *in silico* approach. Compound **8.152** (Figure 8.11) was the most promising MMP-14 inhibitor in this series (IC_{50} = 5 nM).

Shiozaki et al. [119] reported a series of (1S,2R,3R)-2,3-dimethyl-2-phenyl-1-sulfamidocyclopropanecarboxylates as promising and highly aggrecanase-selective inhibitors. Several compounds (compounds **8.153–8.160**, Table 8.11) displayed highly potent MMP-14 inhibitory efficacy.

TABLE 8.8

A Series of Arylsulfonamide-Based Effective MMP-14 Inhibitors (IC_{50} in nM)

Cpd	n	R	R_1	MMP-1	MMP-2	MMP-13	MMP-14
8.129	1	H		720	0.04	0.1	4.0
8.130	2	H		>5,000	10	18	135
8.131	1	H		2,900	0.43	0.65	24
8.132	1	H		11,000	3.4	7.0	71
8.133	1	i-Butyl		>5,000	1.4	1.5	82

Cpd, compound.

Shengule et al. [120] reported some ageladine A-related analogs. Compounds **8.161** and **8.162** (Figure 8.11) were the most effective MMP-14 inhibitors (IC_{50} = 200 nM and 570 nM, respectively). Gooyit et al. [121] reported some water-soluble gelatinase inhibitors. Compounds **8.163**, **8.164**, and **8.165** (Figure 8.11) resulted in effective MMP-14 inhibitory efficacy (K_i of 210 nM, 260 nM, and 680 nM, respectively). These molecules also produced a good pharmacokinetic profile. Testero et al. [122] reported some sulfonate-containing thiiranes as selective gelatinase inhibitors.

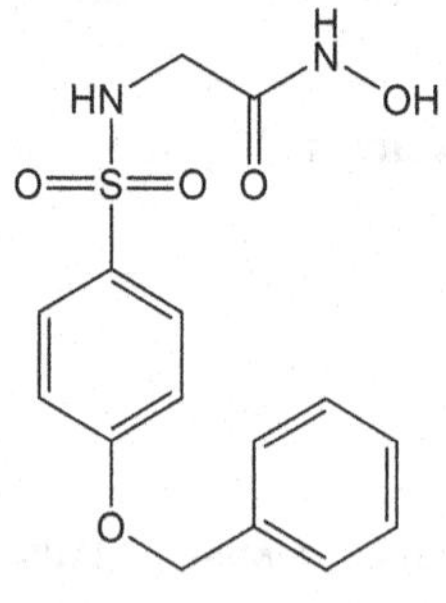

(8.134)
MMP-1 IC_{50} = 27,000 nM
MMP-2 IC_{50} = 3.8 nM
MMP-9 IC_{50} = 96 nM
MMP-14 IC_{50} = 310 nM

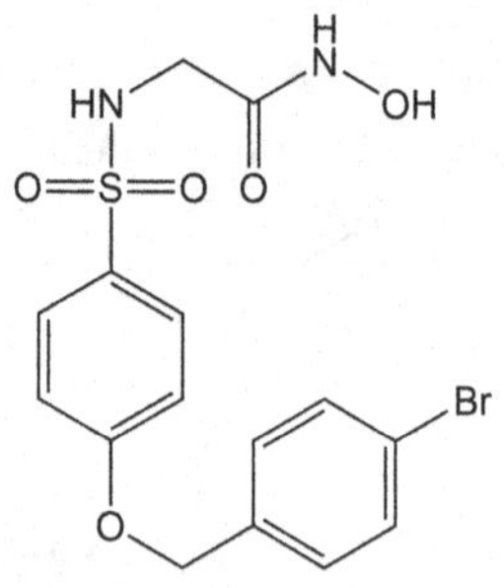

(8.135)
MMP-1 IC_{50} = 1,20,000 nM
MMP-2 IC_{50} = 1.2 nM
MMP-9 IC_{50} = 1.4 nM
MMP-14 IC_{50} = 630 nM

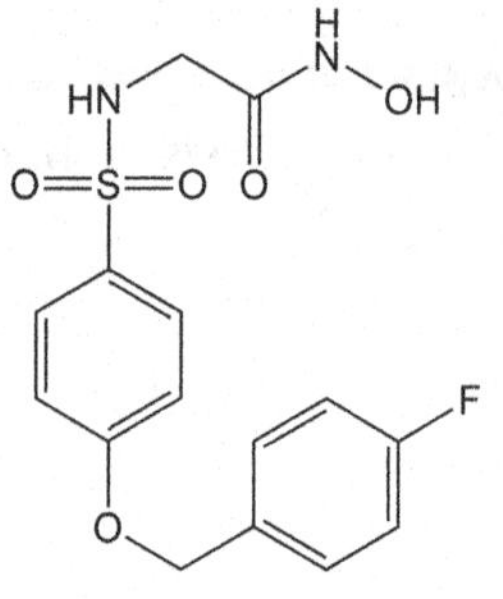

(8.136)
MMP-1 IC_{50} = 32,000 nM
MMP-2 IC_{50} = 3 nM
MMP-9 IC_{50} = 42 nM
MMP-14 IC_{50} = 590 nM

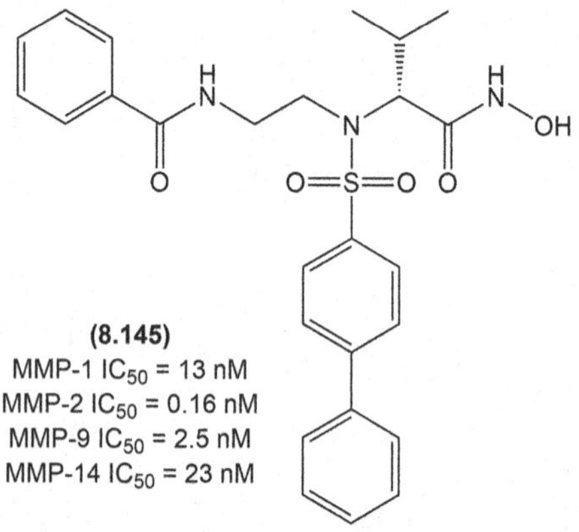

(8.145)
MMP-1 IC_{50} = 13 nM
MMP-2 IC_{50} = 0.16 nM
MMP-9 IC_{50} = 2.5 nM
MMP-14 IC_{50} = 23 nM

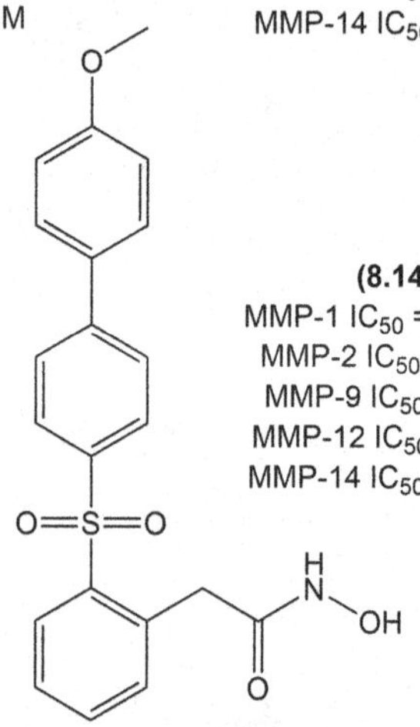

(8.146)
MMP-1 IC_{50} = 8,300 nM
MMP-2 IC_{50} = 9.7 nM
MMP-9 IC_{50} = 94 nM
MMP-12 IC_{50} = 4.8 nM
MMP-14 IC_{50} = 710 nM

FIGURE 8.9 Some more potential MMP-14 inhibitors (compounds **8.134–8.136**, **8.145–8.146**).

Among these molecules, compounds **8.166**, **8.167,** and **8.168** (Figure 8.11) were also found to be highly effective against MMP-14 (K_i of 150 nM, 360 nM, and 240 nM, respectively). All of them exhibited high solubility and good intrinsic clearance but lower half-lives.

Lee et al. [123] reported some potent thiirane-based gelatinase inhibitors. However, many of these molecules (compounds **8.169–8.177**, Table 8.12) exerted promising MMP-14 inhibitory activity. All of them exhibited lower half-lives.

Gooyit et al. [124] reported some *o*-phenyl carbamate and phenyl urea thiiranes as potent MMP-2 inhibitors. Among these molecules, compounds **8.178** and **8.179** (Figure 8.12) were effective MMP-14 inhibitors (K_i = 1.9 μM and 2.1 μM, respectively). However, compound **8.178** exhibited a relatively shorter half-live ($T_{1/2}$ = 24.8 min).

Nguyen et al. [125] reported some potent MMP-9 inhibitors. Compound **8.180** (Figure 8.12) was the most efficacious MMP-14 inhibitor (K_i = 53 nM).

TABLE 8.9

A Series of N-O-Isopropyl Sulfonamido-Based Hydroxamates as Effective MMP-14 Inhibitors (IC$_{50}$ in nM)

(8.137-8.143)   (8.144)

Cpd	R	R$_1$	MMP-1	MMP-2	MMP-3	MMP-9	MMP-13	MMP-14
8.137	H	-CH$_2$CH$_2$NHCOPh	780	1.50	450	9.00	4.60	94
8.138	H	-CH$_2$CH$_2$NHSO$_2$CH$_3$	320	1.00	71	8.60	2.20	95
8.139	H	-CH$_2$CH$_2$NHCOCH$_3$	280	0.33	47	6.50	0.68	41
8.140	H	-CH$_2$CH$_2$NHCOBn	1,300	1.40	120	6.40	1.40	81
8.141	OMe	-CH$_2$CH$_2$NHCOCH$_3$	660	0.13	20	2.00	0.58	23
8.142	OMe	-CH$_2$CH$_2$NHCOBn	1,400	0.37	63	2.90	0.25	25
8.143	H	-CH(CH$_3$)$_2$	490	0.81	50	6.70	4.10	9.8
8.144	-	-	200	0.67	105	0.43	0.19	3.9

Cpd, compound.

Hurst and co-workers reported some mercaptosulphide-based MMP-14 inhibitors. Most of the molecules (compounds **8.181–8.198**, Table 8.13) were highly potent inhibitors of MMP-14 [2, 3].

Jin and co-workers [126] disclosed some MMPIs based on a 3-mercaptopyrrolidine core. Many of these compounds (compounds **8.199–8.210**, Table 8.14) of this series produced potential MMP-14 inhibitory efficacy.

Adhikari et al. [127] designed some selective MMP-2 inhibitors through *in silico* lead identification and a *de novo* lead modification method. Among these molecules, compound **8.211** (Figure 8.12) was the most promising MMP-14 inhibitor (IC$_{50}$ = 427 nM). Matziari et al. [128] disclosed a set of phosphonic peptides as potential selective MMP-11 inhibitors. Compounds **8.212** and **8.213** (Figure 8.12) were found to be highly efficacious MMP-11 inhibitors (K$_i$ of 110 nM and 410 nM, respectively).

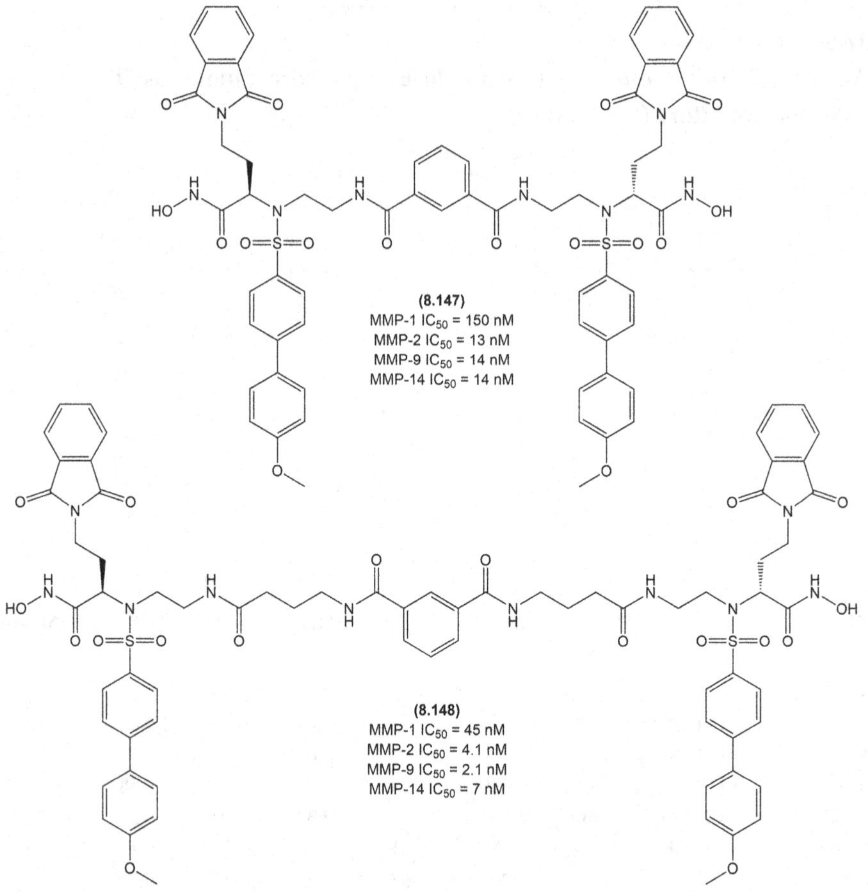

(8.147)
MMP-1 IC_{50} = 150 nM
MMP-2 IC_{50} = 13 nM
MMP-9 IC_{50} = 14 nM
MMP-14 IC_{50} = 14 nM

(8.148)
MMP-1 IC_{50} = 45 nM
MMP-2 IC_{50} = 4.1 nM
MMP-9 IC_{50} = 2.1 nM
MMP-14 IC_{50} = 7 nM

FIGURE 8.10   Various effective MMP-14 inhibitors (compounds **8.147–8.148**).

There are no such promising inhibitors found for other membrane-type MMPs such as MMP-15, MMP-16, MMP-17, MMP-24, and MMP-26. However, MMP-15 is expressed in a variety of human tissues, including leukocytes, endothelial cells, hepatocytes, and placenta. MMP-15 is responsible for cleaving gelatin and can degrade a wide variety of extracellular matrix molecules, including fibronectin and aggrecan. Interestingly, some research suggests that MMP-15 is not involved in the production of soluble endoglin from either placental or endothelial cells [129]. MMP-16 is responsible for diseases like ovarian cancer and asthma [130, 131], but there are no MMP-16 inhibitors for managing those disease conditions. On the other hand, MMP-17, MMP-24, and MMP-26 could be potential biomarkers for different cancers, but very few candidates were tested against these MT-MMPs, especially MMP-15, MMP-16, and MMP-26. The *in vitro* activity of the small molecules of MMP inhibitors evaluated against MMP-15, MMP-16, and MMP-26 are provided in Tables 8.4 to 8.6.

TABLE 8.10

Some Methylated Epigallocatechin Gallate Derivatives as Promising MMP-14 Inhibitors (IC$_{50}$ in nM)

(8.149-8.150)   (8.151)

Cpd	R$_1$	R$_2$	R$_3$	MMP-2	MMP-7	MMP-14
8.149	OH	OMe	OH	8,700	20,000	1,700
8.150	H	OH	OMe	34,000	>1,00,000	3,700
8.151	-	-	-	5,400	20,000	3,100

Cpd, compound.

8.5 SUMMARY

MT1-MMP (or MMP-14) is one of the most important MMPs, which has a crucial role in several major diseases, including cancer, cardiovascular diseases, and neurodegenerative diseases. Research has been conducted exploring the potential roles of MMP-14 in these diseases. However, lacunas in this field exist regarding the design and discovery of MMP-14 inhibitors. The structure of MMP-14 is well-explored, while the catalytic site is well-defined. Therefore, there is a high probability of designing effective and highly selective MMP-14 inhibitors for managing these diseases. However, researchers are focusing on designing other MMP inhibitors (namely collagenase and gelatinase inhibitors) instead of MMP-14. Therefore, there is a great scope for designing potential MMP-14 inhibitors, considering existing MMP-14 inhibitors. In addition, based on X-ray crystallographic data and the application of ligand- and structure-based molecular modeling techniques, potential and selective MMP-14 inhibitors can be designed. Although not much information is available on other membrane-type MMPs, most molecules from this chapter deal with the potential roles of MMP-14 and the respective inhibitors. This can lead to the development of unique ideas for designing effective MMP-14 inhibitors.

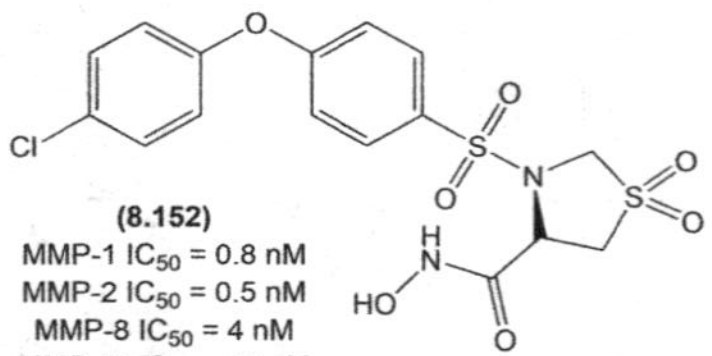

(8.152)
MMP-1 IC$_{50}$ = 0.8 nM
MMP-2 IC$_{50}$ = 0.5 nM
MMP-8 IC$_{50}$ = 4 nM
MMP-12 IC$_{50}$ = 19 nM
MMP-14 IC$_{50}$ = 5 nM

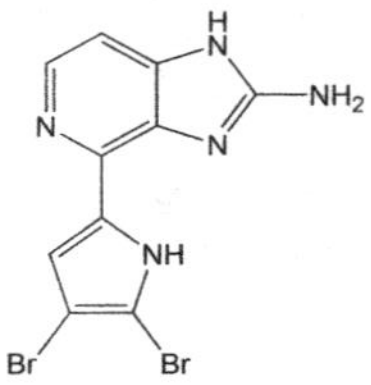

(8.161)
MMP-2 IC$_{50}$ = 1.7 μM
MMP-14 IC$_{50}$ = 0.2 nM

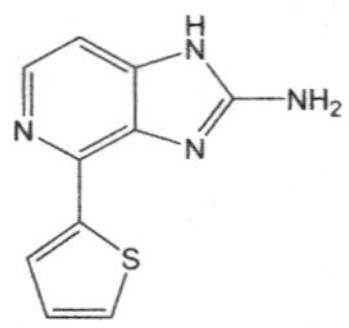

(8.162)
MMP-2 IC$_{50}$ = 3 μM
MMP-14 IC$_{50}$ = 0.57 nM

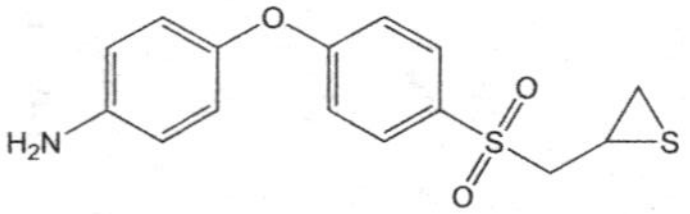

(8.163)
MMP-1 K$_i$ = 10% inhibition at 250 μM
MMP-3 K$_i$ = 23.4 μM
MMP-7 K$_i$ = 16% inhibition at 250 μM
MMP-14 K$_i$ = 210 nM

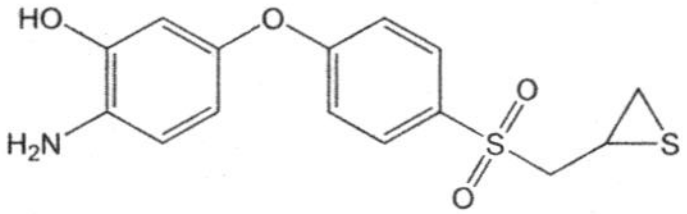

(8.164)
MMP-1 K$_i$ = 11% inhibition at 300 μM
MMP-2 K$_i$ = 78 nM
MMP-3 K$_i$ = 54% inhibition at 300 μM
MMP-7 K$_i$ = 116 μM
MMP-9 K$_i$ = 490 nM
MMP-14 K$_i$ = 260 nM

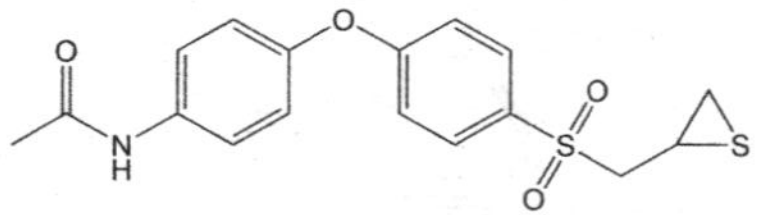

(8.165)
MMP-1 K$_i$ = 5.4 μM
MMP-2 K$_i$ = 110 nM
MMP-3 K$_i$ = 12.2 μM
MMP-7 K$_i$ = 39 μM
MMP-9 K$_i$ = 130 nM
MMP-14 K$_i$ = 680 nM

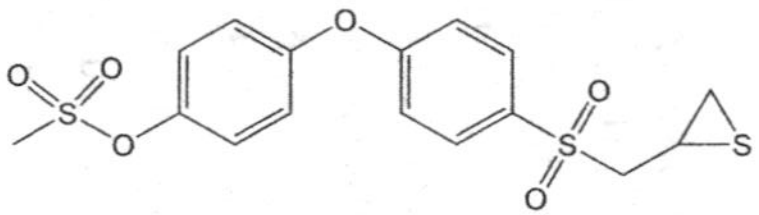

(8.166)
MMP-1 K$_i$ = 1,40,000 nM
MMP-2 K$_i$ = 23 nM
MMP-3 K$_i$ = 600 nM
MMP-7 K$_i$ = 18,000 nM
MMP-9 K$_i$ = 5 nM
MMP-14 K$_i$ = 150 nM

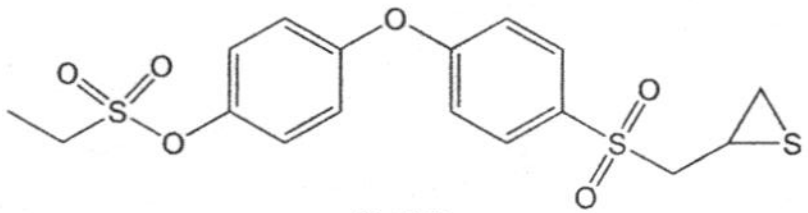

(8.167)
MMP-1 K$_i$ = No Inhibition at 40,000 nM
MMP-2 K$_i$ = 70 nM
MMP-3 K$_i$ = 38% at 20,000 nM
MMP-7 K$_i$ = 8% at 40,000 nM
MMP-9 K$_i$ = 330 nM
MMP-14 K$_i$ = 360 nM

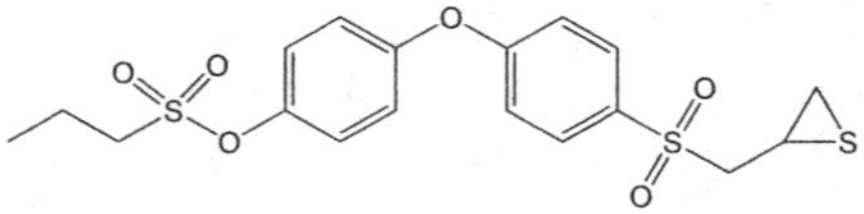

(8.168)
MMP-1 K$_i$ = No Inhibition at 20,000 nM
MMP-2 K$_i$ = 34 nM
MMP-3 K$_i$ = 22% at 20,000 nM
MMP-7 K$_i$ = 5% at 20,000 nM
MMP-9 K$_i$ = 520 nM
MMP-14 K$_i$ = 240 nM

FIGURE 8.11 Another set of potential MMP-14 inhibitors (compounds **8.152**, **8.161–8.168**).

TABLE 8.11
Some Sulfamidocyclopropanecarboxylates Derivatives as Potential MMP-14 Inhibitors (IC$_{50}$ in nM)

Cpd	R	MMP-1	MMP-14
8.153		180	3.4
8.154		33	1.3
8.155		<300	1.2
8.156		4,000	19
8.157		1,000	17

(*Continued*)

TABLE 8.11   (CONTINUED)

Some Sulfamidocyclopropanecarboxylates Derivatives as Potential MMP-14 Inhibitors (IC$_{50}$ in nM)

Cpd	R	MMP-1	MMP-14
8.158	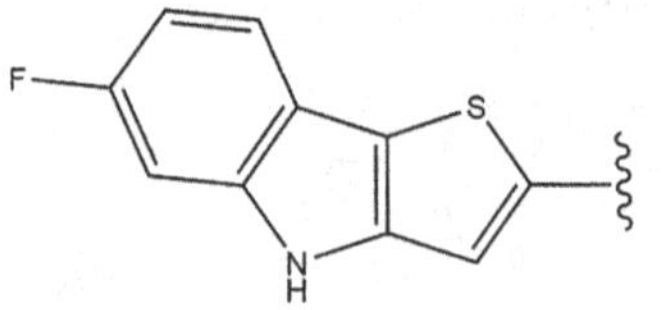	230	8
8.159	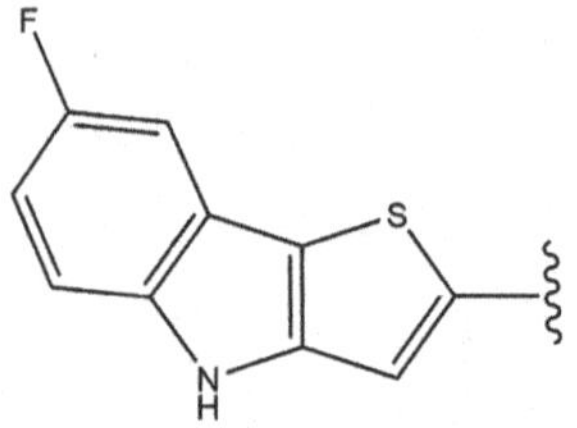	1,300	25
8.160	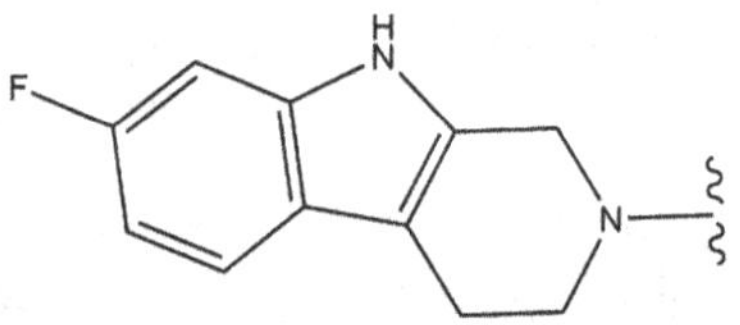	2,300	98

Cpd, compound.

TABLE 8.12

Some Potent Thiirane-Based MMP-14 Inhibitors (K$_i$ in μM)

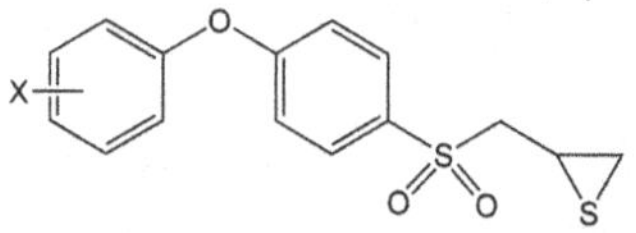

Cpd	X	MMP-1	MMP-2	MMP-3	MMP-7	MMP-9	MMP-14
8.169	p-F	-	0.061	-	-	0.044	0.580
8.170	m-F	-	0.45	27	-	3.0	0.19
8.171	p-CH$_2$OH	205	0.078	4.1	48.5	0.390	0.215
8.172	p-OH	128	0.006	2.2	31.0	0.160	0.090
8.173	p-Oi-Pr	-	0.30	17	-	0.47	0.28
8.174	p-OMOM	-	0.18	12	-	0.16	0.14
8.175	p-OMs	140	0.023	0.575	18.2	0.005	0.145
8.176	p-NH$_2$	-	0.024	23.4	-	0.87	0.22
8.177	p-OCF$_3$	-	0.110	-	-	0.930	5.08

Cpd, compound.

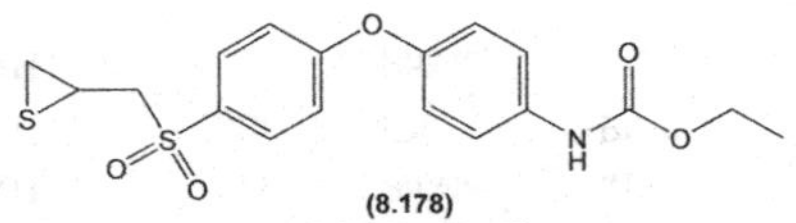

(8.178)
MMP-2 K_i = 290 nM
MMP-9 K_i = 860 nM
MMP-14 K_i = 1,900 nM
MMP-8 K_i = 13,000 nM

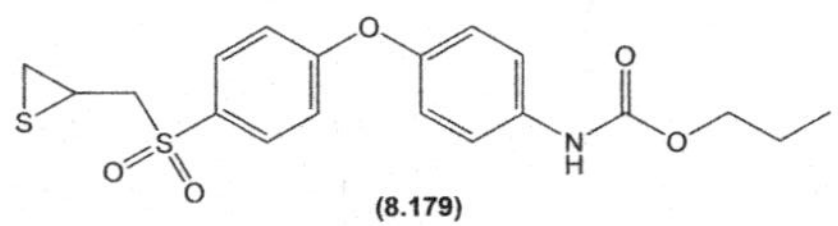

(8.179)
MMP-2 K_i = 490 nM
MMP-9 K_i = 1,100 nM
MMP-14 K_i = 2,100 nM

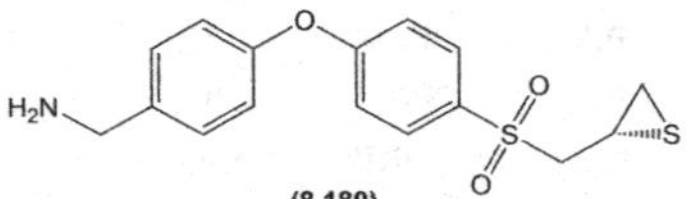

(8.180)
MMP-1 K_i = 24% inhibition at 100 μM
MMP-2 K_i = 37 nM
MMP-3 K_i = 22% at 100 μM
MMP-7 K_i = 15% inhibition at 100 μM
MMP-8 K_i = 2,100 nM
MMP-9 K_i = 190 nM
MMP-14 K_i = 53 nM

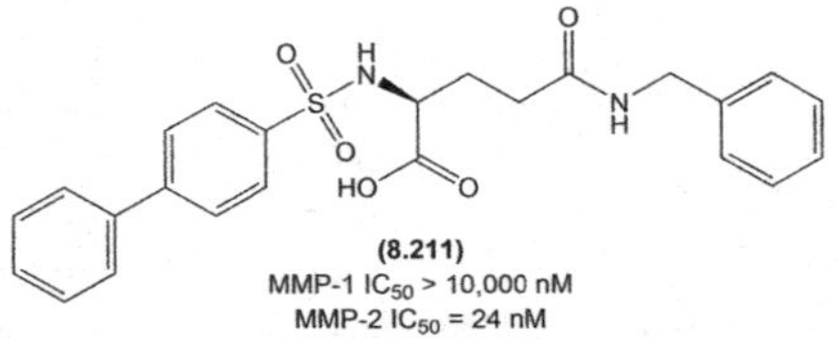

(8.211)
MMP-1 IC_{50} > 10,000 nM
MMP-2 IC_{50} = 24 nM
MMP-8 IC_{50} = 21.30 nM
MMP-9 IC_{50} = 492 nM
MMP-12 IC_{50} = 53.2 nM
MMP-14 IC_{50} = 427 nM

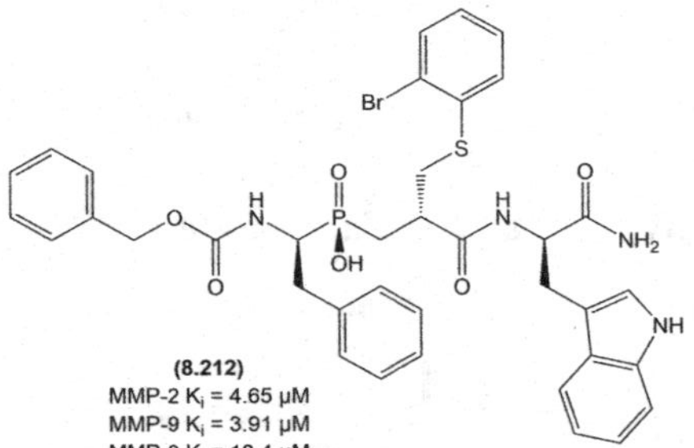

(8.212)
MMP-2 K_i = 4.65 μM
MMP-9 K_i = 3.91 μM
MMP-8 K_i = 18.4 μM
MMP-11 K_i = 0.11 μM
MMP-13 K_i = 4.7 μM
MMP-14 K_i = 30.1 μM

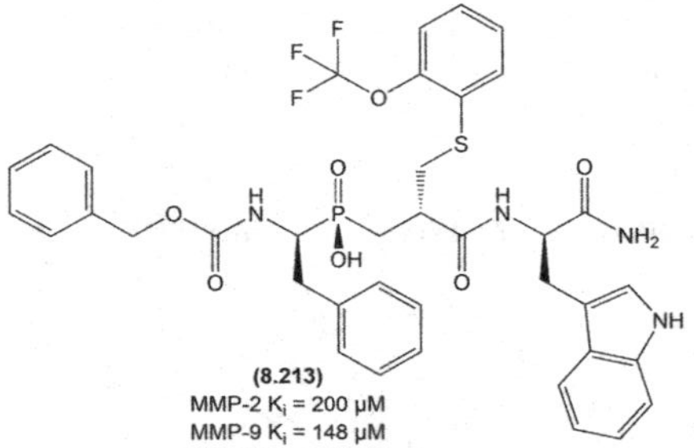

(8.213)
MMP-2 K_i = 200 μM
MMP-9 K_i = 148 μM
MMP-8 K_i = 200 μM
MMP-11 K_i = 0.41 μM
MMP-13 K_i = 200 μM
MMP-14 K_i = 30 μM

FIGURE 8.12 Some more effective MMP-14 inhibitors (compounds **8.178–8.180, 8.211–8.213**).

TABLE 8.13
A Series of Mercaptosulphide-Based MMP-14 Inhibitors (K$_i$ in nM)

Cpd	*	R	R$_1$	R$_2$	R$_3$	MMP-14	MMP-1	MMP-2	MMP-3	MMP-7	MMP-9
8.181	R	H	iBu	-	-	27	52	0.28	250	56	0.43
8.182	S	H	iBu	-	-	160	400	34	3,600	50	17
8.183	S,R	Me	iBu	-	-	18	13	0.35	46	15	0.21
8.184	R,R	Me	iBu	-	-	70	200	110	400	45	18
8.185	S,R	PhtNEt	iBu	-	-	4.5	0.95	0.77	22	15	0.09
8.186	S,R	PhtNBu	iBu	-	-	5.5	20	0.2	10	13	0.11
8.187	S,R	-	iBu	PhMe	Me	24	49	1.1	470	40	0.57
8.188	R,S	-	iBu	PhMe	Me	260	680	85	2,500	710	44
8.189	S,R	-	PhEt	iBu	PMP	16	>12,000	20	100	1,000	8.6
8.190	R,S	-	PhEt	iBu	PMP	380	>12,000	930	150	5,500	180
8.191	S,R	NH$_2$	iBu	PhMe	Me	13	100	6.1	360	26	1.2
8.192	1:1	Me	iBu	PhMe	Me	6.2	99	14	990	91	5.7
8.193	1:1	PhtNMe	iBu	PhMe	Me	70	110	17	300	50	4.9
8.194	1:1	PhtNPr	iBu	PhMe	Me	6	75	8.5	31	12	3.9
8.195	1:1	PhtNPe	iBu	PhMe	Me	7	52	1.7	1.9	11	0.98
8.196	1:1	PhtNEtNH	PhEt	PhMe	Me	3.7	190	1.8	13	250	0.35
8.197	1:1	PhtNEtNH	PhEt	iBu	PMP	3.1	>3,000	31	1.5	76	4.6
8.198	R,S	PhtNEtNH	iBu	PhMe	Me	1.2	8.8	0.7	6	6.5	1.1

Cpd, compound.

TABLE 8.14

A Series of 3-Mercaptopyrrolidine-Based MMP-14 Inhibitors (K_i in nM)

Cpd	*	R	R_1	MMP-1	MMP-2	MMP-3	MMP-7	MMP-9	MMP-13	MMP-14
8.199	cis, 1:1	Me	-	99	14	990	91	5.7	-	6.2
8.200	cis, 1:1	PhtNMe	-	110	17	300	50	4.9	-	70
8.201	cis, 1:1	PhtNPr	-	75	8.5	31	12	3.9	-	6.0
8.202	cis, 1:1	PhtNPent	-	52	1.7	1.9	11	0.98	-	7.0
8.203	1R,2S(+)	-	-	-	430	-	>1,00,000	280	160	68
8.204	(±)	-	-	3,400	18	>2,00,000	>20,000	25	15	18
8.205	1R,2R(-)	-	-	-	67	>1,00,000	36,000	42	10	10
8.206	(±)	NH_2	-	4,100	3.9	460	>25,000	15	50	11
8.207	(±)	NHMe	-	850	2.3	350	>25,000	1.1	28	62
8.208	(±)	PhtEtNH	-	2,800	35	37	12,000	2.4	27	21
8.209	(±)	$MeCONH(CH_2)_5$	-	>6,000	3.8	810	3,000	1.5	1.7	4
8.210	(±)	$NH_2(CH_2)_5$	-	>3,000	3.1	2,000	4,000	3.6	2.0	6.6

Cpd, compound.

REFERENCES

[1]. McCawley LJ, Matrisian LM. Matrix metalloproteinases: They're not just for matrix anymore! *Curr Opin Cell Biol.* 2001;13(5):534–540.

[2]. Hurst DR, Schwartz MA, Ghaffari MA, et al. Catalytic- and ecto-domains of membrane type 1-matrix metalloproteinase have similar inhibition profiles but distinct endopeptidase activities. *Biochem J.* 2004;377(3):775–779.

[3]. Hurst DR, Schwartz MA, Jin Y, et al. Inhibition of enzyme activity of and cell-mediated substrate cleavage by membrane type 1 matrix metalloproteinase by newly developed mercaptosulphide inhibitors. *Biochem J.* 2005;392(3):527–536.

[4]. Hernandez-Barrantes S, Bernardo M, Toth M, et al. Regulation of membrane type-matrix metalloproteinases. *Semin Cancer Biol.* 2002;12(2):131–138.

[5]. Hotary KB, Allen ED, Brooks PC, et al. Membrane type I matrix metalloproteinase usurps tumor growth control imposed by the three-dimensional extracellular matrix. *Cell.* 2003;114(1):33–45.

[6]. Ueda J, Kajita M, Suenaga N, et al. Sequence-specific silencing of MT1-MMP expression suppresses tumor cell migration and invasion: Importance of MT1-MMP as a therapeutic target for invasive tumors. *Oncogene.* 2003;22(54):8716–8722.

[7]. Pei D, Weiss SJ. Transmembrane-deletion mutants of the membrane-type matrix metalloproteinase-1 process progelatinase A and express intrinsic matrix-degrading activity. *J Biol Chem.* 1996;271(15):9135–9140.

[8]. Ohuchi E, Imai K, Fujii Y, et al. Membrane type 1 matrix metalloproteinase digests interstitial collagens and other extracellular matrix macromolecules. *J Biol Chem.* 1997;272(4):2446–2451.

[9]. Zucker S, Drews M, Conner C, et al. Tissue inhibitor of metalloproteinase-2 (TIMP-2) binds to the catalytic domain of the cell surface receptor, membrane type 1-matrix metalloproteinase 1 (MT1-MMP). *J Biol Chem.* 1998;273(2):1216–1222.

[10]. Butler GS, Butler MJ, Atkinson SJ, et al. The TIMP2 membrane type 1 metalloproteinase "receptor" regulates the concentration and efficient activation of progelatinase A. A kinetic study. *J Biol Chem.* 1998;273(2):871–880.

[11]. Nakahara H, Howard L, Thompson EW, et al. Transmembrane/cytoplasmic domain-mediated membrane type 1-matrix metalloprotease docking to invadopodia is required for cell invasion. *Proc Natl Acad Sci USA.* 1997;94(15):7959–7964.

[12]. Yana I, Weiss SJ. Regulation of membrane type-1 matrix metalloproteinase activation by proprotein convertases. *Mol Biol Cell.* 2000;11(7):2387–2401.

[13]. Sternlicht MD, Werb Z. How matrix metalloproteinases regulate cell behavior. *Annu Rev Cell Dev Biol.* 2001;17:463–516.

[14]. Murphy G, Knäuper V. Relating matrix metalloproteinase structure to function: Why the "hemopexin" domain? *Matrix Biol.* 1997;15(8–9):511–518.

[15]. Lauer-Fields JL, Juska D, Fields GB. Matrix metalloproteinases and collagen catabolism. *Biopolymers.* 2002;66(1):19–32.

[16]. Overall CM. Molecular determinants of metalloproteinase substrate specificity: Matrix metalloproteinase substrate binding domains, modules, and exosites. *Mol Biotechnol.* 2002;22(1):51–86.

[17]. Lehti K, Lohi J, Juntunen MM, et al. Oligomerization through hemopexin and cytoplasmic domains regulates the activity and turnover of membrane-type 1 matrix metalloproteinase. *J Biol Chem.* 2002;277(10):8440–8448.

[18]. Mori H, Tomari T, Koshikawa N, et al. CD44 directs membrane-type 1 matrix metalloproteinase to lamellipodia by associating with its hemopexin-like domain. *EMBO J.* 2002;21(15):3949–3959.

[19]. Tam EM, Wu YI, Butler GS, et al. Collagen binding properties of the membrane type-1 matrix metalloproteinase (MT1-MMP) hemopexin C domain. The ectodomain of the 44-kDa autocatalytic product of MT1-MMP inhibits cell invasion by disrupting native type I collagen cleavage. *J Biol Chem.* 2002;277(41):39005–39014.

[20]. Mondal S, Adhikari N, Banerjee S, et al. Matrix metalloproteinase-9 (MMP-9) and its inhibitors in cancer: A minireview. *Eur J Med Chem.* 2020;194:112260.

[21]. Fernandez-Catalan C, Bode W, Huber R, et al. Crystal structure of the complex formed by the membrane type 1-matrix metalloproteinase with the tissue inhibitor of metalloproteinases-2, the soluble progelatinase A receptor. *EMBO J.* 1998;17(17):5238–5248.

[22]. Lang R, Braun M, Sounni NE, et al. Crystal structure of the catalytic domain of MMP-16/MT3-MMP: Characterization of MT-MMP specific features. *J Mol Biol.* 2004;336(1):213–225.

[23]. Baidya SK, Banerjee S, Adhikari N, et al. Selective inhibitors of medium-size s1' pocket matrix metalloproteinases: A stepping stone of future drug discovery. *J Med Chem.* 2022;65(16):10709–10754.

[24]. Zarrabi K, Dufour A, Li J, et al. Inhibition of matrix metalloproteinase 14 (MMP-14)-mediated cancer cell migration. *J Biol Chem.* 2011;286(38):33167–33177.

[25]. Cathcart JM, Banach A, Liu A, et al. Interleukin-6 increases matrix metalloproteinase-14 (MMP-14) levels via down-regulation of p53 to drive cancer progression. *Oncotarget.* 2016;7(38):61107–61120.

[26]. Itoh Y. MT1-MMP: A key regulator of cell migration in tissue. *IUBMB Life.* 2006;58(10):589–596.

[27]. Haage A, Nam DH, Ge X, et al. Matrix metalloproteinase-14 is a mechanically regulated activator of secreted MMPs and invasion. *Biochem Biophys Res Commun.* 2014;450(1):213–218.

[28]. Poincloux R, Lizárraga F, Chavrier P. Matrix invasion by tumour cells: A focus on MT1-MMP trafficking to invadopodia. *J Cell Sci.* 2009;122(17):3015–3024.

[29]. Vos MC, van der Wurff AAM, van Kuppevelt TH, et al. The role of MMP-14 in ovarian cancer: A systematic review. *J Ovarian Res.* 2021;14(1):101.

[30]. Vos MC, Hollemans E, Ezendam N, et al. MMP-14 and CD44 in epithelial-to-mesenchymal transition (EMT) in ovarian cancer. *J Ovarian Res.* 2016;9(1):53.

[31]. Chen N, Zhang G, Fu J, et al. Matrix metalloproteinase-14 (MMP-14) downregulation inhibits esophageal squamous cell carcinoma cell migration, invasion, and proliferation. *Thorac Cancer.* 2020;11(11):3168–3174.

[32]. Kasurinen A, Tervahartiala T, Laitinen A, et al. High serum MMP-14 predicts worse survival in gastric cancer. *PLoS One.* 2018;13(12):e0208800.

[33]. Di D, Chen L, Guo Y, et al. Association of BCSC-1 and MMP-14 with human breast cancer. *Oncol Lett.* 2018;15(4):5020–5026.

[34]. Karamanou K, Franchi M, Vynios D, et al. Epithelial-to-mesenchymal transition and invadopodia markers in breast cancer: Lumican a key regulator. *Semin Cancer Biol.* 2020;62:125–133.

[35]. Wang YZ, Wu KP, Wu AB, et al. MMP-14 overexpression correlates with poor prognosis in non-small cell lung cancer. *Tumour Biol.* 2014;35(10):9815–9821.

[36]. Duan F, Peng Z, Yin J, et al. Expression of MMP-14 and prognosis in digestive system carcinoma: A meta-analysis and databases validation. *J Cancer.* 2020;11(5):1141–1150.

[37]. Kudelski J, Młynarczyk G, Darewicz B, et al. Dominative role of MMP-14 over MMP-15 in human urinary bladder carcinoma on the basis of its enhanced specific activity. *Medicine (Baltimore).* 2020;99(7):e19224.

[38]. Yan TH, Lin ZH, Jiang JH, et al. Matrix metalloproteinase 14 overexpression is correlated with the progression and poor prognosis of nasopharyngeal carcinoma. *Arch Med Res.* 2015;46(3):186–192.

[39]. Wang L, Yuan J, Tu Y, et al. Co-expression of MMP-14 and MMP-19 predicts poor survival in human glioma. *Clin Transl Oncol.* 2013;15(2):139–145.

[40]. Harrison GM, Davies G, Martin TA, et al. The influence of CD44v3-v10 on adhesion, invasion and MMP-14 expression in prostate cancer cells. *Oncol Rep.* 2006;15(1):199–206.

[41]. Morcillo MÁ, García de Lucas Á, Oteo M, et al. MT1-MMP as a PET imaging biomarker for pancreas cancer management. *Contrast Media Mol Imaging.* 2018;2018:8382148.

[42]. Bodnar M, Szylberg L, Kazmierczak W, et al. Differentiated expression of membrane type metalloproteinases (MMP-14, MMP-15) and pro-MMP-2 in laryngeal squamous cell carcinoma. A novel mechanism. *J Oral Pathol Med.* 2013;42(3):267–274.

[43]. Liu M, Qi Y, Zhao L, et al. Matrix metalloproteinase-14 induces epithelial-to-mesenchymal transition in synovial sarcoma. *Hum Pathol.* 2018;80:201–209.

[44]. Kanazawa A, Oshima T, Yoshihara K, et al. Relation of MT1-MMP gene expression to outcomes in colorectal cancer. *J Surg Oncol.* 2010;102(6):571–575.

[45]. Kerkelä E, Ala-aho R, Lohi J, et al. Differential patterns of stromelysin-2 (MMP-10) and MT1-MMP (MMP-14) expression in epithelial skin cancers. *Br J Cancer.* 2001;84(5):659–669.

[46]. Stasiak M, Boncela J, Perreau C, et al. Lumican inhibits SNAIL-induced melanoma cell migration specifically by blocking MMP-14 activity. *PLoS One.* 2016;11(3):e0150226.

[47]. Schmitt R, Tscheuschler A, Laschinski P, et al. A potential key mechanism in ascending aortic aneurysm development: Detection of a linear relationship between MMP-14/TIMP-2 ratio and active MMP-2. *PLoS One.* 2019;14(2):e0212859.

[48]. Miekus N, Luise C, Sippl W, et al. MMP-14 degrades tropoelastin and elastin. *Biochimie.* 2019;165:32–39.

[49]. Abu El-Asrar AM, Mohammad G, Allegaert E, et al. Matrix metalloproteinase-14 is a biomarker of angiogenic activity in proliferative diabetic retinopathy. *Mol Vis.* 2018;24:394–406.

[50]. Dai Q, Lin J, Craig T, et al. Estrogen effects on MMP-13 and MMP-14 regulation of left ventricular mass in dahl salt-induced hypertension. *Gend Med.* 2008;5(1):74–85.

[51]. Li C, Jin XP, Zhu M, et al. Positive association of MMP 14 gene polymorphism with vulnerable carotid plaque formation in a han Chinese population. *Scand J Clin Lab Invest.* 2014;74(3):248–253.

[52]. Schneider F, Sukhova GK, Aikawa M, et al. Matrix-metalloproteinase-14 deficiency in bone-marrow-derived cells promotes collagen accumulation in mouse atherosclerotic plaques. *Circulation.* 2008;117(7):931–939.

[53]. Dahi S, Lee JG, Lovett DH, et al. Differential transcriptional activation of matrix metalloproteinase-2 and membrane type-1 matrix metalloproteinase by experimental deep venous thrombosis and thrombin. *J Vasc Surg.* 2005;42(3):539–545.

[54]. Lin J, Davis HB, Dai Q, et al. Effects of early and late chronic pressure overload on extracellular matrix remodeling. *Hypertens Res.* 2008;31(6):1225–1231.

[55]. Kim JB, Jung MH, Cho JY, et al. The influence of type 2 diabetes mellitus on the expression of inflammatory mediators and tissue inhibitor of metalloproteinases-2 in human chronic periodontitis. *J Periodontal Implant Sci.* 2011;41(3):109–116.

[56]. Ünal A, Baykal O, Öztürk N. Comparison of matrix metalloproteinase 9 and 14 levels in vitreous samples in diabetic and non-diabetic patients: A case control study. *Int J Retina Vitreous.* 2022;8(1):44.

[57]. Candelario-Jalil E, Yang Y, Rosenberg GA. Diverse roles of matrix metalloproteinases and tissue inhibitors of metalloproteinases in neuroinflammation and cerebral ischemia. *Neuroscience*. 2009;158(3):983–994.

[58]. Martins D, Moreira J, Gonçalves NP, et al. MMP-14 overexpression correlates with the neurodegenerative process in familial amyloidotic polyneuropathy. *Dis Model Mech*. 2017;10(10):1253–1260.

[59]. Nishihara T, Remacle AG, Angert M, et al. Matrix metalloproteinase-14 both sheds cell surface neuronal glial antigen 2 (NG2) proteoglycan on macrophages and governs the response to peripheral nerve injury. *J Biol Chem*. 2015;290(6):3693–3707.

[60]. Langenfurth A, Rinnenthal JL, Vinnakota K, et al. Membrane-type 1 metalloproteinase is upregulated in microglia/brain macrophages in neurodegenerative and neuroinflammatory diseases. *J Neurosci Res*. 2014;92(3):275–286.

[61]. Xu I, Thériault M, Brunette I, et al. Matrix metalloproteinases and their inhibitors in Fuchs endothelial corneal dystrophy. *Exp Eye Res*. 2021;205:108500.

[62]. Golubnitschaja O, Yeghiazaryan K, Liu R, et al. Increased expression of matrix metalloproteinases in mononuclear blood cells of normal-tension glaucoma patients. *J Glaucoma*. 2004;13(1):66–72.

[63]. Laudanski P, Szamatowicz J, Ramel P. Matrix metalloproteinase-13 and membrane type-1 matrix metalloproteinase in peritoneal fluid of women with endometriosis. *Gynecol Endocrinol*. 2005;21(2):106–110.

[64]. Wilkinson JM, Davidson RK, Swingler TE, et al. MMP-14 and MMP-2 are key metalloproteases in dupuytren's disease fibroblast-mediated contraction. *Biochim Biophys Acta*. 2012;1822(6):897–905.

[65]. Zigrino P, Brinckmann J, Niehoff A, et al. Fibroblast-derived MMP-14 regulates collagen homeostasis in adult skin. *J Invest Dermatol*. 2016;136(8):1575–1583.

[66]. Hu Z, Gu H, Ni J, et al. Matrix metalloproteinase-14 regulates collagen degradation and migration of mononuclear cells during infection with genotype VII newcastle disease virus. *J Gen Virol*. 2021;102(1). doi: 10.1099/jgv.0.001505.

[67]. Idowu TO, Etzrodt V, Seeliger B, et al. Identification of specific Tie2 cleavage sites and therapeutic modulation in experimental sepsis. *Elife*. 2020;9:e59520.

[68]. Yamamoto M, Tsujishita H, Hori N, et al. Inhibition of membrane-type 1 matrix metalloproteinase by hydroxamate inhibitors: An examination of the subsite pocket. *J Med Chem*. 1998;41(8):1209–1217.

[69]. Xue CB, Voss ME, Nelson DJ, et al. Design, synthesis, and structure-activity relationships of macrocyclic hydroxamic acids that inhibit tumor necrosis factor alpha release in vitro and in vivo. *J Med Chem*. 2001;44(16):2636–2660.

[70]. Aranapakam V, Davis JM, Grosu GT, et al. Synthesis and structure-activity relationship of N-substituted 4-arylsulfonylpiperidine-4-hydroxamic acids as novel, orally active matrix metalloproteinase inhibitors for the treatment of osteoarthritis. *J Med Chem*. 2003;46(12):2376–2396.

[71]. Wu J, Rush TS 3rd, Hotchandani R, et al. Identification of potent and selective MMP-13 inhibitors. *Bioorg Med Chem Lett*. 2005;15(18):4105–4109.

[72]. Park K, Aplasca A, Du MT, et al. Design and synthesis of butynyloxyphenyl beta-sulfone piperidine hydroxamates as TACE inhibitors. *Bioorg Med Chem Lett*. 2006;16(15):3927–3931.

[73]. Condon JS, Joseph-McCarthy D, Levin JI, et al. Identification of potent and selective TACE inhibitors via the S1 pocket. *Bioorg Med Chem Lett*. 2007;17(1):34–39.

[74]. Lombart HG, Feyfant E, Joseph-McCarthy D, et al. Design and synthesis of 3,3-piperidine hydroxamate analogs as selective TACE inhibitors. *Bioorg Med Chem Lett*. 2007;17(15):4333–4337.

[75]. Huang A, Joseph-McCarthy D, Lovering F, et al. Structure-based design of TACE selective inhibitors: Manipulations in the S1'-S3' pocket. *Bioorg Med Chem.* 2007;15(18):6170–6181.

[76]. Park K, Gopalsamy A, Aplasca A, et al. Synthesis and activity of tryptophan sulfonamide derivatives as novel non-hydroxamate TNF-alpha converting enzyme (TACE) inhibitors. *Bioorg Med Chem.* 2009;17(11):3857–3865.

[77]. Hopper DW, Vera MD, How D, et al. Synthesis and biological evaluation of ((4-keto)-phenoxy)methyl biphenyl-4-sulfonamides: A class of potent aggrecanase-1 inhibitors. *Bioorg Med Chem Lett.* 2009;19(9):2487–2491.

[78]. Fray MJ, Dickinson RP, Huggins JP, et al. A potent, selective inhibitor of matrix metalloproteinase-3 for the topical treatment of chronic dermal ulcers. *J Med Chem.* 2003;46(16):3514–3525.

[79]. Reiter LA, Robinson RP, McClure KF, et al. Pyran-containing sulfonamide hydroxamic acids: Potent MMP inhibitors that spare MMP-1. *Bioorg Med Chem Lett.* 2004;14(13):3389–3395.

[80]. Noe MC, Snow SL, Wolf-Gouveia LA, et al. 3-Hydroxy-4-arylsulfonyltetrahydropyranyl-3-hydroxamic acids are novel inhibitors of MMP-13 and aggrecanase. *Bioorg Med Chem Lett.* 2004;14(18):4727–4730.

[81]. Blagg JA, Noe MC, Wolf-Gouveia LA, et al. Potent pyrimidinetrione-based inhibitors of MMP-13 with enhanced selectivity over MMP-14. *Bioorg Med Chem Lett.* 2005;15(7):1807–1810.

[82]. Whitlock GA, Dack KN, Dickinson RP, et al. A novel series of highly selective inhibitors of MMP-3. *Bioorg Med Chem Lett.* 2007;17(24):6750–6753.

[83]. Becker DP, Barta TE, Bedell LJ, et al. Orally active MMP-1 sparing α-tetrahydropyranyl and α-piperidinyl sulfone matrix metalloproteinase (MMP) inhibitors with efficacy in cancer, arthritis, and cardiovascular disease. *J Med Chem.* 2010;53(18):6653–6680.

[84]. Thompson LA, Liauw AY, Ramanjulu MM, et al. Synthesis and evaluation of succinoyl-caprolactam gamma-secretase inhibitors. *Bioorg Med Chem Lett.* 2006;16(9):2357–2363.

[85]. Rosner KE, Guo Z, Orth P, et al. The discovery of novel tartrate-based TNF-alpha converting enzyme (TACE) inhibitors. *Bioorg Med Chem Lett.* 2010;20(3):1189–1193.

[86]. Yu W, Guo Z, Orth P, et al. Discovery and SAR of hydantoin TACE inhibitors. *Bioorg Med Chem Lett.* 2010;20(6):1877–1880.

[87]. Li D, Popovici-Muller J, Belanger DB, et al. Structure and activity relationships of tartrate-based TACE inhibitors. *Bioorg Med Chem Lett.* 2010;20(16):4812–4815.

[88]. Dai C, Li D, Popovici-Muller J, et al. 2-(2-Aminothiazol-4-yl)pyrrolidine-based tartrate diamides as potent, selective and orally bioavailable TACE inhibitors. *Bioorg Med Chem Lett.* 2011;21(10):3172–3176.

[89]. De Savi C, Pape A, Cumming JG, et al. The design and synthesis of novel N-hydroxyformamide inhibitors of ADAM-TS4 for the treatment of osteoarthritis. *Bioorg Med Chem Lett.* 2011;21(5):1376–1381.

[90]. De Savi C, Waterson D, Pape A, et al. Hydantoin based inhibitors of MMP-13-discovery of AZD6605. *Bioorg Med Chem Lett.* 2013;23(16):4705–4712.

[91]. Nara H, Sato K, Naito T, et al. Thieno[2,3-d]pyrimidine-2-carboxamides bearing a carboxybenzene group at 5-position: Highly potent, selective, and orally available MMP-13 inhibitors interacting with the S1' binding site. *Bioorg Med Chem.* 2014;22(19):5487–5505.

[92]. Nara H, Sato K, Kaieda A, et al. Design, synthesis, and biological activity of novel, potent, and highly selective fused pyrimidine-2-carboxamide-4-one-based matrix metalloproteinase (MMP)-13 zinc-binding inhibitors. *Bioorg Med Chem.* 2016;24(23):6149–6165.

[93]. Durham TB, Klimkowski VJ, Rito CJ, et al. Identification of potent and selective hydantoin inhibitors of aggrecanase-1 and aggrecanase-2 that are efficacious in both chemical and surgical models of osteoarthritis. *J Med Chem.* 2014;57(24):10476–10485.

[94]. Durham TB, Marimuthu J, Toth JL, et al. A highly selective hydantoin inhibitor of aggrecanase-1 and aggrecanase-2 with a low projected human dose. *J Med Chem.* 2017;60(13):5933–5939.

[95]. Boiteau JG, Ouvry G, Arlabosse JM, et al. Discovery and process development of a novel TACE inhibitor for the topical treatment of psoriasis. *Bioorg Med Chem.* 2018;26(4):945–956.

[96]. Schröder J, Henke A, Wenzel H, et al. Structure-based design and synthesis of potent matrix metalloproteinase inhibitors derived from a 6H-1,3,4-thiadiazine scaffold. *J Med Chem.* 2001;44(20):3231–3243.

[97]. Krumme D, Tschesche H. Oxal hydroxamic acid derivatives with inhibitory activity against matrix metalloproteinases. *Bioorg Med Chem Lett.* 2002;12(6):933–936.

[98]. Ma D, Wu W, Yang G, et al. Tetrahydroisoquinoline based sulfonamide hydroxamates as potent matrix metalloproteinase inhibitors. *Bioorg Med Chem Lett.* 2004;14(1):47–50.

[99]. Biasone A, Tortorella P, Campestre C, et al. α-Biphenylsulfonylamino 2-methylpropyl phosphonates: Enantioselective synthesis and selective inhibition of MMPs. *Bioorg Med Chem.* 2007;15(2):791–799.

[100]. Tauro M, Laghezza A, Loiodice F, et al. Arylamino methylene bisphosphonate derivatives as bone seeking matrix metalloproteinase inhibitors. *Bioorg Med Chem.* 2013;21(21):6456–6465.

[101]. Moroy G, Denhez C, El Mourabit H, et al. Simultaneous presence of unsaturation and long alkyl chain at P'1 of Ilomastat confers selectivity for gelatinase A (MMP-2) over gelatinase B (MMP-9) inhibition as shown by molecular modelling studies. *Bioorg Med Chem.* 2007;15(14):4753–4766.

[102]. Ledour G, Moroy G, Rouffet M, et al. Introduction of the 4-(4-bromophenyl)benzenesulfonyl group to hydrazide analogs of Ilomastat leads to potent gelatinase B (MMP-9) inhibitors with improved selectivity. *Bioorg Med Chem.* 2008;16(18):8745–8759.

[103]. Rossello A, Nuti E, Carelli P, et al. N-i-Propoxy-N-biphenylsulfonylaminobutylhydroxamic acids as potent and selective inhibitors of MMP-2 and MT1-MMP. *Bioorg Med Chem Lett.* 2005;15(5):1321–1326.

[104]. Rossello A, Nuti E, Catalani MP, et al. A new development of matrix metalloproteinase inhibitors: Twin hydroxamic acids as potent inhibitors of MMPs. *Bioorg Med Chem Lett.* 2005;15(9):2311–2314.

[105]. Marques SM, Nuti E, Rossello A, et al. Dual inhibitors of matrix metalloproteinases and carbonic anhydrases: Iminodiacetyl-based hydroxamate-benzenesulfonamide conjugates. *J Med Chem.* 2008;51(24):7968–7979.

[106]. Nuti E, Casalini F, Avramova SI, et al. N-O-isopropyl sulfonamido-based hydroxamates: Design, synthesis and biological evaluation of selective matrix metalloproteinase-13 inhibitors as potential therapeutic agents for osteoarthritis. *J Med Chem.* 2009;52(15):4757–4773.

[107]. Nuti E, Panelli L, Casalini F, et al. Design, synthesis, biological evaluation, and NMR studies of a new series of arylsulfones as selective and potent matrix metalloproteinase-12 inhibitors. *J Med Chem.* 2009;52(20):6347–6361.

[108]. Nuti E, Casalini F, Avramova SI, et al. Potent arylsulfonamide inhibitors of tumor necrosis factor-alpha converting enzyme able to reduce activated leukocyte cell adhesion molecule shedding in cancer cell models. *J Med Chem.* 2010;53(6):2622–2635.

[109]. Nuti E, Casalini F, Santamaria S, et al. Synthesis and biological evaluation in U87MG glioma cells of (ethynylthiophene)sulfonamido-based hydroxamates as matrix metalloproteinase inhibitors. *Eur J Med Chem.* 2011;46(7):2617–2629.

[110]. Marques SM, Tuccinardi T, Nuti E, et al. Novel 1-hydroxypiperazine-2,6-diones as new leads in the inhibition of metalloproteinases. *J Med Chem.* 2011;54(24):8289–8298.

[111]. Nuti E, Santamaria S, Casalini F, et al. Arylsulfonamide inhibitors of aggrecanases as potential therapeutic agents for osteoarthritis: Synthesis and biological evaluation. *Eur J Med Chem.* 2013;62:379–394.

[112]. Nuti E, Casalini F, Santamaria S, et al. Selective arylsulfonamide inhibitors of ADAM-17: Hit optimization and activity in ovarian cancer cell models. *J Med Chem.* 2013;56(20):8089–8103.

[113]. Nuti E, Cantelmo AR, Gallo C, et al. N-O-isopropyl sulfonamido-based hydroxamates as matrix metalloproteinase inhibitors: Hit selection and in vivo antiangiogenic activity. *J Med Chem.* 2015;58(18):7224–7240.

[114]. Nuti E, Rosalia L, Cuffaro D, et al. Bifunctional inhibitors as a new tool to reduce cancer cell invasion by impairing MMP-9 homodimerization. *ACS Med Chem Lett.* 2017;8(3):293–298.

[115]. Nuti E, Cuffaro D, Bernardini E, et al. Development of thioaryl-based matrix metalloproteinase-12 inhibitors with alternative zinc-binding groups: Synthesis, potentiometric, NMR, and crystallographic studies. *J Med Chem.* 2018;61(10):4421–4435.

[116]. Cuffaro D, Nuti E, Gifford V, et al. Design, synthesis and biological evaluation of bifunctional inhibitors of membrane type 1 matrix metalloproteinase (MT1-MMP). *Bioorg Med Chem.* 2019;27(1):196–207.

[117]. Aihara Y, Yoshida A, Furuta T, et al. Regioselective synthesis of methylated epigallocatechin gallate via nitrobenzenesulfonyl (Ns) protecting group. *Bioorg Med Chem Lett.* 2009;19(15):4171–4174.

[118]. Topai A, Breccia P, Minissi F, et al. In silico scaffold evaluation and solid phase approach to identify new gelatinase inhibitors. *Bioorg Med Chem.* 2012;20(7):2323–2337.

[119]. Shiozaki M, Maeda K, Miura T, et al. Discovery of (1S,2R,3R)-2,3-dimethyl-2-phenyl-1-sulfamidocyclopropanecarboxylates: Novel and highly selective aggrecanase inhibitors. *J Med Chem.* 2011;54(8):2839–2863.

[120]. Shengule SR, Loa-Kum-Cheung WL, Parish CR, et al. A one-pot synthesis and biological activity of ageladine A and analogues. *J Med Chem.* 2011;54(7):2492–2503.

[121]. Gooyit M, Lee M, Schroeder VA, et al. Selective water-soluble gelatinase inhibitor prodrugs. *J Med Chem.* 2011;54(19):6676–6690.

[122]. Testero SA, Lee M, Staran RT, et al. Sulfonate-containing thiiranes as selective gelatinase inhibitors. *ACS Med Chem Lett.* 2010;2(2):177–181.

[123]. Lee M, Ikejiri M, Klimpel D, et al. Structure-activity relationship for thiirane-based gelatinase inhibitors. *ACS Med Chem Lett.* 2012;3(6):490–495.

[124]. Gooyit M, Song W, Mahasenan KV, et al. O-phenyl carbamate and phenyl urea thiiranes as selective matrix metalloproteinase-2 inhibitors that cross the blood-brain barrier. *J Med Chem.* 2013;56(20):8139–8150.

[125]. Nguyen TT, Ding D, Wolter WR, et al. Validation of matrix metalloproteinase-9 (MMP-9) as a novel target for treatment of diabetic foot ulcers in humans and discovery of a potent and selective small-molecule MMP-9 inhibitor that accelerates healing. *J Med Chem.* 2018;61(19):8825–8837.

[126]. Jin Y, Roycik MD, Bosco DB, et al. Matrix metalloproteinase inhibitors based on the 3-mercaptopyrrolidine core. *J Med Chem.* 2013;56(11):4357–4373.

[127]. Adhikari N, Halder AK, Mallick S, et al. Robust design of some selective matrix metalloproteinase-2 inhibitors over matrix metalloproteinase-9 through in silico/fragment-based lead identification and de novo lead modification: Syntheses and biological assays. *Bioorg Med Chem.* 2016;24(18):4291–4309.

[128]. Matziari M, Beau F, Cuniasse P, et al. Evaluation of P1'-diversified phosphinic peptides leads to the development of highly selective inhibitors of MMP-11. *J Med Chem.* 2004;47(2):325–336.

[129]. Kaitu'u-Lino TJ, Palmer K, Tuohey L, et al. MMP-15 is upregulated in preeclampsia, but does not cleave endoglin to produce soluble endoglin. *PLoS One.* 2012;7(6):e39864.

[130]. Duan XJ, Zhang X, Ding N, Zhang JY, Chen YP. LncRNA NEAT1 regulates MMP-16 by targeting miR-200a/b to aggravate inflammation in asthma. *Autoimmunity.* 2021;54(7):439–449.

[131]. Wang W, Liu Y, Yang Y, Huang X, Hou Y. MMP-16 as a new biomarker for predicting prognosis and chemosensitivity of serous ovarian cancer: A study based on bioinformatics analysis. *Crit Rev Eukaryot Gene Expr.* 2021;31(4):1–8.

9 Other MMPs and Their Inhibitors

Suvankar Banerjee, Sandip Kumar Baidya,
Nilanjan Adhikari, and Tarun Jha

CONTENTS

ABSTRACT

Other matrix metalloproteinases (MMPs) are grouped into separate categories, including MMP-12, MMP-19, MMP-20, MMP-21, MMP-27, and MMP-28. These MMPs have yet to undergo substantial research. However, MMP-12 is the most widely explored and studied MMP of other types of MMPs. Also, in many illness states, particularly in COPD, asthma, and respiratory distress, MMP-12 has been identified as a viable biomolecular target. This chapter consists of mechanisms in different disease conditions and related potential inhibitors that will be discussed in detail. X-ray crystallographic data and ligand- and structure-based drug design (LBDD and SBDD) methodologies are considered for creating and developing prospective MMP-12-selective inhibitors as efficient drug candidates due to the significance of MMP-12 in diverse illness situations. Therefore, this chapter might be helpful for future research projects involving the search for different kinds of MMP inhibitors.

Keywords: MMP-12; MMP-19; MMP-20; MMP-21; MMP-27; MMP-28

9.1 INTRODUCTION

A number of matrix metalloproteinases (MMPs) are grouped into a separate category, i.e., other MMPs. This group includes MMP-12, MMP-19, MMP-20, MMP-21, MMP-27, and MMP-28 [1]. However, most of these MMPs have not been studied extensively. Among these MMPs, MMP-12 is the most widely explored and studied MMP. It crucially takes part in several disease conditions [2, 3]. MMP-12 consists of three domains and shares a common structural similarity with other MMPs.

DOI: 10.1201/9781003303282-11

Among these, MMP-1 and MMP-3 have a 49% structural homology with MMP-12. The N-terminal domain I, which is a short signaling peptide, comprises a highly conserved cysteine residue coordinating the Zn^{2+} ion [4–6]. The catalytic domain II comprises the zinc-binding sequence motif HExxHxxGxxH [4, 7, 8]. Domain III, i.e., the hemopexin-like C-terminal domain, shows similarity in sequence with vitronectin and hemopexin [4]. MMP-19, expressed by monocytes, macrophages, fibroblasts, and endothelial cells, comprises some unique residues in the linker portion between the pro-domain and the Zn^{2+} binding domain [9]. It is attached in a non-covalent fashion through its hemopexin domain with cell surface macrophages dependent on cell adhesion. MMP-19 is unique from other MMPs by a C-terminal threonine-rich sequence of 36 residues downstream of the conserved cysteine residue found at the carboxy terminus [10–12]. It is found to hydrolyze various components of the extracellular matrix (ECM) as well as aggrecan, matrix protein, and proteins in cartilage and tendons [10, 13]. MMP-19 also degrades tenascin C, fibronectin, laminin, and nidogen 1 [10, 14, 15]. MMP-19 is also found to process the insulin-like growth factor binding protein-3 (IGFBP-3) in the human epidermis [10, 16]. MMP-20 (also known as enamelysin) has a domain orientation that is similar to other MMPs, including a signal peptide, a pro-domain with the conserved motif PRCGVPD associated with the regulation of enzyme latency, a catalytic domain with a Zn^{2+}-binding site, and a carboxy-terminal fragment similar to the sequence of hemopexin [17]. Again, MMP-28 (also called epilysin) consists of a well-conserved function as 85% of the overall amino acid residues and 97% in the catalytic domain are identical between human and mouse proteins [18, 19]. MMP-28 is a relatively new member of the MMP family, and analysis of the amino acid sequence reveals that it is most related to MMP-19 [18, 20]. Among these other types of MMPs, MMP-12 is well-explored, and much X-ray crystal data has been disclosed to date. The MMP-12 structure bound to a ligand is depicted in Figure 9.1.

9.2 THE PATHOPHYSIOLOGY OF OTHER MMPs

Among these MMPs, MMP-12 is the most widely studied MMP. MMP-12 has been established as an effective biomolecular target for different disease conditions, namely emphysema [21], inflammatory respiratory diseases like COPD [22–27], asthma [28–30], allergic rhinitis [31], allergic airway inflammation [32], chronic rhinosinusitis with nasal polyposis [33], several cancers like endometrial adenocarcinoma [34], oral squamous cell carcinoma [35], non-small cell lung cancer [36], gastric cancer [37], colorectal cancer [38], neuroinflammation and neurological diseases [3, 39], heart-related diseases like chronic heart disease [40], ischemic strokes [41], coronary artery disease [42, 43], abdominal aortic aneurysms [44], osteoarthritis [45], rheumatoid arthritis [46, 47], experimental autoimmune encephalomyelitis [48], Crohn's disease [49], dermatitis [50], and viral infection [51].

MMP-19 expression in fibroblasts is based on ERK1/2 and p38 signaling pathways. Again, MMP-19 has been found to have profibrotic activity in hepatic fibrosis [9]. The absence of MMP-19 has been found to elevate colitis with a reduced survival rate due to enhanced levels of proinflammatory modulators [52]. On the

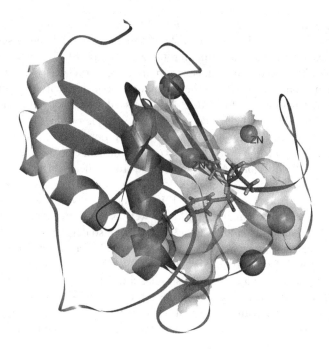

FIGURE 9.1 Ligand-bound crystal structure of MMP-12 (PDB: 1RMZ) (zinc ions are shown as a dark gray ball; calcium ions are shown as a light gray ball; the bound ligand is shown in the dark gray stick; The catalytic surface is shown in light gray).

other hand, both MMP-19 and MMP-28 are found to be downregulated during the malignant conversion of the colon and take part in tissue homeostasis [53]. Again, in the case of mammary gland tumors, there is a disappearance of MMP-19 from tumor cells and blood vessels and a simultaneous increase in MMP-2 level [54]. A deficiency of MMP-19 also influences allergen-induced airway inflammation [55]. MMP-19 is highly expressed in active multiple sclerosis [56]. It is also a prime regulator of lung fibrosis [57]. Again, MMP-19 and MMP-20 are highly expressed in human pancreatic ductal carcinoma [58]. High expression of MMP-19 is related to the poor prognosis of patients having colorectal cancer [59]. Nevertheless, MMP-19 has been found to promote metastasis and subsequently enhance mortality in NSCLC [60]. Moreover, it has been upregulated during the progression and invasion of melanoma [61].

MMP-20 is overexpressed in laryngeal squamous cell carcinoma [62]. It has been found that overexpression of MMP-21 is related to a poor prognosis during colorectal cancer [63]. The abnormal expression of MMP-28 has been associated with the progression of bladder cancer [64]. MMP-28 has been found to be widely expressed in tumors [65]. MMP-28 triggers TGF-β-mediated epithelial-mesenchymal transformation in lung cancer [66]. Overexpression of MMP-28 is a major reason for the poor prognosis of gastric cancer [67]. MMP-28 has also been found to participate in key roles in atrial fibrillation and heart failure [68].

9.3 SELECTIVE MMP-12 INHIBITORS

A variety of MMP-12 inhibitors have been designed, synthesized, and evaluated to date. Jeng and coworkers from Novartis Pharmaceuticals [69] reported a set of sulfonamide-containing hydroxamates as efficacious inhibitors of mouse macrophage metalloelastase (MMP-12). Some of the compounds (like compounds **9.1** and **9.2**, Figure 9.2) exhibited potent MMP-12 inhibition.

Dublanchet and coworkers from Pfizer Global Research and Development [70] reported some thiophene carboxamido derivatives as potent MMP-12 inhibitors. Compound **9.3** (Figure 9.2), containing a 2-morpholine-4-yl-ethyl substitution at the carboxamide moiety, yielded potent MMP-12 inhibition (IC_{50} = 57 nM). Again, the 2-carboxy-1-phenylethyl analog (compound **9.4**, Figure 9.2) resulted in more than four-fold potent MMP-12 inhibition (IC_{50} = 14 nM). The X-ray crystal data of compound **9.4** bound with MMP-12 disclosed that the biaryl moiety positioned into the S1' pocket made several hydrophobic interactions. The thiophene and aromatic rings exhibited hydrophobic interactions with Thr215, His218, and Tyr240. The 4-pyridyl group produced lipophilic interaction with amino acid residues Lys241 and Val235. In addition, the hydrogen bonding interactions were noticed with amino acids Leu181, Ala182, and Tyr240, as well as with a water-mediated hydrogen bonding with Gly179.

Ma and coworkers [71] reported several tetrahydroisoquinoline-containing sulfon-amide hydroxamates as efficacious MMPIs. The 2',5'-dichlorophenyl compound (compound **9.5**, Figure 9.2) yielded potent MMP-12-selective inhibition (IC_{50} = 170 nM) over other MMPs. Ma et al. [72] further disclosed some γ-keto carboxylic acid derivatives as potential MMPIs. Many of them were potent MMP-12-selective inhibitors over other MMPs tested. Compounds with *n*-hexyl (compound **9.6**, Figure 9.2), c-pentyl-methyl (compound **9.7**, Figure 9.2), and benzyl (compound **9.8**, Figure 9.2) substitutions at the methylene moiety adjacent to the carbonyl function resulted in equipotent and equally selective MMP-12 inhibitors. However, smaller alkyl groups and bulky aryl substitutions at the same position decreased the MMP-12 selectivity. Compound **9.9** (Figure 9.2) contained a *p*-chlorophenyl function at the terminal end along with an *n*-hexyl substitution at the methylene function and displayed the highest MMP-12 inhibitory potential, as well as selectivity over other MMPs tested. The molecular docking interaction showed that the *p*-chloro function produced extra polar interactions with Lys241, Thr227, and Arg424 at the bottom of the S1' pocket of MMP-12, MMP-2, and MMP-9, respectively. In the porcine pancreatic elastase (PPE)-induced emphysema hamster model, treatment with selective MMP-12 inhibitor (compound **9.9**) protected the integrity of the alveolar septal walls and elastic fibers from cleaving. It also significantly protected against lung hemorrhage *in vivo* and can be a valuable molecule for optimization against MMP-12-mediated emphysema.

Interestingly, among the pyridylthiol and pyridinone derivatives reported by Hayashi and coworkers [73], the pyridinone analog with a 3-fluorobenzyl substitution (compound **9.10**, Figure 9.3) and pyridylthiol compound with 2,5-difluorobenzyl substitution (compound **9.11**, Figure 9.3) depicted excellent selectivity toward MMP-12. This might indicate the influence of fluorobenzyl substitution of these pyridinone and pyridylthiol analogs for MMP-12 selectivity.

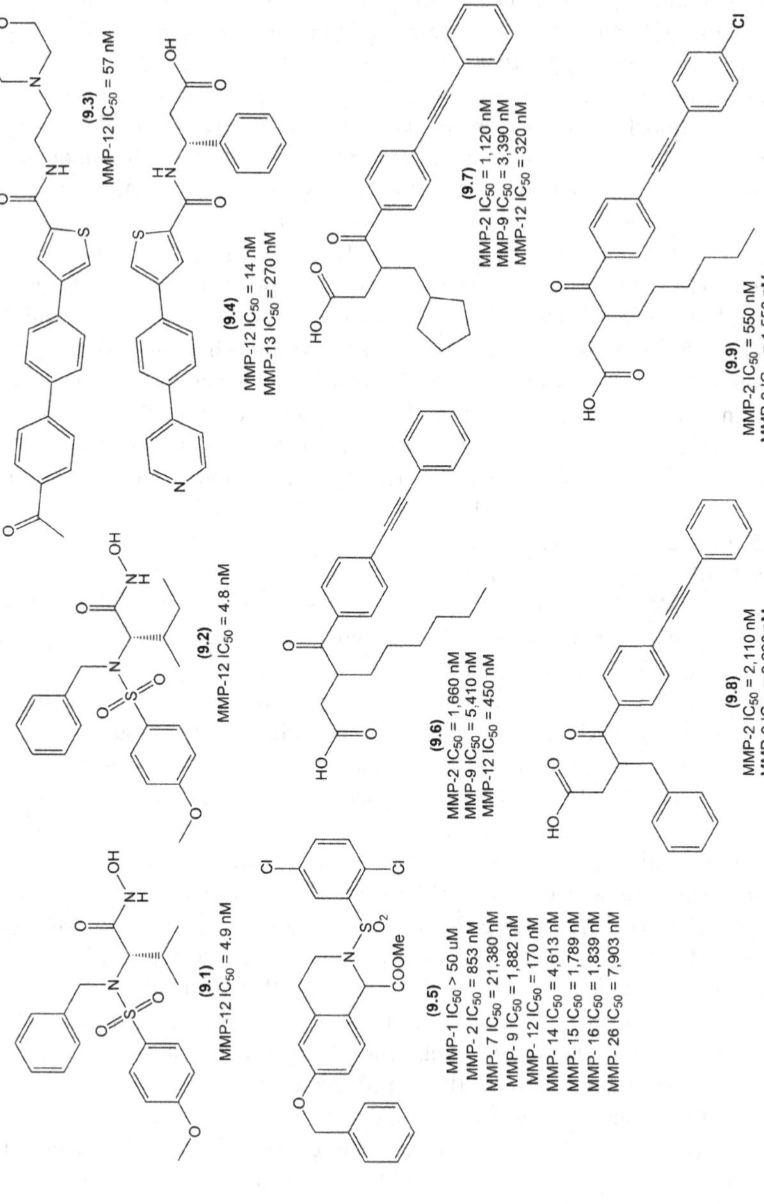

FIGURE 9.2 Some potential MMP-12 inhibitors (compounds 9.1–9.9).

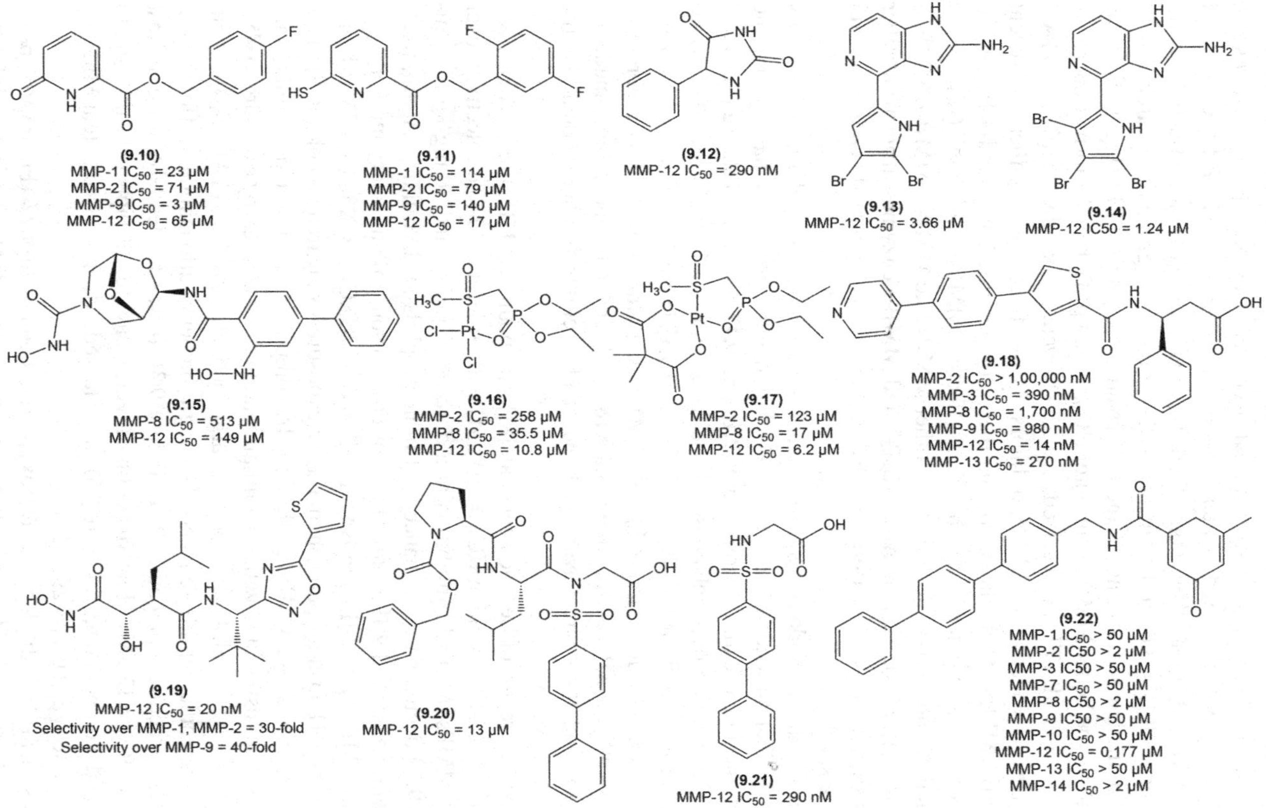

FIGURE 9.3 Various effective MMP-12 inhibitors (compounds 9.10–9.22).

Nordstrom et al. [74] identified some MMP-12 inhibitors by utilizing biosensor-dependent screening of a fragment library. Compound **9.12** (Figure 9.3) exerted competitive inhibition of MMP-12 (IC_{50} = 290 nM) with a ligand efficiency of 0.7 kcal/mol. Ando and Terashima of Kyorin Pharmaceutical Company [75] reported some ageladine A derivatives and evaluated their activity against MMP-12. Compound **9.13** (Figure 9.3) among these compounds was found to be the most effective MMP-12 inhibitor (IC_{50} = 3.66 μM). Further study by the same group of researchers [76] provided another series of ageladine A derivatives. Compound **14** (Figure 9.3) was found to be the better MMP-12 inhibitor (IC_{50} = 1.24 μM) than the former one.

Mannino et al. [77] synthesized a set of bicyclic molecular scaffolds (BTAa) derivatives as selective MMP-12 inhibitors. Most of them were either less potent or inactive MMP-12 inhibitors. Among these compounds, Compound **9.15** (Figure 9.3), although less potent, was the most effective MMP-12 inhibitor (IC_{50} = 149 μM), maintaining good selectivity over other MMPs like MMP-1, MMP-7, MMP-8, MMP-10, and MMP-13. However, MMP-1 and MMP-7 enzymes differ from other MMPs since they have inserted small S1' pockets, which apparently cannot contain the large substituent.

Sasanelli and coworkers [78] investigated some platinum complexes as inhibitors of MMPs. Platinum complexes exhibit DNA-damaging properties, having a unique class of antitumor features. Compounds **9.16** and **9.17** (Figure 9.3) showed selective MMP-12 inhibition over gelatinase. Some metzincin family small molecule-based MMPIs have been disclosed [79, 80]. Compound **9.18** (Figure 9.3) showed promising MMP-12-selective inhibition (IC_{50} = 14 nM) with a minimum of 19-fold more efficacy than other MMPs. Also, compound **9.18** was found to form one water-mediated hydrogen bond, three direct hydrogen bonds, and several hydrophobic contacts at the MMP-12 active site.

As per the report of Le Quement et al. [81], compound **9.19** (Figure 9.3) displayed a strong MMP-12 inhibition (IC_{50} = 20 nM) with at least a 30-fold selectivity over several MMPs. MMP-12 inhibition at a dose of 10 mg/kg and 30 mg/kg by compound **9.19** decreased the enhancement in neutrophils in BAL fluids. Again, treatment with compound **9.19** significantly lowered various inflammatory markers such as TNF-I, MIP-1γ, and IL-6 in BAL fluids and KC/CXCL1, CX3CL1, TIMP-1, and I-TAC/CXCL11 in lung parenchyma after exposure to cigarette smoke (CS). This suggests that selective MMP-12 inhibition by compound **9.19** lowered the inflammatory processes associated with lung inflammation that occurred by exposure to CS.

Cobos-Correa et al. [82] reported a target-activated prodrug (TAP) by using an MMP-12-specific peptide sequence bearing a biphenylsulfonamide scaffold in the backbone structure (compound **9.20**, Figure 9.3). It was moderately active against MMP-12 (IC_{50} = 13 μM). However, upon enzyme cleavage, the biphenyl sulfonamido acetic acid (compound **9.21**, Figure 9.3) was released, which showed potent MMP-12 inhibitory activity (IC_{50} = 290 nM).

Aerts et al. [83] disclosed a hydroxypyrone compound **9.22** (Figure 9.3) bearing a terphenyl scaffold as an efficacious and highly MMP-12-selective inhibitor (IC_{50} = 177 nM) compared with other MMPs. Treatment with compound **9.22** produced a significant lowering in LPS-induced lethality caused by systemic inflammation. It also markedly lowered the loss of blood-cerebrospinal fluid barrier (BCSFB) permeability in endotoxic mice.

Badland et al. [84] from Pfizer Global Research and Development reported a set of arylthiophene-based MMP-12 inhibitors. The biaryl derivatives were more potent compared with the monoaryl derivatives. The α-fluorothiophene analogs (compound **9.23–9.26**, Figure 9.4) were potent MMP-12 inhibitors.

Mori et al. [85] disclosed several MMPIs through structure-based optimization of the arylsulfonamide scaffold. Many of these compounds displayed potent MMP-12 inhibitory potency. Compound **9.27** (Figure 9.4) containing a phenethyl sulfonamido moiety resulted in potency and, to some extent, selective MMP-12 inhibitory efficacy (K_i = 23 nM). However, the incorporation of D-proline substitution enhanced the binding affinity toward MMP-12. Many of them produced dual MMP-12/MMP-13

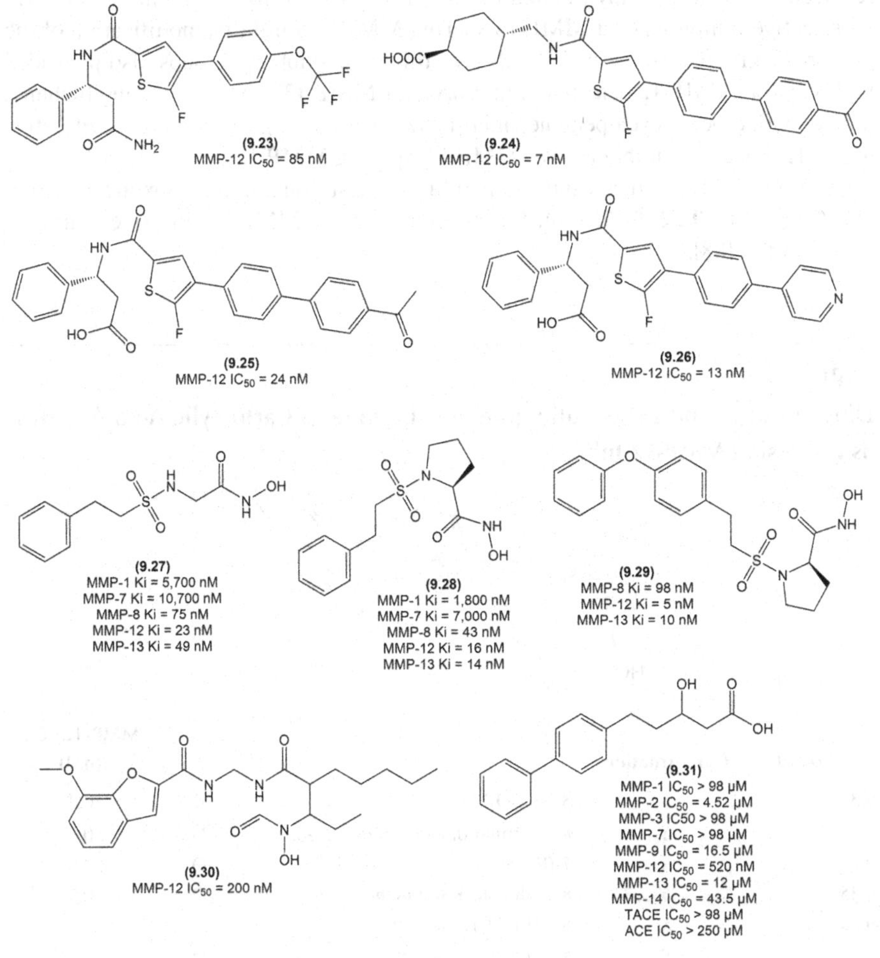

(9.23)
MMP-12 IC_{50} = 85 nM

(9.24)
MMP-12 IC_{50} = 7 nM

(9.25)
MMP-12 IC_{50} = 24 nM

(9.26)
MMP-12 IC_{50} = 13 nM

(9.27)
MMP-1 K_i = 5,700 nM
MMP-7 K_i = 10,700 nM
MMP-8 K_i = 75 nM
MMP-12 K_i = 23 nM
MMP-13 K_i = 49 nM

(9.28)
MMP-1 K_i = 1,800 nM
MMP-7 K_i = 7,000 nM
MMP-8 K_i = 43 nM
MMP-12 K_i = 16 nM
MMP-13 K_i = 14 nM

(9.29)
MMP-8 K_i = 98 nM
MMP-12 K_i = 5 nM
MMP-13 K_i = 10 nM

(9.30)
MMP-12 IC_{50} = 200 nM

(9.31)
MMP-1 IC_{50} > 98 μM
MMP-2 IC_{50} = 4.52 μM
MMP-3 $IC50$ > 98 μM
MMP-7 IC_{50} > 98 μM
MMP-9 IC_{50} = 16.5 μM
MMP-12 IC_{50} = 520 nM
MMP-13 IC_{50} = 12 μM
MMP-14 IC_{50} = 43.5 μM
TACE IC_{50} > 98 μM
ACE IC_{50} > 250 μM

FIGURE 9.4 A set of potential MMP-12 inhibitors (compounds **9.23–9.31**).

inhibitory efficacy (compound **9.28–9.29**, Figure 9.4). Other compounds also showed non-selectivity with MMP-8.

The researchers of GlaxoSmithKline Pharmaceuticals [86] reported some reverse hydroxamate inhibitors. Compound **9.30** (Figure 9.4) was the maximum effective MMP-12 inhibitor (IC_{50} = 200 nM) among these molecules. Holmes and coworkers [87] reported some β-hydroxy carboxylic acid derivatives as potential inhibitors of MMP-12. Compound **9.31** (Figure 9.4), containing the biphenyl group, was an effective MMP-12-selective inhibitor (IC_{50} = 520 nM) over other MMPs. Compound **9.31** was found to coordinate the Zn^{2+} ion through the carboxylic group, and the hydroxy group formed a hydrogen bonding interaction with Leu181. The biphenyl group entered into the S1' pocket of the MMP-12. The respective enantiomers of compound **9.31** were also promising MMP-12-selective inhibitors. Modification of the terminal phenyl group with various substituents like *m*-cyano, *p*-cyano, *p*-thiomethyl, or replacement with 4-pyridyl, benzofuran-2-yl resulted in highly potent and MMP-12-selective inhibitors over MMP-13 sparing MMP-1. Similarly, modification of the β-hydroxy group with methoxy, carbonyl, thio, and sulphoxy groups also produced highly potent MMP-12-selective inhibitors over MMP-13. Again, replacing biphenyl moiety with dibenzocyclopentene and *p*-benzyloxyphenyl groups produced effective MMP-12-selective inhibitors over MMP-13, sparing MMP-1.

A series of dibenzofuran and dibenzothiophene sulfonamido carboxylic acid analogs (compound **9.32–9.37**, Table 9.1) as promising and MMP-12-selective inhibitors was reported [88].

TABLE 9.1

Dibenzofuran and Dibenzothiophene Sulfonamido Carboxylic Acid Analogs as Promising MMP-12 Inhibitors

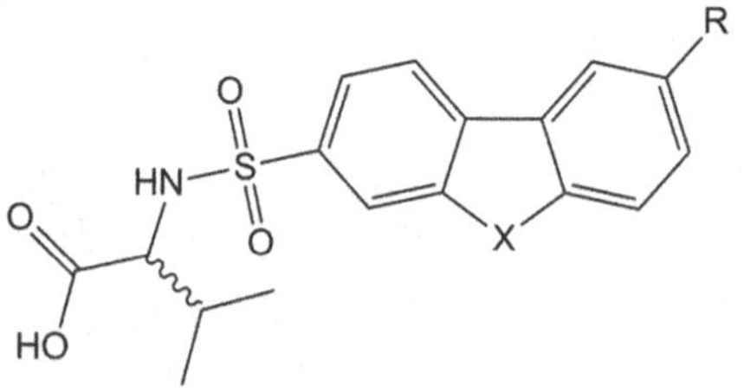

Compound	Conformation	R	X	MMP-12 IC_{50} (nM)
9.32	*S*	8-NHCO$_2$Me	S	0.4
9.33	*S*	8 (3-(trifluoromethyl)-1H-pyrazol-1-yl)	O	0.7
9.34	*R*	7-(1H-pyrrol-1-yl)	O	0.8
9.35	*S*	8-(3-thiophen-3-ylureido)	O	0.9
9.36	*S*	8-CH$_2$CCCH$_2$OCONH$_2$	O	1
9.37	*S*	8-(3-(4-fluorobenzyl)ureido)	O	1

Hagimori et al. [89] reported several dibenzofuran sulfonamide-based carboxylic acid compounds (compound **9.38–9.42**, Table 9.2) as potential and selective MMP-12 inhibitors compared with MMP-13.

In 2009, Nuti and colleagues [90] designed, synthesized, and evaluated a set of arylsulfone derivatives as effective MMP-12 inhibitors. The biphenylsulfonamido-based hydroxamate molecule comprising an *i*-propoxy substitution at the nitrogen atom (compound **9.43**, Figure 9.5) produced a highly potent MMP-12-selective inhibitor ($IC_{50} = 0.2$ nM), whereas its respective carboxylic acid derivative (compound **9.44**, Figure 9.5) significantly reduced MMP-12 inhibition ($IC_{50} = 410$ nM) though being a selective MMP-12 inhibitor.

Structural moderation of the sulfonamide group with the sulfone moiety provided a set of potent MMP-12 inhibitors. In this series, compound **9.45** (Figure 9.5), possessing a *p*-methoxy phenoxyphenyl group associated with the *ortho* position of the *N*-hydroxy-2-phenylacetamido moiety displayed potent MMP-12 inhibition ($IC_{50} = 0.2$ nM), maintaining at least a four-fold selectivity over other MMPs tested. MMP-12 inhibitory activity was lowered several times when the *p*-methoxy phenoxyphenyl moiety was altered with a biphenyl moiety (compound **9.46**, Figure 9.5), although it was also a potent and selective MMP-12 inhibitor. Similarly, equipotent activity and selectivity were noticed for the methyl counterpart of compound **9.46** (compound **9.47**, Figure 9.5), although it was a racemate compound. The molecular docking analysis of compound **9.45** with MMP-12 (PDB ID: 1RMZ) displayed that the *p*-methoxy phenoxyphenyl group was inserted properly into the S1' pocket. Nevertheless, one sulfonyl oxygen atom produced stable hydrogen bonding interactions with Leu181 and Ala182. Also, the amido and hydroxyl groups of the hydroxamate function,

---

TABLE 9.2

Dibenzofuran Sulfonamide-Based Carboxylic Acid Analogs as Potential and Selective MMP-12 Inhibitors (IC_{50} in nM)

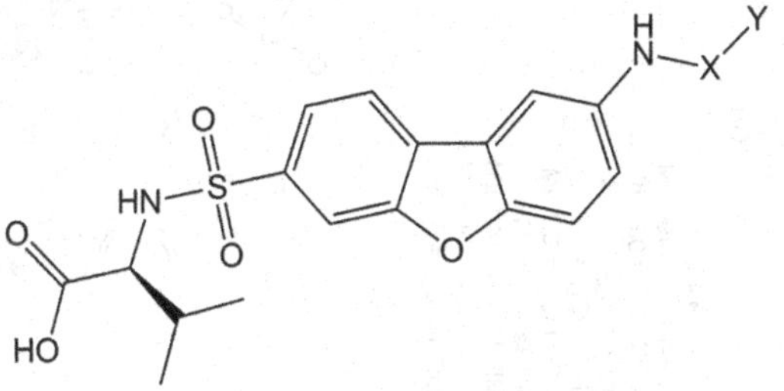

Compound	X	Y	MMP-12	MMP-13
9.38	CO	O-(4-I)Ph	8.5	69
9.39	CO	(4-I)Ph	502	>2,000
9.40	SO_2	(4-I)Ph	297	403
9.41	CO	O-(4-F)Ph	6.2	65
9.42	CO	O-(4-Br)Ph	11	51

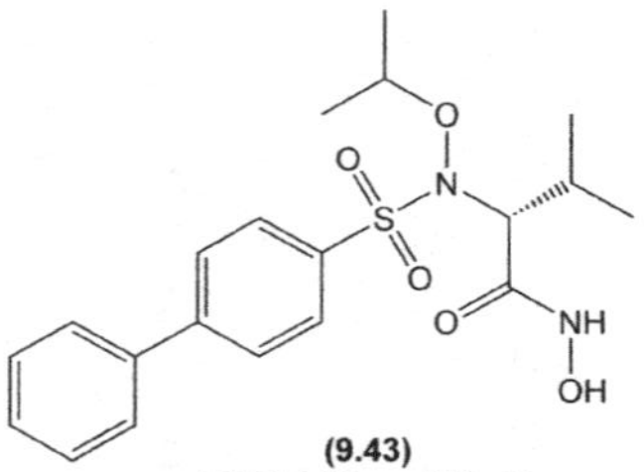

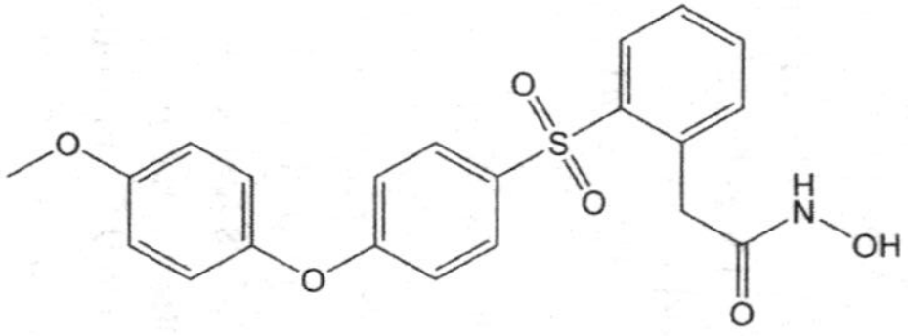

(9.45)
MMP-1 IC_{50} = 3,500 nM
MMP-2 IC_{50} = 3.5 nM
MMP-3 IC_{50} = 21 nM
MMP-8 IC_{50} = 5.1 nM
MMP-9 IC_{50} = 0.80 nM
MMP-12 IC_{50} = 0.20 nM
MMP-13 IC_{50} = 4.1 nM
MMP-14 IC_{50} = 33 nM
MMP-16 IC_{50} = 32 nM

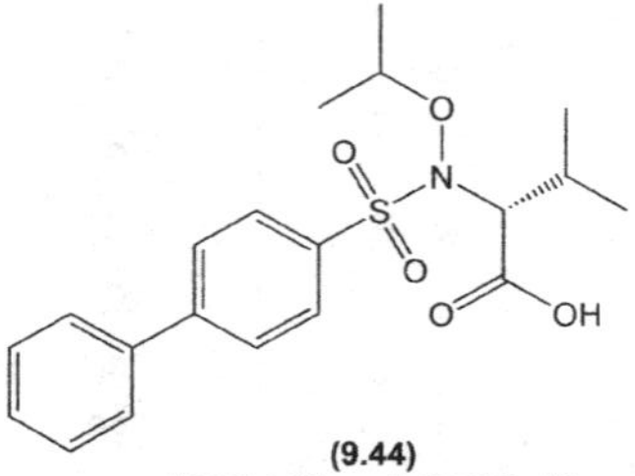

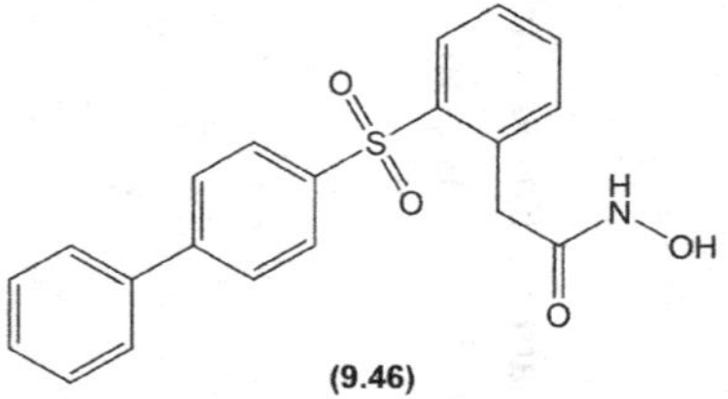

(9.44)
MMP-1 IC_{50} > 1,00,000 nM
MMP-2 IC_{50} = 1,500 nM
MMP-3 IC_{50} = 54,000 nM
MMP-8 IC_{50} = 2,000 nM
MMP-9 IC_{50} = 24,000 nM
MMP-12 IC_{50} = 410 nM
MMP-13 IC_{50} = 7,900 nM
MMP-14 IC_{50} = 10,000 nM
MMP-16 IC_{50} = 18,000 nM

(9.43)
MMP-1 IC_{50} = 490 nM
MMP-2 IC_{50} = 0.80 nM
MMP-3 IC_{50} = 50 nM
MMP-8 IC_{50} = 1.6 nM
MMP-9 IC_{50} = 6.7 nM
MMP-12 IC_{50} = 0.20 nM
MMP-13 IC_{50} = 4.1 nM
MMP-14 IC_{50} = 9.8 nM
MMP-16 IC_{50} = 51 nM

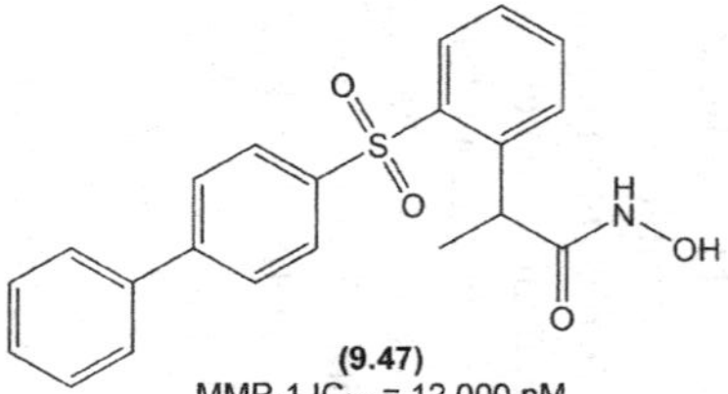

(9.47)
MMP-1 IC_{50} = 12,000 nM
MMP-2 IC_{50} = 73 nM
MMP-3 IC_{50} = 5,600 nM
MMP-8 IC_{50} = 390 nM
MMP-9 IC_{50} = 340 nM
MMP-12 IC_{50} = 6 nM
MMP-13 IC_{50} = 74 nM
MMP-14 IC_{50} = 860 nM
MMP-16 IC_{50} = 470 nM

(9.46)
MMP-1 IC_{50} = 29,000 nM
MMP-2 IC_{50} = 38 nM
MMP-3 IC_{50} = 23,000 nM
MMP-8 IC_{50} = 370 nM
MMP-9 IC_{50} = 310 nM
MMP-12 IC_{50} = 6 nM
MMP-13 IC_{50} = 62 nM
MMP-14 IC_{50} = 940 nM
MMP-16 IC_{50} = 220 nM

FIGURE 9.5   Some potential and selective MMP-12 inhibitors (compounds **9.43–9.47**).

apart from Zn^{2+} chelation, produced hydrogen bonding interactions with Ala182 and Glu219, respectively.

Nuti et al. [91] further modified the earlier reported compounds and designed and developed some thioaryl-based MMP-12 inhibitors. The *para*-methoxy biphenyl derivative attached with the N-hydroxy phenyl acetamido moiety through the thiol group (compound **9.48**, Figure 9.6) produced good inhibition toward MMP-12 with non-selectivity to MMP-2. A similar equipotent molecule (compound **9.49**, Figure 9.6) was produced when the thiol group was replaced with the sulfonamide function. Moderation of the N-hydroxy acetamide group of compounds **9.48** and **9.49** into N-hydroxy piperidine-2,6-dione moiety provided highly efficacious and MMP-12-selective inhibitors **9.50** and **9.51**, respectively (Figure 9.6).

SAR analysis revealed that compounds bearing monocarboxylic acid and dicarboxylic acid moieties also provided effective MMP-12 inhibitors selective over MMP-2 and MMP-9. Molecules bearing a hydroxy piperidine 2,6-dione zinc-binding group (ZBG) (compound **9.50**) exerted potent and MMP-12-selective inhibition (IC_{50} = 33 nM) compared with other MMPs. Alteration of the group of compound **9.50** with the sulfonyl group provided an almost equipotent MMP-12 inhibitor (compound **9.51**, Figure 9.6) having an IC_{50} of 40 nM, although the selectivity is slightly lowered.

Li et al. [92] reported some dibenzofuran analogs as MMP-12-selective inhibitors over MMP-13. Compound **9.52** (Figure 9.6) was a highly effective MMP-12-selective inhibitor (IC_{50} = 2 nM) over other MMPs and aggrecanases-1 and -2. Compound **9.52** also displayed potent human MMP-12 inhibitory efficacy and was selective over mice (IC_{50} = 160 nM), rats (IC_{50} = 320 nM), and sheep (IC_{50} = 22.3 nM). Compound **9.52** was evaluated in a mouse lung inflammatory model in C57BL/6 mice. At 30 mg/kg per oral dose, compound **9.52** provided a good pharmacokinetic profile. Metabolic stability studies revealed that compound **9.52** was stable in liver microsomes in mice, rats, dogs, monkeys, and humans ($t_{1/2}$ > 60 min). Compound **9.52** did not show any Ames toxicity with no LERG activity. Compound **9.52** showed a marked reduction in total BAL inflammation (more than 50%), as well as absolute macrophages (more than 70% inhibition), and the minimum effective dose of compound **9.52** was 5 mg/kg per oral b.i.d. in C57BL/6 mice. MMP-12 crucially takes part in airway inflammation and remodeling. Considering this, Li and coworkers [93] reported some orally effective derivatives as potent MMP-12 inhibitors. Compound **9.53** (Figure 9.6) was found to stabilize the carbamate moiety by elimination of the free amino group through the construction of the cyclic ring. Thus, compound **9.53** may enhance selectivity over other MMPs.

A group of researchers from Pfizer Global Research and Development and NiKem Research [94] discovered some dibenzofuran sulfonamide-containing carboxylic acid compounds as promising MMP-12 inhibitors (**9.54–9.74**, Table 9.3) selective over MMP-8 and MMP-13 for the treatment of COPD.

The N-linked dibenzofuran analogs containing five-membered heterocyclic ring structures like 2-oxazolidinone (compound **9.54**, Table 9.3), pyrazole (compound **9.55**, Table 9.3), and 3-trifluoromethyl pyrazole (compound **9.56**, Table 9.3) yielded 19-fold, 15-fold, and 44-fold MMP-12 selectivity over MMP-8, respectively. MMP-12 selectivity over MMP-8 was drastically reduced for compounds with six-membered

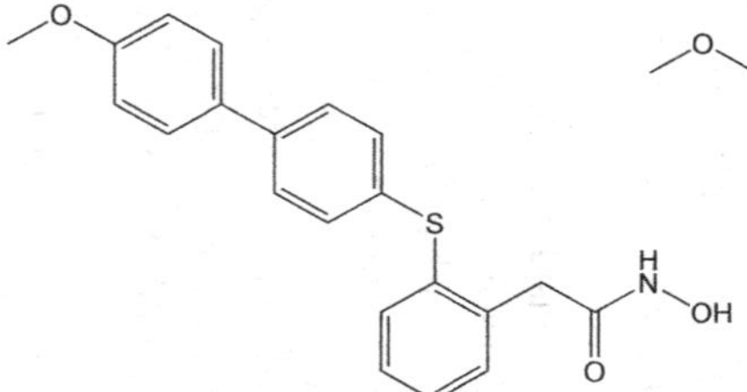

(9.48)
MMP-1 IC$_{50}$ = 2,50,000 nM
MMP-2 IC$_{50}$ = 6.8 nM
MMP-9 IC$_{50}$ = 120 nM
MMP-12 IC$_{50}$ = 4 nM
MMP-14 IC$_{50}$ = 2,000 nM

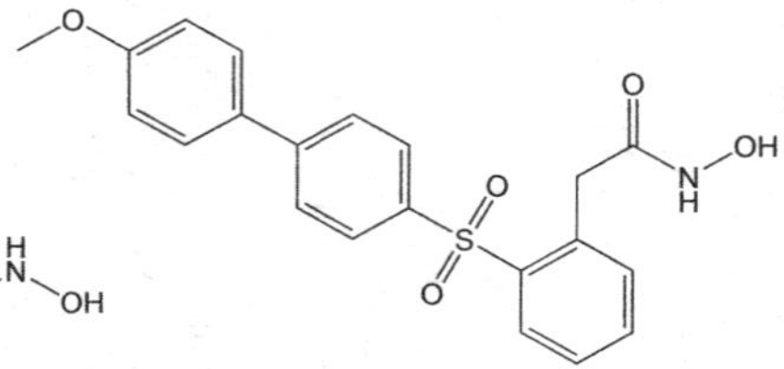

(9.49)
MMP-1 IC$_{50}$ = 8,300 nM
MMP-2 IC$_{50}$ = 9.7 nM
MMP-9 IC$_{50}$ = 94 nM
MMP-12 IC$_{50}$ = 4.8 nM
MMP-14 IC$_{50}$ = 710 nM

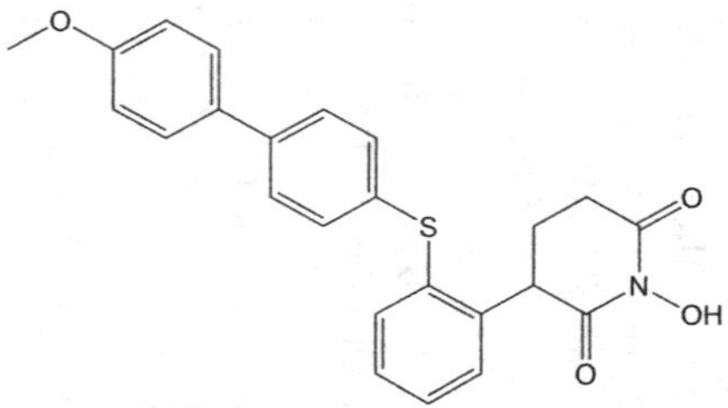

(9.50)
MMP-1 IC$_{50}$ = 2,60,000 nM
MMP-2 IC$_{50}$ = 670 nM
MMP-9 IC$_{50}$ = 5,800 nM
MMP-12 IC$_{50}$ = 33 nM
MMP-14 IC$_{50}$ = 40,000 nM

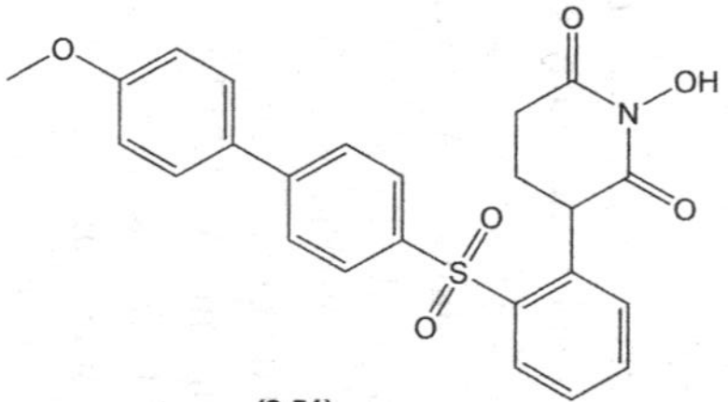

(9.51)
MMP-1 IC$_{50}$ > 10,000 nM
MMP-2 IC$_{50}$ = 414 nM
MMP-9 IC$_{50}$ = 1,430 nM
MMP-12 IC$_{50}$ = 40 nM
MMP-14 IC$_{50}$ = 4,000 nM

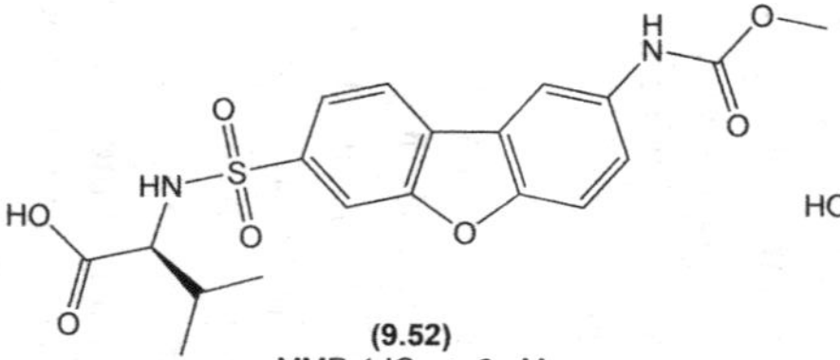

(9.52)
MMP-1 IC$_{50}$ > 6 μM
MMP-3 IC$_{50}$ = 351 nM
MMP-7 IC$_{50}$ > 22 μM
MMP-9 IC$_{50}$ = 1,300 nM
MMP-12 IC$_{50}$ = 2 nM
MMP-13 IC$_{50}$ = 120 nM
MMP-14 IC$_{50}$ = 1,100 nM
TACE IC$_{50}$ > 25 μM
Aggrecanase-1 IC$_{50}$ > 5 μM
Aggrecanase-2 IC$_{50}$ > 10 μM

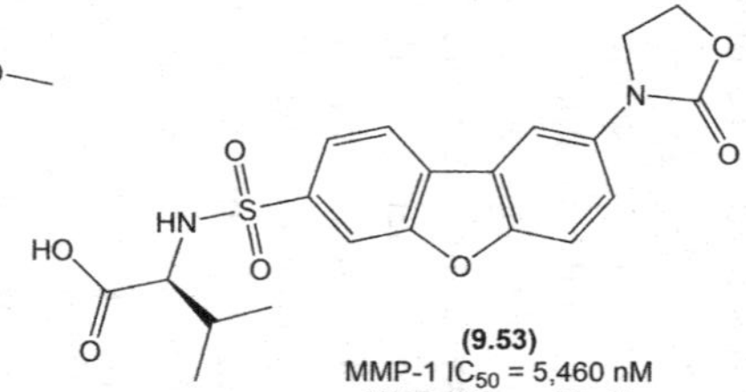

(9.53)
MMP-1 IC$_{50}$ = 5,460 nM
MMP-2 IC$_{50}$ = 66 nM
MMP-3 IC$_{50}$ = 300 nM
MMP-7 IC$_{50}$ = 7,830 nM
MMP-8 IC$_{50}$ = 37 nM
MMP-9 IC$_{50}$ = 318 nM
MMP-12 IC$_{50}$ = 1.4 nM
MMP-13 IC$_{50}$ = 46 nM
MMP-14 IC$_{50}$ = 2,250 nM
TACE IC$_{50}$ = 40,000 nM
Aggrecanase-1 IC$_{50}$ = 18,000 nM
Aggrecanase-2 IC$_{50}$ = 22,600 nM

FIGURE 9.6 Another set of potential and selective MMP-12 inhibitors (compounds **9.48–9.53**).

TABLE 9.3

Dibenzofuran Sulfonamide-Based Carboxylic Acid Derivatives as Potent and Selective MMP-12 Inhibitors (IC_{50} in nM)

Compound	R	MMP-8	MMP-12	MMP-13
9.54	oxazolidine-2-one-3-yl	38	2	176
9.55	1H-pyrazole-1-yl	225	15	555
9.56	3-trifluoromethyl-1H-pyrazole-1-yl	30.80	0.70	244.3
9.57	3-furyl	13.20	0.40	360
9.58	5-methyl-3-furyl	30	0.10	327
9.59	5-chloro-3-furyl	7	0.10	144
9.60	2-thienyl	20	0.20	338
9.61	5-methyl-2-thienyl	25	0.20	240
9.62	Pyrrole-2-yl	57.20	0.40	210
9.63	Thiazole-2-yl	154	1	1,980
9.64	5-methyl-thiazole-2-yl	189.60	1.20	552
9.65	5-i-propyl-1,2,4-oxadiazole-3-yl	85.50	4.50	–
9.66	5-t-butyl-1,2,4-oxadiazole-3-yl	187	17	–
9.67	5-i-butyl-1,2,4-oxadiazole-3-yl	113.40	5.40	–
9.68	5-methoxymethyl-1,2,4-oxadiazole-3-yl	19	1.90	–
9.69	5-trifluoromethyl-1,2,4-oxadiazole-3-yl	99	2.20	–
9.70	5-c-propyl-1,2,4-oxadiazole-3-yl	89.60	1.60	–
9.71	5-c-butyl-1,2,4-oxadiazole-3-yl	101.20	2.30	–
9.72	5-c-hexyl-1,2,4-oxadiazole-3-yl	662.40	7.20	–
9.73	5-phenyl-1,2,4-oxadiazole-3-yl	240	4	–
9.74	5-(tetrahydrofuran-3-yl)-1,2,4-oxadiazole-3-yl	30	0.30	–

heterocyclic ring structures like pyrazine, 4-methyl pyrazine, and morpholine derivatives. However, for all these N-linked derivatives, higher MMP-12 selectivity was maintained over MMP-13. Interestingly, for the C-linked dibenzofuran analogs containing five-membered heterocyclic scaffolds, both MMP-12 inhibitory activity and selectivity over MMP-8 and MMP-13 were greatly improved. Compounds containing 3-furyl (compound **9.57**), 5-methyl-2-furyl (compound **9.58**), 5-chloro-2-furyl (compound **9.59**), 2-thienyl (compound **9.60**), 5-methyl-2-thienyl (compound **9.61**), 2-pyrrolyl (compound **9.62**), 2-thiazolyl (compound **9.63**), and 5-methyl-2-thiazolyl (compound **9.64**) compounds were significantly potent MMP-12 inhibitors (activity in pM) and selective over MMP-8 and MMP-13 (Table 9.3). Among these compounds, remarkable MMP-12 selectivity (> 150-fold) over MMP-8 was observed for compounds **9.58**, **9.63**, and **9.64**, where these three compounds were also more than 450-fold selective over MMP-13. The X-ray crystal structure of compound **9.63** with

MMP-12 explored the dibenzofuran scaffold replaced with the thiazole moiety that completely captured the S1' pocket while the carboxylic acid was found to coordinate with the Zn^{2+} ion. The sulfonyl oxygen atom produced stable hydrogen bonding with the backbone amino acids. Depending on the binding interactions of the crystal structure, it can be presumed that higher hydrophobic interactions at the S1' pocket may improve the efficacy. Therefore, some new oxadiazole derivatives (compound **9.65–9.74**, Table 9.3) were substituted with several alkyl, c-alkyl, aryl, and heteroaryl groups. All of them were highly potent MMP-12 inhibitors where the c-alkyl (compound **9.70–9.72**, Table 9.3), aryl (compound **9.73**, Table 9.3), and heteroaryl (compound **9.74**, Table 9.3) derivatives were highly MMP-12 selective (selectivity > 50-fold over MMP-8) compared with the branched alkyl (compound **9.65–9.67**, Table 9.3) and methoxymethyl (compound **9.68**, Table 9.3) analogs. Compound **9.63** was also tested to check its MMP-12 selectivity over other MMPs and was found to be exceptionally MMP-12-selective over other MMPs (MMP-2 IC_{50} = 501 nM, MMP-3 IC_{50} = 2,530 nM, MMP-7 IC_{50} = 57,700 nM, MMP-8 IC_{50} = 154 nM, MMP-9 IC_{50} = 1,970 nM, MMP-13 IC_{50} = 1,980 nM). Besides human MMP-12, Compound **9.63** yielded equipotency to sheep MMP-12. Again, in the case of other animal species, such as MMP-12 of mice, rabbits, dogs, and monkeys, it was moderately potent. At 2 mg/kg iv dose, compound **9.63** provided a lower clearance (5 mL/min/kg) with a high C_{max} (5550 ng/ml), AUC (20317 h ng/ml), and a higher bioavailability (63%). Not only that, compound **9.63** expressed satisfactory oral efficacy while evaluated in the C57BL/6 mouse ear swelling model (30 mg/kg dose) and lung inflammation model (5 mg/kg PO, BID).

Based on the X-ray crystal structure of compound **9.75** (Figure 9.7) with MMP-12 [95], Nuti et al. [96] inserted suitable spacers between the β-N-acetyl-D-glutamine (GlcNAc) as the P2' substituents and the biphenyl sulphonamido carboxylic acid moiety to design a new series of sugar-containing thioureido and triazole-containing water-soluble potent and MMP-12-selective inhibitors.

Although both types of compounds resulted in a stronger affinity toward MMP-12 than MMP-9, the thioureido-based compounds were better than the triazole analogs. Although compound **9.75** was a potent and MMP-12-selective inhibitor (IC_{50} = 35 nM), the X-ray crystallographic data explored that the benzamidoethyl group directed toward the S2' pocket did not contribute to inhibitor binding. The introduction of a thioureidoethyl chain between the GlcNAc and biphenylsulfonamide scaffold yielded a two-fold more potent MMP-12 inhibitor (**9.76**, Figure 9.7) that was more selective over other MMPs compared with the initial compound **9.75**. The crystallographic results showed that as a result of the highly flexible thiourea linker, the sugar moieties were placed in a completely different orientation compared with the respective compounds with triazole linker. Probably, this might be the reason for the greater MMP-12 affinity of thiourea analogs than the respective triazoles. Therefore, due to the incorporation of a flexible thiourea linker as well as the glycosidic part directed toward the S2' pocket, such types of compounds may offer nanomolar inhibitory potency and selectivity toward MMP-12 as well as improving bioavailability. Compound **9.77** (Figure 9.7) with a slight modification as **9.78** of Figure 9.3 (hydroxyl group in the position of the acetyl function) slightly decreased MMP-12

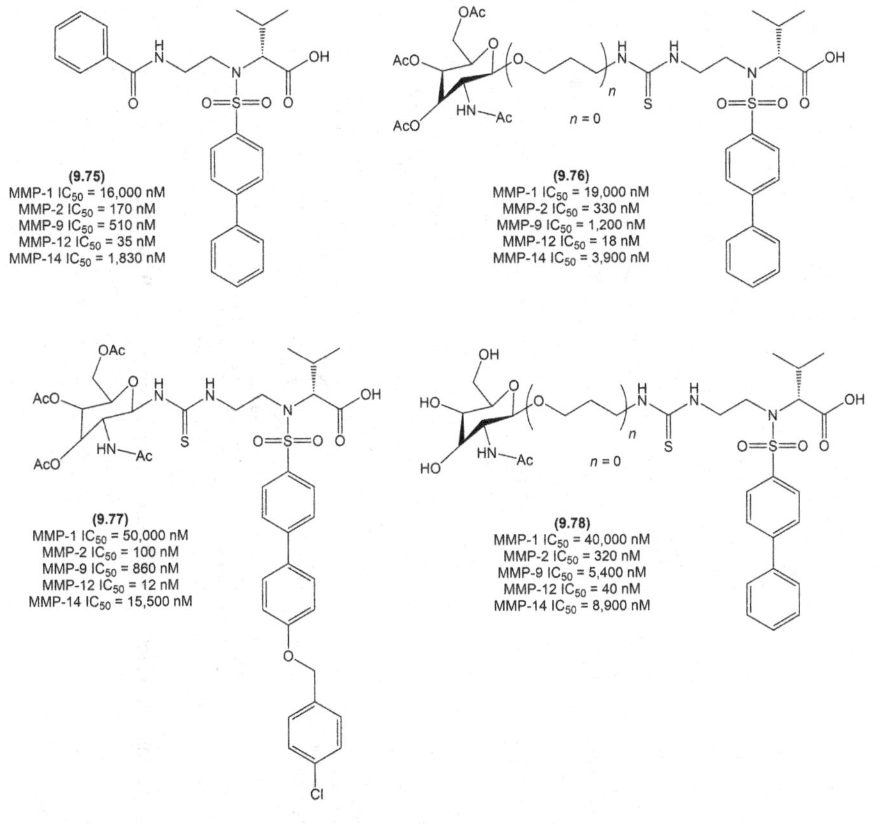

FIGURE 9.7 Some sugar-containing thioureido and triazole-based water-soluble potent and selective MMP-12 inhibitors (compounds **9.75–9.78**).

inhibition ($IC_{50} = 40$ nM) but with greater selectivity compared with compound **9.76**. Replacement of the biphenyl group of compound **9.76** with 4-(4'-chlorobenzyloxy) biphenyl group yielded similar MMP-12 inhibitory potency ($IC_{50} = 12$ nM), but the selectivity over MMP-2 was slightly diminished, and selectivity over MMP-14 was enhanced. Regarding solubility, glycoconjugates 2 and 3 showed increased solubility (> 5 mM). However, due to the bulky P1' substituent of compound **9.78** (Figure 9.7), there was a sharp decrease in solubility (180 µM). Modification of compounds **9.76** and **9.77** [96] with several sugar-based P2' substituents resulted in potential and MMP-12-selective inhibitors over MMP-9 [97]. These molecules showed good initial permeability due to higher lipophilicity and total polar surface area.

Modification of the aryl group of compound **9.75** [96] with a triazole-based cationic scaffold also provided highly potent and MMP-12-selective inhibitors over MMP-2 and MMP-9 (**9.79–9.83**, Figure 9.8) [98]. Compound **9.79** (Figure 9.8) containing a higher group attached to the triazole ring was a potent MMP-12-selective inhibitor ($IC_{50} = 214$ nM) over MMP-2 and MMP-9. Replacement of the thiol group

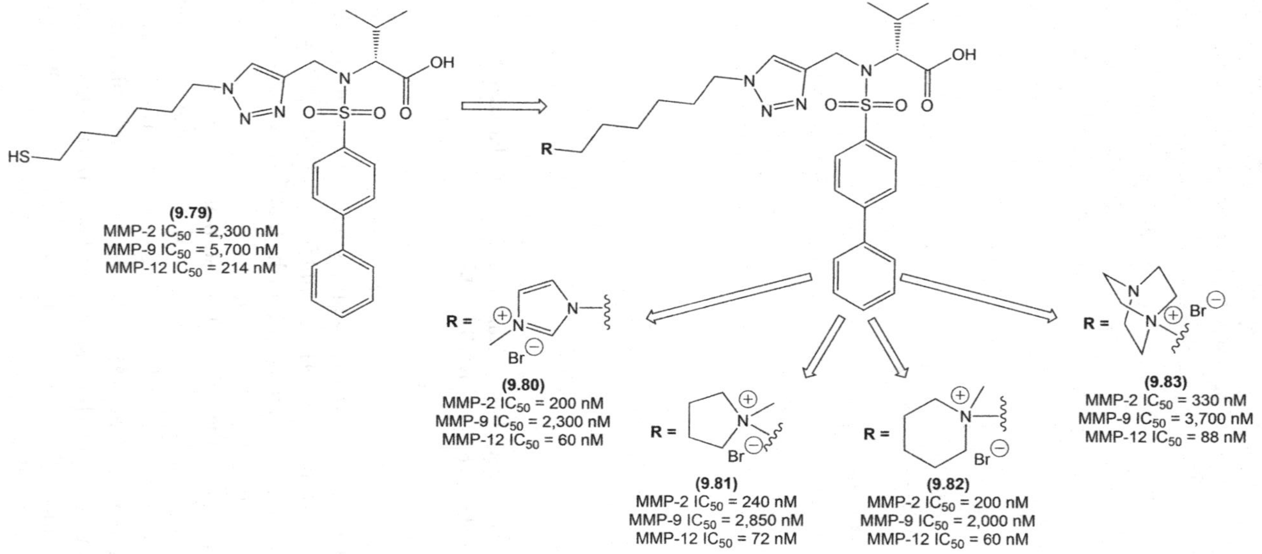

FIGURE 9.8 Some triazole-based cationic scaffold-containing potent and selective MMP-12 inhibitors (compounds **9.79–9.83**).

with heterocyclic ring structures yielded potent MMP-12 inhibitors, but the selectivity over MMP-2 and MMP-9 was diminished.

Devel and coworkers [99] disclosed a set of peptide-containing compounds without any phosphinic ZBG as potent and MMP-12-selective inhibitors (K_i in nM). In this context, compound **9.84** (Figure 9.9) was considered the starting molecule bearing a p-bromo phosphinate moiety at the terminal position, which was a potent and MMP-12-selective inhibitor (K_i = 0.19 nM).

It was highly efficacious as the X-ray crystallographic study showed phosphoryl function interacted strongly with the catalytic Zn^{2+} ion at the active site of MMP-12. Modifying the triaryl group of compound **9.84** with a p-dimethylamino phenylisoxazolyl moiety also produced a potent and highly MMP-12-selective inhibitor (**9.85**, Figure 9.9) [100]. Removal of the phosphinic moiety from compound **9.84** resulted in compounds **9.86** and **9.87** (Figure 9.9), showing the loss of both potency and selectivity, although it was a potent MMP-12-selective inhibitor [99]. Compound **9.86** yielded highly potent MMP-12 inhibition. However, compound **9.87**, containing the carboxylic acid function, produced a reduction in MMP-2 and MMP-13 inhibitory activity with a decrease in MMP-12 inhibitory activities without exhibiting any effect on MMP-3, MMP-8, MMP-9, MMP-10, and MMP-14. Bordenave et al. [101] reported some RXP470-derived probes (**88–92**, Table 9.4), which are highly potent MMP-12-selective inhibitors over other MMPs.

Further moderation of the ZBG phosphoryl function with hydroxamate and carboxylate functions produced potent MMP-12-selective inhibition [102]. Modification of compound **9.93** (Table 9.5) at the side chain aryl groups produced various effective and MMP-12-selective inhibitors [100]. Compound **9.94** (Table 9.5) having a biphenyl isoxazole moiety was a potent and MMP-12-selective inhibitor (K_i = 3.4 nM).

Interestingly, reducing the aryl chain by abolishing the isoxazole ring through replacement with a phenyl function led to the discovery of biphenyl and related compounds that were also effective MMP-12-selective inhibitors. Besides the unsubstituted biphenyl compound (**9.95**, Table 9.5), molecules having substitution at the *meta* position of the terminal phenyl group with hydroxy (**9.96**), nitro (**9.97**), carboxylic acid (**9.98**), chloro (**9.99**), 3,5-dichloro (**9.100**), methoxy (**9.101**), and hydroxymethyl (**9.102**, Table 9.5) yielded highly efficacious MMP-12 inhibition along with good selectivity over other MMPs. In addition, the terphenyl compound (**9.103**, Table 9.5) was also an effective and selective inhibitor. Moreover, the moderation of the terminal phenyl function of compound **9.95** with several heterocyclic moieties produced potential and MMP-12-selective inhibitors. Compounds possessing 2-thienyl (**9.104**), 3-thienyl (**9.105**), pyrrolyl (**9.106**), 5-methyl-2-thienyl (**9.107**), 5-methyl-2-thienyl (**9.108**), 3-methyl-2-thienyl (**9.109**), and 5-methyl-1,2,4-oxadiazole-3-yl (**9.110**) produced highly efficacious and MMP-12-selective inhibitors (Table 9.5). Nevertheless, the introduction of thiophenyl group in between the phenyl groups of the biphenyl moiety resulted in potent and MMP-12-selective inhibitors (**9.111–9.112**, Table 9.5).

The X-ray crystal structure of MMP-12 bound to **9.112** (Table 9.5) showed thienyl producing a higher number of van der Waals interactions with amino acids like Val235, Tyr240, Lys241, Val243, and Phe248. The X-ray crystal structure of

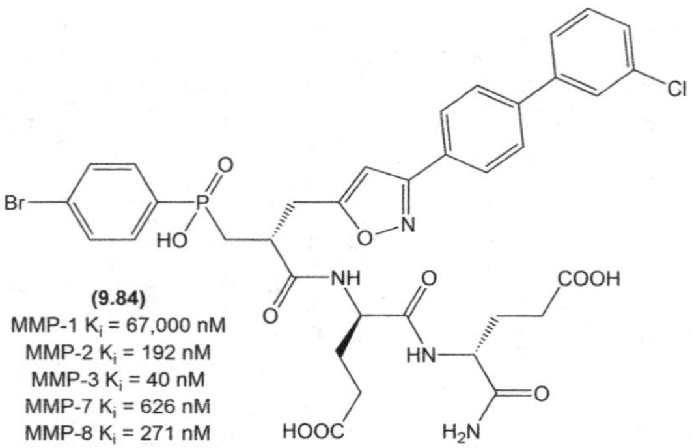

(9.84)

MMP-1 K_i = 67,000 nM
MMP-2 K_i = 192 nM
MMP-3 K_i = 40 nM
MMP-7 K_i = 626 nM
MMP-8 K_i = 271 nM
MMP-9 K_i = 67,000 nM
MMP-10 K_i = 18,400 nM
MMP-12 K_i = 0.19 nM
MMP-13 K_i = 49 nM
MMP-14 K_i = 140 nM

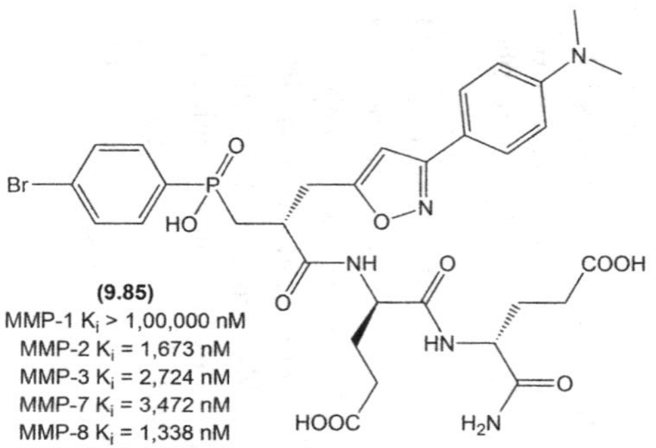

(9.85)

MMP-1 K_i > 1,00,000 nM
MMP-2 K_i = 1,673 nM
MMP-3 K_i = 2,724 nM
MMP-7 K_i = 3,472 nM
MMP-8 K_i = 1,338 nM
MMP-9 K_i = 8,286 nM
MMP-10 K_i = 504 nM
MMP-12 K_i = 4.4 nM
MMP-13 K_i = 6,524 nM
MMP-14 K_i = 871 nM

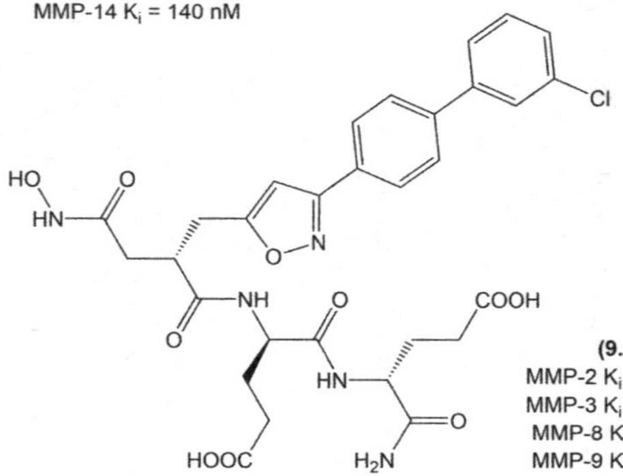

(9.86)

MMP-2 K_i = 0.59 nM
MMP-3 K_i = 0.30 nM
MMP-8 K_i = 8.1 nM
MMP-9 K_i = 8.7 nM
MMP-10 K_i = 1.4 nM
MMP-12 K_i = 0.04 nM
MMP-13 K_i = 0.008 nM
MMP-14 K_i = 2.2 nM

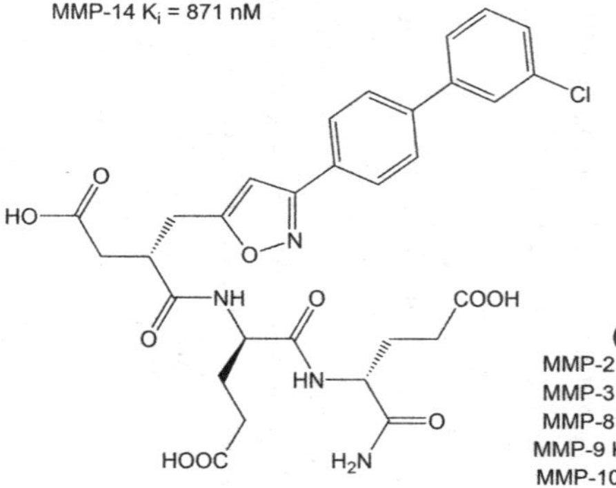

(9.87)

MMP-2 K_i = 290 nM
MMP-3 K_i = 245 nM
MMP-8 K_i = 932 nM
MMP-9 K_i = 3,668 nM
MMP-10 K_i = 318 nM
MMP-12 K_i = 5.8 nM
MMP-13 K_i = 19 nM
MMP-14 K_i = 1,075 nM

FIGURE 9.9   Some peptide-based derivatives as potent and highly selective MMP-12 inhibitors (compounds **9.84–9.87**).

(Continued)

TABLE 9.4
RXP470-Derived Probes as Potent and Selective MMP-12 Inhibitors (Compound 9.88-9.92) (K_i in nM)

TABLE 9.4 (CONTINUED)
RXP470-Derived Probes as Potent and Selective MMP-12 Inhibitors (Compound 9.88-9.92) (K_i in nM)

Cpd	MMP-1	MMP-2	MMP-3	MMP-7	MMP-8	MMP-9	MMP-10	MMP-12	MMP-13	MMP-14
9.88	>10,000	973	31	1,623	2,065	4,167	71	0.90	74	1,133
9.89	4,658	862	187	1,417	1,501	2,172	95	6.7	122	511
9.90	>10,000	1,231	155	821	2,098	3,197	62	5.2	181	1,566
9.91	6,387	2,128	526	944	1,775	3,760	256	5.9	261	1,606
9.92	5,777	860	18	1,273	1,272	2,229	10	0.34	80	445

Cpd, compound.

TABLE 9.5
Several Potential and Selective MMP-12 Inhibitors (K_i in nM)

Cpd	R	MMP-1	MMP-2	MMP-3	MMP-7	MMP-8	MMP-9	MMP-10	MMP-12	MMP-13	MMP-14
9.93	3-Cl	17,900	76	62	1,200	181	565	48	8.3	40	2,060
9.94	H	ND	83	78	ND	383	1,720	114	3.4	60	1,990
9.95	H	>1,00,000	445	6,700	24,700	226	1,090	1,110	18.6	689	5,900
9.96	3-OH	ND	11,400	29,900	ND	1,660	4,340	3,070	176	28,700	28,700
9.97	3-NO$_2$	ND	2,600	24,100	ND	1,250	1,365	3,390	73	463	8,020
9.98	3-COOH	ND	6,380	13,100	ND	4,450	4,150	11,700	91	6,930	26,000
9.99	3-Cl	ND	2,820	55,000	ND	1,890	1,880	6,920	57	1,850	2,370
9.100	3,5-diCl	ND	1,200	1,810	ND	4,820	1,665	2,850	56	1,630	2,340
9.101	3-OMe	ND	8,930	25,300	ND	1,640	8,070	4,170	35	5,460	15,800
9.102	3-CH$_2$OH	ND	7,465	13,300	ND	809	9,100	7,650	52	4,730	12,500
9.103	4-Ph	7,800	53	74	502	132	1,740	76	1.63	20	1,980
9.104	2-Thienyl	>1,00,000	142	2,210	4,000	40	1,540	373	8.6	321	1.10
9.105	3-Thienyl	ND	492	3,070	ND	60	1,790	661	11.9	895	2,630

(Continued)

TABLE 9.5 (CONTINUED)
Several Potential and Selective MMP-12 Inhibitors (K_i in nM)

Cpd	R	MMP-1	MMP-2	MMP-3	MMP-7	MMP-8	MMP-9	MMP-10	MMP-12	MMP-13	MMP-14
9.106	Pyrrolyl	ND	1,370	2,040	ND	373	1,050	1,840	59	1,220	4,850
9.107	5-Me-2-thienyl	ND	97	2,210	ND	10.3	242	353	1.84	564	1,700
9.108	4-Me-2-thienyl	ND	868	3,260	ND	233	2,760	1,415	22	1,300	9,930
9.109	3-Me-2-thienyl	ND	3,380	12,600	ND	766	9,130	2,190	84	1,780	6,310
9.110	5-Me-1,2,4-oxadiazolyl	ND	3,400	6,040	ND	839	2,060	8,320	155	1,090	2,650
9.111	5-Ph-2-Thienyl	ND	279	108	ND	381	874	156	2.58	200	2,280
9.112	4-Ph-2-Thienyl	11,800	1,060	3,880	2,000	410	9,890	872	1.92	684	3,010

Cpd, compound.

compound **9.93** revealed that the chlorophenyl function was moved toward Lys241 and pushed toward the solvent. Again, for the compound **9.112**-MMP-12 complex, the terminal phenyl group was directed toward Phe248. The presence of an additional thienyl ring of compound **9.112** assisted in accommodating the group perfectly at the S1' residues, i.e., Tyr240 and Lys241. However, in the case of compound **9.93**, a large gap produces a bigger void volume between the aryl group and the S1' residues for interaction. Presumably, this might be the reason for the higher efficacy of compound **9.112** with respect to compound **9.93**. Based on the molecular docking analysis performed with compound **9.112** and other MMPs, it was proposed [102] that besides the variations of loop conformation among various MMPs, the variation in the nature of residues at positions 241 and 243 might be the reason for selective inhibition or binding. Nevertheless, the shape of the P1' substituent is also crucial. Here, the linear shape of the P1' substitution of compound **9.93** may occur due to poor selectivity rather than the better selectivity of the bend-shaped P1' substitution of compound **9.112**.

Gona et al. [103] reported some hydroxamate-dependent MMP-12-selective inhibitors and radiotracers. Compound **9.113** (Figure 9.10) exerted potent and highly MMP-12-selective inhibition ($K_i = 1.1$ nM).

Modification of the carboxylic acid function with a glutamic acid moiety produced an equipotent and equi-selective MMP-12 inhibitor (**9.114**, Figure 9.10). Replacement of both acidic groups with amide functions produced potent MMP-12 inhibitors (**9.115**, Figure 9.10), but the selectivity over MMP-2 was greatly lowered. On the other hand, compounds **9.116**, **9.117**, and **9.118** (Figure 9.10), having structural similarities with the earlier compounds, were comparatively less potent but highly effective and selective MMP-12 inhibitors.

As MMP-12 was highly expressed in the abdominal aortic aneurysm (AAA), it was found that ^{99m}Tc-**9.117** and ^{99m}Tc-**9.118** were strongly bound to AAA compared with normal aortic tissue. Again, in C57BL/6J mice, among these two radiolabeled ligands, ^{99m}Tc-**9.118** showed faster blood clearance than ^{99m}Tc-**9.117**. As both these tracers exhibited low uptake in the normal aorta, these may be used effectively for vascular imaging. In the *in vivo* murine model of AAA, ^{99m}Tc-**9.118** revealed a marked uptake of tracer where MMP-12 expression was upregulated. Therefore, specific binding of ^{99m}Tc-**9.118** with molecular imaging may be used for other MMP-12-mediated disease conditions.

A set of fluorinated five-membered heteroaryl-substituted dibenzofuran sulfonamide compounds (**9.119–9.127**, Table 9.6) was designed and evaluated as potential MMP-12-selective inhibitors by Butsch and coworkers [104].

Compound **9.119** (Table 9.6), a fluorinated triazole analog, yielded a potent and highly MMP-12-selective inhibition ($IC_{50} = 0.19$ nM), whereas the respective hydroxamate analog **9.120** (Table 9.6) drastically reduced MMP-12 inhibition ($IC_{50} = 62$ nM), although it was selective. Positional changes of the triazole moiety linked with the fluropropyl and fluroethyl substitutions also produced highly potent MMP-12-selective inhibitors (compounds **9.121–9.122**, Table 9.6). Extremely potent and selective molecules were also observed for fluroethyl-substituted imidazole derivatives (compounds **9.123–9.124**, **Table 9.6**). Nevertheless, highly potent and MMP-12

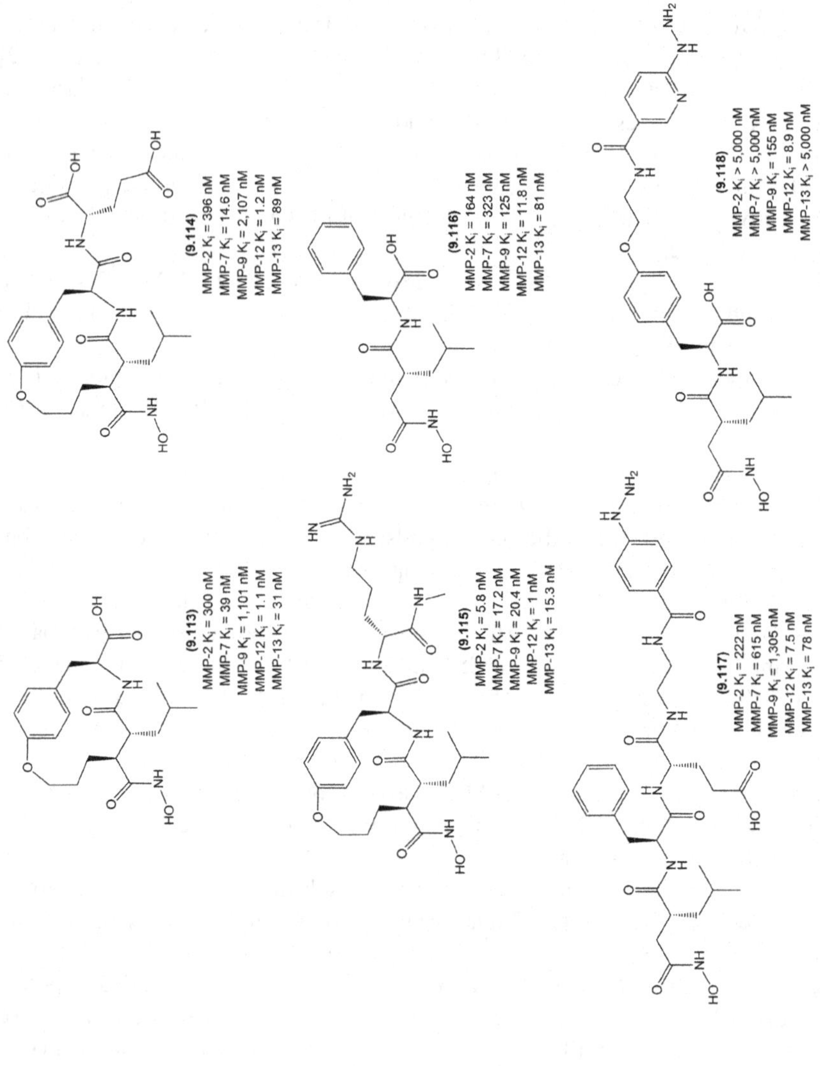

(9.113)
MMP-2 K$_i$ = 300 nM
MMP-7 K$_i$ = 39 nM
MMP-9 K$_i$ = 1,101 nM
MMP-12 K$_i$ = 1.1 nM
MMP-13 K$_i$ = 31 nM

(9.114)
MMP-2 K$_i$ = 396 nM
MMP-7 K$_i$ = 14.6 nM
MMP-9 K$_i$ = 2,107 nM
MMP-12 K$_i$ = 1.2 nM
MMP-13 K$_i$ = 89 nM

(9.115)
MMP-2 K$_i$ = 5.8 nM
MMP-7 K$_i$ = 17.2 nM
MMP-9 K$_i$ = 20.4 nM
MMP-12 K$_i$ = 1 nM
MMP-13 K$_i$ = 15.3 nM

(9.116)
MMP-2 K$_i$ = 164 nM
MMP-7 K$_i$ = 323 nM
MMP-9 K$_i$ = 125 nM
MMP-12 K$_i$ = 11.8 nM
MMP-13 K$_i$ = 81 nM

(9.117)
MMP-2 K$_i$ = 222 nM
MMP-7 K$_i$ = 615 nM
MMP-9 K$_i$ = 1,305 nM
MMP-12 K$_i$ = 7.5 nM
MMP-13 K$_i$ = 78 nM

(9.118)
MMP-2 K$_i$ > 5,000 nM
MMP-7 K$_i$ > 5,000 nM
MMP-9 K$_i$ = 155 nM
MMP-12 K$_i$ = 8.9 nM
MMP-13 K$_i$ > 5,000 nM

FIGURE 9.10 Some hydroxamate-based selective MMP-12 inhibitors (compounds **9.113–9.118**).

TABLE 9.6
Fluorinated Five-Membered Heteroaryl-Substituted Dibenzofuran Sulfonamide Derivatives (IC$_{50}$ in nM)

Compound	R$_1$	R$_2$	MMP-2	MMP-8	MMP-9	MMP-12	MMP-13
9.119	4-(3-fluoropropyl)-1H-1,2,3-triazole-1-yl	OH	81	19	2,230	0.19	288
9.120	4-(3-fluoropropyl)-1H-1,2,3-triazole-1-yl	NHOH	2,670	421	8,760	62	1,170
9.121	N-(3-fluoropropyl)-1H-1,2,3-triazole-4-yl	OH	35	2	>10,000	0.001	16
9.122	N-(3-fluoropropyl)-1H-1,2,3-triazole-4-yl	NHOH	174	27	>10,000	3	62
9.123	1-(2-fluoroethyl)-1H-pyrazole-3-yl	OH	6.5	8.5	413	0.0008	2.4
9.124	1-(2-fluoroethyl)-1H-pyrazole-4-yl	OH	0.84	0.18	151	0.0004	3.2
9.125	4-(2-fluoroethyl)-thiazole-2-yl	OH	55	2	195	0.081	60
9.126	4-(2-fluoroethyl)-5-methyl-thiazol-2-yl	OH	0.49	0.51	200	0.94	12
9.127	5-(2-fluoroethyl)-thiene-2-yl	OH	20	2	58	0.001	20

selective molecules were produced by substituting the pyrazoles with thiazoles (compounds **9.125–9.126**, Table 9.6) and thiophene (compound **9.127**, Table 9.6) analogs.

Azide and -C≡CH substitutions in place of heteroaryl moieties yielded potent MMP-12 inhibition but showed non-selectivity of inhibition among various MMPs. The radiolabeled fluorinated compounds exhibited excellent stability in the *in vitro* and *in vivo* mouse models. Such MMP-12-selective inhibitors may be targeted for treating MMP-12-mediated disease conditions like COPD, irritant contact dermatitis, and collagen-induced arthritis (CIA). Groups of researchers also reported several potential MMP-12 inhibitors that may be effective for managing several disease conditions like COPD [105–107].

9.4 SUMMARY

Among these other MMPs, only MMP-12 has been established as a promising biomolecular target in several disease conditions, especially COPD, asthma, and respiratory distress. Interestingly, among these other types of MMPs, only the mechanisms of MMP-12 have been explored well to date. However, other MMPs (MMP-19, MMP-20, MMP-21, MMP-27, and MMP-28) have not been studied extensively. Various ligand-bound crystal structures of MMP-12 have also been disclosed, revealing the binding pattern of interactions. Importantly, structures of no other type of MMPs mentioned here have crystal structures. The lack of knowledge related to the mechanisms and structures may hinder the discovery of potential inhibitors of other types of MMPs. In this chapter, an outline of other MMPs (especially MMP-12) and their mechanisms in different disease conditions and related potential inhibitors have been discussed in detail. Though little effort has been given to acquire knowledge of other MMPs except for MMP-12, compounds containing various ZBGs may be evaluated to judge their potentiality against other MMPs. Importantly, MMP-12 being a well-established target, several potent and selective inhibitors have been tried. Still, none of them has come out in the market as promising drug candidates, probably because of unwanted adverse effects or unacceptable pharmacokinetic profiles. Considering the importance of MMP-12 in various disease conditions, X-ray crystallographic data with ligand-based drug design and structure-based drug design approaches can be further considered for the design and discovery of potential MMP-12-selective inhibitors as effective drug candidates. In addition, the intuitive designing and binding mode of interaction assessment of the existing inhibitors can also be a fruitful strategy. This chapter may provide useful information regarding future endeavors associated with the discovery of other types of MMP inhibitors.

REFERENCES

[1]. Mondal S, Adhikari N, Banerjee S, et al. Matrix metalloproteinase-9 (MMP-9) and its inhibitors in cancer: A minireview. *Eur J Med Chem.* 2020;194:112260.

[2]. Baggio C, Velazquez JV, Fragai M, et al. Therapeutic targeting of MMP-12 for the treatment of chronic obstructive pulmonary disease. *J Med Chem.* 2020;63(21):12911–12920.

[3]. Chelluboina B, Nalamolu KR, Klopfenstein JD, et al. MMP-12, a promising therapeutic target for neurological diseases. *Mol Neurobiol.* 2018;55(2):1405–1409.

[4]. Nar H, Werle K, Bauer MM, et al. Crystal structure of human macrophage elastase (MMP-12) in complex with a hydroxamic acid inhibitor. *J Mol Biol.* 2001;312(4):743–751.

[5]. Becker JW, Marcy AI, Rokosz LL, et al. Stromelysin-1: Three-dimensional structure of the inhibited catalytic domain and of the C-truncated proenzyme. *Protein Sci.* 1995;4(10):1966–1976.

[6]. Morgunova E, Tuuttila A, Bergmann U, et al. Structure of human pro-matrix metalloproteinase-2: Activation mechanism revealed. *Science.* 1999;284(5420):1667–1670.

[7]. Bode W, Grams F, Reinemer P, et al. The metzincin-superfamily of zinc-peptidases. *Adv Exp Med Biol.* 1996;389:1–11.

[8]. Bode W, Fernandez-Catalan C, Tschesche H, et al. Structural properties of matrix metalloproteinases. *Cell Mol Life Sci.* 1999;55(4):639–652.

[9]. Craig VJ, Zhang L, Hagood JS, et al. Matrix metalloproteinases as therapeutic targets for idiopathic pulmonary fibrosis. *Am J Respir Cell Mol Biol.* 2015;53(5):585–600.

[10]. Mysliwy J, Dingley AJ, Sedlacek R, et al. Structural characterization and binding properties of the hemopexin-like domain of the matrix metalloproteinase-19. *Protein Expr Purif.* 2006;46(2):406–413.

[11]. Pendás AM, Knäuper V, Puente XS, et al. Identification and characterization of a novel human matrix metalloproteinase with unique structural characteristics, chromosomal location, and tissue distribution. *J Biol Chem.* 1997;272(7):4281–4286.

[12]. Mueller MS, Mauch S, Sedlacek R. Structure of the human MMP-19 gene. *Gene.* 2000;252(1–2):27–37.

[13]. Stracke JO, Fosang AJ, Last K, et al. Matrix metalloproteinases 19 and 20 cleave aggrecan and cartilage oligomeric matrix protein (COMP). *FEBS Lett.* 2000;478(1–2):52–56.

[14]. Stracke JO, Hutton M, Stewart M, et al. Biochemical characterization of the catalytic domain of human matrix metalloproteinase 19. Evidence for a role as a potent basement membrane degrading enzyme. *J Biol Chem.* 2000;275(20):14809–14816.

[15]. Titz B, Dietrich S, Sadowski T, et al. Activity of MMP-19 inhibits capillary-like formation due to processing of nidogen-1. *Cell Mol Life Sci.* 2004;61(14):1826–1833.

[16]. Sadowski T, Dietrich S, Koschinsky F, et al. Matrix metalloproteinase 19 regulates insulin-like growth factor-mediated proliferation, migration, and adhesion in human keratinocytes through proteolysis of insulin-like growth factor binding protein-3. *Mol Biol Cell.* 2003;14(11):4569–4580.

[17]. Llano E, Pendás AM, Knäuper V, et al. Identification and structural and functional characterization of human enamelysin (MMP-20). *Biochemistry.* 1997;36(49):15101–15108.

[18]. Illman SA, Lohi J, Keski-Oja J. Epilysin (MMP-28) – Structure, expression and potential functions. *Exp Dermatol.* 2008;17(11):897–907.

[19]. Illman SA, Keski-Oja J, Parks WC, et al. The mouse matrix metalloproteinase, epilysin (MMP-28), is alternatively spliced and processed by a furin-like proprotein convertase. *Biochem J.* 2003;375(Pt 1):191–197.

[20]. Lohi J, Wilson CL, Roby JD, et al. Epilysin, a novel human matrix metalloproteinase (MMP-28) expressed in testis and keratinocytes and in response to injury. *J Biol Chem.* 2001;276(13):10134–10144.

[21]. Gharib SA, Manicone AM, Parks WC. Matrix metalloproteinases in emphysema. *Matrix Biol.* 2018;73:34–51.

[22]. Lagente V, Le Quement C, Boichot E. Macrophage metalloelastase (MMP-12) as a target for inflammatory respiratory diseases. *Expert Opin Ther Targets.* 2009;13(3):287–295.

[23]. Nénan S, Boichot E, Lagente V, Bertrand CP. Macrophage elastase (MMP-12): A pro-inflammatory mediator?. *Mem Inst Oswaldo Cruz.* 2005;100(Suppl 1):167–172.

[24]. Molet S, Belleguic C, Lena H, et al. Increase in macrophage elastase (MMP-12) in lungs from patients with chronic obstructive pulmonary disease. *Inflamm Res.* 2005;54(1):31–36.

[25]. Demedts IK, Morel-Montero A, Lebecque S, et al. Elevated MMP-12 protein levels in induced sputum from patients with COPD. *Thorax.* 2006;61(3):196–201.

[26]. Chaudhuri R, McSharry C, Brady J, et al. Sputum matrix metalloproteinase-12 in patients with chronic obstructive pulmonary disease and asthma: Relationship to disease severity. *J Allergy Clin Immunol.* 2012;129(3):655–663.e8.

[27]. Belvisi MG, Bottomley KM. The role of matrix metalloproteinases (MMPs) in the pathophysiology of chronic obstructive pulmonary disease (COPD): A therapeutic role for inhibitors of MMPs? *Inflamm Res.* 2003;52(3):95–100.

[28]. Abd-Elaziz K, Jesenak M, Vasakova M, Diamant Z. Revisiting matrix metalloproteinase 12: Its role in pathophysiology of asthma and related pulmonary diseases. *Curr Opin Pulm Med.* 2021;27(1):54–60.

[29]. Chiba Y, Yu Y, Sakai H, Misawa M. Increase in the expression of matrix metalloproteinase-12 in the airways of rats with allergic bronchial asthma. *Biol Pharm Bull.* 2007;30(2):318–323.

[30]. Mukhopadhyay S, Sypek J, Tavendale R, et al. Matrix metalloproteinase-12 is a therapeutic target for asthma in children and young adults. *J Allergy Clin Immunol.* 2010;126(1):70-6.e16.

[31]. Zhou Y, Xu M, Gong W, et al. Circulating MMP-12 as potential biomarker in evaluating disease severity and efficacy of sublingual immunotherapy in allergic rhinitis. *Mediators Inflamm.* 2022;2022:3378035.

[32]. Makino A, Shibata T, Nagayasu M, et al. RSV infection-elicited high MMP-12-producing macrophages exacerbate allergic airway inflammation with neutrophil infiltration. *iScience.* 2021;24(10):103201.

[33]. Lygeros S, Danielides G, Kyriakopoulos GC, et al. Evaluation of MMP-12 expression in chronic rhinosinusitis with nasal polyposis. *Rhinology.* 2022;60(1):39–46.

[34]. Yang X, Dong Y, Zhao J, et al. Increased expression of human macrophage metalloelastase (MMP-12) is associated with the invasion of endometrial adenocarcinoma. *Pathol Res Pract.* 2007;203(7):499–505.

[35]. Saleem Z, Shaikh AH, Zaman U, et al. Estimation of salivary matrix metalloproteinases-12 (MMP-12) levels among patients presenting with oral submucous fibrosis and oral squamous cell carcinoma. *BMC Oral Health.* 2021;21(1):205.

[36]. Hofmann HS, Hansen G, Richter G, et al. Matrix metalloproteinase-12 expression correlates with local recurrence and metastatic disease in non-small cell lung cancer patients. *Clin Cancer Res.* 2005;11(3):1086–1092.

[37]. Zheng J, Chu D, Wang D, et al. Matrix metalloproteinase-12 is associated with overall survival in Chinese patients with gastric cancer. *J Surg Oncol.* 2013;107(7):746–751.

[38]. Zucker S, Vacirca J. Role of matrix metalloproteinases (MMPs) in colorectal cancer. *Cancer Metastasis Rev.* 2004;23(1–2):101–117.

[39]. Liu Y, Zhang M, Hao W, et al. Matrix metalloproteinase-12 contributes to neuroinflammation in the aged brain. *Neurobiol Aging.* 2013;34(4):1231–1239.

[40]. Polonskaya YV, Kashtanova EV, Murashov IS, et al. Association of matrix metalloproteinases with coronary artery calcification in patients with CHD. *J Pers Med.* 2021;11(6):506.

[41]. Wang CY, Zhang CP, Li BJ, et al. MMP-12 as a potential biomarker to forecast ischemic stroke in obese patients. *Med Hypotheses.* 2020;136:109524.

[42]. Jguirim-Souissi I, Jelassi A, Slimani A, et al. Matrix metalloproteinase-1 and matrix metalloproteinase-12 gene polymorphisms and the outcome of coronary artery disease. *Coron Artery Dis.* 2011;22(6):388–393.

[43]. Jguirim-Souissi I, Jelassi A, Addad F, et al. Plasma metalloproteinase-12 and tissue inhibitor of metalloproteinase-1 levels and presence, severity, and outcome of coronary artery disease. *Am J Cardiol.* 2007;100(1):23–27.

[44]. Longo GM, Buda SJ, Fiotta N, et al. MMP-12 has a role in abdominal aortic aneurysms in mice. *Surgery.* 2005;137(4):457–462.

[45]. Kaspiris A, Khaldi L, Chronopoulos E, et al. Macrophage-specific metalloelastase (MMP-12) immunoexpression in the osteochondral unit in osteoarthritis correlates with BMI and disease severity. *Pathophysiology.* 2015;22(3):143–151.

[46]. Chen YE. MMP-12, an old enzyme plays a new role in the pathogenesis of rheumatoid arthritis? *Am J Pathol.* 2004;165(4):1069–1070.

[47]. Liu M, Sun H, Wang X, et al. Association of increased expression of macrophage elastase (matrix metalloproteinase 12) with rheumatoid arthritis. *Arthritis Rheum.* 2004;50(10):3112–3117.

[48]. Goncalves DaSilva A, Liaw L, Yong VW. Cleavage of osteopontin by matrix metalloproteinase-12 modulates experimental autoimmune encephalomyelitis disease in C57BL/6 mice. *Am J Pathol.* 2010;177(3):1448–1458.

[49]. Di Sabatino A, Saarialho-Kere U, Buckley MG, et al. Stromelysin-1 and macrophage metalloelastase expression in the intestinal mucosa of Crohn's disease patients treated with infliximab. *Eur J Gastroenterol Hepatol.* 2009;21(9):1049–1055.

[50]. Salmela MT, Pender SL, Reunala T, MacDonald T, Saarialho-Kere U. Parallel expression of macrophage metalloelastase (MMP-12) in duodenal and skin lesions of patients with dermatitis herpetiformis. *Gut.* 2001;48(4):496–502.

[51]. Bassiouni W, Ali MAM, Schulz R. Multifunctional intracellular matrix metalloproteinases: Implications in disease. *FEBS J.* 2021;288(24):7162–7182.

[52]. Brauer R, Tureckova J, Kanchev I, et al. MMP-19 deficiency causes aggravation of colitis due to defects in innate immune cell function. *Mucosal Immunol.* 2016;9(4):974–985.

[53]. Bister VO, Salmela MT, Karjalainen-Lindsberg ML, et al. Differential expression of three matrix metalloproteinases, MMP-19, MMP-26, and MMP-28, in normal and inflamed intestine and colon cancer. *Dig Dis Sci.* 2004;49(4):653–661.

[54]. Djonov V, Högger K, Sedlacek R, et al. MMP-19: Cellular localization of a novel metalloproteinase within normal breast tissue and mammary gland tumours. *J Pathol.* 2001;195(2):147–155.

[55]. Gueders MM, Hirst SJ, Quesada-Calvo F, et al. Matrix metalloproteinase-19 deficiency promotes tenascin-C accumulation and allergen-induced airway inflammation. *Am J Respir Cell Mol Biol.* 2010;43(3):286–295.

[56]. van Horssen J, Vos CM, Admiraal L, et al. Matrix metalloproteinase-19 is highly expressed in active multiple sclerosis lesions. *Neuropathol Appl Neurobiol.* 2006;32(6):585–593.

[57]. Yu G, Kovkarova-Naumovski E, Jara P, et al. Matrix metalloproteinase-19 is a key regulator of lung fibrosis in mice and humans. *Am J Respir Crit Care Med.* 2012;186(8):752–762.

[58]. Zhai LL, Wu Y, Cai CY, et al. High-level expression and prognostic significance of matrix metalloprotease-19 and matrix metalloprotease-20 in human pancreatic ductal adenocarcinoma. *Pancreas.* 2016;45(7):1067–1072.

[59]. Chen Z, Wu G, Ye F, et al. High expression of MMP-19 is associated with poor prognosis in patients with colorectal cancer. *BMC Cancer.* 2019;19(1):448.

[60]. Yu G, Herazo-Maya JD, Nukui T, et al. Matrix metalloproteinase-19 promotes metastatic behavior in vitro and is associated with increased mortality in non-small cell lung cancer. *Am J Respir Crit Care Med.* 2014;190(7):780–790.

[61]. Müller M, Beck IM, Gadesmann J, et al. MMP-19 is upregulated during melanoma progression and increases invasion of melanoma cells. *Mod Pathol.* 2010;23(4):511–521.

[62]. Liu Y, Li Y, Liu Z, et al. Prognostic significance of matrix metalloproteinase-20 overexpression in laryngeal squamous cell carcinoma. *Acta Otolaryngol.* 2011;131(7):769–773.

[63]. Huang Y, Li W, Chu D, et al. Overexpression of matrix metalloproteinase-21 is associated with poor overall survival of patients with colorectal cancer. *J Gastrointest Surg.* 2011;15(7):1188–1194.

[64]. Wang H, Wu JX, Chen XP, et al. Expression and clinical significance of MMP-28 in bladder cancer. *Technol Cancer Res Treat.* 2020;19:1533033820974017.

[65]. Marchenko GN, Strongin AY. MMP-28, a new human matrix metalloproteinase with an unusual cysteine-switch sequence is widely expressed in tumors. *Gene.* 2001;265(1–2):87–93.

[66]. Illman SA, Lehti K, Keski-Oja J, Lohi J. Epilysin (MMP-28) induces TGF-beta mediated epithelial to mesenchymal transition in lung carcinoma cells. *J Cell Sci.* 2006;119(Pt 18):3856–3865.

[67]. Zhang J, Pan Q, Yan W, Wang Y, He X, Zhao Z. Overexpression of MMP-21 and MMP-28 is associated with gastric cancer progression and poor prognosis. *Oncol Lett.* 2018;15(5):7776–7782.

[68]. Zhan G, Wenhua G, Jie H, et al. Potential roles of circulating matrix metalloproteinase-28 (MMP-28) in patients with atrial fibrillation. *Life Sci.* 2018;204:15–19.

[69]. Jeng AY, Chou M, Parker DT. Sulfonamide-based hydroxamic acids as potent inhibitors of mouse macrophage metalloelastase. *Bioorg Med Chem Lett.* 1998;8(8):897–902.

[70]. Dublanchet AC, Ducrot P, Andrianjara C, et al. Structure-based design and synthesis of novel non-zinc chelating MMP-12 inhibitors. *Bioorg Med Chem Lett.* 2005;15(16):3787–3790.

[71]. Ma D, Wu W, Yang G, et al. Tetrahydroisoquinoline based sulfonamide hydroxamates as potent matrix metalloproteinase inhibitors. *Bioorg Med Chem Lett.* 2004;14(1):47–50.

[72]. Ma D, Jiang Y, Chen F, et al. Selective inhibition of matrix metalloproteinase isozymes and in vivo protection against emphysema by substituted gamma-keto carboxylic acids. *J Med Chem.* 2006;49(2):456–458.

[73]. Hayashi R, Jin X, Cook GR. Synthesis and evaluation of novel heterocyclic MMP inhibitors. *Bioorg Med Chem Lett.* 2007;17(24):6864–6870.

[74]. Nordström H, Gossas T, Hämäläinen M, et al. Identification of MMP-12 inhibitors by using biosensor-based screening of a fragment library. *J Med Chem.* 2008;51(12):3449–3459.

[75]. Ando N, Terashima S. Synthesis and matrix metalloproteinase (MMP)-12 inhibitory activity of ageladine A and its analogs. *Bioorg Med Chem Lett.* 2007;17(16):4495–4499.

[76]. Ando N, Terashima S. Synthesis of novel ageladine A analogs showing more potent matrix metalloproteinase (MMP)-12 inhibitory activity than the natural product. *Bioorg Med Chem Lett.* 2009;19(18):5461–5463.

[77]. Mannino C, Nievo M, Machetti F, et al. Synthesis of bicyclic molecular scaffolds (BTAa): An investigation towards new selective MMP-12 inhibitors. *Bioorg Med Chem.* 2006;14(22):7392–7403.

[78]. Sasanelli R, Boccarelli A, Giordano D, et al. Platinum complexes can inhibit matrix metalloproteinase activity: Platinum-diethyl[(methylsulfinyl)methyl]phosphonate complexes as inhibitors of matrix metalloproteinases 2, 3, 9, and 12. *J Med Chem.* 2007;50(15):3434–3441.

[79]. Georgiadis D, Yiotakis A. Specific targeting of metzincin family members with small-molecule inhibitors: Progress toward a multifarious challenge. *Bioorg Med Chem.* 2008;16(19):8781–8794.

[80]. Morales R, Perrier S, Florent JM, et al. Crystal structures of novel non-peptidic, non-zinc chelating inhibitors bound to MMP-12. *J Mol Biol.* 2004;341(4):1063–1076.

[81]. Le Quément C, Guénon I, Gillon JY, et al. The selective MMP-12 inhibitor, AS111793 reduces airway inflammation in mice exposed to cigarette smoke. *Br J Pharmacol.* 2008;154(6):1206–1215.

[82]. Cobos-Correa A, Stein F, Schultz C. Target-activated prodrugs (TAPs) for the auto-regulated inhibition of MMP-12. *ACS Med Chem Lett.* 2012;3(8):653–657.

[83]. Aerts J, Vandenbroucke RE, Dera R, et al. Synthesis and validation of a hydroxypy-rone-based, potent, and specific matrix metalloproteinase-12 inhibitor with anti-inflammatory activity in vitro and in vivo. *Mediators Inflamm.* 2015;2015:510679.

[84]. Badland M, Compère D, Courté K, et al. Thiophene and bioisostere derivatives as new MMP-12 inhibitors. *Bioorg Med Chem Lett.* 2011;21(1):528–530.

[85]. Mori M, Massaro A, Calderone V, et al. Discovery of a new class of potent MMP inhibitors by structure-based optimization of the arylsulfonamide scaffold. *ACS Med Chem Lett.* 2013;4(6):565–569.

[86]. Kallander LS, Washburn D, Hilfiker MA, et al. Reverse hydroxamate inhibitors of bone morphogenetic protein 1. *ACS Med Chem Lett.* 2018;9(7):736–740.

[87]. Holmes IP, Gaines S, Watson SP, et al. The identification of beta-hydroxy carboxylic acids as selective MMP-12 inhibitors. *Bioorg Med Chem Lett.* 2009;19(19):5760–5763.

[88]. Norman P. Selective MMP-12 inhibitors: WO-2008057254. *Expert Opin Ther Pat.* 2009;19(7):1029–1034.

[89]. Hagimori M, Temma T, Kudo S, et al. Synthesis of radioiodinated probes targeted toward matrix metalloproteinase-12. *Bioorg Med Chem Lett.* 2018;28(2):193–195.

[90]. Nuti E, Panelli L, Casalini F, et al. Design, synthesis, biological evaluation, and NMR studies of a new series of arylsulfones as selective and potent matrix metal-loproteinase-12 inhibitors. *J Med Chem.* 2009;52(20):6347–6361.

[91]. Nuti E, Cuffaro D, Bernardini E, et al. Development of thioaryl-based matrix metal-loproteinase-12 inhibitors with alternative zinc-binding groups: Synthesis, potentio-metric, NMR, and crystallographic studies. *J Med Chem.* 2018;61(10):4421–4435.

[92]. Li W, Li J, Wu Y, et al. A selective matrix metalloprotease 12 inhibitor for potential treatment of chronic obstructive pulmonary disease (COPD): Discovery of (S)-2-(8-(methoxycarbonylamino)dibenzo[b,d]furan-3-sulfonamido)-3-methylbutanoic acid (MMP-408). *J Med Chem.* 2009;52(7):1799–1802.

[93]. Li W, Li J, Wu Y, et al. Identification of an orally efficacious matrix metalloprotease 12 inhibitor for potential treatment of asthma. *J Med Chem.* 2009;52(17):5408–5419.

[94]. Wu Y, Li J, Wu J, et al. Discovery of potent and selective matrix metalloprotease 12 inhibitors for the potential treatment of chronic obstructive pulmonary disease (COPD). *Bioorg Med Chem Lett.* 2012;22(1):138–143.

[95]. Antoni C, Vera L, Devel L, et al. Crystallization of bi-functional ligand protein com-plexes. *J Struct Biol.* 2013;182(3):246–254.

[96]. Nuti E, Cuffaro D, D'Andrea F, et al. Sugar-based arylsulfonamide carboxylates as selective and water-soluble matrix metalloproteinase-12 inhibitors. *ChemMedChem.* 2016;11(15):1626–1637.

[97]. Cuffaro D, Camodeca C, D'Andrea F, et al. Matrix metalloproteinase-12 inhibitors: Synthesis, structure-activity relationships and intestinal absorption of novel sugar-based biphenylsulfonamide carboxylates. *Bioorg Med Chem.* 2018;26(22):5804–5815.

[98]. D'Andrea F, Nuti E, Becherini S, et al. Design and synthesis of ionic liquid-based matrix metalloproteinase inhibitors (MMPIs): A simple approach to increase hydrophilicity and to develop MMPI-coated gold nanoparticles. *ChemMedChem.* 2019;14(6):686–698.

[99]. Devel L, Rogakos V, David A, et al. Development of selective inhibitors and substrate of matrix metalloproteinase-12. *J Biol Chem.* 2006;281(16):11152–11160.

[100]. Devel L, Garcia S, Czarny B, et al. Insights from selective non-phosphinic inhibitors of MMP-12 tailored to fit with an S1' loop canonical conformation. *J Biol Chem.* 2010;285(46):35900–35909.

[101]. Bordenave T, Helle M, Beau F, et al. Synthesis and in vitro and in vivo evaluation of MMP-12 selective optical probes. *Bioconjug Chem.* 2016;27(10):2407–2417.

[102]. Rouanet-Mehouas C, Czarny B, Beau F, et al. Zinc-metalloproteinase inhibitors: Evaluation of the complex role played by the zinc-binding group on potency and selectivity. *J Med Chem.* 2017;60(1):403–414.

[103]. Gona K, Toczek J, Ye Y, et al. Hydroxamate-based selective macrophage elastase (MMP-12) inhibitors and radiotracers for molecular imaging. *J Med Chem.* 2020;63(23):15037–15049.

[104]. Butsch V, Börgel F, Galla F, et al. Design, (radio) synthesis, and in vitro and in vivo evaluation of highly selective and potent matrix metalloproteinase 12 (MMP-12) inhibitors as radiotracers for positron emission tomography. *J Med Chem.* 2018;61(9):4115–4134.

[105]. Baggio C, Cerofolini L, Fragai M, et al. HTS by NMR for the identification of potent and selective inhibitors of metalloenzymes. *ACS Med Chem Lett.* 2018;9(2):137–142.

[106]. Schiødt CB, Buchardt J, Terp GE, et al. Phosphinic peptide inhibitors of macrophage metalloelastase (MMP-12). Selectivity and mechanism of binding. *Curr Med Chem.* 2001;8(8):967–976.

[107]. Baggio C, Velazquez JV, Fragai M, Nordgren TM, Pellecchia M. Therapeutic targeting of MMP-12 for the treatment of chronic obstructive pulmonary disease. *J Med Chem.* 2020;63(21):12911–12920.

Part C

Modeling of MMP Inhibitors

10 Modeling Inhibitors of Collagenases

Sandip Kumar Baidya, Suvankar Banerjee,
Nilanjan Adhikari, Balaram Ghosh, and Tarun Jha

CONTENTS

ABSTRACT

Collagenases (especially MMP-1, MMP-8, and MMP-13) play crucial roles in several diseases, such as cancer, arthritis, periodontal disease, and cardiovascular disease.

Considering their implication in various disease conditions, collagenases can be regarded as promising biomolecular targets for designing effective collagenase inhibitors. Depending on different crystallographic data and existing collagenase inhibitors, ligand- and structure-based drug design (LBDD and SBDD) methodologies can be applied to designing and discovering new collagenase inhibitors. In this chapter, various drug-designing approaches conducted on existing collagenase inhibitors are discussed in detail. Applying these LBDD and SBDD methodologies to collagenase inhibitors may unveil novel collagenase inhibitors.

Keywords: Collagenases; MMP-1; MMP-8; MMP-13; QSAR studies; Molecular docking

DOI: 10.1201/9781003303282-13

10.1 INTRODUCTION

Among the various classes of MMPs, collagenase is one of the prime classes participating in several pathophysiological and cellular functions [1]. Four collagenases are known to date, namely collagenase-1 or fibroblast collagenase (MMP-1), collagenase-2 or neutrophil collagenase (MMP-8), collagenase-3 (MMP-13), and collagenase-4 (MMP-18) [2]. A number of studies have been conducted on the first three collagenases (i.e., MMP-1, MMP-8, and MMP-13), and these are well-established, whereas little work has been carried out to date regarding collagenase-4 (MMP-18). Collagenase-1 (MMP-1) has a direct correlation with the progression and cellular invasion of several cancers [1], including breast cancer [3, 4], ovarian cancer [5, 6], melanoma [7, 8], pancreatic cancer [9, 10], esophageal cancer [11, 12], gastric cancer [13, 14], and colorectal cancer [15, 16]. MMP-8 is also linked to various cancers, including oral squamous cell carcinoma [17], prostate cancer [18], head and neck squamous cell carcinoma [17, 19], gastric cancer [20], bladder cancer [21], and breast cancer [22]. Again, MMP-13 is associated with various cancers, namely squamous cell carcinoma [23, 24], lung cancer [25, 26], gastric cancer [27, 28], bladder cancer [29], colorectal cancer [30, 31], thyroid cancer [32], prostate cancer [33], breast cancer [34, 35], head and neck cancer [36, 37], and non-small cell lung cancer (NSCLC) [38]. In addition, MMP-13 is related to several other neoplastic conditions such as hepatocellular carcinoma [39], squamous cell carcinoma [23], tumor angiogenesis [40], malignant peripheral nerve sheath tumors [41], melanoma [42], cutaneous malignant melanoma [43], glioma [44, 45], eyelid basal carcinoma [46], fibrosarcoma [47], osteosarcoma [48], chondrosarcoma [49, 50], and nasopharyngeal carcinoma [51].

Besides cancer, collagenases are also related to the pathophysiology of other disease conditions. MMP-1 has a good correlation with diseases such as cardiovascular disorders [52, 53], chronic obstructive pulmonary disease (COPD) [54], periodontal diseases [55], Parkinson's disease [56], rheumatoid arthritis [57, 58], and osteoarthritis [59, 60]. Again, MMP-8 is associated with diseases like rheumatoid arthritis [61, 62], cardiovascular disorders [63, 64], atherosclerosis [65], gingival growth, periodontal disease [66, 67], chronic tonsillitis [68], obesity and insulin resistance [69], and sepsis [70, 71]. MMP-13 has a direct connection with osteoarthritis and rheumatoid arthritis [72–74], periodontal diseases [75, 76], cardiovascular disorders [77], brain injury [78], diabetes [79], liver fibrosis [80], asthma and COPD [81], and atherosclerosis [82, 83]. Therefore, these collagenases can be targeted for the design and development of potential collagenase inhibitors to combat such disease conditions.

10.2 STRUCTURAL ASPECTS OF COLLAGENASES

Collagenases have a canonical multidomain structure, including an N-terminal signal peptide, propeptide, catalytic domain, proline-rich hinge region, and hemopexin domain [1]. Regarding the structures of collagenases, the N-terminal signal peptide plays a crucial role in guiding the newly synthesized preprocollagenase for secretion [1, 84]. The propeptide comprises a conserved cysteine amino acid residue, also called cysteine switch. Propeptide also produces a covalent linkage with the catalytic

Zn^{2+} ion. The catalytic domain comprises a highly conserved zinc-binding sequence (i.e., HEXXHXXGXXH) that is essential for the proteolytic activity of these MMPs [1]. Collagenases comprise the hemopexin domain and depict sequence similarity to hemopexin, which is highly conserved among MMPs [1]. It is connected to the catalytic region through the proline-rich hinge region. Two cysteine residues flanking the hemopexin domain subsequently produce a disulfide bridge, folding the domain and looking like a four-bladed propeller-like structure [1]. The hemopexin domain is crucial for recognizing the substrate specificity, controlling the proteolytic activity, and assisting in binding tissue inhibitors of metalloproteinases (TIMPs). However, collagenases do not possess any additional fibronectin-II-like inserts [1]. The representative structure of various types of collagenases is depicted in Figure 10.1.

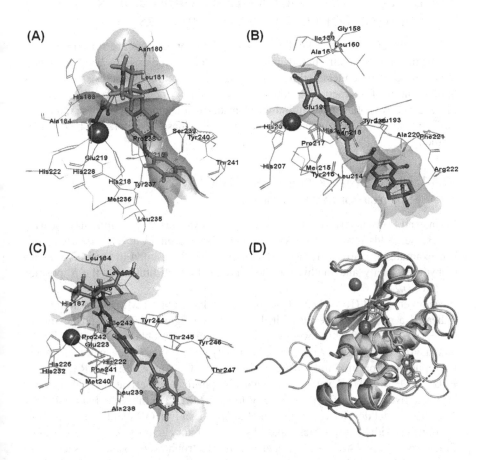

FIGURE 10.1   (A) Active site of MMP-1 with hydroxamate ZBG containing inhibitor (PDB: 966C); (B) Active site of MMP-8 with non-zinc binding inhibitor (PDB: 4DPE); (C) Active site of MMP-13 with non-zinc binding inhibitor (PDB: 3I7I); (D) Alignment of all the collagenases catalytic domains with inbound ligands.

10.3　X-RAY CRYSTAL STRUCTURE AND NMR SOLUTION STRUCTURES OF COLLAGENASES

To date, a high number of X-ray crystallographic structures and NMR solution structures of various collagenases have been reported [85]. Among these collagenase structures, several collagenases are ligand-bound; thus, the ligand's binding pattern into the active site can be explored. Not only that, the crucial catalytic site amino acid residues for ligand binding have also been recognized. Depending on the binding pattern of ligands at the collagenase active site, newer effective and selective inhibitors of collagenases can be designed. Details of the X-ray crystal structures and NMR solution structures of these collagenases are provided in Table 10.1.

10.4　LIGAND- AND STRUCTURE-BASED DRUG DESIGN STRATEGIES OF COLLAGENASE INHIBITORS

As far as the crucial roles of collagenases in different diseases are concerned, various ligand- and structure-based molecular modeling studies have been conducted to date for a better understanding of the essential structural attributes as well as the binding mode of interactions modulating the inhibitory potential of collagenases by these respective collagenase inhibitors. Considering the outcomes of these molecular modeling studies, newer potent and selective collagenase inhibitors can be designed further.

10.4.1　Ligand- and Structure-Based Drug Design Strategies of MMP-1 Inhibitors

Verma and Hansch performed QSAR analyses on various MMP-1 inhibitors bearing diverse scaffolds [86]. The QSAR model performed on 13 acyclic α-sulfonamide hydroxamate derivatives (I) ($R^2 = 0.849$; $Q^2 = 0.727$) resulted in a positive impact of hydrophobicity and methyl and 3-pyridylmethyl substitution at the Y position (Figure 10.2A).

Another model ($R^2 = 0.827$, $Q^2 = 0.731$) conducted on 11 MMP-1 inhibitors (II) indicated a positive influence of hydrophobicity (Figure 10.2B). A further model ($R^2 = 0.973$, $Q^2 = 0.939$) developed on eight human fibroblast collagenase inhibitors, having P1' modified *t*-butyl glycine moiety (III), produced a negative impact of hydrophobicity on inhibitory efficacy (Figure 10.2C). Again, the QSAR model ($R^2 = 0.848$, $Q^2 = 0.747$) developed on eight phosphinic acid derivatives (IV) resulted in a negative impact of hydrophobicity toward MMP-1 inhibition (Figure 10.2D). A QSAR model developed on 20 quinolinone derivatives (V) exhibited a parabolic relationship with hydrophobicity and MMP-1 inhibitory activity, where the optimum ClogP value was 2.481. It suggested that the hydrophobicity value of such types of molecules should be within the range; beyond that value, the MMP-1 inhibitory activity further decreased (Figure 10.2E). In addition, the presence of the methoxy group at the *para* position of the arylsulfonamide moiety was favorable for MMP-1

TABLE 10.1

Details of the X-Ray Crystal Structures and NMR Solution Structures of Collagenases [85]

PDB ID	Collagenases	Type	Structure	Resolution (Å)	Sequence length	Substrate/inhibitor	Year of release
3AYK	MMP-1	Solution NMR	Catalytic domain	–	169	N-hydroxy-2(R)-[[(4-methoxyphenyl)sulfonyl](3-picolyl)a mino]-3-methylbutanamide hydrochloride	1999
4AYK	MMP-1	Solution NMR	Catalytic domain	–	169	N-hydroxy-2(R)-[[(4-methoxyphenyl)sulfonyl](3-picolyl)a mino]-3-methylbutanamide hydrochloride	1999
2CLT	MMP-1	X-ray	Catalytic domain	2.67	367	–	2006
1AYK	MMP-1	Solution NMR	Catalytic domain	–	169	–	1998
2AYK	MMP-1	Solution NMR	Catalytic domain	–	169	–	1998
3SHI	MMP-1	X-ray	Catalytic domain	2.20	156	–	2012
966C	MMP-1	X-ray	Catalytic domain	1.90	157	N-hydroxy-2-[4-(4-phenoxy-benzenesulfonyl)-tetrahydro-p yran-4-yl]-acetamide	1999
4AUO	MMP-1	X-ray	–	3.00	367	–	2012
1FBL	MMP-1	X-ray	C-terminal domain	2.50	370	N-[3-(N'-hydroxycarboxamido)-2-(2-methylpropyl)-propano yl]-O-tyrosine-N-methylamide	1995
1SU3	MMP-1	X-ray	–	2.20	450	4-(2-hydroxyethyl)-1-piperazine ethanesulfonic acid	2005
2J0T	MMP-1	X-ray	Catalytic domain	2.54	170	–	2007
1FLS	MMP-13	Solution NMR	Catalytic domain	–	165	N-hydroxy-2-[(4-methoxy-benzenesulfonyl)-pyridin-3-ylme thyl-amino]-3-methyl-benzamide	2000
1FM1	MMP-13	Solution NMR	Catalytic domain	–	165	N-hydroxy-2-[(4-methoxy-benzenesulfonyl)-pyridin-3-ylme thyl-amino]-3-methyl-benzamide	2000
2E2D	MMP-13	X-ray	–	–	180	–	2007
1YOU	MMP-13	X-ray	Catalytic domain	2.30	168	5-(2-ethoxyethyl)-5-[4-(4-fluorophenoxy)phenoxy]pyrimid ine-2,4,6(1H,3H,5H)-trione	2005

(Continued)

TABLE 10.1 (CONTINUED)
Details of the X-Ray Crystal Structures and NMR Solution Structures of Collagenases [85]

PDB ID	Collagenases	Type	Structure	Resolution (Å)	Sequence length	Substrate/inhibitor	Year of release
456C	MMP-13	X-ray	Catalytic domain	2.40	168	2-{4-[4-(4-chloro-phenoxy)-benzenesulfonyl]-tetrahydro-pyran-4-yl}-n-hydroxy-acetamide	1999
830C	MMP-13	X-ray	Catalytic domain	1.60	168	4-[4-(4-chloro-phenoxy)-benzenesulfonylmethyl]-tetrahydro-pyran-4-carboxylic acid hydroxyamide	1999
5UWK	MMP-13	X-ray	–	1.60	172	(S)-3-methyl-2-(4'-(((4-oxo-4,5,6,7-tetrahydro-3h-cyclopenta[d]pyrimidin-2-yl)thio)methyl)-[1,1'-biphenyl]-4-ylsulfonamido)butanoic acid	2017
5UWL	MMP-13	X-ray	–	2.55	172	(S)-N-(3-methyl-1-(methylamino)-1-oxobutan-2-yl)-5-(4-(((4-oxo-4,5,6,7-tetrahydro-3H-cyclopenta[d]pyrimidin-2-yl)thio)methyl)phenyl)furan-2-carboxamide	2017
5UWM	MMP-13	X-ray	–	1.62	172	(R)-N-(3-methyl-1-(methylamino)-1-oxobutan-2-yl)-5-(4-(((4-oxo-4,5,6,7-tetrahydro-3H-cyclopenta[d]pyrimidin-2-yl)thio)methyl)phenyl)furan-2-carboxamide	2017
3ELM	MMP-13	X-ray	–	1.90	171	(2R)-{[5-(4-ethoxyphenyl)thiophen-2-yl]sulfonyl}amino){1-[(1-methylethoxy)carbonyl]piperidin-4-yl}ethanoic acid	2009
2D1N	MMP-13	X-ray	Catalytic domain	2.37	166	–	2006
5B5O	MMP-13	X-ray	Catalytic domain	1.20	172	N-phenyl-4-[(4H-1,2,4-triazol-3-ylsulfanyl)methyl]-1,3-thiazol-2-amine	2017
5B5P	MMP-13	X-ray	Catalytic domain	1.60	172	4-oxo-N-{3-[2-(1H-1,2,4-triazol-3-ylsulfanyl)ethoxy]benzyl}-3,4-dihydroquinazoline-2-carboxamide	2017
5UWN	MMP-13	X-ray	–	3.20	172	N-(2-aminoethyl)-4'-(((4-oxo-4,5,6,7-tetrahydro-3H-cyclopenta[d]pyrimidin-2-yl)thio)methyl)-[1,1'-biphenyl]-4-sulfonamide	2017

(Continued)

TABLE 10.1 (CONTINUED)

Details of the X-Ray Crystal Structures and NMR Solution Structures of Collagenases [85]

PDB ID	Collagenases	Type	Structure	Resolution (Å)	Sequence length	Substrate/inhibitor	Year of release
3WV1	MMP-13	X-ray	Catalytic domain	1.98	171	4-[2-((6-fluoro-2-[(3-methoxybenzyl)carbamoyl]-4-oxo-3,4-dihydroquinazolin-5-yl]oxy)ethyl]benzoic acid	2014
4FU4	MMP-13	X-ray	–	2.85	368	–	2013
3WV3	MMP-13	X-ray	Catalytic domain	1.60	171	N-(3-methoxybenzyl)-4-oxo-3,4-dihydrothieno[2,3-d]pyrimidine-2-carboxamide	2014
1XUC	MMP-13	X-ray	–	1.70	171	N,N'-bis(3-methylbenzyl)pyrimidine-4,6-dicarboxamide	2005
3WV2	MMP-13	X-ray	Catalytic domain	2.30	171	N-(3-methoxybenzyl)-4-oxo-3,4-dihydroquinazoline-2-carboxamide	2014
5BOT	MMP-13	X-ray	–	1.85	171	ethyl 5-carbamoyl-1H-indole-2-carboxylate	2009
3I71	MMP-13	X-ray	–	2.21	171	N-[4-(5-[[(1S)-1-cyclohexyl-2-(methylamino)-2-oxoethyl]carbamoyl]furan-2-yl)phenyl]-1-benzofuran-2-carboxamide	2009
1PEX	MMP-13	X-ray	–	2.70	207	–	1996
1XUR	MMP-13	X-ray	–	1.85	171	N,N'-bis(pyridin-3-ylmethyl)pyrimidine-4,6-dicarboxamide	2004
3O2X	MMP-13	X-ray	–	1.90	164	N-hydroxy-1-(2-methoxyethyl)-4-[[4-(3-[5-[4-(trifluoromethoxy)phenyl]-2H-tetrazol-2-yl]propoxy)phenyl]sulfonyl]piperidine-4-carboxamide	2010
1CXV	MMP-13	X-ray	–	2.00	164	2-[4-[4-(4-chloro-phenoxy)-benzenesulfonyl]-tetrahydro-pyran-4-yl]-N-hydroxy-acetamide	1999
2PJT	MMP-13	X-ray	Catalytic domain	2.80	165	tert-butyl 4-([[4-(but-2-YN-1-ylamino)phenyl]sulfonyl]methyl)-4-[(hydroxyamino)carbonyl]piperidine-1-carboxylate	2007
7JU8	MMP-13	X-ray	–	2.00	171	Tetraethylene Glycol	2020

(Continued)

TABLE 10.1 (CONTINUED)
Details of the X-Ray Crystal Structures and NMR Solution Structures of Collagenases [85]

PDB ID	Collagenases	Type	Structure	Resolution (Å)	Sequence length	Substrate/inhibitor	Year of release
3KRY	MMP-13	X-ray	—	1.90	164	1-(2-methoxyethyl)-N-oxo-4-({4-[4-(trifluoromethoxy)phe noxy]phenyl}sulfonyl)piperidine-4-carboxamide	2009
2YIG	MMP-13	X-ray	—	1.70	171	4-(4-{[(3S)-3-hydroxy-1-azabicyclo[2.2.2]oct-3-yl]ethynyl} phenoxy)-N-(pyridin-4-ylmethyl)benzamide	2011
4FVL	MMP-13	X-ray	—	2.44	368	di(hydroxyethyl)ether; glycerol; S-1,2-propanediol	2012
4G0D	MMP-13	X-ray	—	2.54	368	di(hydroxyethyl)ether; glycerol; S-1,2-propanediol	2012
3ZXH	MMP-13	X-ray	—	1.30	171	N-hydroxy-N^2-(3-methylbutyl)-N^2-(naphthalen-2-ylsul fonyl)-D-valinamide	2011
3TVC	MMP-13	X-ray	—	2.43	169	N-2-[3-(1,1':4',1''-terphenyl-4-yl)propanoyl]-L-alpha-gluta mine; di(hydroxyethyl)ether	2011
4JP4	MMP-13	X-ray	—	1.43	173	N-[(2S)-4-(5-fluoropyrimidin-2-yl)-1-({4-[5-(2,2,2-trifluoro ethoxy)pyrimidin-2-yl]piperazin-1-yl}sulfonyl)butan-2-y l]-N-hydroxyformamide	2013
4JPA	MMP-13	X-ray	—	2.00	173	3-[[(2-[4-([[(4S)-4-methyl-2,5-dioxoimidazolidin-4-yl]m ethyl]sulfonyl)piperazin-1-yl]sulfonyl)pyrimidin-5-yl]oxy)methyl] benzonitrile	2013
2OW9	MMP-13	X-ray	Catalytic domain	1.74	170	benzyl 6-benzyl-5,7-dioxo-6,7-dihydro-5H-[1,3] thiazolo[3,2-C]pyrimidine-2-carboxylate	2007
2OZR	MMP-13	X-ray	Catalytic domain	2.30	170	4-{[1-methyl-2,4-dioxo-6-(3-phenylprop-1-yn-1-yl)-1,4-d ihydroquinazolin-3(2h)-yl]methyl}benzoic acid	2007
4L19	MMP-13	X-ray	—	1.66	171	2-[(4-methylbenzyl)sulfanyl]-3,5,6,7-tetrahydro-4H-cycl openta[d]pyrimidin-4-one	2013
6HV2	MMP-13	X-ray	—	1.71	168	glycerol	2018

(Continued)

TABLE 10.1 (CONTINUED)

Details of the X-Ray Crystal Structures and NMR Solution Structures of Collagenases [85]

PDB ID	Collagenases	Type	Structure	Resolution (Å)	Sequence length	Substrate/inhibitor	Year of release
1ZP5	MMP-8	X-ray	Catalytic domain	1.80	163	N-{2-[(4'-cyano-1,1'-biphenyl-4-yl)oxy]ethyl}-N'-hydroxy-N-methylurea	2005
3DNG	MMP-8	X-ray	—	2.00	163	(5S)-5-(2-amino-2-oxoethyl)-4-oxo-N-[(3-oxo-3,4-dihydro-2H-1,4-benzoxazin-6-yl)methyl]-3,4,5,6,7,8-hexahydro[1]benzothieno[2,3-d]pyrimidine-2-carboxamide	2008
3DPE	MMP-8	X-ray	—	1.60	163	N-{[2-(2-amino-3,4-dioxocyclobut-1-en-1-yl)-1,2,3,4-tetrahydroisoquinolin-7-yl]methyl}-4-oxo-3,5,6,8-tetrahydro-4H-thiopyrano[4',3':4,5]thieno[2,3-d]pyrimidine-2-carboxamide 7,7-dioxide	2008
3DPF	MMP-8	X-ray	—	2.10	163	N-{[2-(2-amino-3,4-dioxocyclobut-1-en-1-yl)-1,2,3,4-tetrahydroisoquinolin-7-yl]methyl}-4-oxo-3,5,6,8-tetrahydro-4H-thiopyrano[4',3':4,5]thieno[2,3-d]pyrimidine-2-carboxamide 7,7-dioxide	2008
1JH1	MMP-8	X-ray	—	2.70	158	but-3-enyl-[5-(4-chloro-phenyl)-3,6-dihydro-[1,3,4]thiadiazin-2-ylidene]-amine	2001
1ZS0	MMP-8	X-ray	—	1.56	163	(1S)-1-{[(4'-methoxy-1,1'-biphenyl-4-yl)sulfonyl]amino}-2-methylpropylphosphonic acid	2005
1ZVX	MMP-8	X-ray	—	1.87	163	(1R)-1-{[(4'-methoxy-1,1'-biphenyl-4-yl)sulfonyl]amino}-2-methylpropylphosphonic acid	2005
1BZS	MMP-8	X-ray	—	1.70	165	2-(biphenyl-4-sulfonyl)-1,2,3,4-tetrahydro-isoquinoline-3-carboxylic acid	1998

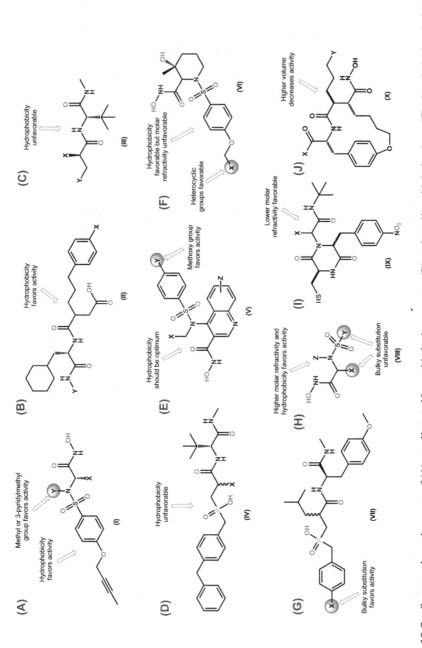

FIGURE 10.2 Structural requirements of (A) acyclic α-sulfonamide hydroxamates; (B) carboxylic acid derivatives; (C) t-butyl glycine derivatives; (D) phosphinic acid derivatives; (E) quinolinone derivatives; (F) 3-hydroxy,3-methylpipecolic hydroxamates; (G) phosphinic acid derivatives; (H) sulfonylated amino acid hydroxamates; (I) diketopiperazine derivatives; (J) macrocyclic hydroxamates for MMP-1 inhibition.

inhibition ($R^2 = 0.891$, $Q^2 = 0.724$). A QSAR model ($R^2 = 0.846$, $Q^2 = 0.761$) constructed on 16 3-hydroxy,3-methylpipecolic hydroxamate derivatives (VI) disclosed a positive impact of hydrophobicity and the presence of heterocyclic groups at the X position, whereas molar refractivity was found to contribute negatively toward MMP-1 inhibition (Figure 10.2F). On the other hand, the QSAR model ($R^2 = 0.850$, $Q^2 = 0.747$) built on nine phosphinic acid derivatives (VII) revealed that bulky substitution at the X position may favor MMP-1 inhibition (Figure 10.2G). Again, the QSAR model ($R^2 = 0.884$, $Q^2 = 0.838$) generated on 31 sulfonylated amino acid hydroxamates (VIII) showed that higher molar refractivity or higher hydrophobicity favored MMP-1 inhibition, whereas bulky substitutions at both X and Y positions were unfavorable for MMP-1 inhibition (Figure 10.2H). Further, the QSAR model ($R^2 = 0.973$, $Q^2 = 0.941$) developed on eight diketopiperazines (IX) reflected a negative impact of molar refractivity toward MMP-1 inhibition (Figure 10.2I). Again, the QSAR model ($R^2 = 0.912$, $Q^2 = 0.857$) developed on eight macrocyclic hydroxamates (X) revealed that a higher volume of such compounds may have a detrimental effect on MMP-1 inhibition (Figure 10.2J).

Kumar and Gupta [87] performed a QSAR study (Figure 10.3A) on 28 sulfonamido hydroxamates having MMP-1 inhibitory efficacy ($R^2 = 0.689$, $R^2_A = 0.66$). The QSAR model revealed the positive impact of electrotopological state atom indices of the sulfonamido nitrogen atom, suggesting that the nitrogen may take part positively in some favorable charge transfer reactions with MMP-1 inhibition. Moreover, the presence of pentafluorophenyl moiety and the *m*-trifluoromethyl phenyl group at the molecular structure may have a positive influence on MMP-1 inhibition.

Gupta et al. [88] conducted a QSAR study (Figure 10.3B) on 19 arylsulfonamide derivatives having MMP-1 inhibitory efficacy ($R^2 = 0.811$, $R^2_A = 0.79$). It was noticed that Kier's first-order valence molecular connectivity index of R substituents ($^1\chi\ ^vR$) contributed negatively toward MMP-1 inhibition. It also suggested that the degree of branching, atom connectivity, and unsaturation in the molecular structure may be detrimental to MMP-1 inhibition. Apart from that, substitution at the W position contributed positively toward MMP-1 inhibition.

Another QSAR model (Figure 10.3C) performed on a total of heteroaryl-containing and hydantoin-based arylsulfonamido hydroxamates disclosed a parabolic relationship between the Kier's first-order valence molecular connectivity index of R substituents and the MMP-1 inhibitory activity ($R^2 = 0.870$, $R^2_A = 0.850$). The availability of π or a lone pair of electrons around the sulfur atom may be favorable for MMP-1 inhibition. Again, the sulfonyl or carbonyl group at the Y position may be beneficial for MMP-1 inhibition.

Verma et al. [89] performed a QSAR model (Figure 10.3D) on some diverse MMP-1 inhibitors. It was noticed that the number of valence electrons contributed positively toward MMP-1 inhibition ($R^2 = 0.956$, $Q^2 = 0.887$). The further model performed on some MMP-1 inhibitors also disclosed a favorable contribution of the number of valence electrons (NVE) toward MMP-1 inhibition.

Jamloki and co-workers [90] performed a QSAR study on 27 MMP-1 inhibitors bearing a 5-amino-2-mercapto-1,3,4-thiadiazole scaffold. The QSAR model

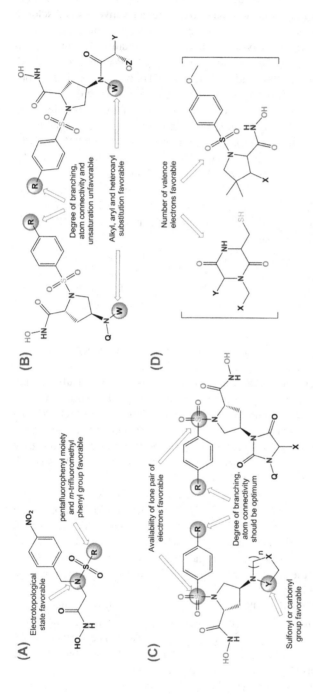

FIGURE 10.3   Structural requirements of (A) sulfonamido hydroxamates; (B) arylsulfonamide derivatives; (C) heteroaryl-containing and hydantoin-based arylsulfonamido hydroxamates; (D) diverse MMP-1 inhibitors for MMP-1 inhibition.

($R^2 = 0.834$, $Q^2 = 0.734$) revealed the positive influence of the carbon valence connectivity index of order 1, the third alpha-modified shape index, and the number of fluorine atoms for MMP-1 inhibition. It further suggested that higher branching may favor MMP-1 inhibition. Moreover, fluorene atoms may be involved in forming favorable hydrogen bonding interactions at the MMP-1 active site (Figure 10.4).

Gupta and Kumaran [91] performed a QSAR study on some anthranilic acid-based MMP-1 inhibitors (**I**) ($R = 0.960$, $Q^2 = 0.800$) (Figure 10.5). The first model revealed a parabolic relationship between lipophilicity (logP) and MMP-1 inhibition. The optimum value of logP was found to be 1.13. These models also expressed that the higher hydrophobicity of such molecules may be responsible for higher MMP-1 inhibition. Similarly, another QSAR model ($R = 0.919$, $Q^2 = 0.670$) performed on another set of anthranilates (**II**) disclosed that higher hydrophobicity may be unfavorable for MMP-1 inhibition (Figure 10.5). However, 3-pyridyl methyl substitution at the R_2 position and aromatic substitution at the R_3 position were favorable for MMP-1 inhibition. Again, another QSAR model ($R = 0.935$, $Q^2 = 0.740$) on another set of anthranilates (**III**), apart from the importance of lower hydrophobicity, aromatic substituent at the R_4 position, and 3-pyridyl methyl substitution a the R_3 position, exhibited the positive influence of bromine substitution at the R_4 position and benzyloxy substitution at the R_1 position (Figure 10.5). Finally, another QSAR model ($R = 0.916$, $Q^2 = 0.670$) on another set of anthranilates (**IV**) disclosed that lower hydrophobicity may be crucial for higher MMP-1 inhibition (Figure 10.5).

Gupta and co-workers [92] conducted a comparative QSAR study on 31 sulphonylated amino acids hydroxamates (**I**) having potential MMP-1 inhibitory activity (Figure 10.6). The QSAR model revealed that the degree of brunching, connectivity of atoms, and unsaturation in molecules may favor MMP-1 inhibition. On the other hand, the eloctrotopological state atom indices of the sulfur atom were favorable, but the eloctrotopological state atom indices of the nitrogen atom were unfavorable for MMP-1 inhibition. Nevertheless, pentafluoro phenyl substitution at the R position had a positive impact on MMP-1 inhibition.

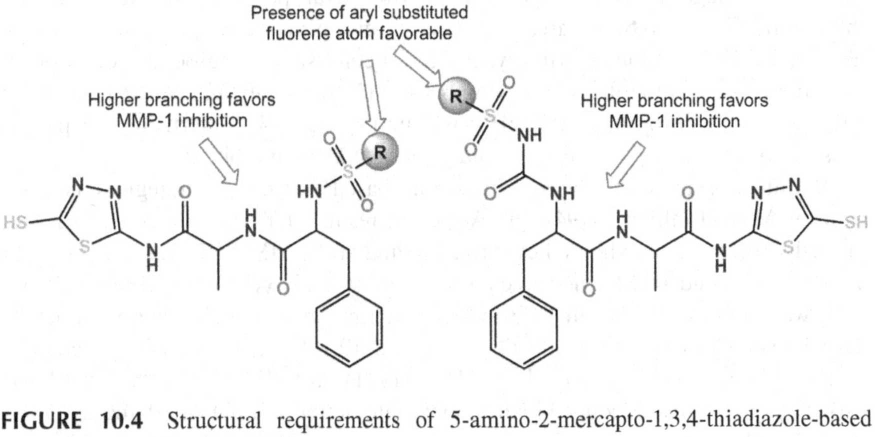

FIGURE 10.4 Structural requirements of 5-amino-2-mercapto-1,3,4-thiadiazole-based compounds for MMP-1 inhibition.

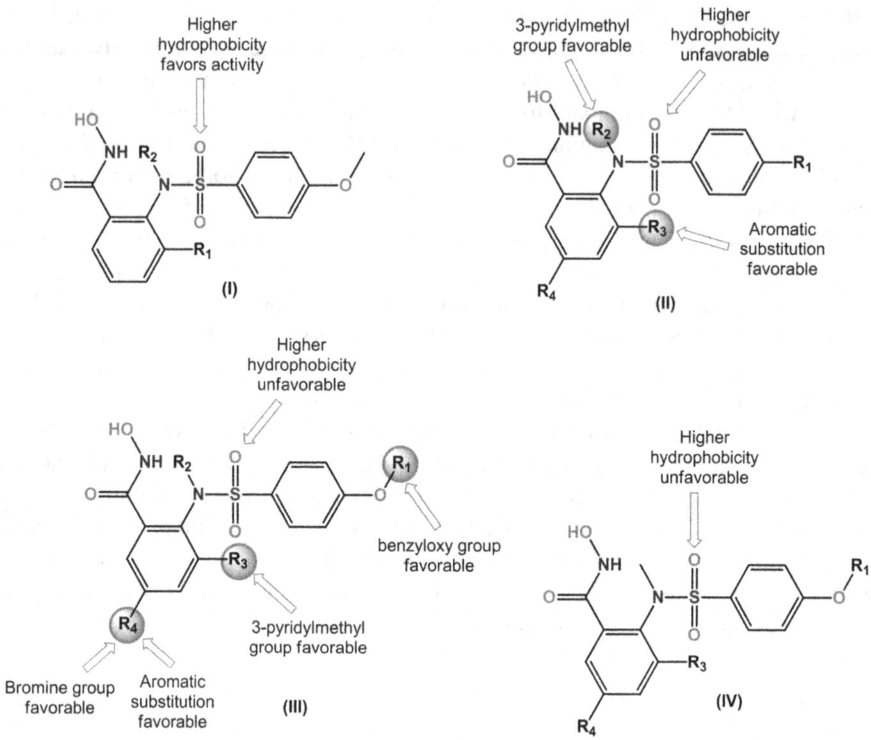

FIGURE 10.5 Structural requirements of some (A) *p*-methoxy phenylsulfonylanthranilates; (B) p-substituted phenylsulfonyl anthranilates; (C) substituted anthranilates; (D) substituted anthranilates for MMP-1 inhibition.

Gupta and Kumaran [93] further performed a QSAR study on some bicyclic heteroaryl hydroxamates having potential MMP-1 inhibitory activity. For the first set of quinoline analogs (II), it was observed that lower hydrophobicity may favor MMP-1 inhibition (Figure 10.6). Again, the methoxy group at the R_2 position was favorable for MMP-1 inhibitory efficacy. For the second set of heterocyclic compounds (III), there was a parabolic relationship between lipophilicity and MMP-1 inhibition (Figure 10.6). The optimum ClogP was found to be 1.14. Nevertheless, 3-pyridyl substitution at the R_1 position was conducive to MMP-1 inhibition.

A number of studies disclosed the structure-based drug design strategies conducted by using MMP-1 inhibitors [94–101]. As per the results of Yuan et al. [94], a derivative of methylrosmarinate exhibited effective binding at the MMP-1 active site (PDB ID: 966C). Compound **10.1** formed zinc chelation to the carboxylic group (Figure 10.7).

It was stabilized through hydrophobic interaction in the S1′ and S3′ pockets. The 4-(benzyloxy)phenyl group of compound **10.1** formed hydrophobic contacts with amino acid residues, namely Val215, Arg214, and His218. On the other hand, 3-(benzyloxy)phenyl produced hydrophobic interactions with Tyr240 and Tyr210 at the S3′ pocket (Figure 10.7). The group at the *para* position of the benzene ring was

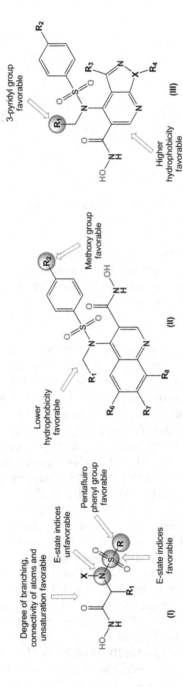

FIGURE 10.6 Structural requirements of (I) sulphonylated amino acids hydroxamates; (II) bicyclic heteroaryl hydroxamates; (III) heterocyclic compounds (IV) for MMP-1 inhibition.

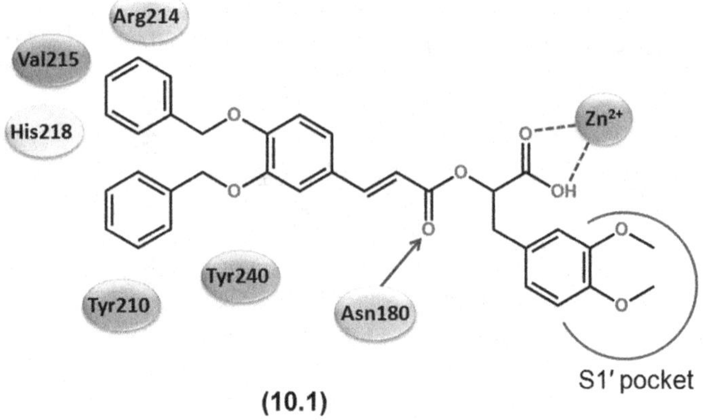

FIGURE 10.7 Binding mode of interaction of compound **10.1** at the MMP-1 active site (PDB ID: 966C).

inserted into the S1' pocket. The carbonyl group formed a hydrogen bonding interaction with Asn180. Smaller hydrophobic groups such as 4-methoxyphenyl, 4-trifluromethylphenyl, and 4-nitrophenyl decreased MMP-1 inhibitory activity, indicating the importance of hydrophobic interaction at the S1' pocket.

Parta et al. [96], through scaffold-based screening and MD simulation, showed that phenolic compounds may be potential MMP-1 inhibitors. Naturally occurring compounds such as berberine, magnolol, epigallocatechin gallate (EGCG), curcumin, phloretin, and quercetin were the most effective MMP-1 inhibitors as per the structure-based design analysis. The molecular modeling study with MMP-1 (PDB ID: 1HFC) showed that EGCG displayed both high MMP-1 inhibition and binding affinity (−8.43 kcal/mol) toward MMP-1, probably due to the formation of hydrogen bonding interactions with Leu181, Ala184, Glu219, Tyr237, and Tyr240. Curcumin exhibited binding affinity toward MMP-1 (-8.61 kcal/mol), forming four hydrogen bonds with active site amino acids Asn180, Leu181, Ala184, and Arg214. Again, phloretin displayed high binding affinity (−8.91 kcal/mol) with MMP-1 by producing hydrogen bonds with amino acids residues Leu181, Ala182, Arg214, His218, Glu219, Leu235, Tyr237, and Pro238. Based on the molecular modeling study, two compounds (ZINC02436922 and ZINC03075557) were finally screened, showing far better binding affinity (i.e., −10.01 kcal/mol and −9.57 kcal/mol, respectively) with MMP-1 (Figure 10.8). Compound ZINC02436922 formed six hydrogen bonding interactions with Asn180, Leu181, Ala182, Ala184, Glu219, and Tyr240 at MMP-1 active site, whereas compound ZINC03075557 formed only one hydrogen bond with Try240 (Figure 10.8).

Yasmeen and Gupta [97] examined the binding pattern of some terpenoid derivatives obtained from *Dalbergia sissoo* into the active site of MMP-1 (PDB ID: 2CLT). Lupeol showed the highest binding free energy (−8.24 kcal/mol) and exhibited hydrogen bonding interactions with Thr204, Asn211, and Leu212.

Priya et al. [98] performed a molecular docking study of some phytochemicals to screen the potential inhibitors of MMP-1. These results disclosed several

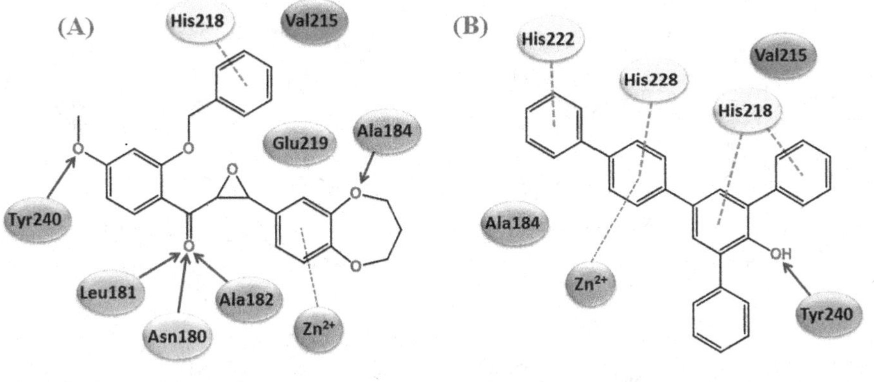

FIGURE 10.8 Binding mode of interaction of (A) ZINC02436922 and (B) ZINC03075557 at the MMP-1 active site (PDB ID: 1HFC).

phytochemicals with zinc binding groups (ZBGs) and non-zinc binding groups (non-ZBGs) as effective MMP-1 inhibitors. Several compounds, such as quercetin, myricetin, luteolin, EGCG, epigallocatechin, and butein, were found as promising MMP-1 inhibitors while docked into the active site of MMP-1 (PDB ID: 1HFC) (Figure 10.9). Quercetin and myricetin both displayed effective hydrogen bonding with amino acid residues Glu219, Tyr240, and Pro238. Importantly, myricetin formed another hydrogen bonding with Tyr210 (Figure 10.9A and B). Luteolin produced two π-π stacking interactions with His218 and His228 and one hydrogen bond with Tyr237 (Figure 10.9C). EGCG, apart from the π-π stacking interaction with His228, formed a π-cationic interaction with the Zn^{2+} ion and three hydrogen bonding with Glu219 (Figure 10.9D). Again, epigallocatechin formed several hydrogen bonding interactions with Asn180, Tyr240, Tyr210, and Glu209 (Figure 10.9E). Butein formed monodentate chelation with Zn^{2+} ion through one phenolic OH group (Figure 10.9F). It also produced two π-π stacking interactions with His218 and His222. In addition, hydrogen bonds were found with Ala184 and Tyr237.

As per the report of Lee et al. [99], (-)-epicatechin and proanthocyanidin B2 were found to be effective MMP-1 inhibitors. The MD simulation study expressed that hydrogen bonding and ionic interactions with amino acid residues such as His218, Glu219, His222, and His228 stabilized the binding with MMP-1. The MM/GBSA analysis revealed the importance of Coulomb interactions and van der Waals interactions for the stabilization of these flavonol-MMP-1 complexes.

10.4.2 LIGAND- AND STRUCTURE-BASED DRUG DESIGN STRATEGIES OF MMP-8 INHIBITORS

A QSAR model [90] produced (R^2 = 0.840, Q^2 = 0.773) on 25 5-amino-2-mercapto-1,3,4-thiadiazole derivatives. MMP-8 inhibitory potential revealed the third

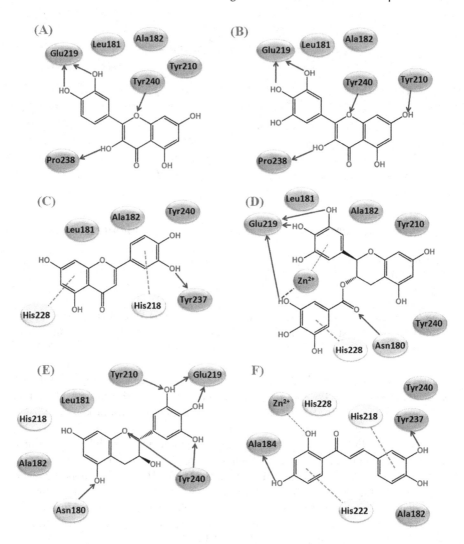

FIGURE 10.9 Binding mode of interaction of (A) quercetin, (B) myricetin, (C) luteolin, (D) EGCG, (E) epigallocatechin, and (F) butein at the MMP-1 active site (PDB ID: 1HFC).

alpha-modified shape index, the number of fluorine atoms, and the presence of an amide function in the vicinity of sulfonamide moiety in these derivatives. It suggested that higher branching at the molecular terminus may favor MMP-8 inhibition. Nevertheless, fluorine atoms may be beneficial for MMP-8 inhibition by forming favorable hydrogen bonding at the active site of MMP-8.

Kumar and Gupta [87] performed a QSAR study ($R^2 = 0.690$, $R^2_A = 0.690$) on 31 MMP-8 inhibitors (Figure 10.10A). The negative coefficient of electrotopological state atom indices of the sulfonamido nitrogen atom negatively contributed to MMP-8 inhibition. Moreover, compounds having pentafluorophenyl moiety and meta-trifluoromethyl phenyl moiety displayed a positive effect on MMP-8 inhibitory activity.

Verma and Hansch [86] performed a QSAR study on 17 sulfonamide derivatives ($R^2 = 0.841$, $Q^2 = 0.739$) (Figure 10.10B). It resulted in the implication of higher hydrophobicity for effective MMP-8 inhibition. Moreover, the presence of the methyl group at the R_2 position was found detrimental to MMP-8 inhibition. Another QSAR model [86] performed on 15 carboxylic acid-based MMP-8 inhibitors ($R^2 = 0.906$, $Q^2 = 0.881$) reflected that bulky substitution having good polarizability as X substituents may favor MMP-8 inhibition (Figure 10.10C). Similarly, the QSAR model [86] performed on 12 nonpeptidic malonic acid hydroxamates ($R^2 = 0.923$, $Q^2 = 0.889$) reflected that higher MMP-8 inhibition was dependent on polarizable Y substituents (Figure 10.10D).

Guti et al. [102] performed a classification-based molecular modeling study of 88 biphenyl sulfonamide MMP-8 inhibitors. A Bayesian classification modeling study revealed that the L-glutamate and L-valine substitutions at the sulfonamide end were unfavorable (Figure 10.11).

Furthermore, the 3-methyl benzofuran 2-carboxamide group at the para position of the biphenyl ring had a negative impact on MMP-8 inhibition. However, bulky substituents, namely N-hydroxy-1,2,3,4-tetrahydroisoquinoiline 3-carboxamide and (1-amino-2-methylpropyl) phosphonic acid groups at the sulfonamido terminal, were found beneficial for MMP-8 inhibitory activity (Figure 10.11). Linear discriminant analysis (LDA) study pointed out that at the sulfonamide moiety, several moieties (such as N-hydroxy 2-carboxamide, t-butyl formate, 2-amino acetamide, and phosphonic

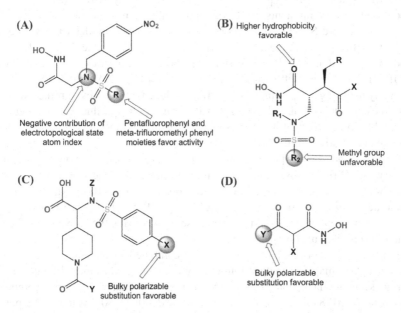

FIGURE 10.10 Structural requirements of (A) arylsulfonamido hydroxamates, (B) sulfonamides, (C) carboxylic acids, and (D) malonic acid hydroxamates for MMP-8 inhibitory activity.

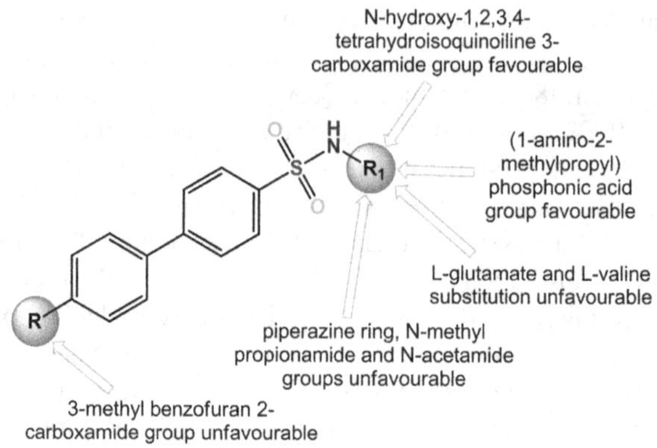

FIGURE 10.11 Structural requirements of biphenyl sulfonamide derivatives for MMP-8 inhibitory activity.

acid) were favorable. However, at the same position, the presence of several groups was found unfavorable (such as piperazine ring, N-methyl propionamide, and N-acetamide) (Figure 10.11). Similarly, the SARpy analysis resulted in 2-amino N-hydroxy prope-namide, piperazine-1-carbaldehyde, and (1-amino-2-methylpropyl) phosphonic acid groups at the sulfonamido end being conducive to MMP-8 inhibition (Figure 10.11).

Matter and co-workers [103] performed a 3D-QSAR CoMFA CoMSIA analysis on 90 1,2,3,4-tetrahydroisoqunoline-3-carboxylates and hydroxamates. The CoMFA model with five components produced statistically significant results ($R^2 = 0.905$, $R^2_{CV} = 0.569$, and SD = 0.321), whereas another CoMFA model with five compo-nents with different grid spacing slightly reduced the R^2_{CV} value (0.516). Both these models exhibited more or less 50% steric and 50% electrostatic contributions toward MMP-8 inhibitory activity. Similarly, in the case of CoMSIA models, these models (either by using a grid spacing of 2Å or 1Å) produced more or less similar outcomes. Both these models exhibited a high R^2 value, but the R^2_{CV} value was just below the acceptable limit (<0.500). Both these CoMSIA models revealed the importance of steric, electrostatic, and hydrophobic contributions.

Cortes-Pacheco et al. [104] examined the binding mode of some bisphosphonic esters with MMP-8. Most of these compounds chelated to the Zn^{2+} ion through the phosphonate group. Hydrogen bonds were observed with the oxygen atoms and amino acid residues, namely His162, Ile159, Tyr219, Leu160, Ala161, and Arg222. Moreover, hydrophobic interactions were also found during the enzyme-ligand inter-action to stabilize this complex.

Kalva and co-workers [105] performed a combined ligand- and structure-based pharmacophore mapping analysis followed by virtual screening and subsequent molec-ular docking and molecular dynamic (MD) simulation analysis to screen compounds as possible MMP-8 inhibitors. The compound ZINC00673680 was found as a possible MMP-8 inhibitor, showing several hydrogen bonding interactions (Arg222), includ-ing water-mediated hydrogen bonding with active site amino acid residues (Ala213, Pro211, Ser228) and π-π stacking interactions with Phe221 (Figure 10.12).

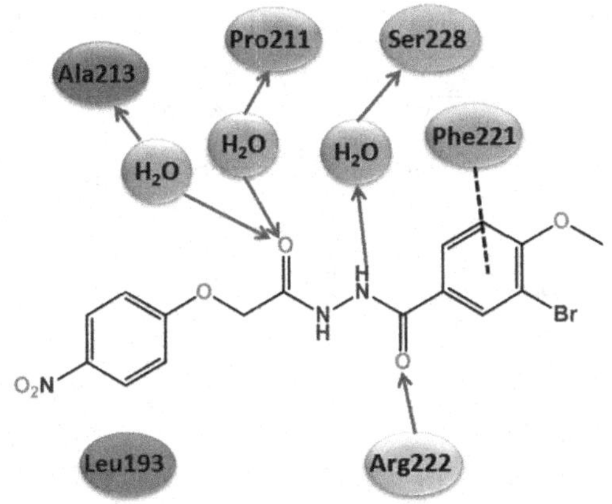

(ZINC00673680)

FIGURE 10.12 Binding mode of interaction of ZINC00673680 at the MMP-8 active site.

10.4.3 LIGAND- AND STRUCTURE-BASED DRUG DESIGN STRATEGIES OF MMP-13 INHIBITORS

A QSAR model [86] developed ($R^2 = 0.959$, $Q^2 = 0.925$) on 14 sulfonamide derivatives (**I**) (Figure 10.13) depicted the importance of higher hydrophobicity and the absence of the methyl group at the R_2 position toward potential MMP-13 inhibition.

Similarly, a QSAR model [86] on six spirobarbiturates (**II**) (Figure 10.13) ($R^2 = 0.871$, $Q^2 = 0.728$) reflected the importance of hydrophobic parameters at X substituents for higher MMP-13 inhibition. Again, the QSAR model [86] developed on nine 3-substituted anthranilate hydroxamic acids (**III**) (Figure 10.13) ($R^2 = 0.952$, $Q^2 = 0.922$) provided the negative implication of hydrophobicity toward higher MMP-13 inhibition. Another QSAR model [86] constructed on ($R^2 = 0.925$, $Q^2 = 0.824$) ten diazepine hydroxamates (**IV**) (Figure 10.13) revealed the importance of a hydrophobic parameter toward Y substituents and the phenyl carbonyl group at Y substituents for higher MMP-13 inhibition. Another QSAR model developed [86] on 15 carboxylic acid derivatives ($R^2 = 0.906$, $Q^2 = 0.799$) (**V**) (Figure 10.13) exhibited the positive influence of molar refractivities imparted by substituents at the X and Y axis and the negative impact of hydrophobic substituents toward the X axis for higher MMP-13 inhibition. Again, the QSAR model developed on [86] ten amide-substituted piperazine derivatives (**VI**) (Figure 10.13) ($R^2 = 0.925$, $Q^2 = 0.842$) disclosed the positive effect of hydrophobicity and the negative effect of molar refractivity toward MMP-13 inhibition. A QSAR model developed [86] on eight 1,4-diazepine-5-hydroxamic acids (**VII**) (Figure 10.13) ($R^2 = 0.889$, $Q^2 = 0.812$) resulted in a positive influence of molar refractivity toward MMP-13 inhibition.

Kumaran and Gupta [106] reported a QSAR study on 22 piperidine sulfonamide aryl hydroxamic acid analogs (Figure 10.14A) as MMP-13 inhibitors ($R^2 = 0.910$, $Q^2 = 0.860$). The study showed that MMP-13 inhibitors were correlated with the

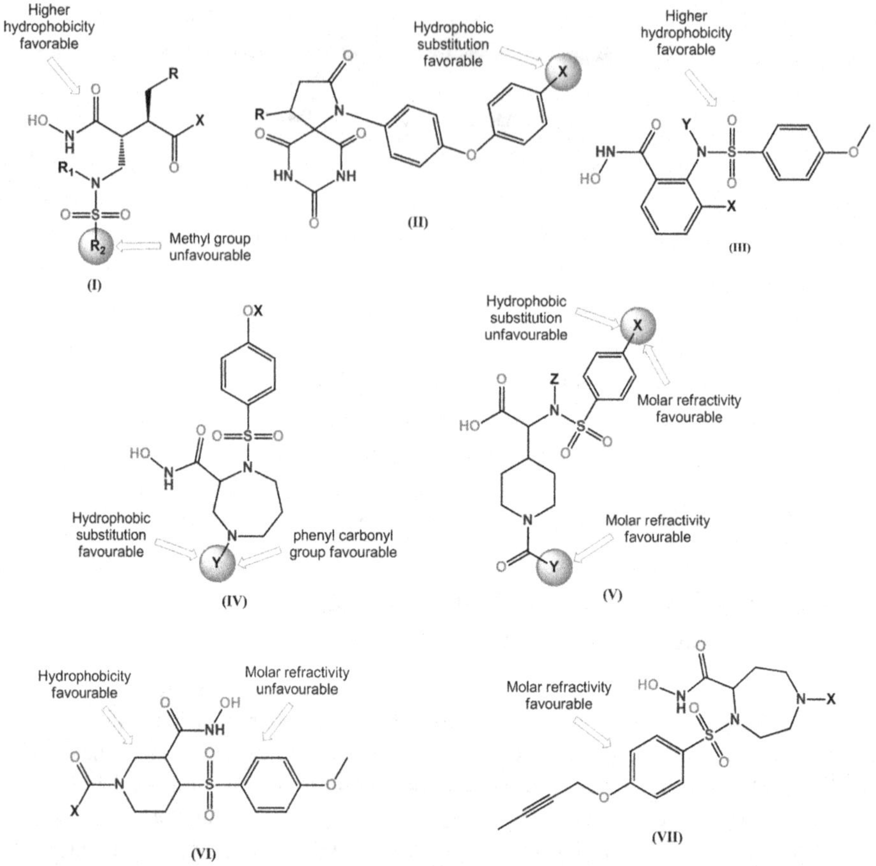

FIGURE 10.13 Structural requirements of (A) sulfonamide derivatives, (B) spirobarbiturates, (C) 3-substituted anthranilate hydroxamic acids, (D) diazepine hydroxamates, (E) carboxylic acid derivatives, (F) amide-substituted piperazine derivatives, and (G) 1,4-diazepine-5-hydroxamic acids for MMP-13 inhibitory activity.

hydrophobicity of these compounds through a parabolic relationship. The optimum value of ClogP was 2.05. Moreover, higher hydrophobicity was not conducive to MMP-13 inhibitory potency. Again, the 4-substituted phenoxy piperidinyl group at the R_1 position expressed a conducive effect toward MMP-13 inhibition.

Further QSAR study reported on 16 MMP-13 inhibitors (Figure 10.14B) from the same group of researchers [107]. The results indicated that MMP-13 inhibition was primarily regulated by the polarizability of these compounds ($R = 0.947$, $Q^2 = 0.720$). Moreover, c-pentyl substitution at the R position and the methyl group at the R_2 position were favorable for the MMP-13 inhibitory activity of these molecules. Another model performed on some arylsulfonamide derivatives (Figure 10.14C) showed the positive influence of hydrophobicity and butynyloxy substitution at the R position ($R = 0.890$, $Q^2 = 0.680$).

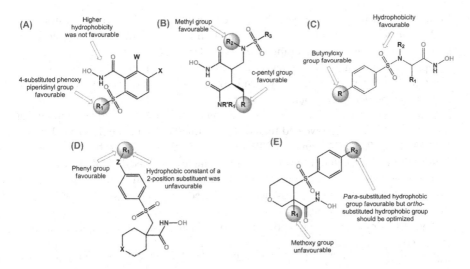

FIGURE 10.14 Structural requirements of (A) piperidine sulfonamide aryl hydroxamic acids, (B) arulsulfonyl hydroxamates, (C) arylsulfonamides, (D) pyranyl hydroxamic acids, and (E) pyran-containing hydroxamates for MMP-13 inhibitory activity.

Kumaran et al. [108] reported a QSAR study conducted on a series of pyranyl hydroxamic acid analogs as MMP-13 inhibitors ($R = 0.884$, $Q^2 = 0.690$) (Figure 10.14D). The QSAR model showed the positive impact of the phenyl group at the R_1 position for higher MMP-13 inhibition. However, the hydrophobic constant of a 2-position substituent at the R_1 position was not conducive to MMP-13 inhibition. Another QSAR model ($R = 0.926$, $Q^2 = 0.680$) performed on another set of pyran-containing hydroxamates revealed that the methoxy group was unfavorable at the R_1 position (Figure 10.14E). The *para*-substituted hydrophobic group at the R_2 position was favorable for MMP-13 inhibition. Again, the *ortho*-substituted hydrophobic group at the R_2 position showed a parabolic relation with MMP-13 inhibition.

A further QSAR study from the same group of researchers [88] on a series of functionalized 4-aminoproline-based hydroxamates as potential MMP-13 inhibitors disclosed the positive impact of Kier's first-order valence molecular connectivity index of the 4-amide group and the R-substituted phenyl ring and the negative impact of the electrotopological state atom index of the sulfur atom on MMP-13 inhibition.

Huang and co-workers [109] performed a QSAR study on 53 quinazolinones as MMP-13 inhibitors. In this work, they systematically studied 3D-QSAR, such as CoMFA, CoMSIA, and Topomer CoMFA, molecular docking, and MD simulations. The key structural features obtained exhibited a great contribution toward MMP-13 inhibitory activity. Both the CoMFA and CoMSIA models qualified internal and external cross-validation (CoMFA: $Q^2 = 0.646$, $R^2 = 0.992$, and $R^2_{pred} = 0.829$; CoMSIA: $Q^2 = 0.704$, $R^2 = 0.992$ and $R^2_{pred} = 0.839$). Similarly, the Topomer CoMFA model produced a Q^2 of 0.592 and an R^2 of 0.714. The 3D-QSAR study disclosed that a small hydrogen bond acceptor group in place of fluoro substitution was favorable for activity. Again, the hydrogen bond acceptor group at the terminal carboxylic acid group was also favorable. Further, the bulky hydrophilic and hydrogen bond acceptor group was found favorable at the phenyl ring attached to the carboxylic acid group. Again, the small electronegative hydrophobic group in place of the oxyethyl function was favorable for activity. Similarly, the electropositive, hydrophilic, and hydrogen bond acceptor group was preferred in place of the methoxy group substituted at the phenyl ring. The molecular docking study of the best active compound at the MMP-13 active site revealed that several amino acids, namely Lys140, Asn215, Met253, Thr247, Thr245, and Ala238, formed effective hydrogen bonding interactions with the functional groups present in the molecule. Based on 3D-QSAR models and molecular docking observations, eight new quinazolinone-based molecules (compounds **10.2–10.9**) were designed. These predicted well as per the CoMFA and CoMSIA models (Figure 10.15).

The MD simulation study showed that the ligand-drug complex maintained a U-shaped conformation. The quinazoline ring formed electrostatic interactions with Gly248, Tyr245, Tyr246, and Tyr247 to maintain stability. In addition, newer designed compounds produced additional hydrogen bonding with Ser250 and Gly248.

Hadizadeh and Shamsara [110] conducted a 3D-QSAR and molecular docking study on a series of 46 carboxylic acid-based MMP-12 and MMP-13 inhibitors. Several alignment principles were used to develop CoMFA/CoMSIA models. In this approach, the best-docked poses were followed by alignment based on their zinc-binding group. From this study, the CoMSIA contour maps suggested that the flexibility of residues Val194, Leu214, and Thr220 had a crucial role directly or indirectly in the ligand binding site of the MMP-13 enzyme, which exhibited intrinsic flexibility toward the S1' pocket.

Kalva et al. [111] reported a ligand and protein-based pharmacophore 3D-QSAR model and molecular docking studies on a series of non-zinc binding 32 human MMP-13 inhibitors. These pharmacophore models were used to screen compounds from ZINC databases to obtain novel MMP-13 inhibitors. The lead molecule was further refined with the help of a docking study. Furthermore, the novel lead compounds were validated with the crystal ligand bind pose, different scoring functions, E-model energies, and ROC curve. Interestingly, the binding mode interaction disclosed that four lead compounds obtained from the ZINC database, i.e., ZINC02535232, ZINC08399795, ZINC12419118, and ZINC00624580, interacted with the specific amino acid residues such as Lys249 and Phe252 through hydrophobic interaction responsible for MMP-13 selectivity and favored strong binding with the side chain residues Leu218, Tyr246, Phe252, and Pro255.

Xi and co-workers [112] reported *in silico* combined docking and QSAR methods conducted on a series of carboxylic acid-based MMP-13 inhibitors. A molecular docking study was initially performed and based on the docked complex, and the descriptors characterizing enzyme-ligand interactions were estimated. Furthermore, the genetic algorithm (GA) and multiple linear regression (MLR) were conducted

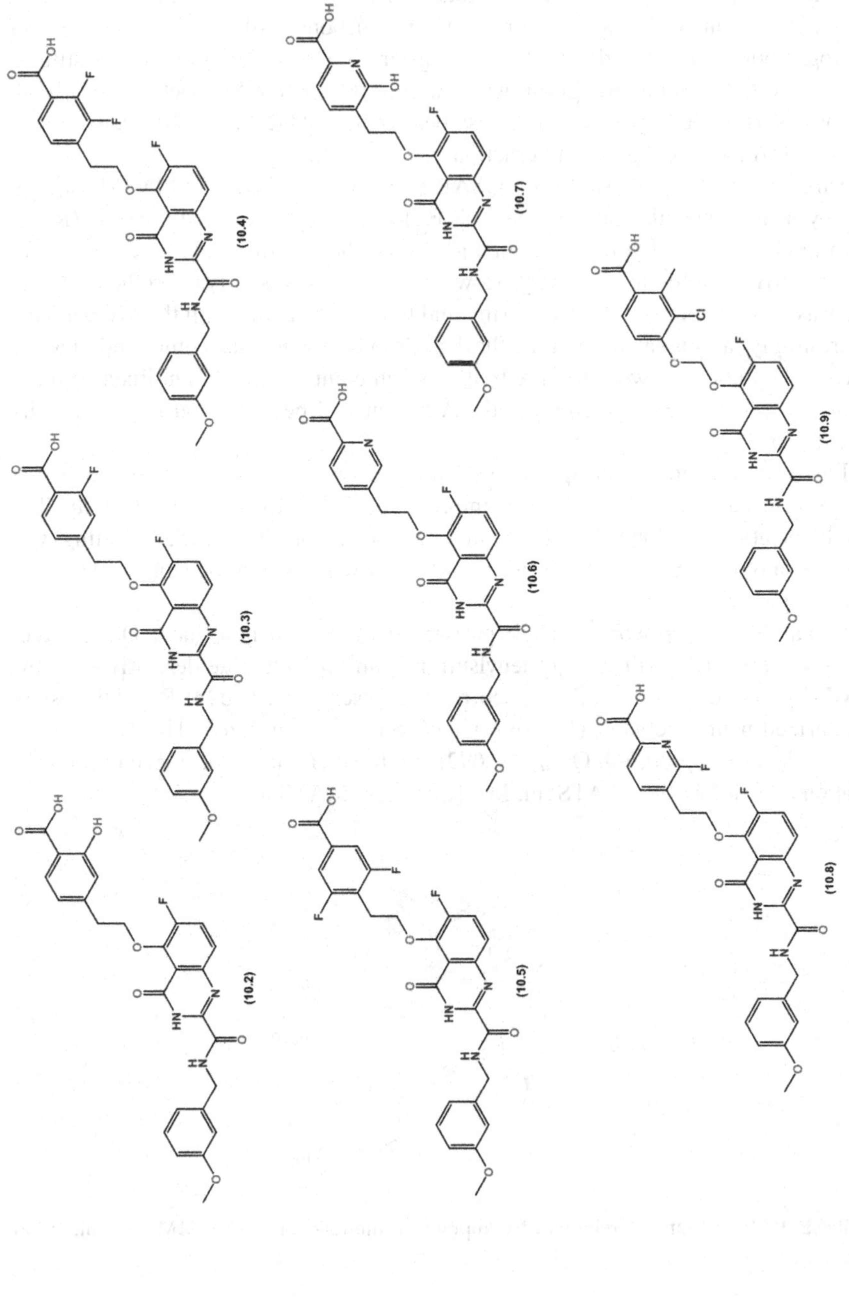

FIGURE 10.15   Newly designed probable potential MMP-13 inhibitors (compounds **10.2–10.9**).

to obtain the crucial descriptors associated with the MMP-13 inhibitory activity. The binding mode of the best active compound in the MMP-13 enzyme active site displayed three important residues, His222, His226, and His232, at the catalytic domain, which is responsible for coordinating with the Zn^{2+} ion. Again, in the ZBG, one oxygen atom was found to form a hydrogen bond with Glu223, and another hydrogen bond was formed with the amide group and Pro242. Again, the substituent adjacent to the sulfonamide group was found to occupy the S1' pocket of MMP-13 and was surrounded by amino acid residues, namely Ala219, Leu218, Ala221, and Leu239, through hydrophobic interaction.

Sarma et al. [113] reported a 3D-QSAR model on a series of 39 MMP-13 inhibitors by using molecular field analysis (MFA) and receptor surface analysis (RSA). Both models revealed similar information about the substitutional requirement for better MMP-13 inhibitory activity. However, the RSA model was predicted better and was in agreement with the experimental results compared with the MFA model. Interestingly, an explanation from the RSA model found that compounds having linear substitution showed better activities when compared with non-linear groups. Again, the electronegative group at the A region will be beneficial for the activity (Figure 10.16).

Furthermore, some electropositive substitution over an aromatic ring attached to the -SO_2 group at the B region may improve the MMP-13 inhibitory activity. The middle position was found conserved and may be responsible for their binding with the Zn^{2+} atom. Again, flexibility in the A and B regions may benefit the MMP-13 inhibitory activity.

Fernández and co-workers [114] performed linear and non-linear QSAR studies on a series of N-hydroxy-2[(phenylsulfonyl)amino]acetamide derivatives having MMP-13 inhibition by using 2D autocorrelation descriptors. The MLR and Bayesian-regularized neural network (BRANN) approaches were utilized. The MLR model ($R^2 = 0.787$, $Q^2_{LOO} = 0.703$, $Q^2_{L3O} = 0.692$) exhibited crucial importance of autocorrelation descriptors like MATS4m, MATS8m, and MATS3v.

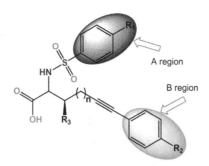

FIGURE 10.16 A and B regions of compound inhibitors for higher MMP-13 inhibitory activity.

Fernández and Caballero [115] further reported QSAR modeling to determine the selectivity of a series of 80 N-hydroxy-phenylsulfonylacetamide derivatives as promising MMP-13 inhibitors by using linear and non-linear predictive models. The QSAR models were built by using MLR combined with a GA. Moreover, the authors conducted a Bayesian regularized genetic neural network (BRGNN) for non-linear modeling. From the QSAR study, it was found that 2D autocorrelation descriptors were crucial for higher MMP-13 inhibitory activity. The autocorrelation descriptors such as MATs6v and GATS6v provided sufficient structural details to yield promising MMP-13 inhibitory activity.

A QSAR study was reported on two novel series of selective non-zinc binding MMP-13 inhibitors [116]. In this work, a significant correlation was found with MMP-13 inhibitory activity and 2D-descriptor, obtained through the combinational protocol in multiple linear regression (CP-MLR) computational procedures. The identified descriptor MPC10 highlighted the role of the molecular path count of order 10, and increasing the value of MPC10 may improve MMP-13 inhibitory activity. Furthermore, the descriptors N-075 or C-030, which correspond to the aromatic ring structural fragments CH-N-CH or N-CH-N, respectively, exhibited a detrimental effect on inhibitory activity.

El Ashry et al. [117] performed a structure-based design and optimization of some pyrimidine-based dual inhibitors of MMP-10/13. One of these compounds showed a π-π stacking interaction with the phenyl ring and Thr245 at the MMP-13 active site (PDB ID: 456C). El-Kashef et al. [118] reported that sulochrin bound to the MMP-13 active site (PDB ID: 1XUD) by forming hydrogen bonding with Pro236, π-π stacking interaction with Phe252, and van der Waals interaction with Leu239, Phe241, and Gly237, as well as hydrophobic interaction with Lys249 and His222.

Ramezani and Shamsara [119] performed a virtual screening to identify new inhibitors of MMP-13. Compound **10.10** produced zinc chelation through the carboxylic acid group, whereas the amide group produced hydrogen bonding with side chain amino acid Glu223, and the hydroxyl group produced hydrogen bonding with backbone amino acids Ala186 and Leu185 (Figure 10.17A). Moreover, a π-π stacking interaction with the phenyl group and His222 was also noticed. Again, compound **10.11** exhibited zinc chelation through the carboxylic group, whereas the adjacent amide and ether functions formed hydrogen bonding with Ala186. Furthermore, the terminal methoxy oxygen produced hydrogen bonding with the side chain amino acid Thr245 (Figure 10.17B). On the other hand, compound **10.12**, without showing zinc chelation, displayed hydrogen bonding with several backbone amino acid residues, namely Leu185, Ala186, Thr245, Ile243, and Phe241 (Figure 10.17C).

As per the report of Nuti et al. [120], one of the potent MMP-13 inhibitors, while binding to the MMP-13 active site, the *para*-chloro benzyloxy diphenyl moiety inserts deep into the large S1' pocket. Again, the *para*-chloro benzyl ring produced a T-shaped interaction with Phe252 and formed a hydrophobic interaction with Leu218 and Leu239. The phenyl ring adjacent to the sulfonamide moiety was flanked by lipophilic residues Leu185 and Val219.

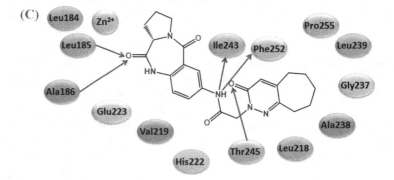

FIGURE 10.17   Binding mode of interaction of (A) compound **10.11**, (B) compound **10.12**, and (C) compound **10.13** at the MMP-13 active site.

10.5 SUMMARY

Collagenases (particularly MMP-1, MMP-8, and MMP-13) are one of the prime members of the MMP family and crucially participate in several diseases, including various cancers, asthma, COPD, osteoarthritis, rheumatoid arthritis, periodontal disease, diabetes, cardiovascular diseases, and atherosclerosis. To date, research has been conducted exploring the crucial roles of these collagenases in various disease conditions. Moreover, many collagenase inhibitors have also been designed, synthesized, and biologically tested. However, due to a lack of selectivity or broad-spectrum MMP inhibition, such collagenase inhibitors are not yet available in the market. Considering their crucial implication in these disease conditions, there is still huge scope to design and discover novel and selective collagenase inhibitors as drug candidates for the management of such disease states. In this context, a huge number of X-ray crystal structures and NMR solution structures, along with the binding orientation of respective collagenase inhibitors, have been disclosed. This can be an added advantage as X-ray crystallographic data provide the 3D orientation of the inbound ligands and explore the crucial binding mode of interaction with key amino acid residues at the active site of respective collagenases. Keeping in mind useful information, structure-based drug design (SBDD) strategies can be applied to obtain fruitful outcomes in terms of the discovery of novel collagenase inhibitors. A variety of molecular modeling studies have been conducted on diverse collagenase inhibitors. Furthermore, various ligand-based drug design (LBDD) methodologies can be considered for the design of selective collagenase inhibitors. In this chapter, several LBDD and SBDD methodologies already carried out on various collagenase inhibitors have been discussed in detail, which can provide crucial information related to the future design of novel collagenase inhibitors. Therefore, considering the abovementioned aspects obtained by these molecular modeling methodologies, there should be a huge scope for designing novel molecules more effective than existing ones. They may open a new horizon in the future design and development of selective collagenase inhibitors.

REFERENCES

[1]. Adhikari N, Amin SA, Jha T. Collagenases and gelatinases and their inhibitors as anticancer agents. In *Cancer-Leading Proteases*. Academic Press, 2020, pp. 265–294.

[2]. Yadav MR, Murumkar PR, Zambre VP. Advances in studies on collagenase inhibitors. *Exp Suppl*. 2012;103:83–135.

[3]. Argote Camacho AX, González Ramírez AR, Pérez Alonso AJ, et al. Metalloproteinases 1 and 3 as potential biomarkers in breast cancer development. *Int J Mol Sci*. 2021;22(16):9012.

[4]. Zhu Y, Tao Z, Chen Y, et al. Exosomal MMP-1 transfers metastasis potential in triple-negative breast cancer through PAR1-mediated EMT. *Breast Cancer Res Treat*. 2022;193(1):65–81.

[5]. Wang FQ, Fisher J, Fishman DA. MMP-1-PAR1 axis mediates LPA-induced epithelial ovarian cancer (EOC) invasion. *Gynecol Oncol*. 2011;120(2):247–255.

[6]. Brinckerhoff CE, Rutter JL, Benbow U. Interstitial collagenases as markers of tumor progression. *Clin Cancer Res*. 2000;6(12):4823–4830.

[7]. Iida J, McCarthy JB. Expression of collagenase-1 (MMP-1) promotes melanoma growth through the generation of active transforming growth factor-beta. *Melanoma Res*. 2007;17(4):205–213.

[8].   Huntington JT, Shields JM, Der CJ, et al. Overexpression of collagenase 1 (MMP-1) is mediated by the ERK pathway in invasive melanoma cells: Role of BRAF mutation and fibroblast growth factor signaling. *J Biol Chem.* 2004;279(32):33168–33176.

[9].   Ito T, Ito M, Shiozawa J, et al. Expression of the MMP-1 in human pancreatic carcinoma: Relationship with prognostic factor. *Mod Pathol.* 1999;12(7):669–674.

[10].   Endo H, Watanabe T, Sugioka Y, et al. Activation of two distinct MAPK pathways governs constitutive expression of matrix metalloproteinase-1 in human pancreatic cancer cell lines. *Int J Oncol.* 2009;35(6):1237–1245.

[11].   Peng HH, Zhang X, Cao PG. MMP-1/PAR-1 signal transduction axis and its prognostic impact in esophageal squamous cell carcinoma. *Braz J Med Biol Res.* 2012;45(1):86–92.

[12].   Murray GI, Duncan ME, O'Neil P, et al. Matrix metalloproteinase-1 is associated with poor prognosis in oesophageal cancer. *J Pathol.* 1998;185(3):256–261.

[13].   Bao W, Fu HJ, Jia LT, et al. HER2-mediated upregulation of MMP-1 is involved in gastric cancer cell invasion. *Arch Biochem Biophys.* 2010;499(1–2):49–55.

[14].   Cai QW, Li J, Li XQ, et al. Expression of STAT3, MMP-1 and TIMP-1 in gastric cancer and correlation with pathological features. *Mol Med Rep.* 2012;5(6):1438–1442.

[15].   Jonsson A, Falk P, Angenete E, et al. Plasma MMP-1 expression as a prognostic factor in colon cancer. *J Surg Res.* 2021;266:254–260.

[16].   Bendardaf R, Buhmeida A, Ristamäki R, et al. MMP-1 (collagenase-1) expression in primary colorectal cancer and its metastases. *Scand J Gastroenterol.* 2007;42(12):1473–1478.

[17].   Kazmi A, Abbas Z, Saleem Z, et al. Relation of salivary MMP-8 with oral submucous fibrosis and oral squamous cell carcinoma: A cross sectional analytical study. *BMJ Open.* 2022;12(12):e060738.

[18].   Memon MA, Aleem B, Memon HA, et al. Assessing salivary matrix metalloproteinase-8 in prostate cancer patients undergoing androgen deprivation therapy. *Clin Exp Dent Res.* 2022;8(5):1277–1283.

[19].   Moilanen M, Pirilä E, Grénman R, et al. Expression and regulation of collagenase-2 (MMP-8) in head and neck squamous cell carcinomas. *J Pathol.* 2002;197(1):72–81.

[20].   Laitinen A, Hagström J, Mustonen H, et al. Serum MMP-8 and TIMP-1 as prognostic biomarkers in gastric cancer. *Tumour Biol.* 2018;40(9):1010428318799266.

[21].   Zhang LF, Zhu LJ, Zhang W, et al. MMP-8 C-799 T, Lys460Thr, and Lys87Glu variants are not related to risk of cancer. *BMC Med Genet.* 2019;20(1):162.

[22].   Thirkettle S, Decock J, Arnold H, et al. Matrix metalloproteinase 8 (collagenase 2) induces the expression of interleukins 6 and 8 in breast cancer cells. *J Biol Chem.* 2013;288(23):16282–16294.

[23].   Wang H, Li H, Yan Q, et al. Serum matrix metalloproteinase-13 as a diagnostic biomarker for cutaneous squamous cell carcinoma. *BMC Cancer.* 2021;21(1):816.

[24].   Mahmoudian RA, Gharaie ML, Abbaszadegan MR, et al. Crosstalk between MMP-13, CD44, and TWIST1 and its role in regulation of EMT in patients with esophageal squamous cell carcinoma. *Mol Cell Biochem.* 2021;476(6):2465–2478.

[25].   Li Y, Sun B, Zhao X, et al. MMP-2 and MMP-13 affect vasculogenic mimicry formation in large cell lung cancer. *J Cell Mol Med.* 2017;21(12):3741–3751.

[26].   Yan HQ, Zhang D, Shi YY, et al. Ataxia-telangiectasia mutated activation mediates tumor necrosis factor-alpha induced MMP-13 up-regulation and metastasis in lung cancer cells. *Oncotarget.* 2016;7(38):62070–62083.

[27].   Sheibani S, Mahmoudian RA, Abbaszadegan MR, et al. Expression analysis of matrix metalloproteinase-13 in human gastric cancer in the presence of Helicobacter pylori infection. *Cancer Biomark.* 2017;18(4):349–356.

[28].   Elnemr A, Yonemura Y, Bandou E, et al. Expression of collagenase-3 (matrix metalloproteinase-13) in human gastric cancer. *Gastric Cancer.* 2003;6(1):30–38.

[29]. Boström PJ, Ravanti L, Reunanen N, et al. Expression of collagenase-3 (matrix metal-loproteinase-13) in transitional-cell carcinoma of the urinary bladder. *Int J Cancer.* 2000;88(3):417–423.

[30]. Yan Q, Yuan Y, Yankui L, et al. The expression and significance of CXCR5 and MMP-13 in colorectal cancer. *Cell Biochem Biophys.* 2015;73(1):253–259.

[31]. Yamada T, Oshima T, Yoshihara K, et al. Overexpression of MMP-13 gene in colorectal cancer with liver metastasis. *Anticancer Res.* 2010;30(7):2693–2699.

[32]. Wang JR, Li XH, Gao XJ, et al. Expression of MMP-13 is associated with inva-sion and metastasis of papillary thyroid carcinoma. *Eur Rev Med Pharmacol Sci.* 2013;17(4):427–435.

[33]. Wang SW, Tai HC, Tang CH, et al. Melatonin impedes prostate cancer metastasis by suppressing MMP-13 expression. *J Cell Physiol.* 2021;236(5):3979–3990.

[34]. Zhang B, Cao X, Liu Y, et al. Tumor-derived matrix metalloproteinase-13 (MMP-13) correlates with poor prognoses of invasive breast cancer. *BMC Cancer.* 2008;8:83.

[35]. Kotepui M, Punsawad C, Chupeerach C, et al. Differential expression of matrix metalloproteinase-13 in association with invasion of breast cancer. *Contemp Oncol (Pozn).* 2016;20(3):225–228.

[36]. Ansell A, Jerhammar F, Ceder R, et al. Matrix metalloproteinase-7 and −13 expres-sion associate to cisplatin resistance in head and neck cancer cell lines. *Oral Oncol.* 2009;45(10):866–871.

[37]. Luukkaa M, Vihinen P, Kronqvist P, et al. Association between high collagenase-3 expression levels and poor prognosis in patients with head and neck cancer. *Head Neck.* 2006;28(3):225–234.

[38]. Hsu CP, Shen GH, Ko JL. Matrix metalloproteinase-13 expression is associated with bone marrow microinvolvement and prognosis in non-small cell lung cancer. *Lung Cancer.* 2006;52(3):349–357.

[39]. Jin D, Tao J, Li D, et al. Golgi protein 73 activation of MMP-13 promotes hepatocel-lular carcinoma cell invasion. *Oncotarget.* 2015;6(32):33523–33533.

[40]. Kudo Y, Iizuka S, Yoshida M, et al. Matrix metalloproteinase-13 (MMP-13) directly and indirectly promotes tumor angiogenesis. *J Biol Chem.* 2012;287(46):38716–38728.

[41]. Holtkamp N, Atallah I, Okuducu AF, et al. MMP-13 and p53 in the progression of malignant peripheral nerve sheath tumors. *Neoplasia.* 2007;9(8):671–677.

[42]. Zhao X, Sun B, Li Y, et al. Dual effects of collagenase-3 on melanoma: Metastasis pro-motion and disruption of vasculogenic mimicry. *Oncotarget.* 2015;6(11):8890–8899.

[43]. Corte MD, Gonzalez LO, Corte MG, et al. Collagenase-3 (MMP-13) expression in cutaneous malignant melanoma. *Int J Biol Markers.* 2005;20(4):242–248.

[44]. Yeh WL, Lu DY, Lee MJ, et al. Leptin induces migration and invasion of glioma cells through MMP-13 production. *Glia.* 2009;57(4):454–464.

[45]. Wang J, Li Y, Wang J, et al. Increased expression of matrix metalloprotein-ase-13 in glioma is associated with poor overall survival of patients. *Med Oncol.* 2012;29(4):2432–2437.

[46]. Mercuţ IM, Simionescu CE, Stepan AE, et al. The immunoexpression of MMP-1 and MMP-13 in eyelid basal cell carcinoma. *Rom J Morphol Embryol.* 2020;61(4):1221–1226.

[47]. Ala-Aho R, Johansson N, Baker AH, et al. Expression of collagenase-3 (MMP-13) enhances invasion of human fibrosarcoma HT-1080 cells. *Int J Cancer.* 2002;97(3):283–289.

[48]. Zapico JM, Acosta L, Pastor M, et al. Design and synthesis of water-soluble and potent MMP-13 inhibitors with activity in human osteosarcoma cells. *Int J Mol Sci.* 2021;22(18):9976.

[49]. Tang CH, Chen CF, Chen WM, et al. IL-6 increases MMP-13 expression and motility in human chondrosarcoma cells. *J Biol Chem.* 2011;286(13):11056–11066.

[50]. Uría JA, Balbín M, López JM, et al. Collagenase-3 (MMP-13) expression in chondrosarcoma cells and its regulation by basic fibroblast growth factor. *Am J Pathol.* 1998;153(1):91–101.

[51]. Shan Y, You B, Shi S, et al. Hypoxia-induced matrix metalloproteinase-13 expression in exosomes from nasopharyngeal carcinoma enhances metastases. *Cell Death Dis.* 2018;9(3):382.

[52]. Ghaffarzadeh A, Bagheri M, Khadem-Vatani K, et al. Association of MMP-1 (rs1799750)-1607 2G/2G and MMP-3 (rs3025058)-1612 6A/6A genotypes with coronary artery disease risk among Iranian turks. *J Cardiovasc Pharmacol.* 2019;74(5):420–425.

[53]. Kondapalli MS, Galimudi RK, Gundapaneni KK, et al. MMP-1 circulating levels and promoter polymorphism in risk prediction of coronary artery disease in asymptomatic first degree relatives. *Gene.* 2016;595(1):115–120.

[54]. Geraghty P, Dabo AJ, D'Armiento J. TLR4 protein contributes to cigarette smoke-induced matrix metalloproteinase-1 (MMP-1) expression in chronic obstructive pulmonary disease. *J Biol Chem.* 2011;286(34):30211–30218.

[55]. Popat R, Bhavsar NV, Popat PR. Gingival crevicular fluid levels of matrix metalloproteinase-1 (MMP-1) and tissue inhibitor of metalloproteinase-1 (TIMP-1) in periodontal health and disease. *Singapore Dent J.* 2014;35:59–64.

[56]. Gupta V, Singh MK, Garg RK, et al. Evaluation of peripheral matrix metalloproteinase-1 in Parkinson's disease: A case-control study. *Int J Neurosci.* 2014;124(2):88–92.

[57]. Zhang C, Chen L, Gu Y. Polymorphisms of MMP-1 and MMP-3 and susceptibility to rheumatoid arthritis. A meta-analysis. *Z Rheumatol.* 2015;74(3):258–262.

[58]. Riley GP, Harrall RL, Watson PG, et al. Collagenase (MMP-1) and TIMP-1 in destructive corneal disease associated with rheumatoid arthritis. *Eye (Lond).* 1995;9(6):703–718.

[59]. Liu J, Wang G, Peng Z. Association between the MMP-1-1607 1G/2G polymorphism and osteoarthritis risk: A systematic review and meta-analysis. *Biomed Res Int.* 2020;2020:5190587.

[60]. Liang L, Zhu DP, Guo SS, et al. MMP-1 gene polymorphism in osteoporosis. *Eur Rev Med Pharmacol Sci.* 2019;23(3):67–72.

[61]. Mattey DL, Nixon NB, Dawes PT. Association of circulating levels of MMP-8 with mortality from respiratory disease in patients with rheumatoid arthritis. *Arthritis Res Ther.* 2012;14(5):R204.

[62]. Tchetverikov I, Lard LR, DeGroot J, et al. Matrix metalloproteinases-3, -8, -9 as markers of disease activity and joint damage progression in early rheumatoid arthritis. *Ann Rheum Dis.* 2003;62(11):1094–1099.

[63]. Aquilante CL, Beitelshees AL, Zineh I. Correlates of serum matrix metalloproteinase-8 (MMP-8) concentrations in nondiabetic subjects without cardiovascular disease. *Clin Chim Acta.* 2007;379(1–2):48–52.

[64]. Cárcel-Márquez J, Cullell N, Muiño E, et al. Causal effect of MMP-1 (matrix metalloproteinase-1), MMP-8, and MMP-12 levels on ischemic stroke: A Mendelian randomization study. *Stroke.* 2021;52(7):e316–e320.

[65]. Lenglet S, Mach F, Montecucco F. Role of matrix metalloproteinase-8 in atherosclerosis. *Mediators Inflamm.* 2013;2013:659282.

[66]. Orozco-Páez J, Rodríguez-Cavallo E, Díaz-Caballero A, et al. Quantification of matrix metalloproteinases MMP-8 and MMP-9 in gingival overgrowth. *Saudi Dent J.* 2021;33(5):260–267.

[67]. Romero-Castro NS, Vázquez-Villamar M, Muñoz-Valle JF, et al. Relationship between TNF-α, MMP-8, and MMP-9 levels in gingival crevicular fluid and the subgingival microbiota in periodontal disease. *Odontology.* 2020;108(1):25–33.

[68]. Ilmarinen T, Lont T, Hagström J, et al. Systemic matrix metalloproteinase-8 response in chronic tonsillitis. *Infect Dis (Lond)*. 2017;49(4):302–307.

[69]. Lauhio A, Färkkilä E, Pietiläinen KH, et al. Association of MMP-8 with obesity, smoking and insulin resistance. *Eur J Clin Invest*. 2016;46(9):757–765.

[70]. Zhou X, Lu J, Chen D, et al. Matrix metalloproteinase-8 inhibitors mitigate sepsis-induced myocardial injury in rats. *Chin Med J (Engl)*. 2014;127(8):1530–1535.

[71]. Sivula M, Hästbacka J, Kuitunen A, et al. Systemic matrix metalloproteinase-8 and tissue inhibitor of metalloproteinases-1 levels in severe sepsis-associated coagulopathy. *Acta Anaesthesiol Scand*. 2015;59(2):176–184.

[72]. Burrage PS, Mix KS, Brinckerhoff CE. Matrix metalloproteinases: Role in arthritis. *Front Biosci*. 2006;11:529–543.

[73]. Hu Q, Ecker M. Overview of MMP-13 as a promising target for the treatment of osteoarthritis. *Int J Mol Sci*. 2021;22(4):1742.

[74]. Wan Y, Li W, Liao Z, et al. Selective MMP-13 inhibitors: Promising agents for the therapy of osteoarthritis. *Curr Med Chem*. 2020;27(22):3753–3769.

[75]. Guimaraes-Stabili MR, de Medeiros MC, Rossi D, et al. Silencing matrix metalloproteinase-13 (Mmp-13) reduces inflammatory bone resorption associated with LPS-induced periodontal disease in vivo. *Clin Oral Investig*. 2021;25(5):3161–3172.

[76]. de Aquino SG, Guimaraes MR, Stach-Machado DR, et al. Differential regulation of MMP-13 expression in two models of experimentally induced periodontal disease in rats. *Arch Oral Biol*. 2009;54(7):609–617.

[77]. Zhang CY, Li XH, Zhang T, Fu J, et al. Hydrogen sulfide suppresses the expression of MMP-8, MMP-13, and TIMP-1 in left ventricles of rats with cardiac volume overload. *Acta Pharmacol Sin*. 2013;34(10):1301–1309.

[78]. Ueno M, Chiba Y, Matsumoto K, et al. Blood-brain barrier damage in vascular dementia. *Neuropathology*. 2016;36(2):115–124.

[79]. Waldron AL, Schroder PA, Bourgon KL, et al. Oxidative stress-dependent MMP-13 activity underlies glucose neurotoxicity. *J Diabetes Complications*. 2018;32(3): 249–257.

[80]. Uchinami H, Seki E, Brenner DA, et al. Loss of MMP 13 attenuates murine hepatic injury and fibrosis during cholestasis. *Hepatology*. 2006;44(2):420–429.

[81]. Howell C, Smith JR, Shute JK. Targeting matrix metalloproteinase-13 in bronchial epithelial repair. *Clin Exp Allergy*. 2018;48(9):1214–1221.

[82]. Quillard T, Tesmenitsky Y, Croce K, et al. Selective inhibition of matrix metalloproteinase-13 increases collagen content of established mouse atherosclerosis. *Arterioscler Thromb Vasc Biol*. 2011;31(11):2464–2472.

[83]. Quillard T, Araújo HA, Franck G, et al. Matrix metalloproteinase-13 predominates over matrix metalloproteinase-8 as the functional interstitial collagenase in mouse atheromata. *Arterioscler Thromb Vasc Biol*. 2014;34(6):1179–1186.

[84]. Ala-aho R, Kähäri VM. Collagenases in cancer. *Biochimie*. 2005;87(3–4):273–286. https://www.rcsb.org/. Accessed April 2023.

[85]. RCSB Protein Data Bank. Available at: https://www.rcsb.org.

[86]. Verma RP, Hansch C. Matrix metalloproteinases (MMPs): Chemical-biological functions and (Q)SARs. *Bioorg Med Chem*. 2007;15(6):2223–2268.

[87]. Kumar D, Gupta SP. A quantitative structure-activity relationship study on some matrix metalloproteinase and collagenase inhibitors. *Bioorg Med Chem*. 2003;11(3):421–426.

[88]. Gupta SP, Kumar D, Kumaran S. A quantitative structure-activity relationship study of hydroxamate matrix metalloproteinase inhibitors derived from functionalized 4-aminoprolines. *Bioorg Med Chem*. 2003;11(9):1975–1981.

[89]. Verma RP, Kurup A, Hansch C. On the role of polarizability in QSAR. *Bioorg Med Chem*. 2005;13(1):237–255.

[90]. Jamloki A, Karthikeyan C, Hari Narayana Moorthy NS, Trivedi P. QSAR analysis of some 5-amino-2-mercapto-1,3,4-thiadiazole based inhibitors of matrix metalloproteinases and bacterial collagenase. *Bioorg Med Chem Lett*. 2006;16(14):3847–3854.

[91]. Gupta SP, Kumaran S. A quantitative structure-activity relationship study on some series of anthranilic acid-based matrix metalloproteinase inhibitors. *Bioorg Med Chem*. 2005;13(18):5454–5462.

[92]. Gupta SP, Maheswaran V, Pande V, et al. A comparative QSAR study on carbonic anhydrase and matrix metalloproteinase inhibition by sulfonylated amino acid hydroxamates. *J Enzyme Inhib Med Chem*. 2003;18(1):7–13.

[93]. Gupta SP, Kumaran S. Quantitative structure-activity relationship studies on matrix metalloproteinase inhibitors: Bicyclic heteroaryl hydroxamic acid analogs. *Lett Drug Des Discov*. 2005;2(7):522–528.

[94]. Yuan H, Lu W, Wang L, et al. Synthesis of derivatives of methyl rosmarinate and their inhibitory activities against matrix metalloproteinase-1 (MMP-1). *Eur J Med Chem*. 2013;62:148–157.

[95]. Tuccinardi T, Martinelli A, Nuti E, et al. Amber force field implementation, molecular modelling study, synthesis and MMP-1/MMP-2 inhibition profile of (R)- and (S)-N-hydroxy-2-(N-isopropoxybiphenyl-4-ylsulfonamido)-3-methylbutanamides. *Bioorg Med Chem*. 2006;14(12):4260–4276.

[96]. Patra S, Saravanan P, Das B, et al. Scaffold-based screening and molecular dynamics simulation study to identify two structurally related phenolic compounds as potent MMP-1 inhibitors. *Comb Chem High Throughput Screen*. 2020;23(8):757–774.

[97]. Yasmeen S, Gupta P. Interaction of selected terpenoids from *Dalbergia sissoo* with catalytic domain of matrix metalloproteinase-1: An in silico assessment of their anti-wrinkling potential. *Bioinform Biol Insights*. 2019;13:1177932219896538.

[98]. Shunmuga Priya V, Pradiba D, Aarthy M, et al. *In-silico* strategies for identification of potent inhibitor for MMP-1 to prevent metastasis of breast cancer. *J Biomol Struct Dyn*. 2021;39(18):7274–7293.

[99]. Lee KE, Bharadwaj S, Yadava U, et al. Computational and in vitro investigation of (-)-epicatechin and proanthocyanidin B2 as inhibitors of human matrix metalloproteinase 1. *Biomolecules*. 2020;10(10):1379.

[100]. Alamzeb M, Setzer WN, Ali S, et al. Spectral, anti-inflammatory, anti-pyretic, leishmanicidal, and molecular docking studies, against selected protein targets, of a new bisbenzylisoquinoline alkaloid. *Front Chem*. 2021;9:711190.

[101]. Wongrattanakamon P, Nimmanpipug P, Sirithunyalug B, et al. Molecular modeling of non-covalent binding of Ligustrum lucidum secoiridoid glucosides to AP-1/matrix metalloproteinase pathway components. *J Bioenerg Biomembr*. 2018;50(4):315–327.

[102]. Guti S, Baidya SK, Banerjee S, et al. A robust classification-dependent multi-molecular modelling study on some biphenyl sulphonamide based MMP-8 inhibitors. *SAR QSAR Environ Res*. 2021;32(10):835–861.

[103]. Matter H, Schwab W, Barbier D, et al. Quantitative structure-activity relationship of human neutrophil collagenase (MMP-8) inhibitors using comparative molecular field analysis and X-ray structure analysis. *J Med Chem*. 1999;42(11):1908–1920.

[104]. Cortes-Pacheco A, Jiménez-Arellanes MA, Palacios-Can FJ, et al. Synthesis, antiinflammatory activity, and molecular docking studies of bisphosphonic esters as potential MMP-8 and MMP-9 inhibitors. *Beilstein J Org Chem*. 2020;16:1277–1287.

[105]. Kalva S, Vinod D, Saleena LM. Combined structure- and ligand-based pharmacophore modeling and molecular dynamics simulation studies to identify selective inhibitors of MMP-8. *J Mol Model*. 2014;20(5):2191.

[106]. Kumaran S, Gupta SP. A quantitative structure-activity relationship study on matrix metalloproteinase inhibitors: Piperidine sulfonamide aryl hydroxamic acid analogs. *J Enzyme Inhib Med Chem.* 2007;22(1):23–27.

[107]. Gupta SP, Kumaran S. Quantitative structure-activity relationship studies on matrix metalloproteinase inhibitors: Hydroxamic acid analogs. *Med Chem.* 2006;2(3):243–250.

[108]. Kumaran S, Gupta SP. A quantitative structure-activity relationship study on some novel series of hydroxamic acid analogs acting as matrix metalloproteinase inhibitors. *Med Chem.* 2007;3(2):167–173.

[109]. Huang S, Feng K, Ren Y. Molecular modelling studies of quinazolinone derivatives as MMP-13 inhibitors by QSAR, molecular docking and molecular dynamics simulations techniques. *Medchemcomm.* 2018;10(1):101–115.

[110]. Hadizadeh F, Shamsara J. Receptor-based 3D-QSAR approach to find selectivity features of flexible similar binding sites: Case study on MMP-12/MMP-13. *Int J Bioinform Res Appl.* 2015;11(4):326–346.

[111]. Kalva S, Saranyah K, Suganya PR, et al. Potent inhibitors precise to S1' loop of MMP-13, a crucial target for osteoarthritis. *J Mol Graph Model.* 2013;44:297–310.

[112]. Xi L, Li S, Yao X, et al. In silico study combining docking and QSAR methods on a series of matrix metalloproteinase 13 inhibitors. *Arch Pharm (Weinheim).* 2014;347(11):825–833.

[113]. Sarma JA, Rambabu G, Srikanth K, et al. Analogue based design of MMP-13 (Collagenase-3) inhibitors. *Bioorg Med Chem Lett.* 2002;12(19):2689–2693.

[114]. Fernández M, Caballero J, Tundidor-Camba A. Linear and nonlinear QSAR study of N-hydroxy-2-[(phenylsulfonyl)amino]acetamide derivatives as matrix metalloproteinase inhibitors. *Bioorg Med Chem.* 2006;14(12):4137–4150.

[115]. Fernández M, Caballero J. QSAR modeling of matrix metalloproteinase inhibition by N-hydroxy-alpha-phenylsulfonylacetamide derivatives. *Bioorg Med Chem.* 2007;15(18):6298–6310.

[116]. Singh P. A quantitative structure-activity relationship study on a series of selective non-zinc binding inhibitors of MMP-13. *Med Chem.* 2014;10(2):174–188.

[117]. El Ashry ESH, Awad LF, Teleb M, et al. Structure-based design and optimization of pyrimidine- and 1,2,4-triazolo[4,3-a]pyrimidine-based matrix metalloproteinase-10/13 inhibitors via Dimroth rearrangement towards targeted polypharmacology. *Bioorg Chem.* 2020;96:103616.

[118]. El-Kashef DH, Youssef FS, Reimche I, et al. Polyketides from the marine-derived fungus Aspergillus falconensis: In silico and in vitro cytotoxicity studies. *Bioorg Med Chem.* 2021;29:115883.

[119]. Ramezani M, Shamsara J. Virtual screening on MMP-13 led to discovering new inhibitors including a non-zinc binding and a micro molar one: A successful example of receptor selection according to cross-docking results for a flexible enzyme. *Comb Chem High Throughput Screen.* 2017;20(8):719–725.

[120]. Nuti E, Casalini F, Avramova SI, et al. N-O-isopropyl sulfonamido-based hydroxamates: Design, synthesis and biological evaluation of selective matrix metalloproteinase-13 inhibitors as potential therapeutic agents for osteoarthritis. *J Med Chem.* 2009;52(15):4757–4773.

11 Modeling Inhibitors of Gelatinases

Samima Khatun, Sk. Abdul Amin, Suvankar Banerjee, Shovanlal Gayen, and Tarun Jha

CONTENTS

ABSTRACT

Matrix metalloproteinases are extracellular zinc-containing proteolytic metalloenzymes that play a significant role in numerous pathological and physiological processes. Gelatinase A (MMP-2) and gelatinase B (MMP-9) play a crucial role in cancer progression, the pathogenesis of heart diseases, and inflammation. Overexpression of these gelatinases can lead to a number of inflammatory, cancerous, and degenerative disorders. Several computational techniques have been employed to understand their selective inhibition to tackle serious and widespread diseases. This chapter highlights the various molecular modeling approaches used to design MMP-2 and MMP-9 inhibitors. It offers a critical perspective for investigating the many options for the structure-based drug design of highly potent novel MMP-2 and MMP-9 inhibitors.

Keywords: Matrix metalloproteinase-2 (MMP-2); Matrix metalloproteinase-9 (MMP-9); Gelatinase; Cancer; Molecular modeling; QSAR; Molecular docking

11.1 INTRODUCTION

Matrix metalloproteinases (MMPs) are zinc-dependent peptidases categorized into subgroups [1]. Depending on the matrix component, degraded MMPs can be

DOI: 10.1201/9781003303282-14

categorized into four types: collagenases (MMP-1, MMP-8, MMP-13), gelatinases (MMP-2, MMP-9), stromelysins (MMP-3, MMP-10, MMP-11), and membrane-type MMPs (MT-MMPs) [2]. To date, hydroxamates, thiols, carbamoylphosphonates, hydroxyureas, β-lactam, squaric acids, and other nitrogenous compounds have all been discovered as MMP inhibitors [3]. The majority of these are composed of a metal-coordinating moiety known as a zinc-binding group (ZBG), which binds to the catalytic zinc ion of these MMPs.

Matrix metalloproteinase-2 (gelatinase A) belongs to the MMP family and has a strong correlation with cancer progression, metastasis of cancer cells, and angiogenesis [2]. MMP-2 is secreted by a variety of cells as the latent precursor, pro-gelatinase A (proMMP-2) [4]. MMP-2 is essential for controlling growth factors like vascular endothelial growth factor (VEGF) and insulin-like growth factor (IGF), which are necessary for the invasion of cancerous tissue into circulation as well as for the development of new blood vessels or angiogenic events. The activity of MMP-2 to degrade the extracellular matrix (ECM) has a direct impact on angiogenesis [5]. MMP-2 is also involved in ischemic stroke and cardiovascular manifestations. Additionally, the presence of MMP-2 is necessary for the regulation of several cytokines and chemokines, such as TNF-α, to have an anti-inflammatory effect [6]. Although type IV and type V collagen, as well as vitronectin, elastin, and other proteins, can all be considered appropriate substrates for MMP-2 and MMP-9. Type I collagen is the only type of collagen that MMP-2 can break down.

Matrix metalloproteinase-9 (gelatinase B) is one of the most crucial MMPs in the gelatinases category. It plays significant roles in several pathophysiological conditions and can break down ECM components. MMP-9 dysregulation and overexpression are linked to several diseases [7]. Therefore, MMP-9 modulation and inhibition are crucial therapeutic strategies for treating different diseases, including cancer. During tissue remodeling, MMP-9 leads to the breakdown of gelatin and type IV, V, XI, and XVI collagens, which are necessary for metastasis and the invasion of tumors [8]. It also contributes to the delaying of wound healing by deteriorating extracellular matrices linked to typical tissue remodeling processes. MMP-9 is typically found in the cerebellum, cerebral cortex, and hippocampus [9]. MMP-9 production typically takes place in the bone marrow during the process of granulocyte differentiation [10]. Fibroblasts, macrophages, leukocytes, neutrophils, and endothelial cells all release MMP-9 as zymogens or inactive forms. VEGF has also been reported to activate MMP-9 during lung metastasis; hence, MMP-9 deficiency aids in reducing metastasis [11]. Additionally, MMP-9 plays a critical role in several malignancies related to inflammation [12].

The availability of 3D protein structures is one of the most significant prerequisites in structural drug development. Structural elucidation can be done by either spectral analysis (X-ray diffraction study and solution NMR spectroscopy) or electron microscopy. Since 1995, several studies have been conducted to elucidate the structure of MMP-2. In all, 11 entries can be found in the Protein Data Bank (PDB) of the Research Collaboratory for Structural Bioinformatics (RSCB) for MMP-2 [13]. 1CK7, 1EAK, 1GEN, 1GXD, 1QIB, 1RTG, 3AYU, 1CXW, 1HOV, 1JVM, and

1KSO are the crystal structures available for MMP-2, where few structures (1QIB, 3AYU, and 1HOV) are the most suitable for structure-based drug designing. These 11 structures can offer a detailed knowledge of the overall MMP-2 structures and their functional roles. Unless otherwise specified, the RSCB PDB structures can be seen using the NGL viewer. It has been funded by the US National Science Foundation (NSF), the National Institutes of Health (NIH), and the Department of Energy (DOE). Further, in the UniProt database, MMP-2 holds an ID of P08253 [14] and has a molecular weight of 72 kDa.

The PDB contains at least 23 MMP-9 crystal structures that can be utilized for structure-based drug discovery. These are 1GKC, 1GKD, 1L6J, 2OW0, 2OW1, 2OW2, 2OVX, 2OVZ, 4H1Q, 4H2E, 4H3X, 4H82, 4HMA, 4JIJ, 4JQG, 4XCT, 4WZV, 5CUH, 5I12, 5TH9, 5UE3, 5UE4, and 6ESM. Wild-type MMP-9 (PDB 1GKC) and its mutant-active site (PDB 1GKD), which were identified at 2.3 and 2.1 of the resolution, respectively, were the first holoprotein crystal structures of human MMP-9. In combination with a peptidic reverse hydroxamate, both proteins acquire the usual MMP folds. The catalytic center of MMP-9 is coordinated by a glutamic acid residue (402) and a histidine triad (401, 405, and 411). Most significantly, MMP-9 can be distinguished from other MMPs at the S1′ pocket, which is present on the opposite side of the smaller pockets found in collagenase, matrilysin, and fibroblast [15].

MMPs are multidomain enzymes comprising catalytic, pro-peptide, and hemo-pexin (except matrilysin and MMP-7) domains. In all MMPs, the cysteine residue, which is strictly conserved in the pro-peptide domain, has been demonstrated to be critical for keeping MMPs inactive. The sulfhydryl group of this cysteine residue is believed to be linked to the catalytic Zn^{2+} ion, which is required for activation through the cysteine switch mechanism [16]. The 3D structure of MMP-2 and MMP-9 is unique compared with all other MMPs [17]. MMP-2 and MMP-9 each have three fibronectin type II-like domains incorporated into their catalytic domains that mediate contact with the substrates (type I and type IV collagen, gelatin, and laminin) [18–20]. The catalytic domain of both MMP-2 and MMP-9 has five calcium ions, in addition to two zinc ions, which make them structurally similar. However, MMP-9 varies from MMP-2 in terms of structural and functional features, such as in the lengthy, highly O-glycosylated linker between the hemopexin and the catalytic domain [21].

MMP-2 and MMP-9 are found to affect angiogenesis and tumor growth by increasing apoptosis during tissue remodeling and neo-angiogenesis, as well as decreasing apoptosis through an increase in the bioavailability of VEGF [22]. Clinical studies explored that MMP-2 and MMP-9 inhibitors are effective in treating the aforementioned diseases [23–24]. Therefore, more research related to designing MMP-2 and MMP-9 inhibitors is crucial for further modifying these inhibitors to have the desired activity. Various computational techniques have recently been employed to explore MMPs and their inhibitors. This chapter provides a detailed insight into the various modeling approaches applied recently for designing gelatinase inhibitors.

11.2 DESIGN STRATEGIES FOR GELATINASE INHIBITORS

Drug design has the potential to lower the costs related to financial, operational, and human resources. As a result, rational drug design has become a popular option in both academia and industry. In this context, molecular modeling using QSAR and molecular docking studies, as well as molecular dynamic (MD) simulation and virtual screening, can be fruitful options. Gelatinases are also given thorough multi-modal inputs in the form of ligand- and structure-based design strategies, as they are a plausible target for reducing cell proliferation. The structure-based technique, in particular, can be broken down into two types, as indicated in Figure 11.1.

11.2.1 CATALYTIC DOMAIN BINDING

Gelatin, collagens (type 3 and type 4), elastin, aggrecan, and cartilage linkages are the major substrates for gelatinases, which are required for maintaining the integrity of a normal ECM [25]. The catalytic portion is where the protein binds to the enzyme. As a result, competitive inhibition of gelatinases becomes the most effective strategy. Similarly, the Zn^{2+} ion and its surrounding pockets (S1, S2, S3 and S1', S2', S3') are also crucial for inhibition.

11.2.1.1 Zinc Binding

The catalytic domain of gelatinase contains two different zinc ions, each of which is linked to the protein by three histidine residues. The catalytic zinc is critical because the substrate protein is hydrolyzed at the glutamine residue, and this ion stabilizes it in the intermediate stage by forming a gemdiolate. As a result, many chemists have decided to target the zinc ion by inhibiting it with a peptidomimetic (specifically, a glutamine mimetic) small molecule. When it comes to designing a specific inhibitor, however, a problem arises. Since the Zn^{2+} ion is shared by all MMPs, it is challenging to build a particular inhibitor that does not attach to the Zn^{2+} ion. The unique feature of the gelatinase is the variable S1' pocket that is hydrophobic and comparatively longer.

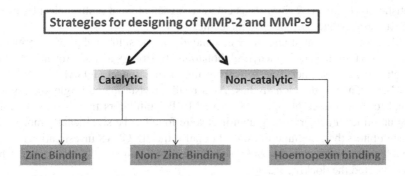

FIGURE 11.1 Designing strategies for MMP-2 and MMP-9.

11.2.1.2 Non-Zinc Binding

Regarding the binding of the catalytic Zn^{2+} ion, researchers tend to divide it into areas of conflict. It has been discovered that the majority of inhibitors with a ZBG are nonselective inhibitors, causing more detrimental effects. As a result, a non-zinc binding compound that fits neatly into the S1' pocket of gelatinases may be comparatively more selective than a compound bearing a ZBG.

11.2.2 NON-CATALYTIC INHIBITORS

The MMP exosite, particularly the hemopexin domain, could represent a prominent target for non-catalytic suppression. The main disadvantage is that this group has a poor affinity for inhibitors, making it difficult to design a suitable inhibitor. From a different viewpoint, it is possible that this area could be accessible for additional exploration. The exosite of the collagen-binding domain of gelatinase is inhibited by a specific oligopeptide [26].

11.3 QSAR APPROACHES IN THE DESIGNING OF GELATINASE (MMP-2 AND MMP-9) INHIBITORS

Several molecular modeling studies have been conducted on diverse sets of MMP-2 and MMP-9 inhibitors. Finding a target-specific gelatinase inhibitor with acceptable pharmacodynamic features remains a challenge. QSAR approaches may be one of the prospective drug design strategies to explore the critical structural aspects that would help find viable MMP-2/MMP-9 inhibitors.

Jha et al. [27] focused on the generation of several QSAR models on training set molecules, followed by prediction and validation on the test set and validation sets. This group synthesized and biologically evaluated a total of 67 glutamate-based derivatives to explore the major structural requirements for potential MMP-2 inhibition, employing robust multiple molecular modeling techniques (2D-QSAR, LDA-QSAR, Bayesian classification, HQSAR, 3D-QSAR CoMFA, and CoMSIA, as well as Open3DQSAR). Individually, each of these QSAR investigations was validated statistically. Figure 11.2 shows a schematic representation of multi-molecular modeling studies on glutamate-derived molecules.

Multiple molecular studies have concluded that the sulphonyl group is preferable to the acetyl group. The biphenyl sulphonamide function was also proven to be more beneficial than the phenyl acetyl carboxamido function in HQSAR, LDA-QSAR, and Bayesian classification studies. As a result, arylsulfonamido glutamines were found to be considerably more effective MMP-2 inhibitors than arylcarboxamido isoglutamines. Furthermore, glutamines were found to be significantly more effective inhibitors than isoglutamines. Additionally, the 2D-QSAR investigation revealed the relevance of the arylcarboxamido group at the glutamic acid's γ-terminus, which corroborated the docking studies.

Furthermore, Jha and coworkers [28] also synthesized and evaluated 59 glutamine and isoglutamine derivatives, subjecting them to a robust *in silico* multiple molecular modeling study that included several ligand-based (regression and classification-based 2D-QSARs and 3D-QSARs) and structure-based techniques (molecular docking study) for the further development of selective MMP-2 inhibitor designing. Individual S-MLR models were generated on 44 training set molecules and 15 different types of descriptors and then validated using 15 test set compounds. The 2D-QSAR study revealed that the arylsulfonamide scaffold was better than the aryl carboxamide function, which was validated by HQSAR, CoMFA, and CoMSIA.

The HQSAR model revealed the significance of one of the sulfonyl oxygen atoms and the adjacent phenyl ring in enhanced MMP-2 inhibition, which was in agreement with the results obtained from the 3D-QSAR CoMFA and CoMSIA analyses and so verified each other's results. The QAAR study demonstrated the

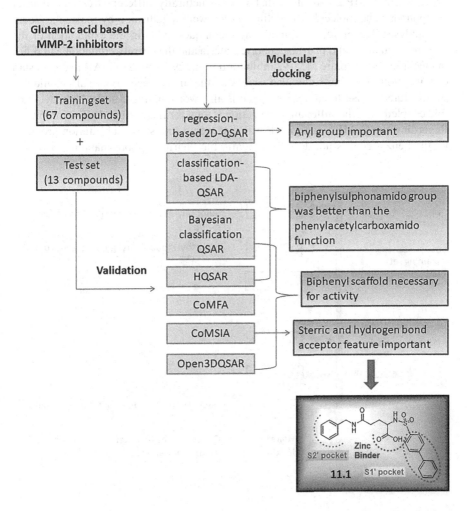

FIGURE 11.2 Multiple molecular modeling studies on some derivatives and analogs of glutamic acid as matrix metalloproteinase-2 inhibitors.

significance of the hydrophobicity of these compounds that may favor MMP-2 inhibition. In terms of MMP-2 selectivity, glutamines outperformed isoglutamines according to QAAR and molecular docking studies. Overall, the results of the various multi-QSARs corroborated each other along with the SAR observations (Figure 11.3). Therefore, these findings may shed light on future designing aspects of selective MMP-2 inhibitors [28].

Jha and coworkers [29] 2017 performed multi-chemometric modeling approaches (namely S-MLR, LDA-QSAR, Bayesian classification modeling, pharmacophore mapping, 3D-QSAR CoMFA, and CoMSIA) on a large dataset containing 222 diverse MMP-2 inhibitors for exploring the structural requirements to design higher active MMP-2 inhibitors. The reliability of these models was validated to predict 24 *in-house* MMP-2 inhibitors that were structurally different from the dataset compounds. The molecular modeling results were adjudicated by molecular docking analysis. Therefore, these modeling techniques aided in the exploration of the required structural and pharmacophoric criteria and the overall validation and refining techniques for future MMP-2 inhibitor design [29]. The 2D-QSAR and Bayesian classification modeling study also suggested the importance of arylsulfonamide or *p*-substituted arylsulfonamide groups. It is also worth noting that the biphenyl scaffold coupled with the sulfonamide function is vital for increasing MMP-2 inhibition. Regarding the CoMFA analysis, it was discovered that steric substitution provided by the benzyl ring is not desirable. Again, the pharmacophore mapping exhibited

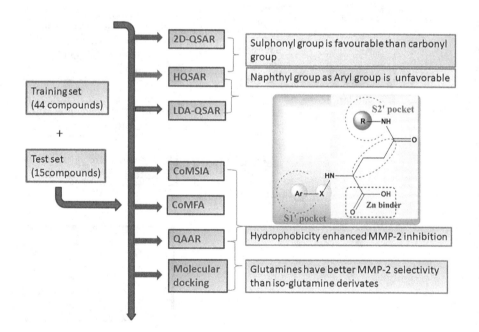

FIGURE 11.3 Exploring in-house glutamate inhibitors of matrix metalloproteinase-2 through validated robust chemical-biological quantitative approaches.

several excluded volumes near the benzyl ring, implying that bulky steric substituents are not ideal in this situation (Figure 11.4).

During the last two decades, many synthetic small-molecule MMP inhibitors have been tested in clinical trials, but none of these achieved satisfactory outcomes for further research. One key explanation could be the lack of understanding of the structural and physicochemical requirements for MMP inhibition. The first report published by Halder et al. [30] combines four different molecular modeling approaches (regression QSAR, classification QSAR, pharmacophore mapping, and 3D QSAR) to comprehend the structural and physicochemical requirements of diverse selective MMP-2 inhibitors. This study highlighted the structural and physicochemical requirements of structurally varied selective MMP-2 inhibitors using chemometric and molecular modeling methods. For molecular modeling, 202 compounds with considerable structural and activity variations were utilized. Regression QSAR analysis was used to extract detailed information on the impact of various structural and physicochemical factors on MMP-2 inhibition. Five-membered rings, fractional positively charged surface area, lipophilicity, and other characteristics were shown to be important in QSAR models. A higher molecular volume was discovered to be unfavorable. Hypogen and PHASE were used to perform pharmacophore mapping. One hydrophobic and three hydrogen bond acceptor characteristics were required in both models. Internal (Q^2) and external (R^2_{Pred}) cross-validation

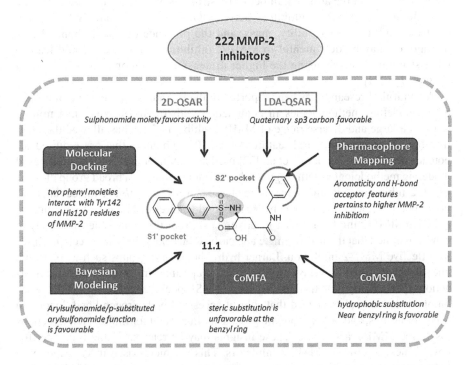

FIGURE 11.4 Anticancer matrix metalloproteinase-2 inhibitor designing through robust, validated multi-QSAR modeling approaches.

parameters were used to justify the quality of the regression models. The linear model was developed using stepwise regression ($Q^2 = 0.822$, $R^2_{Pred} = 0.667$). Linear ($Q^2 = 0.845$, $R^2_{Pred} = 0.638$) and spline models ($Q^2 = 0.882$, $R^2_{Pred} = 0.644$) were developed using a genetic algorithm. The Bayesian models and recursive partitioning (RP) showed a cross-validated area under the receiver operating characteristic curve (AUC_{ROC_CV}) of 0.979 and 0.805, respectively [30].

Finding a target-specific MMP-2 inhibitor with acceptable pharmacodynamic features, despite using many approaches, remains a difficult challenge. Regression QSAR methodologies could be one of the drug design methods used to explore the key structural properties needed to find a promising MMP-2 inhibitor. Sanyal et al. [31] reported a ligand-based chemometric approach that has been thoroughly explored for arylsulfonamide-based hydroxamates having potential MMP-2 inhibition. The PaDEL descriptors and stepwise multiple linear regression were used to explore 72 compounds (S-MLR). A workable statistical model with an acceptable metric related to these models was also developed using the partial least squares (PLS) approach. The models were compared with those previously published on the same endpoint. A QSAR model was fabricated that gave insight into the structural manipulation of novel compounds. For model building and model validation, a training set of 54 compounds and a test set of 18 compounds were used. A few descriptors indicated that the relative van der Waals volume and the atomic number of these atoms present in the molecule may be preferable for MMP-2 inhibitory activity. Other features, namely Sanderson electronegativity, polarizability, mass, and the presence of double-bonded carbon atoms, may be detrimental to MMP-2 inhibition. This study could lead to more structure analysis using the higher dimensional chemometric and *de novo* drug design [31].

A handful of research has been reported in the literature on using classification-based modeling methodologies in conjunction with fragment-based data mining tools on a large and diverse range of MMP-2 inhibitors. This has allowed the identification of critical structural features of MMP-2 inhibitors that are required for potency and efficacy. Banerjee et al. [32] used a combination of classification-based modeling methodologies with fragment-based data mining on a broad group of 4,151 MMP-2 inhibitors. Significantly, parameters such as *MW*, *AlogP*, molecular fractional polar surface area, and the hydrogen bond features can be used to distinguish effective MMP-2 inhibitors from inactive ones. From this comprehensive study, it can be assumed that the hydroxamate and carboxylic acid groups are excellent ZBGs for effective MMP-2 inhibition. Larger hydrophobic aryl groups such as biphenyl, phenoxy phenyl, and 3-pyridyl carboxamido groups are significant for possible interactions (particularly with the His120) inside the S1' pocket for efficient MMP-2 inhibition. This study also showed that solvent accessibility, hydrogen bond donor and acceptor groups, and bulky aromatic groups are important for improved interactions inside the MMP-2 active site. These insights may be relevant in the future for the development of efficient MMP-2 inhibitors. This fragment-based investigation will help us to uncover the aspects that can offer compound selectivity for MMP-2 when compared with other medium-size S1' pocket MMPs [32].

In 2003, Gupta et al. [33] reported a QSAR analysis on four series of 4-amino-proline-based hydroxamates, namely, substituted amines, lactic acid amide derivatives, inhibitors including hydantoin moieties, and various other structural scaffolds (Figure 11.5). An attempt has been made to correlate the inhibition activities of the compounds with Kier's first-order valence molecular connectivity index ($^1\chi^v$) of substituents/molecules and the electrotopological state (E-state) indices (Si) of the atoms. The correlations obtained for the inhibition of the MMP-2 enzyme suggested substituents at the amide nitrogen may be conducive to activity for all MMPs except for MMP-2, even if the entire amide group is sterically unfavorable. Likewise, substituents at the phenyl moiety have been discovered to be crucial for inhibitory efficacy, and the electronic involvement of the SO_2 group of the sulfonyl phenyl moiety has also been elucidated. It is also worth noting that, with the exception of MMP-2, all the enzymes may have the same active site to accommodate the W-substituent [33].

Kumar et al. [34] introduced a few hydroxamate inhibitors of MMPs for the progression of MMP-2 and MMP-9 inhibitor design and development. A QSAR study has been made on 33 compounds employing $^1\chi^v$ of the substituents and E-state indices of the individual atoms (Figure 11.6). The enzyme inhibition constant (Ki) of these inhibitors in nanomolar (nM) concentration was obtained from Easson–Stedman plots [35] using a linear regression algorithm. For correlation purposes, log(1/Ki) values were extracted and correlated with $^1\chi^v$; $^1\chi^v$ of a molecule can be largely correlated with the hydrophobicity (log P) of the molecules. It represents the molecule's degree of branching, atom connection, and unsaturation in the molecule.

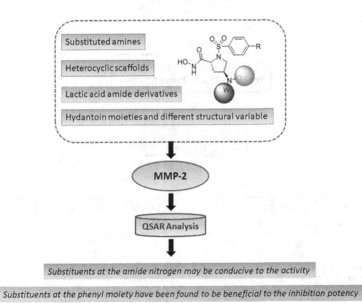

FIGURE 11.5 QSAR study on the inhibitions of some MMPs by functionalized 4-aminoproline-based hydroxamates.

The results showed that MMP-2 and MMP-9 inhibition is significantly influenced by the hydrophobicity of the R-group. A multiple regression analysis was performed, and the results showed that a positive coefficient of D implies that an R substituent containing a fluorine atom will be more pertinent to the activity than any other type of R substituent. Groups such as C_6F_5 or $3\text{-}CF_3\text{-}C_6H_4$ are thought to form hydrogen bonds with the Zn^{2+} ion of the enzyme or with any hydrogen bonding site of the enzyme via the fluorine atom. In addition to charge-charge or hydrogen bonding interactions, these groups might affect the activity significantly due to their hydrophobic properties [34].

Gupta et al. [36] published a QSAR study on the inhibitory effects of 39 sulfonylated amino acid hydroxamates on MMP-2 and MMP-9. The hydroxamates' inhibitory potency was found to be highly correlated with the $^1\chi^v$ of the molecule and E-state indices of specific atoms. As per findings, hydroxamate-gelatinase binding entails some hydrophobic interactions. A group such as C_6F_5 in the sulfonyl moiety has been demonstrated to be effective in MMP-2 and MMP-9 inhibition and will enhance the inhibitory efficacy of the compounds, which is thought to be owing to the interaction of this group with the Zn^{2+} ion present in the enzyme's catalytic site. Excellent correlations were obtained using multiple regression analysis between the activity and $^1\chi^v$ of the molecules and the E-state indices of some atoms. The positive dependence of gelatinases on $^1\chi^v$ suggests that less polar molecules will have better activity that might have some hydrophobic interactions with the enzymes. Lastly, the

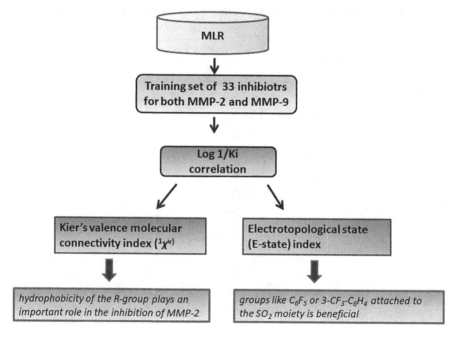

FIGURE 11.6   A quantitative structure-activity relationship study on some MMP inhibitors based on hydroxamic acid.

QSAR study revealed that hydroxamate-like gelatinase inhibitors may have polar or hydrophobic interactions with certain polar and hydrophobic sites available within the enzyme.

Adhikari et al. [37] designed a series of novel potent and selective MMP-2 inhibitors over MMP-9 inhibitors through the concepts of molecular modeling. On a dataset of 214 structurally diverse compounds, two types of molecular modeling techniques were used: regression analyses (2D and 3D QSAR studies) and the pharmacophore mapping technique, with the goal of understanding the mechanistic activity of the designed molecules. In addition, classification analyses (Bayesian modeling and recursive partitioning techniques) were carried out to ensure the selectivity of the compounds toward MMP-2/MMP-9. In terms of the predictability of the lead compound, the results of several regression models were found to be similar. The most potent MMP-2 inhibitor was compound **11.2**, whereas compound **11.3** had the highest MMP-2 selectivity (Figure 11.7). The docking poses, binding energies, *in silico* ADME features, and molecular dynamics simulation results of major compounds demonstrated that the majority of these designed molecules are non-cytotoxic even at high concentrations in the A549 cell line. The most active MMP-2 inhibitor (compound **11.2**) exhibited an IC_{50} of 24 nM, whereas the best selective inhibitor (compound **11.3**, $IC_{50} = 51$ nM) showed at least four times selectivity to MMP-2 over all other MMPs tested. Molecular docking and dynamics indicated that the 3,5-difluoro benzene molecule had a better binding with Zn^{2+}. The biphenyl moiety served as an

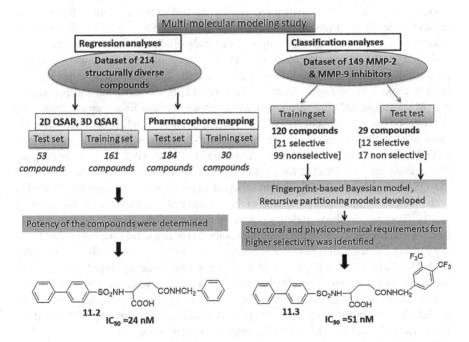

FIGURE 11.7 A multi-molecular study for developing potent and selective MMP-2 inhibitors over MMP-9.

excellent P1 pocket substitute. The active derivatives did not affect the human lung cancer cell line A549. These inhibitors inhibited intracellular MMP-2 expression by up to 78% at non-cytotoxic dosages and had good anti-migration and anti-invasive capabilities against A549 cells [37].

Fernandez et al. [38] constructed linear and non-linear QSAR models for linking inhibitor structural features with their biological activity against MMP-2 and MMP-9. The inhibitory activity (IC_{50}) of a dataset of 32 N-hydroxy-2-[(phenylsulfonyl) amino]acetamide derivatives (HPSAAs) against MMP-2 and MMP-9 was investigated using a multiple linear regression approach. A diverse set of 2D autocorrelation descriptors was used to screen the important structural information where linear correlations for inhibitory actions of HPSAAs were developed using MLR models with appropriate statistical significance and predictive capacity. This study demonstrated linear relationships between molecular properties and inhibitory activities using hydrophobicity-related descriptors ($^1\chi^v$ or logP) and E-state indices. Consequently, the authors described the importance of electrostatic interactions and hydrophobicity as the key features in determining inhibitor-enzyme affinities. It was observed that atomic van der Waals volumes have significant roles in the inhibition of MMP-2 and MMP-9 (Cv = 43%). Furthermore, the study concluded that spatial and hydrophobic-related effects guide HPSAA anchoring in gelatinase active sites [38].

MMP inhibitors have previously failed in clinical studies due to off-target effects in solid tumors. As a result, novel MMP inhibitors are becoming crucial. Das et al. [39] presented regression-based 2D-QSARs (S-MLR, ANN, and SVM), topomer CoMFA, and Bayesian classification models to refine the structural features for achieving better gelatinase (MMP-2 and MMP-9) inhibitory activity. A library of diverse aryl sulphonamide-based derivatives with binding affinity values (Ki) was collected for the preparation of the dataset. The structural requirements of aryl sulphonamides were investigated using MLR-based 2D-QSAR models, which showed high statistical significance. Moreover, the top MLR models from the two datasets (MMP-2 and MMP-9 inhibitors) were chosen for non-linear approaches. The descriptors, such as PubchemFP629, SHBint6, SHBint7, and nsssN, were directly associated with the binding affinities of MMP-2, whereas SHBint10, nsssN, and AATS2i were directly related to binding affinities of MMP-9. The aryl hydrophobic scaffold fits well into the S1' pocket. This result is based on observations using 2D-QSAR and Naive Bayes. The presence of two aryl sulphonyl groups connected with the ureido function is preferable to the presence of a single aryl sulphonyl group as P1'. Topomer CoMFA models support this observation. The S1' pocket is stabilized by the ureido group. This is an important factor in modulating gelatinase binding affinity. Tertiary nitrogen atoms connected to P1', P2', and a ZBG are required for MMP-2 and MMP-9 binding affinities. According to the topomer CoMFA study, the 4-nitrobenzyl group is preferable as a P2' fragment, whereas the benzyl group is not. These modeling experiments show that the hydroxamate moiety has a beneficial effect on both MMP-2 and MMP-9. According to the topomer CoMFA data, the steric and electrostatic fields play important roles in gelatinase inhibition. As a result, these findings may be useful for future research on aryl sulfonamide-based gelatinase inhibitors [39].

Further, Das et al. [40] used molecular modeling techniques to explore a pool of 110 compounds with MMP-2 and MMP-9 inhibitory activities with structural diversity and variable potencies to explore several important structural requirements to design better active inhibitors. The study highlighted the importance of arylsulfonamido hydrophobic function to fit well into the S1' pocket of gelatinases. The tertiary nitrogen atom was also advantageous for binding with MMP-2 and MMP-9. The hydroxamate moiety's positive influence was also observed in the modeling study. The key findings of the research indicate that the $-PO_3H_2$ feature shows a poor zinc-binding property. The insertion of an aromatic ring between the ZBG and the sulphonyl group significantly decreased activity. Notably, N-O-isopropyl sulfonamido-based compounds containing the sulfonamido fragment inhibited gelatinase well. MMP-2 inhibitory action of ethynylthiophene sulfonamido-based hydroxamates (compounds **11.4–11.8**, Figure 11.8B) was promising (IC_{50} range: 1.3–17 nM). The N-alkyloxy substituent had a negative impact on MMP-2 and MMP-9 inhibition, most likely because MMP-2 and MMP-9 inhibition is dependent on multiple replacements, and drugs will not achieve adequate inhibition unless the substitutions are properly optimized for size, shape, hydrophobicity, and so on. Furthermore, applying conventional QSAR equations in combination with non-linear models enabled rapid screening and prediction of various derivatives of MMP-2 and MMP-9 inhibitors. The modeling analysis will assist medicinal chemists in speeding up anticancer drug design and discovery research in the future [40].

Gupta and Kumaran [41] reported several QSAR studies on MMP-9 inhibitors. From the MLR model of ten p-methoxy sulfonamide derivatives, the model

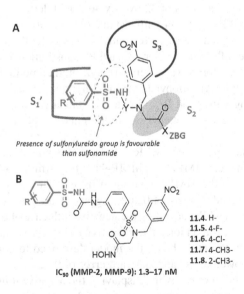

11.4. H-
11.5. 4-F-
11.6. 4-Cl-
11.7. 4-CH3-
11.8. 2-CH3-

IC_{50} (MMP-2, MMP-9): 1.3–17 nM

FIGURE 11.8 (A) Structural requirements for screening more desirable inhibitors for gelatinases and (B) ethynylthiophene sulfonamido-based hydroxamates (compounds **11.4-11.8**) as promising inhibitors of MMP-2 and MMP-9.

displayed an R and R^2_{CV} of 0.954 and 0.86 with a standard error of 0.15. This model also suggested a negative contribution of the lipophilicity (logP) values for these sulfonamide analogs for their MMP-9 inhibition. Another MLR model developed using 19 p-oxyaryl/alkyl substituted sulfonamide-based MMP-9 inhibitors yielded an R of 0.882 with a standard error of 0.64 and an R^2_{CV} of 0.5. The model also indicated the negative contribution of the logP and the p-methoxy benzyl group substitution at the P_1' substituent of these compounds. Again, the model developed on 16 MMP-9 inhibitors with an R and standard error of 0.920 and 0.37, respectively, showed an R^2_{CV} of 0.64 while depicting the positive correlation between the polarizability and acetylene-containing substituents with MMP-9 inhibition, indicating the negative influence of nitrogen-containing substituents. Another MLR model developed using 19 MMP-9 inhibitors showed an R-value of 0.935 with a standard error and R^2_{CV} of 0.13 and 0.74, respectively. This model suggested the positive influence of substitutions at the P_2' pocket substituents of these molecules while indicating the lipophilicity as a negative influencer for their MMP-9 inhibitory activity.

In another study, Gupta and Kumaran [42] attempted to correlate the MMP-9 inhibitory activity of 17 hydroxamate-containing benzodiazepine derivatives with their molecular properties and substitutions. This MLR model with an R of 0.932 and an R^2_{CV} of 0.65 with a standard error of 0.25 showed a positive influence of the E-state index of a nitrogen atom attached to the sulfonyl group for MMP-9 inhibition. This indicates the presence of loan pair/π electrons can produce higher MMP-9 inhibitory activity. The model also identified the positive contribution of acetylene-derived substituent and the negative influence of the aliphatic ring for the MMP-9 inhibitory activity of these benzodiazepine derivatives.

The QSAR study of a series of 42 hydroxamic acid derivatives [43] delivered an R-value of 0.891 and R^2_{CV} of 0.74 with a standard error of 0.31 for the MLR model. The model also suggested the negative contribution of ClogP and $ClogP^2$ while suggesting the positive influence of chloro phenyl P_1' substitution as a beneficial feature for these MMP-9 inhibitors toward their activity. Another model developed using ten N-p-substituted oxyphenyl sulfonyl diazepine-2-hydroxamic acid derivatives showed an R of 0.914 along with good R^2_{CV} and a low standard error while indicating the positive influence of carboxy phenyl substitution and lipophilicity for their MMP-9 inhibitory activity.

Roy and coworkers performed MLR-based QSAR studies on a series of 18 gelatinase inhibitors with their MMP-2 and MMP-9 binding affinity [44]. The MLR model developed to correlate the MMP-2 binding affinity of those compounds showed an R^2 of 0.830 with a standard error of 0.202, suggesting the positive influence of electronic parameter (σ_m) while indicating the negative influence of σ_m^2, hydrophobicity of the substituents (π_x), and molecular refractivity of substituents (MR_x) for MMP-2 binding affinity. On the other hand, the model developed to correlate the MMP-9 binding affinity showed an R^2 and standard error of 0.828 and 0.237 and indicated the positive contribution of σ_m while displaying the negative influence of molecular refractivity and σ_m^2 toward the binding affinity of these compounds.

Gupta and Kumaran performed linear regression analysis on a set of acyclic hydroxamate analogs to correlate their gelatinase inhibitory activity with their physicochemical properties [45]. The model developed on 19 MMP-2 inhibitors showed an R-value of 0.971, along with an R^2_{CV} and standard error of 0.90 and 0.19, respectively. On the other hand, the model developed using 17 MMP-9 inhibitors delivered R and R^2_{CV} values of 0.994 and 0.80, respectively, with a standard error of 0.29. The models identified the positive contribution of polarizability, methyl group, and c-pentyl ring substitution for MMP-2 inhibition and suggested the positive influence of ClogP (lipophilicity) and substitution at the aryl ring for higher MMP-9 inhibition.

Fernandez and Caballero [46] performed Bayesian regularized genetic neural network (BRGNN) and multiple linear regression (MLR) analysis on a series of N-hydroxy-α-phenylsulfonyl acetamide analogs. The MLR model developed using 66 MMP-9 inhibitors identified the positive influence of the descriptors ATS3e, MATS2e, GATS1e, and GATS6p, while suggesting MATS4e, ATS6m, and GATS1v as negative regulators of the activity. The MLR model also displayed R^2 and R^2_{CV} values of 0.731 and 0.605, with a standard error of 0.416 for the training set. The model also showed an R^2_{Pred} of 0.713 for the 12 test set molecules. Also, the BRGNN model developed using the aforementioned descriptors displayed R^2 and Q^2 values of 0.844 and 0.601 with 0.224 standard error for the training set while producing an R^2_{Pred} of 0.814 for the test set compounds.

Field-based and Gaussian-based 3D-QSAR studies have been performed on a series of barbiturate-based MMP-9 inhibitors [47]. The field-based 3D-QSAR model was developed using the partial least square (PLS) method. The field-based PLS model has shown a standard deviation (SD) of 0.130 with an R^2, R^2_{CV}, R^2 scramble (R^2Sc), and Q^2 values of 0.845, 0.582, 0.896, and 0.771, whereas the Gaussian-based PLS model showed an SD of 0.175 with an R^2, R^2_{CV}, R^2 scramble (R^2Sc), and Q^2 values of 0.928, 0.563, 0.0.854, and 0.850. The analysis of contour maps for these two models indicated that a molecule with incremental bond length in the fourth position of homopiperazine and piperazine analogs suggests that increased bulk at that position may decrease the activity.

Rathee and coworkers performed a pharmacophore and field-based 3D-QSAR study on a series of hydroxamate-containing gelatinase inhibitors [48]. The field-based 3D-QSAR study showed an R^2 of 0.67, SD of 0.2, and Q^2 of 0.51 with a stability value of 0.23 for the MMP-2 inhibitory activity. On the other hand, for the MMP-9 inhibitory activity of the molecules, the 3D-QSAR study showed an R^2 of 0.77, SD of 0.2, and Q^2 of 0.59 with a stability value of 0.30. In contrast, the best pharmacophore hypothesis with three aromatic and two ring aromatic features delivered a site score of 0.91, a vector score of 0.991, and a volume score of 0.842. The field contour maps explained the extent of hydrophobic, electron-withdrawing, and hydrogen bond donor groups in the molecular structure that influenced the MMP-2 and MMP-9 inhibitory potential of the dataset compounds. The volume occluded contours suggested that MMP-2 and MMP-9 inhibitory activity can be increased if the electron-withdrawing feature near the phenyl ring of hydroxamate was supplemented by suitable functional groups and by assimilating the hydrogen bond donor and hydrophobic and positive ionic groups at particular positions of these hydroxamate derivatives.

A QSAR-mediated structural analysis of arylsulfonamide-based carboxylic acid derivatives was performed by Mondal and colleagues [49]. In this study, several conventional and modern QSAR approaches were adopted to correlate the MMP-9 inhibitory potency of 135 carboxylic acid-containing MMP-9 inhibitors with their structural attributes. In this study, linear QSAR methods such as MLR models, non-linear regression-models such as support vector machine (SVM) and artificial neural network (ANN), and classification-based Bayesian classification and recursive partitioning studies were performed to identify the crucial structural attributes of these MMP-9 inhibitors that regulate their MMP-9 inhibitory potency. The MLR model showed R^2 and Q^2 values of 0.685 and 0.602, respectively, for the training set compounds while producing an R^2_{Pred} value of 0.610 for the test set compounds. The ANN and the SVM models developed using the same descriptor set used for the MLR study showed an R-value of 0.909 and 0.815 for the training set while producing Q^2 values of 0.723 and 0.700, respectively. Additionally, the SVM and ANN models also delivered R_{Pred} values of 0.695 and 0.792 for the test set. Also, for the classification-based QSAR studies, the Bayesian classification study showed $AUCROC_{LOO-CV}$ and $AUCROC_{5-CV}$ values of 0.834 and 0.839 with sensitivity, specificity, precision, and accuracy scores of 0.959, 0.776, 0.758, and 0.853, respectively, for the training set. For the test set, the Bayesian classification model delivered an $AUCROC_{Pred}$ value of 0.905, along with sensitivity, specificity, precision, and accuracy scores of 0.923, 0.760, 0.667, and 0.816, respectively. Additionally, the best tree-based recursive partitioning model showed an AUCROC of 0.800 and $AUCROC_{5-CV}$ of 0.710 for the internal cross-validation while having sensitivity, specificity, precision, and accuracy scores of 0.0.777, 0.761, 0.704, and 0.767, respectively, for the training set. The recursive partitioning model also showed an $AUCROC_{Pred}$ value of 0.803 with sensitivity, specificity, precision, and accuracy scores of 0.0.737, 0.846, 0.680, and 0.579, respectively, for the test set compounds.

These studies suggested that groups like tetrazole derivatives, biphenyloxy, and piperidine, as well as molecular properties like the number of rotatable bonds (nRB) and hydrogen bond acceptor (nHBA), can provide positive contributions toward MMP-9 inhibitory potency. The recursive partitioning study suggested an important contribution of the molecular weight (MW) of these molecules toward their activity. Furthermore, the regression-based study suggested poor contribution of the substituted and/or unsubstituted 3-pyridyl methyl group of these compounds toward MMP-9 inhibition. Similar suggestions were made by the Bayesian classification study. Also, the p-nitrophenyl group was found to be detrimental to MMP-9 inhibition from the analysis of both the MLR and Bayesian classification studies. Analysis of the regression-based QSAR studies suggested the detrimental effect of the p-bromo biphenyl moiety on MMP-9 inhibitory potency. Besides, the descriptors of the MLR model hinted at the negative effects of n-alkyl chain-containing compounds, which were further supported by the Bayesian classification study. In addition, the MLR study suggested a negative impact of bulky groups on MMP-9 inhibition.

Apart from these, a few Hansch analyses and Free-Wilson-related approaches were used to correlate the gelatinase inhibitory activity/gelatinase binding affinity through MLR model development, which was performed to correlate fundamental molecular properties [49–50].

11.4 DESIGNING GELATINASE (MMP-2 AND MMP-9) INHIBITORS USING THE MOLECULAR DOCKING TECHNIQUE

In recent years, a lot of research on MMP-2 and MMP-9 inhibition has been performed by implementing molecular docking techniques by researchers with promising results. Durrant et al. [51] used a few pyrone-based derivatives and docked them into multiple structures extracted from matrix metalloproteinase molecular dynamics simulations. All protein preparation methods were completed prior to docking, and partial charges were added. The *Ab initio* Hartree Fock method [52] was used to calculate the electrostatic potential (HF/6-31G*) partial charges for zinc, and all the flanking histidine residues were given using the RESP tool. AMBER-99SB was utilized as a preferred docking tool [53]. The study revealed that the ligand has two possible conformers, one in which the S1' pocket remains deeply occupied and the other in which the ligand is not susceptible to the MMP-2 enzyme's deep pocket. According to this study, the fickle nature of the S1' pocket has led to many of its inhibitors performing at suboptimal potency. Further, the dynamics of the S1' binding pocket show receptor switches in three major conformational states: (a) fully closed (incompatible with binding docking; (b) semi-open (compatible with weak binding); and (c) fully open (compatible with strong binding) [51].

ZBGs target the catalytic zinc ion in the active site of MMP to block the active site and enzymatic activity of the MMP. *In vitro* and *in vivo* studies have shown that chemically modified tetracyclines (CMTs) are effective MMP inhibitors. To gain a better understanding of the interaction of CMTs with the catalytic site of MMPs, Marcial et al. [54] focused on the direct interaction of CMTs with the active site of the MMP-2 using various computational techniques like molecular docking, MD simulations, and free energy calculations for seven CMT derivatives.

Molecular docking indicated that all CMTs bind to the catalytic zinc of the MMP-2 enzyme at the O11–O12 site except the CMT-3 analog. The CMT-3 analog (also known as COL-3) appears inside the S1' subsite, facilitating van der Waals and hydrophobic contacts with the hydrophobic S1' pocket. The CMT-3 molecule (compound **11.9**) is perhaps the simplest tetracycline derivative, with no bulky substituents at the C4, C6, and C7 positions (Figure 11.9). This implies that steric hindrance caused by the bulky groups at position C6 determines how CMTs interact with the MMP-2 target and plays a significant role in protein-ligand binding. Following molecular docking, the compounds were subjected to MD simulation to assess the strength of the binding poses of these molecules, which revealed CMT-3 as the most active molecule. Furthermore, the binding energy calculated in the solution indicates that the CMT-3 complexes are the most favorable. Quantum mechanics (QM) calculations [55] were also carried out using the Gaussian 09 suite, with potential energy curves generated from the fully optimized geometry of the model using the hybrid B3LYP functional and 6-31G(d) basis sets for ligand atoms and Stuttgart/Dresden effective core potentials (ECPs) and the corresponding SDD valence basis set for Zn atoms. Restrained electrostatic potential (RESP) charges for zinc ions and their chemical surroundings were calculated at the B3LYP/6-311++G(3df,2pd) level. This study is the first step toward understanding the molecular mechanism of CMTs as MMP inhibitors.

Fabre et al. [56] synthesized a new series of α-piperidine-α-sulfone hydroxamic acids to improve water solubility and explore their inhibitory activity against the MMP-2 enzyme. The computational docking method was utilized to support the SAR of the selected triazole-based compounds; 19 different molecules having MMP-2 inhibitory activity were docked into the active site of the protein (the tenth isoform of the 1HOV). The click approach enabled the discovery of compound **11.10** (Figure 11.10), a promising lead compound with potent inhibition of MMP-2 (IC$_{50}$ = 1.7 nM), promising MMP-2 selectivity (~26), improved LE index, and drug-like properties (solubility in the mg/mL range). Glide was the software of choice for molecular docking. Water LOGSY [57] and STD [58] intermolecular interaction experiments were used in the characterization of novel inhibitors binding MMP-2. Both are ligand-based techniques that provide equivalent binding information. UV spectroscopy was used to determine the kinetic solubility of the derivatives in water, as described by Mobashery [59]. Further, the cytotoxicity and anti-invasive activity of the molecules were determined on highly metastatic human fibrosarcoma tumor cells (HT1080) using a fluorimetric QCM ECMatrix Cell Invasion Assay (Millipore).

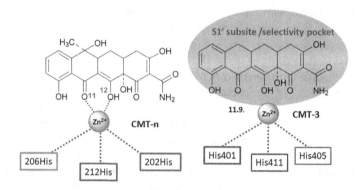

FIGURE 11.9 Molecular docking of CMT (10) with MMP-2 (PDB ID:1QIB) showing the bond formation of CMT with the catalytic zinc ion of the MMP-2 protein.

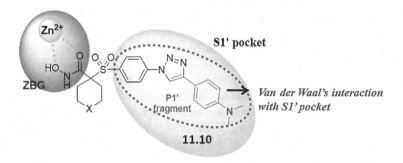

FIGURE 11.10 Docking interaction of the promising lead compound (triazole-based hydroxamate, compound **11.11**) with the MMP-2 (PDB: 1HOV). The gray dashed line shows van der Waals group interaction with the S1' pocket of the MMP-2.

Several nutraceuticals, for example, curcumin (diferuloylmethane) obtained from the plant *Curcuma longa*, have been extensively investigated for their beneficial effects against various human cancers. However, its entry into clinical practice has been severely limited due to poor bioavailability and rapid metabolism [60]. To overcome such limitations, Ahmed et al. [61] synthesized a novel analog, viz. 3,4-difluorobenzylidene curcumin, which is commonly referred to as CDF, with dramatically improved bioavailability and *in vivo* anticancer efficacy. Binding characteristics of curcumin and CDF were assessed with MMP-2 using *in silico* docking studies to further emphasize the differences in the behavior of CDF. Utilizing AutoDock 4.2, it was docked onto the NMR structure of MMP-2 1HOV and optimized using self-docking of the co-crystallized ligand. The docking interactions for curcumin could lead to two important conclusions. The catalytic Zn^{2+} ion binds to the curcumin methoxy group of the curcumin molecule at one end with a 1.9 Å distance and Arg149 at the other end with a 2Å distance. The ligand was discovered to be within the S1 pocket. Interactions with S1' residue Ala84 (1.8 Å), Leu83 (2.0 Å), and active site His 120 (2.1 Å) were observed for difluorobenzyl curcumin (Figure 11.11). It was also noticed that difluorobenzyl curcumin binding with the co-crystal hydroxamic acid of the 1HOV crystal structure (SC-74020) had similar overlapping. Biological experiments such as gelatin zymography, miRNA analysis, invasion assays, and ELISA were also used to evaluate them. In A549 and H1299 NSCLC cells, CDF inhibited MMP-2 expression and activity considerably more efficiently than curcumin, validating the molecular modeling results. CDF induced the activity of miR-874,

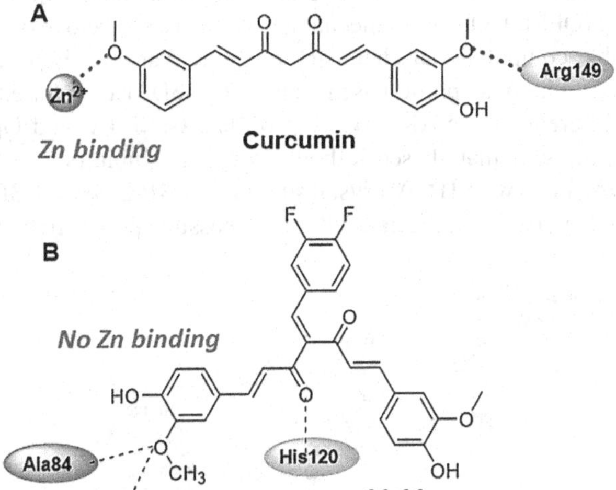

FIGURE 11.11   (A) Two-dimensional interaction of curcumin and MMP-2 (PDB: 1HOV) enzyme showing that the zinc ion binds with one of the methoxy groups in Curcumin. (B) The second figure depicts the interaction between CDF (compound **11.11**) and various MMP-2 residues, with no Zn binding.

an MMP-2-targeting miRNA. As a result, it appears that CDF inhibits MMP-2 via multiple pathways. and is more effective than curcumin, indicating that it should be investigated further as an anticancer drug [61].

Mukherjee et al. [62] highlighted MMP-2 targeted pentanoic acid as the lead compound (compound **11.12**) with good cytotoxicity against leukemia cell lines. Molecular docking data indicated that this compound showed significant interactions with MMP-2 (Figure 11.12). However, the enzymatic study indicated that this compound possesses varying degrees of inhibitory activity on MMP-2. Since gelatinase inhibition is primarily dependent on the bulky hydrophobic aryl group directed toward the S1′ pocket, its gelatinase inhibitory activity is lower. The molecules exhibit gelatinase inhibition due to the presence of a carboxylic acid function as a zinc-binding group, but due to the presence of a *p*-nitrophenyl group rather than a bulky higher aryl function, it exhibits lower gelatinase inhibition. As a result, the reduced hydrophobic character is the primary determinant of its cytotoxicity. Fluorescence imaging revealed that compound **11.12** induced nicked DNA of the K562 cell line, which is a hallmark of apoptosis. The compound-induced cytotoxicity was also found to be apoptotic in nature, according to flow cytometric analysis. In addition, flow cytometry and western blot analysis demonstrated that compound **11.12** exposure inhibits MMP-2 expression in the K562 cell line.

As a result, this research could help to confirm how MMP-2 inhibition causes cytotoxicity in a chronic myeloid leukemia cell line (K562). Further, this study could be used to conduct further research on the lead candidate in order to develop a better MMP-2 inhibitor with a higher cytotoxic profile in the future [62].

Adhikari et al. [63] implemented several methods, including quantum polarized ligand docking (QPLD). Quantum mechanics has proven to be one of the most accurate and reliable computational chemistry methods. Various alignment techniques (docking-based, pharmacophore-based, and Open3DALIGN-based) were used to construct different 3D-QSAR models (CoMFA, CoMSIA, and Open3DQSAR) on some potential glutamate-based in-house MMP-2 inhibitors to understand their molecular interactions with 1HOV crystal structure MMP-2. Several 3D-QSAR studies were carried out based on the dataset's many possible poses. To better understand

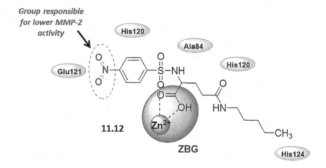

FIGURE 11.12 Interaction between pentanoic acid-based lead compound **11.12** and MMP-2 crystal structure 1HOV.

the interactions between the ligands and the protein, some of the compounds were docked at the same time. These were zinc-binding molecules with a carboxylic group as the primary ZBG. Isoglutamates were discovered to be less active due to their inability to fit into the S1' pocket. The sulphonyl group's oxygen atom served as a hydrogen bond donor, binding to both leucine and alanine. The docking-based alignment method provided the best 3D-QSAR model; 3D-QSAR models were correlated with molecular docking study and pharmacophore mapping. The biphenyl moiety of glutamines enters the S1' pocket and forms π-π interactions with Tyr142 and His120, whereas none of the phenylacetyl/naphthylacetyl isoglutamines interacts with Tyr142. Hydrophobicity and steric features of biphenyl function are also important for higher MMP-2 inhibition, according to 3D-QSAR models. The sulfonyl oxygen may form H-bonds with Leu83 and Ala84 of S1' pocket. Figure 11.13 shows the binding state of glutamine derivatives (compounds **11.13** and **11.14**) with MMP-2 (1HOV). This study indicated that biphenylsulfonyl glutamines are more effective at inhibiting MMP-2 than phenylacetyl/naphthylacetyl isoglutamines. These findings could be used to develop more effective MMP-2 inhibitors in the future [63].

Novel MMP-2 inhibitors based on imidazole and thiazole scaffolds were developed by Benscik et al. [1] for acute cardioprotection. A pharmacophore was generated using some of the most well-known and important MMP-2 inhibitors. InstatJChem, a computational tool for identifying similarities and forming a screening library of similar compounds, was used to conduct a computational substructural search. Finally, the screened compounds were docked with the MMP-2 enzyme's crystal structure (1QIB) and NMR structure (1HOV) using genetically optimized

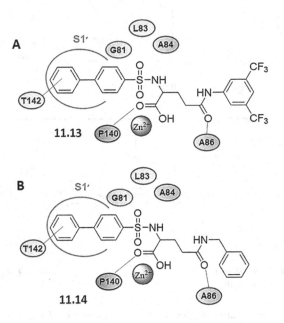

FIGURE 11.13 Binding state of glutamine derivatives with MMP-2 (1HOV).

ligand docking (GOLD) software [64] to quantify the binding interaction between the ligands and the crystal structure (1QIB) and NMR structure (1HOV). The results indicated imidazole and thiazole carboxylic acid-based compounds are more effective at inhibiting MMPs than the conventional hydroxamic acid derivatives of the same molecules. Based on these findings, a 568-membered focused library of imidazole and thiazole compounds was developed *in silico*. Molecular docking of library members into the 3D model of MMP-2 was performed, followed by an *in vitro* medium throughput screening (MTS) based on a fluorescent assay utilizing the MMP-2 catalytic domain. A total of 45 compounds had a docking score greater than 70, with 30 of them being successfully synthesized. This is the first proof that carboxylic acid-based imidazole and thiazole inhibitors are more effective than hydroxamic acid derivatives at inhibiting MMP-2 [1].

Moroy et al. [65] synthesized structural analogs of a well-known broad-spectrum MMP inhibitor, Ilomastat (galardin). The synthesized compounds were analyzed for their inhibitory activity toward MMP-2 and MMP-9 by molecular docking studies. The S1' sub-pocket of MMPs exhibits different chemical and structural differences and is hence taken into account for designing inhibitors with high selectivity. Compounds **11.15** and **11.16** with a phenyl group (Figure 11.14) inhibited MMP-9

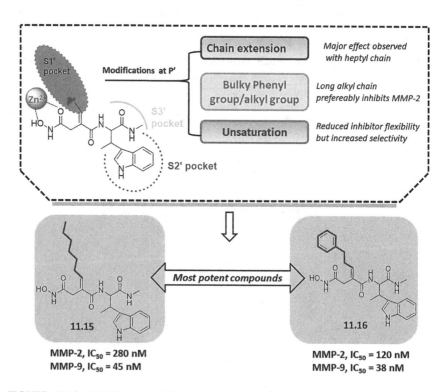

FIGURE 11.14   Modification of Ilomastat at P1' flexible alkyl chain or bulky block-like phenyl groups.

preferentially with IC_{50} values of 45 nM and 38 nM, respectively. However, they also exhibited MMP-2 inhibitory activity with IC_{50} values of 280 and 120 nM, respectively. In order to obtain specific gelatinase A inhibitory activity, P1' of Ilomastat was modified with unsaturation(s) and chain extension carrying a bulky phenyl group or alkyl moieties. The P1' group at Ilomastat, which fits into the distinctive S1' pocket of the MMP-2 enzyme, is fully accountable for its selectivity toward MMP-2. Therefore, docking studies revealed that the presence of unsaturation at P1' reduces the compound's inhibitory efficacy but enhances its selectivity for gelatinase A [65].

Furthermore, Moroy et al. [66] investigated the interactions of oleic acid (compound **11.17**) and its galardin-based derivatives (compound **11.18**) (OL-GALS) with matrix metalloproteinases. Blind docking was used on the crystal structure of MMP-2 (PDB ID: 1CK7) to demonstrate that oleic acid could occupy both the S1' pocket and the Fn(II)3 domain of MMP-2 by utilizing a large grid box that enveloped nearly the entire protein (96×126×120 with 0.64 Å spacing). Molecular docking revealed that oleic acid may bind to the protein in two different ways. In the first case, the hydrophobic chain occupies the S1' pocket, whereas, in the second, the carboxylic acid chelates with the Zn^{2+} ion. The ligand was found to be bound to the third fibronectin-type site of the enzyme in another pose. In the case of the galardin derivative, the –CONHOH group, on the other hand, was unable to provide adequate Zn^{2+} binding activity (Figure 11.15). However, in various biological assays, the activity was in the micromolar range (~4.3 µM). OL-GALS demonstrated less potent gelatinase activity compared with galardin, and no selectivity was found for MMP-2 or MMP-9.

In order to improve the potency of gelatinases, there is a need to discover novel ZBG-containing compounds. Nicolotti et al. [67] discovered a series of 5-hydroxy, 5-substituted pyrimidine-2,4,6-triones as MMP-2 and MMP-9 inhibitors to avoid the shortcomings of hydroxamate MMP inhibitors while keeping a more appealing drug-like appearance. A hydroxyl group was inserted at C5 to achieve better pharmacokinetics by ensuring a higher log P, enhanced aqueous solubility, and limited binding to human serum albumin, while suitably substituted biaryl molecular

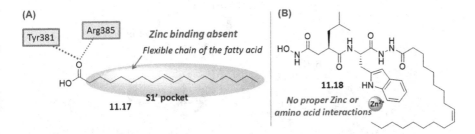

FIGURE 11.15 (A) Interaction of oleic acid (compound **11.17**) with MMP-2 (PDB: 1CK7). The interaction shows that oleic acid can form two hydrogen bonds with Tyr381 and Arg385. (B) Interaction of oleic acid derivative of galardin (compound **11.18**) with MMP-2 showing no proper zinc or amino acid interaction.

fragments were attached to position 5 via a ketomethylene linker to examine the potential of interactions at the S1' subsite (Figure 11.16).

QSAR and docking studies were utilized for the identification of the important determinants that led to the high affinity of the 5-hydroxy, 5-substituted-pyrimidine-2,4,6-trione derivatives. An electronic database with a chemical library of >2,000 compounds was considered in this study. A knowledge-based approach was used to obtain several compounds inhibiting MMP-2 and MMP-9. Binding interactions driving the binding of the active drugs to their preferred MMP target were elucidated using molecular docking simulations. A genetic algorithm-based program was employed, with GOLDSCORE and CHEMPLP as scoring and rescoring functions, respectively. Further, inhibitory activities were determined by a fluorimetric assay, which revealed that biphenyl derivatives with $COCH_3$ and OCF_3 substituents at the *para* position could inhibit MMP-2 and MMP-9 with IC_{50} values as low as 30 nM and 21 nM.

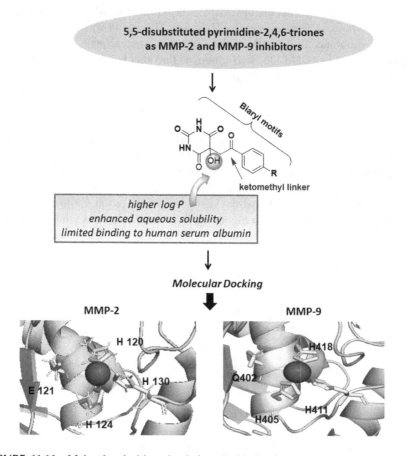

FIGURE 11.16 Molecular docking simulation elucidating important residues of MMP-2 and MMP-9 interacting with the best active compound.

Studies have indicated that inhibition of MMP-2 and MMP-9 is therapeutically important for the treatment of stroke. Elevated levels of gelatinases (MMP-2 and MMP-9) in the brain after stroke play a detrimental role in hemorrhagic stroke, ischemic stroke, and perinatal hypoxic-ischemic brain injury. Kumar et al. [68] investigated whether *Withania somnifera* (WS) phytochemicals inhibit MMP-2 and MMP-9 using *in silico* analysis. Molecular docking was performed to compare the gelatinase-inhibitory capacity of 36 WS phytochemicals with standard gelatinase inhibitors viz quercetin, doxycycline, minocycline, hydroxamic acid, and reverse hydroxamate. Atomic coordinates for the crystal structure of MMP-2 (PDB ID: 1HOV) and MMP-9 (PDB ID: 1GKC) were taken from the RCSB PDB and docking was performed using Auto Dock Tools 1.5.6 (ADT) [69]. A grid box was generated that covers the complete S1' pocket of the MMP-2 binding site and has room for both the rotational and translational movements of the ligands. For MMP-2, the values for the center grid box were preserved at 4.656, 16.977, and 13.903 for the X, Y, and Z-centers with 0.375 Å spacing and 80, 80, and 80 points in the X, Y, and Z dimensions.

While for MMP-9, the grid box center possessed values of 59.039, 23.888, and 116.225 with a 0.375 Å spacing and contained points in the X, Y, and Z dimensions of 80, 80, and 80, respectively. The Lamarckian genetic algorithm (LGA) was employed for 30 runs and 150 maximum population sizes with a maximum of 27,000 generations and 2,500,000 maximum energy evaluations. The final visualization was established with the LigPlot+ tool. The results indicated that 28 out of the 36 compounds exhibited higher affinity for MMP-2 due to their ability to bind with the active site residues of the S1' pocket with lower binding energy and a lower Ki than other inhibitors. Additionally, in comparison with reverse hydroxamate inhibitors, afastuosin E and anolide G showed a stronger affinity for MMP-9. These phytochemicals possess neuroprotective potential as an inherently useful oral drug to combat gelatinase-mediated ischemic and hemorrhagic stroke. Anolide G had the lowest binding energy (−11.10 kcal/mol) and the lowest K_i value of the steroids (11.10 nM). Somniferine, a non-steroid molecule, indicated acceptable binding energy (−10.58 kcal/mol).

Tauro et al. [70] described a novel series of bisphosphonate bone-seeking MMP inhibitors (BP-MMPIs) capable of selective bone targeting and disrupting the vicious cycle of bone tumor growth to overcome undesired side effects of broad-spectrum MMPIs. *In vitro* activity (IC_{50} values) for each inhibitor against MMP-2 and MMP-9 revealed that BP-MMPIs had IC_{50} values in the low micromolar range. Computational investigations, which were utilized to explain some of the observed inhibitory patterns, reveal that MMP-2 has a distinct binding mechanism that explains the isoform's selective inhibition. The binding activity of these compounds was predicted by docking them onto the crystal structure of MMP-2 and MMP-9. The best active compound **11.19** displayed zinc binding through only one phosphonic group; the other group remained H-bonded to Leu164 and Ala165 (Figure 11.17A). Surprisingly, it was discovered that both large hydrophobic and small hydrophilic molecules were able to inhibit the enzyme, however, most compounds did not bind to the S1' pocket but into the S1 and S2 pockets instead. The UV spectrophotometry technique was

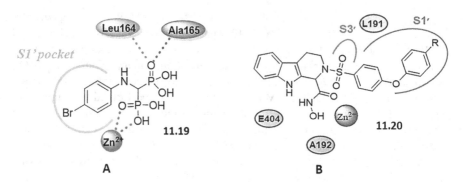

FIGURE 11.17 (A) Docking interaction of biphosphonic acid derivative (compound **11.19**) against the MMP-2 inhibitor. One of the phosphonic acid groups has bidentate chelation with a Zn^{2+} ion, while the other one was found to interact with Leu164 and Ala165; (B) 2D representation of the docking interactions between the tetrahydro β-carboline derivative (compound **11.20**) with MMP-2 protein (PDB ID: 1HOV).

utilized to determine the relative binding affinity of this new set of bisphosphonates to hydroxyapatite [70].

Mangiatordi et al. [71] discovered a series of novel tetrahydro-β-carboline derivatives with strong inhibitory activity against MMP-2 and MMP-9. These compounds possess 2,3,4,9-tetrahydro-1H-pyrido[3,4-b] indole (tetrahydro β-carboline) as their common scaffold, as given in Figure 11.17B (compound **11.20**). Four of the series' most active compounds showed high selectivity toward gelatinases when docked onto the crystal structure of MMP-2 and MMP-9. All four of these compounds were aryl sulphonyl hydroxamates in nature. The 4-substituted phenoxy phenyl group fits into the S1' pocket, while the oxygen atom of the sulphonyl group can fit into the S3' pocket. The hydroxamate group binds to the Zn2+ ion and two different amino acid residues (Glu404 and Ala192). Molecular docking simulations using quantum mechanics-based partial charges reflected the rationale behind binding involving specific interactions with key residues of S1' and S3' domains. Overall, this study suggested that tetrahydro-β-carboline is an important scaffold for the design of novel inhibitors capable of targeting gelatinases selectively across the desired pharmacokinetic range. This study points to tetrahydro-β-carboline as a new molecular scaffold candidate for developing potent and selective gelatinase inhibitors with favorable ADME profiles [71].

11.5 SUMMARY

MMPs have been identified as interesting targets for cancer therapy, especially MMP-2 and MMP-9, due to their extreme up-regulation in cancerous tissues and specialized capacity to break down extracellular matrix components. The selective inhibition of gelatinases continues to be a challenging problem even though many inhibitors have been reported and high-resolution X-ray crystal structures of MMP inhibitor complexes have been revealed. Researchers have discovered different types of scaffolds for the inhibition of MMP-2 and MMP-9, but no effective drug has been found. This research includes different design strategies using various modeling approaches to pinpoint the effective design of selective gelatinase inhibitors. This kind of information may be helpful in the discovery of target-specific inhibitors using robust and reliable modeling approaches in the future.

REFERENCES

[1]. Bencsik P, Kupai A, Görbe É, et al. Development of matrix metalloproteinase-2 inhibitors for cardioprotection. *Front. Pharmacol.* 2018;9:1–14.

[2]. Feng Y, Likos JJ, Zhu L, et al. Solution structure and backbone dynamics of the catalytic domain of matrix metalloproteinase-2 complexed with a hydroxamic acid inhibitor. *Biochim. Biophys. Acta – Proteins Proteom.* 2002;1598:10–23.

[3]. De Oliveira F, Durrant JD, Mccammon JA. Including receptor flexibility and induced fit effects into the design of MMP-2 inhibitors. *J Mol Recognit.* 2010;23:173–182.

[4]. Gohlke U, Gomis-Rüth FX, Crabbe T, et al. The C-terminal (haemopexin-like) domain structure of human gelatinase A (MMP-2): Structural implications for its function. *FEBS Lett.* 1996;378:126–130.

[5]. Gimeno A, Beltran-Debon R, Mulero M, et al. Understanding the variability of the S10 pocket to improve matrix metalloproteinase inhibitor selectivity profiles. *Drug Discov Today.* 2020; 25:38–57.

[6]. Briknarová K, Grishaev A, Bányai L, et al. The second type II module from human matrix metalloproteinase 2: Structure, function and dynamics. *Structure.* 1999;7:1235–1245.

[7]. Mondal S, Adhikari N, Banerjee S, et al. Matrix metalloproteinase-9 (MMP-9) and its inhibitors in cancer: A mini review, *Eur J Med Chem.* 2020;194:112260.

[8]. Liu Y, Liu H, Luo X, et al. Over expression of SMYD3 and matrix metalloproteinase-9 are associate with poor prognosis of patients with gastric cancer. *Tumor Biol.* 2015;36:4377–4386.

[9]. Bronisz E, Kurkowska-Jastrzebska I. Matrix metalloproteinase 9 in epilepsy: The role of neuroinflammation in seizure development. *Mediat Inflamm.* 2016;2:1–14.

[10]. Yabluchanskiy A, Yonggang M, Iyer RP, et al. Matrix metalloproteinase-9: Many shades of function in cardiovascular disease. *Physiology.* 2013;28:391–403.

[11]. Hiratsuka S, Nakamura K, Iwai S, et al. MMP-9 induction by vascular endothelial growth factor receptor-1 is involved in lung specific metastasis. *Cancer Cell.* 2002;2:289–300.

[12]. Bjorklund M, Koivunen E. Gelatinase-mediated migration and invasion of cancer cells. *Biochim Biophys Acta.* 2006;1755:37–69.

[13]. Research Collaboratory for Structural Bioinformatics Protein Data Bank. https://www.rcsb.org/. Accessed October 2022.

[14]. UniProt, UniProtKB - P08253 (MMP-2_HUMAN). https://www.uniprot.org/uniprot/P08253. Accessed October 2022.

[15]. Hariono M, Yuliani SH, Istyastono EP, et al. Matrix metalloproteinase 9 (MMP-9) in wound healing of diabetic foot ulcer: Molecular target and structure-based drug design. *Wound Med.* 2018;22:1–3.

[16]. Morgunova E, Tuuttila A, Bergmann U, et al. Structure of human pro-matrix metalloproteinase-2: Activation mechanism revealed. *Science.* 1999;284:1667–1670.

[17]. Tochowicz A, Maskos K, Huber R, et al. Crystal structures of MMP-9 complexes with five inhibitors: Contribution of the flexible Arg424 side-chain to selectivity, *J Mol Biol* 2007;371:989–1006.

[18]. Morgunova, E, Tuuttila A, Bergmann U, et al. Structure of human pro-matrix metal-loproteinase-2: activation mechanism revealed. *Science.* 1999;284:1667–1670.

[19]. Collier IE, Krasnov PA, Strongin AY, et al. Alanine scanning mutagenesis and func-tional analysis of the fibronectin-like collagen-binding domain from human 92-kDa type IV collagenase. *J Biol Chem.* 1992;267:6776–6781.

[20]. Xu X, Chen Z, Wang Y, et al. Functional basis for the overlap in ligand interac-tions and substrate specificities of matrix metalloproteinases-9 and -2. *Biochem J.* 2005;392:127–134.

[21]. Opdenakker G, Van den Steen PE, Dubois B, et al. Gelatinase B functions as regulator and effector in leukocyte biology. *J Leukoc Biol.* 2001;69:851–859.

[22]. Bergers G, Brekken R, McMahon G, et al. Matrix metalloproteinase-9 triggers the angiogenic switch during carcinogenesis. *Nat Cell Biol.* 2000;2:737–44.

[23]. Hu J, Van den Steen PE, Sang QX, et al. Matrix metalloproteinase inhibitors as therapy for inflammatory and vascular diseases. *Nat Rev Drug Discov.* 2007;6:480–98.

[24]. Sang QX, Jin Y, Newcomer RG, et al. Matrix metalloproteinase inhibitors as prospec-tive agents for the prevention and treatment of cardiovascular and neoplastic diseases. *Curr Top Med Chem.* 2006;6:289–316.

[25]. Mukherjee A, Adhikari N, Jha T. A pentanoic acid derivative targeting matrix metal-loproteinase-2 (MMP-2) induces apoptosis in a chronic myeloid leukemia cell line. *Eur J Med Chem.* 2017;141:37–50.

[26]. Xu X, Chen Z, Wang Y, et al. Inhibition of MMP-2 gelatinolysis by targeting exodo-main-substrate interactions. *Biochem. J.* 2007;406:147–155.

[27]. Jha T, Adhikari N, Saha A, et al. Multiple molecular modelling studies on some deriva-tives and analogues of glutamic acid as matrix metalloproteinase-2 inhibitors. *SAR QSAR Environ Res.* 2018;29:43–68.

[28]. Adhikari N, Amin SA, Saha A, et al. Exploring in house glutamate inhibitors of matrix metalloproteinase-2 through validated robust chemico-biological quantitative approaches. *Struct Chem.* 2018;29:285–297.

[29]. Adhikari N, Amin SA, Saha A, et al. Structural exploration for the refinement of anti-cancer matrix metalloproteinase-2 inhibitor designing approaches through robust vali-dated multi-QSARs. *J Mol Struct.* 2018;1156:501–515.

[30]. Halder AK, Saha A, Jha T. Exploring QSAR and pharmacophore mapping of struc-turally diverse selective matrix metalloproteinase-2 inhibitors. *J Pharm Pharmacol.* 2013;65:1541–1554.

[31]. Sanyal S, Amin SA, Adhikari N, et al. QSAR modelling on a series of arylsulfon-amide-based hydroxamates as potent MMP-2 inhibitors. *SAR QSAR Environ Res.* 2019;30:247–263.

[32]. Banerjee S, Amin SA, Jha T. A fragment-based structural analysis of MMP-2 inhibi-tors in search of meaningful structural fragments. *Comput Biol Med.* 2022;144:105360.

[33]. Gupta SP, Kumar D, Kumaran S. A quantitative structure-activity relationship study of hydroxamate matrix metalloproteinase inhibitors derived from funtionalized 4-amino-prolines. *Bioorg Med Chem.* 2003;11:1975–1981.

[34]. Kumar D, Gupta SP. A quantitative structure-activity relationship study on some matrix metalloproteinase and collagenase inhibitors. *Bioorg Med Chem.* 2003;11:421–426.

[35]. Bieth JG. Theoretical and practical aspects of proteinase inhibition kinetics, *Methods Enzymol.* 1995;248:59–84.

[36]. Gupta SP, Maheswaran V, Pande V, et al. A comparative QSAR study on carbonic anhydrase and matrix metalloproteinase inhibition by sulfonylated amino acid hydrox-amates. *J Enzyme Inhib Med Chem.* 2003;18:7–13.

[37]. Adhikari N, Halder AK, Mallick S, et al. Robust design of some selective matrix metal-loproteinase-2 inhibitors over matrix metalloproteinase-9 through in silico/fragment-based lead identification and de novo lead modification: Syntheses and biological assays. *Bioorg Med Chem.* 2016;24:4291–4309.

[38]. Fernández M, Caballero J, Tundidor-Camba A. Linear and nonlinear QSAR study of N-hydroxy-2-[(phenylsulfonyl)amino] acetamide derivatives as matrix metalloprotein-ase inhibitors. *Bioorg Med Chem.* 2006;14:4137–4150.

[39]. Das S, AminSA, Jha T, Insight into the structural requirement of aryl sulphonamide based gelatinases (MMP-2 and MMP-9) inhibitors-part I: 2D-QSAR, 3D-QSAR topomer CoMFA and Naïve Bayes studies-first report of 3D-QSAR Topomer CoMFA analysis for MMP-9 inhibitors and jointly inhibitors of gelatinases together. *SAR QSAR Environ Res.* 2021;32:655–687.

[40]. Das S, Amin SA, Gayen S, et al. Insight into the structural requirements of gelati-nases (MMP-2 and MMP-9) inhibitors by multiple validated molecular modelling approaches: Part II. *SAR QSAR Environ Res.* 2022;33:167–192.

[41]. Gupta SP, Kumaran S. A quantitative structure–activity relationship study on some series of anthranilic acid-based matrix metalloproteinase inhibitors. *Bioorg Med Chem.* 2005;13:5454–5462.

[42]. Gupta SP, Kumaran S. Quantitative structure-activity relationship studies on benzo-diazepine hydroxamic acid inhibitors of matrix metalloproteinase and tumor necrosis factor α converting enzyme. *Asian J. Biochem.* 2006;1:47–56.

[43]. Gupta SP, Kumaran S. Quantitative structure-activity relationship studies on matrix metalloproteinase inhibitors: Piperazine and diazepine hydroxamic acid analogs. *Asian J Biochem.* 2006;1:211–223.

[44]. Roy K, Pal DK, De AU, et al. QSAR of matrix metalloproteinase inhibitor N-[(substituted phenyl)sulfonyl]-N-4-nitrobenzylglycine hydroxamates using LFER model. *Drug Des Discov.* 2001;17:315–323.

[45]. Gupta SP, Kumaran S. Quantitative structure-activity relationship studies on matrix-metalloproteinase inhibitors: Hydroxamic acid analogs. *Med Chem.* 2006;2:243–250.

[46]. Fernandeza M, Caballerob J. QSAR modeling of matrix metalloproteinase inhi-bition by N-hydroxy-α-phenylsulfonylacetamide derivatives. *Bioorg Med Chem.* 2007;15:6298–6310.

[47]. Kalva S, Vinod D, Saleena LM. Field- and Gaussian-based 3D-QSAR studies on barbi-turate analogs as MMP-9 inhibitors. *Med Chem Res.* 2013;22:5303–5313.

[48]. Rathee D, Lather V, Dureja H. Pharmacophoremodeling and 3D QSAR studies for prediction of matrix metalloproteinases inhibitory activity of hydroxamate derivatives. *Biotechnol Res Innov.* 2017;1:112–122.

[49]. Mondal S, Banerjee S, Amin SA, Jha T. Structural analysis of arylsulfonamide-based carboxylic acid derivatives: A QSAR study to identify the structural contributors toward their MMP-9 inhibition. *Struct Chem.* 2021;32:417–430.

[50]. Gupta SP (ed.). Matrix metalloproteinase inhibitors. *Experientia Supplementum* 2012;103. Springer Basel AG.

[51]. Durrant J, de Oliveira CAF, McCammon JA. Pyrone-based inhibitors of metallopro-teinase types 2 and 3 may work as conformation-selective inhibitors. *Chem Biol Drug Des.* 2011;78:191–198.

[52]. Friesner RA. Ab initio quantum chemistry: Methodology and applications. *Proc Natl Acad Sci.* 2005;102:6648–6653.

[53]. Hornak V, Abel R, Okur A, et al. Simmerling, comparison of multiple amber force fields and development of improved protein backbone parameters. *Proteins.* 2006;65:712–725.

[54]. Marcial BL, Sousa SF, Barbosa IL, et al. Chemically modified tetracyclines as inhibitors of MMP-2 matrix metalloproteinase: A molecular and structural study. *J Phys Chem B*. 2012;116:13644–13654.

[55]. Van Mourik T, Bühl M, Gaigeot MP. Density functional theory across chemistry, physics and biology. *Philos Trans R Soc A Math Phys Eng Sci*. 2014;372:20120488.

[56]. Fabre B, Filipiak K, Zapico JM, et al. Progress towards water-soluble triazole-based selective MMP-2 inhibitors. *Org Biomol Chem*. 2013;11:6623–6641.

[57]. Dalvit C, Pevarello P, Tatò M, et al. Identification of compounds with binding affinity to proteins via magnetization transfer from bulk water. *J Biomol NMR*. 2000;18:65–68.

[58]. Meyer B, Peters T. NMR spectroscopy techniques for screening and identifying ligand binding to protein receptors. *Chem Inform*. 2003;34:864–890.

[59]. Gooyit M, Lee M, Schroeder VA, et al. Selective water-soluble gelatinase inhibitor prodrugs. *J Med Chem*. 2011;54:6676–6690.

[60]. Anand P, Kunnumakkara AB, Newman RA, et al. Bioavailability of curcumin: Problems and promises. *Mol Pharm*. 2007;4:807–818.

[61]. Ahmad A, Sayed A, Ginnebaugh KR, et al. Molecular docking and inhibition of matrix metalloproteinase-2 by novel difluorinatedbenzylidene curcumin analog. *Am J Transl Res*. 2015;7:298–308.

[62]. Mukherjee A, Adhikari N, Jha T. A pentanoic acid derivative targeting matrix metalloproteinase-2 (MMP-2) induces apoptosis in a chronic myeloid leukemia cell line. *Eur J Med Chem*. 2017;141:37–50.

[63]. Adhikari N, Amin SA, Saha A, et al. Understanding chemico-biological interactions of glutamate MMP-2 inhibitors through rigorous alignment-dependent 3D-QSAR Analyses. *ChemistrySelect*. 2017;2:7888–7898.

[64]. GOLD - Protein Ligand Docking Software. https://www.ccdc.cam.ac.uk/solutions/csd-iscovery/components/gold/. Accessed October 2022.

[65]. Moroy G, Denhez C, El Mourabit H, et al. Simultaneous presence of unsaturation and long alkyl chain at P1′ of Ilomastat confers selectivity for gelatinase A (MMP-2) over gelatinase B (MMP-9) inhibition as shown by molecular modelling studies. *Bioorganic Med Chem*. 2007;15:4753–4766.

[66]. Moroy G, Bourguet E, Decarme M, et al. Inhibition of human leukocyte elastase, plasmin and matrix metalloproteinases by oleic acid and oleoyl-galardin derivative(s). *Biochem Pharmacol*. 2011;81:626–635.

[67]. Nicolotti O, Catto M, Giangreco I, et al. Design, synthesis and biological evaluation of 5-hydroxy, 5-substituted-pyrimidine-2,4,6-triones as potent inhibitors of gelatinases MMP-2 and MMP-9. *Eur J Med Chem*. 2012;58:368–376.

[68]. Kumar G, Patnaik R. Inhibition of gelatinases (MMP-2 and MMP-9) by Withania somnifera phytochemicals confers neuroprotection in stroke: An in silico analysis. *Interdiscip Sci Comput Life Sci*. 2018;10:722–733.

[69]. Trott O, Olson AJ. AutoDockVina: Improving the speed and accuracy of docking with a new scoring function, efficient optimization, and multithreading. *J Comput Chem*. 2009;31:455–461.

[70]. Tauro M, Laghezza A, Loiodice F, et al. Arylamino methylene bisphosphonate derivatives as bone seeking matrix metalloproteinase inhibitors. *Bioorg Med Chem*. 2013;21:6456–6465.

[71]. Mangiatordi GF, Guzzo T, Rossano EC, et al. Design, synthesis, and biological evaluation of tetrahydro-β-carboline derivatives as selective sub-nanomolar gelatinase inhibitors. *ChemMedChem*. 2018;13:1343–1352.

12 Modeling Inhibitors of Stromelysins

*Sandip Kumar Baidya, Suvankar Banerjee,
Nilanjan Adhikari, and Tarun Jha*

CONTENTS

ABSTRACT

Stromelysins (namely MMP-3, MMP-10, and MMP-11) are zinc-dependent endopeptidases that are a subclass of MMPs that help with tissue remodeling and extracellular matrix (ECM) proteolysis. In addition to their roles in modulating various disease conditions, these stromelysins have been associated with several disease conditions outside their normal physiological functions. In this context, stromelysins have undergone extensive study regarding their X-ray crystallographic and NMR solution structures. This chapter discusses in detail a variety of ligand- and structure-based drug development (LBDD and SBDD) tactics that have already been undertaken on stromelysin inhibitors that might holistically convey some ideas linked to the future design and discovery of novel stromelysin inhibitors.

Keywords: Stromelysin; Cancer; Hydroxamates; Phosphonamide; Phosphinamide; Thiazepine

12.1 INTRODUCTION

Among various MMPs, MMP-3, MMP-10, and MMP-11 are known as stromelysin 1, stromelysin 2, and stromelysin 3, respectively. Apart from other MMPs, these stromelysins belong to a class of zinc-dependent endopeptidases and assist in the proteolysis of the extracellular matrix (ECM) and tissue remodeling [1–3]. Apart from their normal physiological functions, all these stromelysins (MMP-3, MMP-10, and MMP-11) are associated with several disease conditions. MMP-3 is found to

DOI: 10.1201/9781003303282-15

take part crucial roles in major disease conditions including cardiovascular disorders [4, 5], carotid artery-related complications related to arthritis [6], acute respiratory distress syndrome [7], idiopathic pulmonary fibrosis [8], intervertebral disc disease [9], gastric ulcers [10, 11], rheumatoid arthritis [12, 13], neuronal inflammation [14], schizophrenia [15], periodontitis [16], and virus-induced inflammation [17]. Apart from its crucial role in such diverse diseases, MMP-3 also participates in modulating several cancer conditions, namely lung cancer [8], breast cancer [18, 19], bladder cancer [20], esophageal cancer [21], and nasopharyngeal carcinoma [22]. MMP-10 has a direct correlation with urinary bladder carcinoma [23, 24] and breast carcinoma. MMP-10 has also been associated with idiopathic pulmonary fibrosis [24], atherothrombosis and cardiac diseases [25], asthma [26], as well as Fuchs endothelial corneal dystrophy (FECD) [27]. Similarly, MMP-11 relates to several cancers like cancers of breast, gastric, colorectal, cervical, hepatocellular, and pancreatic, as well as head and neck [28, 29].

12.2 STRUCTURAL ASPECTS OF STROMELYSINS

Regarding the structure and substrate specificity, MMP-3 and MMP-10 display a resemblance (82% structural homology), whereas MMP-11 varies with the former [30, 31]. MMP-3 comprises about 475–478 amino acids, which are found conserved among several species [32, 33]. MMP-3 retains several key domains, i.e., a propeptide domain, a catalytic domain, and a variable ligating peptide with a heme protein domain. On the other hand, MMP-10 is released as a proenzyme that is further activated to produce the active enzyme [30]. Again, MMP-11 is found widely in both normal and disease states [1]. The representative structure of these stromelysins is depicted in Figure 12.1.

12.3 X-RAY CRYSTAL STRUCTURE AND NMR
SOLUTION STRUCTURES OF STROMELYSINS

Several X-ray crystal structures and NMR solution structures of different stromelysins have been reported. Among these structures, several stromelysins are ligand-bound. Therefore, one can explore the binding pattern of the ligand, i.e., how it binds to the catalytic site amino acid residues. Depending on the binding pattern, newer effective and selective inhibitors of stromelysins can be designed. Details of the crystal structures of stromelysins are listed in Table 12.1.

12.4 LIGAND- AND STRUCTURE-BASED DRUG DESIGN
STRATEGIES ON STROMELYSIN INHIBITORS

Considering the crucial roles of stromelysins in various disease conditions, several ligand- and structure-based molecular modeling studies have been carried out to better understand the key structural aspects and the binding pattern of interactions regulating the inhibitory potential of stromelysins. Mostly, MMP-3 has been considered

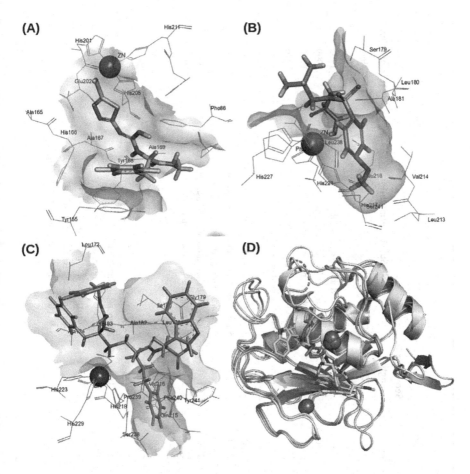

FIGURE 12.1   (A) The catalytic domain of MMP-3 (PDB: 1USN); (B) the catalytic domain of MMP-10 (PDB: 1Q3A); (C) the catalytic domain of MMP-11 (PDB: 1HV5); (D) alignment of all the stromelysins catalytic domains with inbound ligands.

for ligand- and structure-based drug design strategies. Other stromelysins (namely MMP-10 and MMP-11) are not considered for drug design.

As per the report of Hanessian et al. [35], the *p*-methoxy phenylsulfonamido moiety of compound **12.1** (Figure 12.2) oriented properly into the narrow hydrophobic S1′ pocket, and the *i*-butyl group fitted into the S2′ pocket, whereas the benzylthioethyl group accommodated properly into the S1 pocket of MMP-3 enzyme.

In another study, the same group of researchers [36] showed that cyclization of the tertiary nitrogen atom into the pyrrolidine scaffold of compound **12.2** resulted in an almost similar binding mode of interaction at the MMP-3 active site compared with compound **12.1** (Figure 12.2). On the other hand, replacing the benzylthiomethyl group with hydroxymethyl moiety yielded an additional hydrogen bonding interaction with Ala165 at the MMP-3 active site for compound **12.3** (Figure 12.2).

TABLE 12.1

Details of the Crystal Structures of Stromelysins [34]

PDB ID	Type	Structure	Resolution	Sequence length	Substrate/inhibitor	Year of release
1SLM	X-ray	Catalytic domain	1.90	255	—	1996
1SLN	X-ray	Catalytic domain	2.27	173	—	1996
2SRT	Solution NMR	Catalytic domain	—	173	N-carboxyl alkyl-based inhibitor	1995
1B3D	X-ray	Catalytic domain	2.30	173	Hydroxamate-based inhibitor	1999
1UMS	Solution NMR	Catalytic domain	—	174	Hydrophobic peptidic inhibitor	1996
1UMT	Solution NMR	Catalytic domain	—	174	Hydrophobic peptidic inhibitor	1996
1BM6	Solution NMR	Catalytic domain	—	173	Nonpeptidic inhibitor	1999
1C3I	X-ray	Catalytic domain	1.83	173	—	1999
1USN	X-ray	Catalytic domain	1.80	165	5-substituted-1,3,4-thiadiazole-2-thione	1998
2USN	X-ray	Catalytic domain	2.20	165	5-substituted-1,3,4-thiadiazole-2-thione	1998
3USN	Solution NMR	Catalytic domain	—	168	Thiadiazole inhibitor	1999
1HFS	X-ray	Catalytic domain	1.70	160	Biphenylylethyl carboxyalkyl-based inhibitor	1998
1CQR	X-ray	Catalytic domain	2.00	173	Hydroxamate-based inhibitor	2000
1B8Y	X-ray	Catalytic domain	2.00	167	—	1999
1C8T	X-ray	Catalytic domain	2.60	167	—	2000
1QIA	X-ray	Catalytic domain	2.00	165	—	2003
1QIC	X-ray	Catalytic domain	2.00	161	—	2003
1CAQ	X-ray	Catalytic domain	1.80	168	Nonpeptidic inhibitor	1999
1CIZ	X-ray	Catalytic domain	1.64	168	Nonpeptidic inhibitor	1999
2D1O	X-ray	Catalytic domain	2.02	171	Hydroxamic acid inhibitor SM-25453	2006
4DPE	X-ray	—	1.96	173	Platinum-based inhibitor (K[PtCl$_3$(DMSO)])	2013
4G9L	X-ray	—	1.88	173	N-isobutyl-N-[4-methoxyphenylsulfonyl]glycyl hydroxamic acid (NNGH)	2013

(Continued)

TABLE 12.1 (CONTINUED)
Details of the Crystal Structures of Stromelysins [34]

PDB ID	Type	Structure	Resolution	Sequence length	Substrate/inhibitor	Year of release
4JA1	X-ray	–	1.96	173	Platinum-based inhibitor (K[PtCl₃(DMSO)])	2013
1D8M	X-ray	–	2.44	173	Heterocyclic sulfonamides-based inhibitor	2000
1G05	X-ray	–	2.45	173	Heterocyclic sulfonamides-based inhibitor	2001
1BIW	X-ray	–	2.50	173	–	1999
1D5J	X-ray	Catalytic domain	2.60	173	Thiazine- and thiazepine-based inhibitor	2000
1D7X	X-ray	Catalytic domain	2.00	173	Proline scaffold-based inhibitor	2000
1HY7	X-ray	Catalytic domain	1.50	173	Carboxylic acid-based inhibitor	2002
3OHL	X-ray	Catalytic domain	2.36	167	N-hydroxy-2-(4-methoxy-N-(pyridine-3-ylmethyl) phenylsulfonamido)acetamide	2011
3OHO	X-ray	Catalytic domain	2.50	169	N-hydroxy-2-(4-methylphenylsulfonamido)acetam ide	2011
1BQO	X-ray	–	2.30	173	Arylsulfonamido hydroxamate inhibitor	1999
1D8F	X-ray	Catalytic domain	2.40	173	N-hydroxy-1-(4-methoxyphenyl)sulfonyl-4-benzy loxycarbonyl-piperazine-2-carboxamide	2000
2JNP	Solution NMR	Catalytic domain	–	161	N-isobutyl-N-[4-methoxyphenylsulfonyl]glycyl hydroxamic acid (NNGH)	2007
2JT5	Solution NMR	Catalytic domain	–	161	N-hydroxy-2-[N-(2-hydroxyethyl)biphenyl-4-sul fonamide] hydroxamic acid (MLC88)	2008
2JT6	Solution NMR	Catalytic domain	–	161	3-4'-cyanobyphenyl-4-yloxy)-N-hdydroxypropion amide	2008

(Continued)

TABLE 12.1   (CONTINUED)
Details of the Crystal Structures of Stromelysins [34]

PDB ID	Type	Structure	Resolution	Sequence length	Substrate/inhibitor	Year of release
1G49	X-ray	–	1.90	173	(1N)-4-N-butoxyphenylsulfonyl-(2R)-N-hydroxyc arboxamido-(4S)-methanesulfonylamino-pyrrolidine	2001
1UEA	X-ray	Catalytic domain	2.80	173	–	1998
3MFK	X-ray	–	3.00	162	–	2010
1G4K	X-ray	Catalytic domain	2.00	168	5-methyl-5-(4-phenoxy-phenyl)-pyrimidine-2,4,6-tri one	2001
1OO9	Solution NMR	Catalytic domain	–	168	–	2003
6MAV	X-ray	Catalytic domain	2.37	168	–	2019
1Q3A#	X-ray	Catalytic domain	2.10	165	N-isobutyl-N-[4-methoxyphenylsulfonyl]glycyl hydroxamic acid (NNGH)	2004
3V96#	X-ray	Catalytic domain	1.90	184	–	2012
4ILW#	X-ray	Catalytic domain	2.10	194	–	2013
1HV5$	X-ray	Catalytic domain	2.60	165	Phosphonic acid-based inhibitor	2001

#Structure of MMP-10 (stromelysin-2); $structure of MMP-11 (stromelysin-2).

Therefore, the (R)-hydroxy group and the effective interaction with the S1 pocket due to the presence of benzylthiomethyl moiety have been found crucial for MMP-3 inhibition.

Pikul et al. [37] of Procter and Gamble Pharmaceuticals disclosed the binding mode of interaction of compound **12.4** at the MMP-3 active site (Figure 12.3A). The X-ray crystal data (PDB: 163D) displayed that the hydroxamate moiety formed bidentate chelation with the Zn^{2+} ion. Not only that, but the terminal hydroxy group

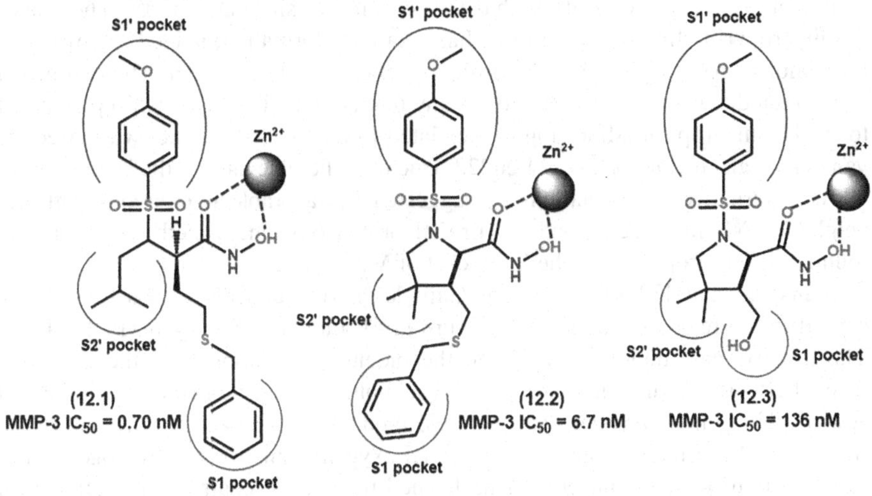

FIGURE 12.2 The binding pattern of compounds **12.1-12.3** at the catalytic site of MMP-3.

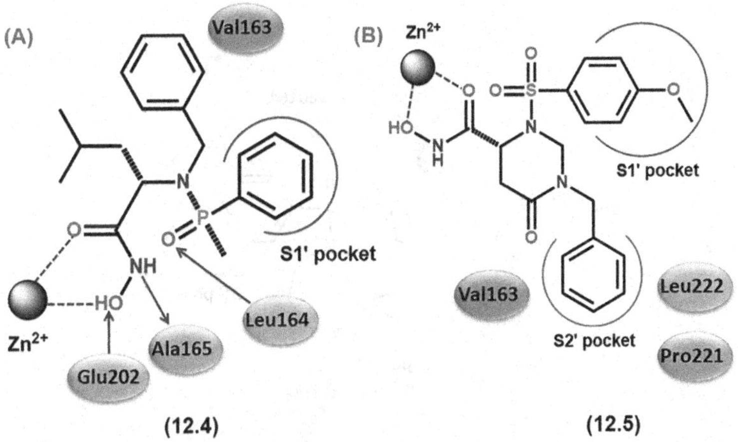

FIGURE 12.3 (A) Binding mode of interaction of compound **12.4** (PDB: 163D) at the stromelysin active site; (B) binding mode of interaction of compound **12.5** (PDB: 1G05) at the stromelysin active site.

also formed a hydrogen bonding interaction with Glu202, and the amide group formed hydrogen bonding with Ala165. The phosphonic acid oxygen atom formed hydrogen bonding with Leu164, and the adjacent methyl group formed a suitable van der Waals interaction with Leu164. The phenyl ring bound to the phosphorus atom fitted nicely into the S1′ pocket, whereas the N-benzyl and the *i*-butyl group formed favorable van der Waals interactions with the hydrophobic side chains of Val163, Leu164, and His166, respectively.

Pikul and co-workers [38] further showed the X-ray co-crystallographic data of compound **12.5** (Figure 12.3B) with truncated stromelysin (PDB: 1G05). The 6-oxo-hexahydropyrimidine ring, due to its half-chair conformation, helped the hydroxa-mate moiety bind to the Zn^{2+} ion through a pseudo-axial position. The oxo group was directed toward the solvent without any interactions. The benzyl group attached to the hexahydropyrimidine ring extrapolated toward the S2′ pocket with effective van der Waals interactions with Leu222. Due to its flexible nature, the benzyl group allows alternative conformations as suggested by favorable interactions with the neighborhood amino acid residues (Pro221 or Val163). The *p*-methoxy group was found to insert properly into the S1′ pocket of MMP-3.

Almstead et al. [39] of Procter and Gamble Pharmaceuticals disclosed the X-ray crystal structure of compound **12.6** (Figure 12.4) bound to stromelysin (PDB: 1D5J). The hydroxamate moiety, apart from the bidentate chelation with the Zn^{2+} ion, formed effective hydrogen bonding with backbone amino acid residues Glu202 and Ala165. The *p*-methoxyphenylsulfonamido moiety accommodated deep inside the S1′ pocket. Nevertheless, one of the sulfonyl oxygen atoms formed hydrogen bond-ing with Leu164. The thiazepine ring formed the pseudo-chair conformation with ring sulfur and methyl groups directed toward the Val163 near the S2′ pocket. The potency of compound **12.6** was mainly dependent on the strong hydrophobic interac-tion with Pro221 and Val163.

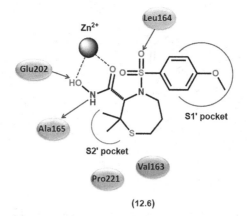

(12.6)

FIGURE 12.4 Binding mode of interaction of compound **12.6** (PDB: 1D5J) at the MMP-3 active site.

Cheng and co-workers [40] from Procter and Gamble Pharmaceuticals disclosed the binding pattern of compound **12.7** (Figure 12.5A) and stromelysin I (PDB: 1D7X). Apart from the strong bidentate chelation between the Zn^{2+} ion and the hydroxamate moiety, there are favorable hydrogen bonding interactions with backbone amino acid residues Glu202 and Ala165 with the hydroxyl and amide functions, respectively. One of the sulfonyl oxygen atoms formed a suitable hydrogen bonding interaction with Leu164. The orientation of the sulfonamido group helped to fit the adjacent *p*-methoxyphenyl group at the S1' pocket. Moreover, the oxime group was extended into the hydrophobic S2' pocket. The sp^2 orientation at the C-4 atom of the pyrrolidine moiety may modulate the higher inhibitory activity of compound **12.7**.

Cheng et al. [41] further analyzed the binding pattern of compound **12.8** (Figure 12.5B) with truncated MMP-3 (PDB: 1D8F). The hydroxamate moiety formed a strong bidentate chelation with the catalytic Zn^{2+} ion, along with two hydrogen bonding interactions with Glu202 and Ala165 through the hydroxyl and amido groups, respectively. In addition, one of the sulfonyl oxygen atoms formed hydrogen bonding interactions with the amido groups of Leu164 and Ala165. The *p*-methoxyphenyl group was inserted deep inside the S1' pocket. Moreover, the carboxybenzyl group was located in an intermediate position between the S1 and S2' pockets, forming hydrophobic interactions with Phe210 and Phe186.

Natchus and co-workers [42] from Procter and Gamble Pharmaceuticals reported the crystal structure of compound **12.9** (Figure 12.6A) with stromelysin (PDB: 1G49). This binding pattern agreed with earlier observations [40, 41]. The *p-n*-butoxy phenyl sulfonamido group fitted nicely into the S1' pocket as well as the hydroxamate moiety strongly bound to the Zn^{2+} ion. Apart from that, the hydroxy and amide groups of the hydroxamate moiety formed hydrogen bonding interactions with Glu202 and Ala165, respectively. On the other hand, one of the oxygen atoms of the sulfonyl group formed hydrogen bonding with Ala165 and Leu164. Not only that, but another hydrogen bonding interaction was also noticed between one of the sulfonyl oxygen atoms of the *p*-methoxyphenyl sulfonamido moiety.

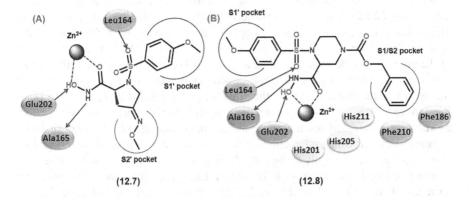

FIGURE 12.5 (A) Binding mode of interaction of compound **12.7** (PDB: 1D7X); (B) binding mode of interaction of compound **12.8** (PDB: 1D8F).

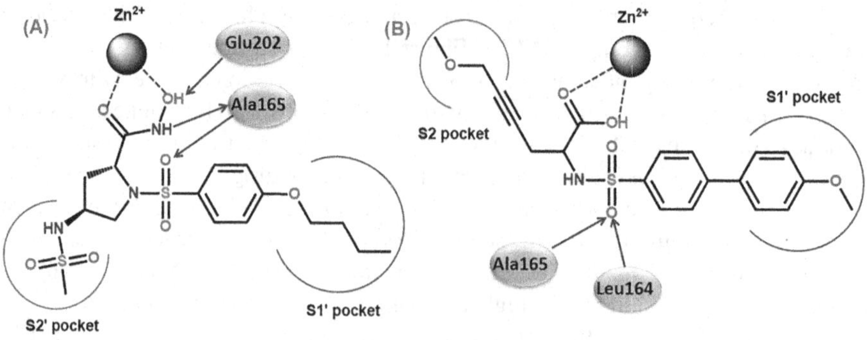

FIGURE 12.6   (A) Binding mode of interaction of compound **12.9** (PDB: 1G49); (B) binding mode of interaction of compound **12.10** (PDB: 1HY7).

Natchus et al. [43] further revealed the crystallographic data of compound **12.10** (Figure 12.6B) with stromelysin I (PDB: 1HY7). It displayed that the biphenyl moiety fitted properly into the S1′ pocket. One of the sulfonyl oxygen atoms formed hydrogen bonding interactions with Leu164 and Ala165, whereas the carboxylic acid moiety formed chelation with the catalytic Zn^{2+} ion. The alkynyl side chain entered into the S2 cleft to make stable interactions.

As per the molecular modeling study of O'Brien et al. [44], the 4′-bromophenyl group of compound **12.11** (Figure 12.7A) entered deep inside the S1′ pocket at the active site of MMP-3 (PDB: 1B8Y). The carboxylic acid moiety was found to chelate to the Zn^{2+} ion as well as the hydroxy group of carboxylic acid moiety, forming a hydrogen bonding interaction with Glu202. On the other hand, one of the sulfonyl oxygen atoms formed hydrogen bonding interactions with Leu164 and Ala165. Due to the electron-withdrawing substituent, the phenyl ring produced π-π stacking interactions with His201 and Tyr223.

Sawa et al. [45] exhibited the phosphonamide-based hydroxamate derivative (compound **12.12**, Figure 12.7B) while binding to the MMP-3 active site (PDB: 1B3D); the hydroxamate function strongly bound to the catalytic Zn^{2+} ion and the p-methoxyphenyl moiety entered inside the S1′ pocket of MMP-3. The oxygen atom of the phosphonamide moiety formed a hydrogen bonding interaction with Ala165. Nevertheless, Ala165 was found to form hydrogen bonding with the amide group of the hydroxamate function. Again, the ethyloxy group resided along with the binding groove of the substrate backbone and formed the van der Waals interaction. Moreover, the tetrahydroisoquinoline moiety interacted at the S1/S2 subsite with favorable van der Waals interactions. The molecular docking study also disclosed that the (R)-isomer was only active, and the respective (S)-isomer was inactive.

Foley and co-workers [46] from Hoffmann-La Roche proposed the X-ray crystal structure of compound **12.13** (Figure 12.8A) with the catalytic site of stromelysin-1. The phenoxyphenyl group was located deep into the S1′ pocket. The nitrogen atom at the third position of the 2,4,6-pyrimidinedione moiety formed chelation with the

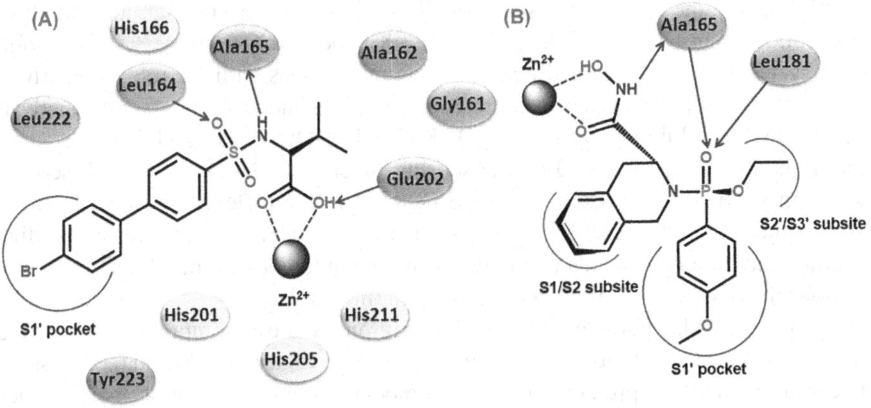

FIGURE 12.7 (A) Binding mode of interaction of compound **12.11** (PDB: 1B8Y); (B) binding mode of interaction of compound **12.12** (PDB: 1B3D).

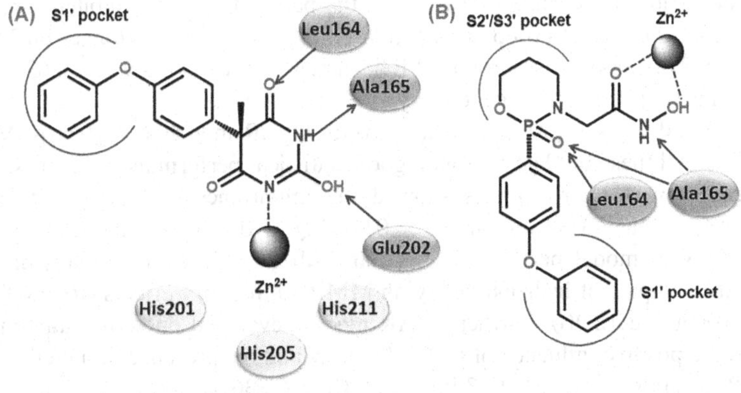

FIGURE 12.8 (A) Binding mode of interaction of compound **12.13** at the MMP-3 active site; (B) binding mode of interaction of compound **12.14** at the MMP-3 active site.

catalytic Zn^{2+} ion that is stabilized by interactions with three histidine residues, namely His201, His205, and His211. On the other hand, the oxygen atom at the second position formed a bidentate hydrogen bonding interaction with Glu202, whereas the oxygen atom at the sixth position produced hydrogen bonding with Leu164 and Ala165.

Sorensen et al. [47] from LEO Pharma proposed the binding mode of interaction for the study of cyclophosphonamides and cyclophosphinamides. The aryl group of compound **12.14** (Figure 12.8B) attached to the phosphorus atom entered into the S1′ pocket. Again, an increase in the size with hydrophobicity drastically enhanced the affinity toward the deep S1' pocket of MMP-3. The cyclic phosphonamide and phosphinamide moiety may lie closer to the S2' or S3' pockets. Nevertheless, the phosphinyl oxygen atom produced hydrogen bonding interactions with Ala165 and Leu164.

Ha et al. [48] performed a comparative binding mode of interaction analysis of 61 MMP-3 inhibitors by using DOCK4/PMF, DOCK4/FF, and FlexX scoring and ranked the ligands based on the scoring functions. The DOCK4/PMF scoring function yielded better results than the DOCK4/FF and FlexX scoring functions. Importantly, the DOCK4/PMF scoring function was able to correlate the binding affinity and predicted scores in a better fashion. On the other hand, FlexX was able to offer the best "fine tuning" in predicted binding modes.

Gupta et al. [49] performed a QSAR study on a dataset comprising 20 MMP-3 inhibitors. This QSAR model produced R^2_{Adj} and Q^2 values of 0.80 and 0.65, respectively, implying good predictability of this model. It noted Kier's first-order valence molecular connectivity index for the aminoproline nitrogen atom ($1_\chi^v N$) as well as the electrotopological state-atom index of the sulfur atom of the sulfonamide moiety. Both parameters contributed negatively to MMP-3 inhibitory activity. Interestingly, it was noticed that molecules having alkyl or heteroaryl substitutions at the functionalized aminoproline moiety favored MMP-3 inhibition. In another QSAR model performed with 26 hydantoin derivatives, the parameter $1_\chi^v N$ exhibited a negative contribution, but the R-group substitution exhibited a positive impact on MMP-3 inhibition. This model also produced R^2_{Adj} and Q^2 values of 0.69 and 0.63, respectively, reflecting good statistical quality.

Verma and Hansch [50] performed several QSAR models on effective MMP-3 inhibitors. All these models exhibited good statistical performance. The first model performed on 11 hydroxamates showed the importance of hydrophobic effects conducive to MMP-3 inhibition ($R^2 = 0.904$, $Q^2 = 0.848$) (Figure 12.9A). Again, another QSAR model performed on 12 arylsulfonamido hydroxamates displayed the positive impact of hydrophobicity on MMP-3 inhibitory effects ($R^2 = 0.857$, $Q^2 = 0.806$) (Figure 12.9B). Further QSAR model developed on some sulphonamide showed the positive influence of hydrophobicity and the presence of a methyl group at the R_1 position toward MMP-3 inhibition ($R^2 = 0.836$, $Q^2 = 0.745$) (Figure 12.9C). Another QSAR model developed on 18 homophenylaniline derivatives, from a positive impact on hydrophobicity, also exhibited a negative impact of steric substituents on biological efficacy ($R^2 = 0.893$, $Q^2 = 0.834$) (Figure 12.9D). Nevertheless, the presence of leucine moiety was found to modulate MMP-3 inhibition. Another model on 15 succinyl hydroxamates resulted in a parabolic relationship with MMP-3 inhibition and hydrophobic substituents at the X position (optimum hydrophobicity = 4.936) (Figure 12.9E). On the other hand, hydrophobic substituents at the Y position had unfavorable MMP-3 inhibition ($R^2 = 0.906$, $Q^2 = 0.842$). The further model performed on 25 succinyl hydroxamates resulted in the positive impact of hydrophobicity and hydroxamate function for higher MMP-3 inhibition ($R^2 = 0.895$, $Q^2 = 0.860$) (Figure 12.9F). Another model performed on eight thiadiazole urea methylamides resulted in the positive influence of molar refractivity toward MMP-3 inhibition ($R^2 = 0.836$, $Q^2 = 0.718$) (Figure 12.9G). A further model developed on some

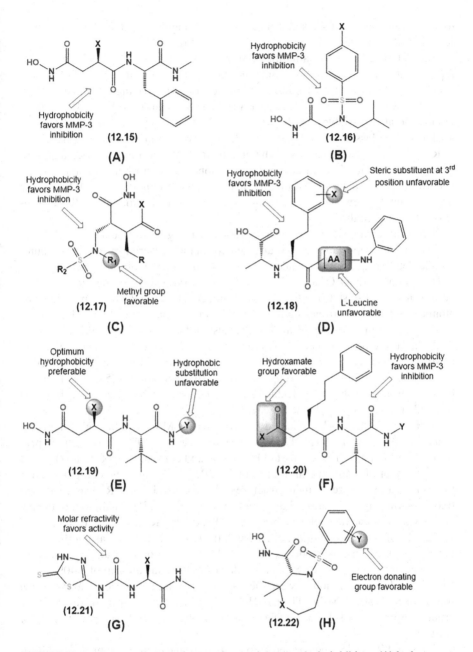

FIGURE 12.9 Structural requirements of potential stromelysin inhibitors (A) hydroxamate derivatives, (B) arylsulfonamido hydroxamates, (C) sulphonamide derivative, (D) homophenylaniline derivatives, (E) succinyl hydroxamates, (F) succinyl hydroxamates, (G) thiadiazole urea methylamides, and (H) thiazepine derivatives.

thiazepine derivatives disclosed that electron-donating groups at the Y position may favor MMP-3 inhibition ($R^2 = 0.860$, $Q^2 = 0.759$) (Figure 12.9H).

Bursi et al. [51] tried to attempt CoMFA models produced by docking flexible representatives into the MMP-3 enzyme. Different conformations of fields were tried to build various CoMFA models with several grid spacing combinations. By using the H-bond field, the best CoMFA model was obtained ($Q^2 = 0.41$, $s = 0.61$, number of latent variables = 4, $R^2 = 0.90$, $F = 98.4$). However, the steric field generated a slightly less good model ($Q^2 = 0.35$, $s = 0.64$, number of latent variables = 5, $R^2 = 0.87$, $F = 59.8$). However, the electrostatic field did not produce a significant model. Among these three fields, the H-bond field contributed the most (64%) toward biological activity. Around the hydroxamate group, the favorability of the donor group was revealed. The presence of acceptor fields around the P1' substituents may enhance the activity.

Fernandez et al. [52] performed a multiple linear regression model on 30 MMP-3 inhibitors. The importance of Moran's autocorrelation descriptors and Geary autocorrelation descriptors was revealed to modulate the MMP-3 inhibitory activity. This model produced LOO-Q^2 and L30-Q^2 values of 0.581 and 0.544, respectively, suggesting it to be the statistically validated model. The QSAR model revealed that atomic Sanderson electronegativities were the major contributor to MMP-3 inhibition. Again, atomic van der Waals volumes also influenced MMP-3 inhibition.

As far as the binding mode of interaction of the N-hydroxyurea compound with MMP-3 is concerned, it was stabilized to form hydrogen bonding with the ethereal oxygen atom and amide group of both Leu164 and Ala165 [53]. The terminal hydroxy group formed monodentate Zn^{2+} chelation. The bulky p-cyano biphenyl scaffold entered deep inside the S1' cavity.

Amin and Welsh [54] conducted CoMFA and CoMSIA studies on some compounds bearing a wide range of MMP-3 inhibitory activity. The CoMFA study produced an acceptable cross-validated R^2 (0.582) and conventional R^2 (0.807) with a standard error of 0.467 and an F ratio of 33.391. Removing some compounds due to conformationally restrained structures, the cross-validated R^2 was increased (0.607) with a higher F ratio (55.304) and a lower SEE (0.471). Again, removing the carboxylate derivatives yielded a better CoMFA model ($R^2_{CV} = 0.614$, $R^2 = 0.968$, $F = 132.103$, SEE = 0.180). On the other hand, the CoMSIA model was not that much better than the CoMFA model. The CoMSIA model produced an R^2_{CV} value of 0.608, a conventional R^2 of 0.835, an F value of 21.986, and an SEE of 0.409. These CoMFA and CoMSIA models were successful in predicting a series of arylsulfonyl isoquinoline-based MMPIs. The CoMFA and CoMSIA contour maps revealed the crucial importance of the steric, electrostatic, hydrogen bond donor, and acceptor features.

Amin and Welsh [55] performed a CoMFA study and designed some 2-phthalimidine glutaric acid analogs. Many of these molecules were predicted as highly active potent MMP-3 inhibitors (predicted $pIC_{50} > 9.2$). The molecular docking interaction of a compound at the MMP-3 active site revealed that the β-phenylethylamine group formed two hydrophobic interactions with Phe186 and Phe210. Two carbonyl oxygen atoms formed the bidentate chelation with the Zn^{2+} ion. The amido group formed hydrogen bonding with Glu202, whereas the other carbonyl oxygen atom formed hydrogen bonding interaction with Leu164. Amin et al. [56] again performed the 3D-QSAR CoMFA study, resulting in a conventional R^2 of 0.989 and a cross-validated R^2 of 0.592. Some important steric and electrostatic features were identified, modulating the MMP-3 inhibitory activity of these compounds.

Amadasi and co-workers [57] conducted the molecular modeling study of some amidinobenzisothiazoles with MMP-3. All compounds placed their amidine group at the S1′ subsite in such a manner that it can form potential hydrogen bonding interactions in an almost similar binding orientation with the side chain amino acids coordinating the benzisothiazole ring and other hydrophobic substituents into the hydrophobic pockets at the entrance and bottom of the cavity, respectively. The amidino group of compound **12.23** formed hydrogen bonding with the carbonyl oxygens of Ala216 and Tyr220, as well as with the imidazole nitrogen of His224 within 3.5Å (Figure 12.10A).

Similarly, compound **12.24** formed hydrogen bonding with amino acids Tyr220, Ala217, and His224, whereas compound **12.25** formed hydrogen bonding interactions with Ala217 and His224 (Figure 12.10B and 12.10C). Both the benzamidine (**12.23**) and *p*-chloro benzamidine (**12.24**) derivatives interacted with the hydrophobic side chains formed by Leu164, Val198, and Tyr223 and resided at the entrance of the cavity. However, the *p*-chloro benzamidine compound (**12.24**) interacted more strongly, interacting deeply with the amino acids Leu197 and Leu226.

Tuccinardi et al. [58] considered 54 training MMP-3 inhibitors for ligand-based 3D-QSAR modeling and validated it on 15 test MMP-3 inhibitors considering nine X-ray crystal structures for a multi-template alignment (MTA) approach. The best MTA 3D-QSAR model resulted in an R^2 of 0.92, a Q^2 of 0.77, and an SDEP$_{test}$ of 0.64. The external set comprising 106 MMP-3 inhibitors also confirmed the predictive ability of the 3D-QSAR model. Interestingly, based on the outcomes of the 3D-QSAR model, some iminodiacetyl-based hydroxamate derivatives were predicted to be effective MMP-3 inhibitors. These compounds were tried further for *in vitro* MMP-3 inhibition and some of them (compounds **12.26**–**12.29**) exerted highly potent MMP-3 inhibitory activity (Figure 12.11).

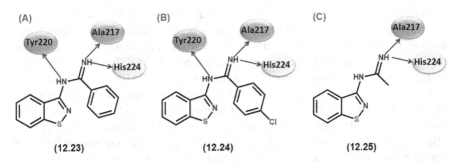

FIGURE 12.10 Binding mode of interactions of (A) compound **12.23**, (B) compound **12.24**, and (C) compound **12.25** at the MMP-3 active site.

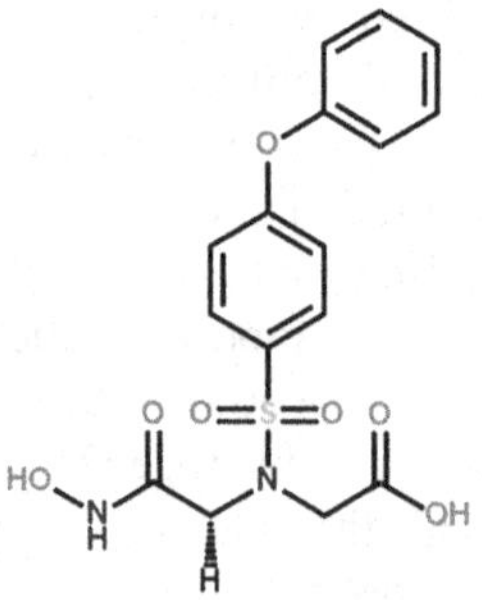

(12.26)
MMP-3 IC_{50} = 37.2 nM

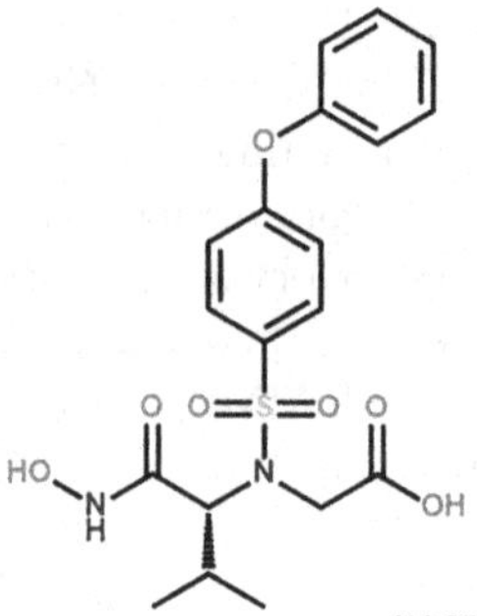

(12.27)
MMP-3 IC_{50} = 6.7 nM

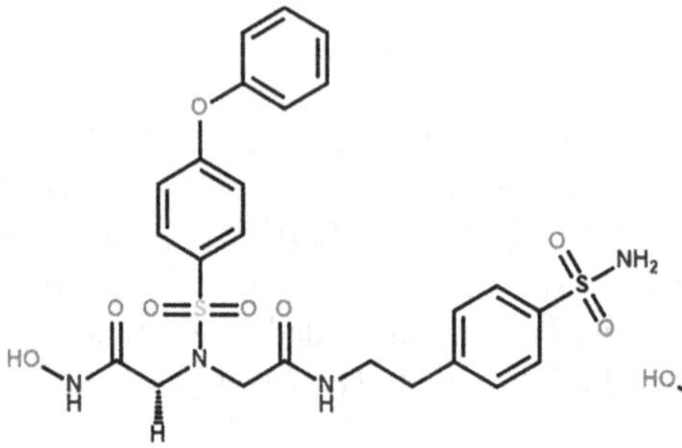

(12.28)
MMP-3 IC_{50} = 6.1 nM

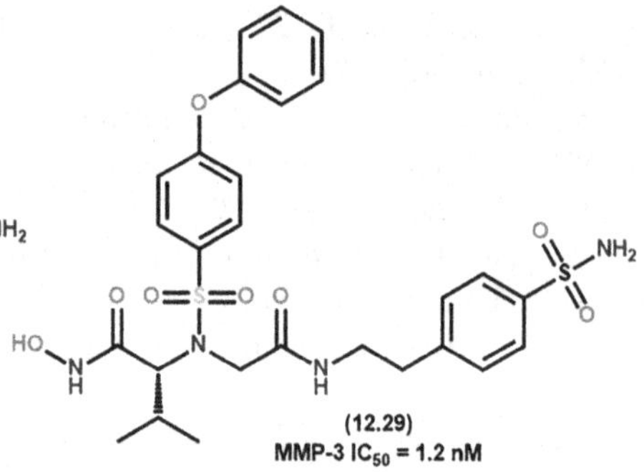

(12.29)
MMP-3 IC_{50} = 1.2 nM

FIGURE 12.11 Designed highly potent MMP-3 inhibitors (compounds **12.26–12.29**).

Durrant and co-workers [59] predicted some conformationally selective pyrone-based inhibitors of MMP-3 through the LUDI docking program. The structure-based molecular dynamics (MD) simulation study was able to evaluate the binding pattern of these molecules as better and more selective MMP-3 inhibitors than MMP-2. This ensemble-based docking study was also able to correlate the differences in the dynamic behavior of MMP-3 and MMP-2 to explain the selectivity of compounds toward MMP-3 over MMP-2.

Senn and co-workers [60] designed some dual MMP-10/MMP-13 selective inhibitors through a molecular docking study. The phenyloxazole moiety was found to be inserted into the S1′ pocket. Similarly, the arylcarboxamide moiety fitted nicely into the S1′ pocket of MMP-3. Amino acid residues, namely Phe242 and Phe248, were found to play crucial roles in aromatic interactions at the MMP-10 active site.

Crasci et al. [61] showed that some flavonoid compounds, namely apigenin-7-O-glucuronide, apigenin-7-O-rutinoside, apigenin-7-O-glucoside, apigenin, luteolin-7-O-glucuronide, luteolin-7-O-glucoside, luteolin-7-O-rutinoside, and luteolin, effectively bind at the MMP-3 active site (PDB: 1HY7), forming several hydrogen bonding interactions. The key amino acid residues involved are Ala165, Leu222, Gly192, Leu218, Asn194, Pro221, Tyr220, Glu216, Arg231, Arg233, and His201.

He et al. [62] reported the molecular modeling study of 6,6'-bieckol obtained from *Ecklonia cava*. The molecular docking interaction of 6,6'-bieckol with MMP-3 (PDB ID: 2JT6) revealed that this molecule (compound **12.30**) exhibited a good docking score (CDOCKER interaction energy = −57.91 kcal/mol). This molecule formed several hydrogen bonding interactions with amino acid residues Thr215, Glu216, Leu218, His201, and Ala165, along with a π-π stacking interaction with His201 (Figure 12.12).

Jerah et al. [63] reported the molecular docking study of curcumin (compound **12.31**) and human MMP-3 (PDB ID: 1BBY) (Figure 12.13). It was found to bind at the active site of MMP-3, whereas the two phenyl rings of curcumin formed a π-π stacking interaction with His201 and His224 as well as Tyr223. Moreover, the hydroxy group formed a hydrogen bonding interaction with Leu218. Again, hydrogen bonding interaction was found between the phenolic hydroxy group and amino acid residues Leu164 and Ala165.

Chin et al. [64] reported the binding mode of interactions of harmine (compound **12.32**), a natural β-carboline alkaloid from *Peganum harmala* with the active site of MMP-3 (PDB: 1HFS). The pyridine nitrogen atom formed Zn^{2+} chelation, and the adjacent methyl group formed π-alkyl interaction with His205 and His211 (Figure 12.14). Nevertheless, the phenyl ring formed π-alkyl interaction with Val163 at the active site. Again, van der Waals interaction was noticed with Glu202.

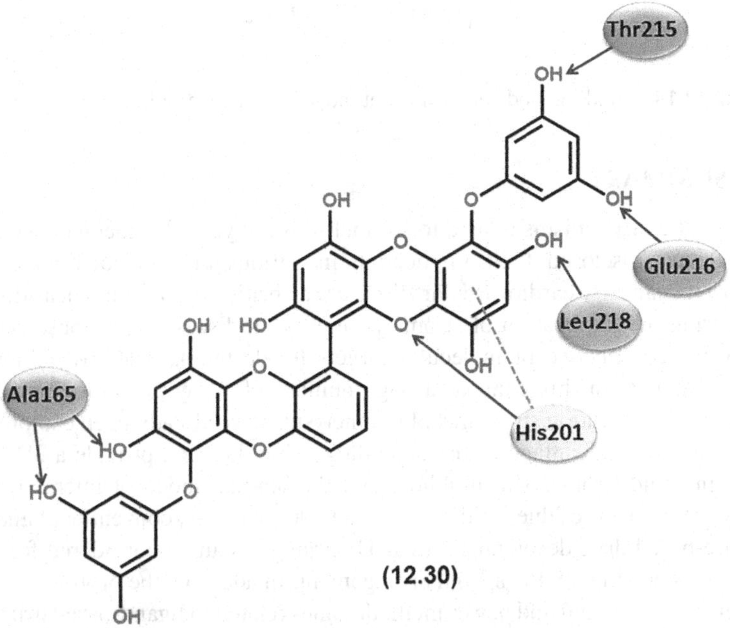

(12.30)

FIGURE 12.12 Binding mode of 6,6'-bieckol at the MMP-3 active site.

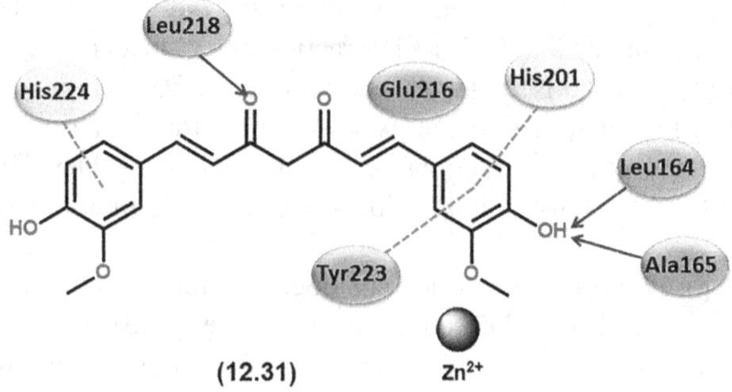

FIGURE 12.13 Binding mode of curcumin at the MMP-3 active site.

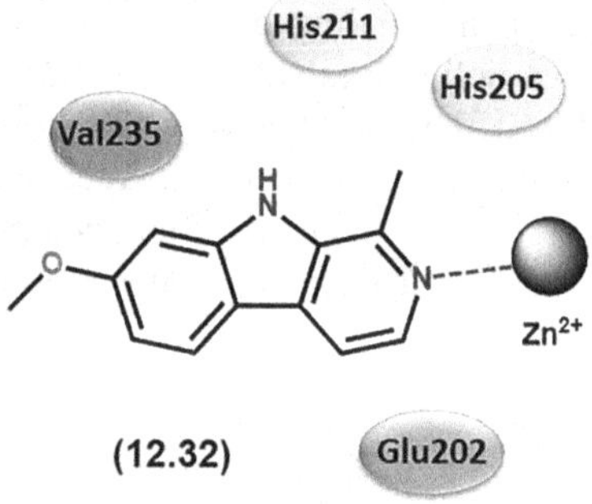

FIGURE 12.14 Binding mode of harmine at the MMP-3 active site.

12.5 SUMMARY

Although the mechanisms related to stromelysins are yet to be adequately explored, evidence has disclosed their implication in various disease conditions, including various cancers, cardiovascular diseases, arthritis, and neurological disorders. Considering the implication of stromelysins in such disease conditions, these may be targeted as effective biomolecular targets for designing selective inhibitors as drug candidates. In this context, a huge number of X-ray crystallographic structures and NMR solution structures of stromelysins have already been explored. This can be an added advantage as the crystallographic data can provide a 3D orientation of inbound stromelysin inhibitors and the binding mode of interactions with the key amino acid residues at the active site. Nevertheless, conventional and newer structure-based drug development (SBDD) strategies can be considered for fruitful outcomes depending on the spatial arrangement. In addition, the prolific application of several conventional and newer methodologies related to ligand-based drug design (LBDD) can also be applied to designing effective and selective stromelysin inhibitors. In this chapter, a number of LBDD and SBDD strategies already conducted on stromelysin inhibitors were discussed in detail, holistically depicting some ideas related to the future design and discovery of novel stromelysin inhibitors. Therefore, considering the abovementioned aspects, there is huge scope for designing novel molecules that are more effective than existing ones. This may be a stepping stone for future drug design and development related to the inhibition of stromelysins.

REFERENCES

[1]. Matziari M, Dive V, Yiotakis A. Matrix metalloproteinase 11 (MMP-11; stromelysin-3) and synthetic inhibitors. *Med Res Rev* 2007;27(4):528–552.

[2]. Nagase H, Visse R, Murphy G. Structure and function of matrix metalloproteinases and TIMPs. *Cardiovasc Res* 2006;69(3):562–573.

[3]. Laronha H, Caldeira J. Structure and function of human matrix metalloproteinases. *Cells* 2020;9(5):1076.

[4]. Eyyupkoca F, Sabanoglu C, Altintas MS, et al. Higher levels of TWEAK and matrix metalloproteinase-3 during the acute phase of myocardial infarction are associated with adverse left ventricular remodeling. *Postepy Kardiol Interwencyjnej* 2021;17(4):356–365.

[5]. Wang X, Han W, Han L, et al. Levels of serum sST2, MMP-3, and Gal-3 in patients with essential hypertension and their correlation with left ventricular hypertrophy. *Evid Based Complement Alternat Med* 2021;2021:7262776.

[6]. Klimontov VV, Koroleva EA, Khapaev RS, et al. Carotid artery disease in subjects with type 2 diabetes: Risk factors and biomarkers. *J Clin Med* 2021;11(1):72.

[7]. Artham S, Verma A, Newsome AS, et al. Patients with acute respiratory distress syndrome exhibit increased stromelysin1 activity in the blood samples. *Cytokine* 2020;131:155086.

[8]. Kreus M, Lehtonen S, Skarp S, et al. Extracellular matrix proteins produced by stromal cells in idiopathic pulmonary fibrosis and lung adenocarcinoma. *PLOS ONE* 2021;16(4):e0250109.

[9]. Ravichandran D, Pillai J, Krishnamurthy K. Genetics of intervertebral disc disease: A review. *Clin Anat* 2022;35(1):116–120.

[10]. Choudhary P, Roy T, Chatterjee A, et al. Melatonin rescues swim stress induced gastric ulceration by inhibiting matrix metalloproteinase-3 via down-regulation of inflammatory signaling cascade. *Life Sci* 2022;297:120426.

[11]. Ming S, Yin H, Li X, et al. GITR promotes the polarization of TFH-like cells in *helicobacter pylori*-positive gastritis. *Front Immunol* 2021;12:736269.

[12]. Kvacskay P, Yao N, Schnotz JH, et al. Increase of aerobic glycolysis mediated by activated T helper cells drives synovial fibroblasts towards an inflammatory phenotype: New targets for therapy? *Arthritis Res Ther* 2021;23(1):56.

[13]. Mirtaheri E, Khabbazi A, Nazemiyeh H, et al. Stachys schtschegleevii tea, matrix metalloproteinase, and disease severity in female rheumatoid arthritis patients: A randomized controlled clinical trial. *Clin Rheumatol* 2022;41(4):1033–1044.

[14]. Lefevere E, Salinas-Navarro M, Andries L, et al. Tightening the retinal glia limitans attenuates neuroinflammation after optic nerve injury. *Glia* 2020;68(12):2643–2660.

[15]. Ordak M, Libman-Sokolowska M, Nasierowski T, et al. Matrix metalloproteinase-3 serum levels in schizophrenic patients. *Int J Psychiatry Clin Pract* 2022:1–7.

[16]. Hashimoto H, Hashimoto S, Shimazaki Y. Functional impairment and periodontitis in rheumatoid arthritis. *Int Dent J* 2022;S0020-6539(22)00022-3.

[17]. Sengupta S, Addya S, Biswas D, et al. Matrix metalloproteinases and tissue inhibitors of metalloproteinases in murine β-coronavirus-induced neuroinflammation. *Virology* 2022;566:122–135.

[18]. Argote Camacho AX, González Ramírez AR, Pérez Alonso AJ, et al. Metalloproteinases 1 and 3 as potential biomarkers in breast cancer development. *Int J Mol Sci* 2021;22(16):9012.

[19]. Suhaimi SA, Chan SC, Rosli R. Matrix metallopeptidase 3 polymorphisms: Emerging genetic markers in human breast cancer metastasis. *J Breast Cancer* 2020; 23(1):1–9.

[20]. Ay A, Alkanli N, Cevik G. Investigation of the relationship between MMP-1 (-1607 1G/2G), MMP-3 (-1171 5A/6A) gene variations and development of bladder cancer. *Mol Biol Rep* 2021;48(12):7689–7695.

[21]. Sharma R, Chattopadhyay TK, Mathur M, et al. Prognostic significance of stromelysin-3 and tissue inhibitor of matrix metalloproteinase-2 in esophageal cancer. *Oncology* 2004;67(3–4):300–309.

[22]. Allen DZ, Aljabban J, Silverman D, et al. Meta-analysis illustrates possible role of lipopolysaccharide (LPS)-induced tissue injury in nasopharyngeal carcinoma (NPC) pathogenesis. *PLOS ONE* 2021;16(10):e0258187.

[23]. Kudelski J, Młynarczyk G, Gudowska-Sawczuk M, et al. Enhanced expression but decreased specific activity of matrix metalloproteinase 10 (MMP-10) in comparison with matrix metalloproteinase 3 (MMP-3) in human urinary bladder carcinoma. *J Clin Med* 2021;10(16):3683.

[24]. Sokai A, Handa T, Tanizawa K, et al. Matrix metalloproteinase-10: A novel biomarker for idiopathic pulmonary fibrosis. *Respir Res* 2015;16:120.

[25]. Rodriguez JA, Orbe J, Martinez de Lizarrondo S, et al. Metalloproteinases and atherothrombosis: MMP-10 mediates vascular remodeling promoted by inflammatory stimuli. *Front Biosci* 2008;13:2916–2921.

[26]. Kuo CS, Pavlidis S, Zhu J, et al. Contribution of airway eosinophils in airway wall remodeling in asthma: Role of MMP-10 and MET. *Allergy* 2019;74(6):1102–1112.

[27]. Xu I, Thériault M, Brunette I, et al. Matrix metalloproteinases and their inhibitors in Fuchs endothelial corneal dystrophy. *Exp Eye Res* 2021;205:108500.

[28]. Ma B, Ran R, Liao HY, et al. The paradoxical role of matrix metalloproteinase-11 in cancer. *Biomed Pharmacother* 2021;141:111899.

[29]. Matziari M, Dive V, Yiotakis A. Matrix metalloproteinase 11 (MMP-11; stromelysin-3) and synthetic inhibitors. *Med Res Rev* 2007;27(4):528–552.

[30]. Piskór BM, Przylipiak A, Dąbrowska E, et al. Matrilysins and stromelysins in pathogenesis and diagnostics of cancers. *Cancer Manag Res* 2020;12:10949–10964.

[31]. Klein T, Bischoff R. Physiology and pathophysiology of matrix metalloproteases. *Amino Acids* 2011;41(2):271–290.

[32]. Wan J, Zhang G, Li X, et al. Matrix metalloproteinase 3: A promoting and destabilizing factor in the pathogenesis of disease and cell differentiation. *Front Physiol* 2021;12:663978.

[33]. Adamcova M, Šimko F. Multiplex biomarker approach to cardiovascular diseases. *Acta Pharmacol Sin* 2018;39(7):1068–1072.

[34]. https://www.rcsb.org/ as accessed in September 2022.

[35]. Hanessian S, Bouzbouz S, Boudon A, et al. Picking the S1, S1' and S2' pockets of matrix metalloproteinases: A niche for potent acyclic sulfonamide inhibitors. *Bioorg Med Chem Lett* 1999;9(12):1691–1696.

[36]. Hanessian S, MacKay DB, Moitessier N. Design and synthesis of matrix metalloproteinase inhibitors guided by molecular modeling. Picking the S(1) pocket using conformationally constrained inhibitors. *J Med Chem* 2001;44(19):3074–3082.

[37]. Pikul S, Dunham KM, Almstead NG, et al. Design and synthesis of phosphinamide-based hydroxamic acids as inhibitors of matrix metalloproteinases. *J Med Chem* 1999;42(1):87–94.

[38]. Pikul S, Dunham KM, Almstead NG, et al. Heterocycle-based MMP inhibitors with P2' substituents. *Bioorg Med Chem Lett* 2001;11(8):1009–1013.

[39]. Almstead NG, Bradley RS, Pikul S, et al. Design, synthesis, and biological evaluation of potent thiazine- and thiazepine-based matrix metalloproteinase inhibitors. *J Med Chem* 1999;42(22):4547–4562.

[40]. Cheng M, De B, Almstead NG, et al. Design, synthesis, and biological evaluation of matrix metalloproteinase inhibitors derived from a modified proline scaffold. *J Med Chem* 1999;42(26):5426–5436.

[41]. Cheng M, De B, Pikul S, et al. Design and synthesis of piperazine-based matrix metalloproteinase inhibitors. *J Med Chem* 2000;43(3):369–380.

[42]. Natchus MG, Bookland RG, De B, et al. Development of new hydroxamate matrix metalloproteinase inhibitors derived from functionalized 4-aminoprolines. *J Med Chem* 2000;43(26):4948–4963.

[43]. Natchus MG, Bookland RG, Laufersweiler MJ, et al. Development of new carboxylic acid-based MMP inhibitors derived from functionalized propargylglycines. *J Med Chem* 2001;44(7):1060–1071.

[44]. O'Brien PM, Ortwine DF, Pavlovsky AG, et al. Structure-activity relationships and pharmacokinetic analysis for a series of potent, systemically available biphenylsulfonamide matrix metalloproteinase inhibitors. *J Med Chem* 2000;43(2):156–166.

[45]. Sawa M, Kiyoi T, Kurokawa K, et al. New type of metalloproteinase inhibitor: Design and synthesis of new phosphonamide-based hydroxamic acids. *J Med Chem* 2002;45(4):919–929.

[46]. Foley LH, Palermo R, Dunten P, et al. Novel 5,5-disubstitutedpyrimidine-2,4,6-triones as selective MMP inhibitors. *Bioorg Med Chem Lett* 2001;11(8):969–972.

[47]. Sørensen MD, Blaehr LK, Christensen MK, et al. Cyclic phosphinamides and phosphonamides, novel series of potent matrix metalloproteinase inhibitors with antitumour activity. *Bioorg Med Chem* 2003;11(24):5461–5484.

[48]. Ha S, Andreani R, Robbins A, et al. Evaluation of docking/scoring approaches: A comparative study based on MMP-3 inhibitors. *J Comput Aid Mol Des* 2000;14(5):435–448.

[49]. Gupta SP, Kumar D, Kumaran S. A quantitative structure-activity relationship study of hydroxamate matrix metalloproteinase inhibitors derived from functionalized 4-aminoprolines. *Bioorg Med Chem* 2003;11(9):1975–1981.

[50]. Verma RP, Hansch C. Matrix metalloproteinases (MMPs): Chemical-biological functions and (Q)SARs. *Bioorg Med Chem* 2007;15(6):2223–2268.

[51]. Bursi R, Sawa M, Hiramatsu Y, et al. A three-dimensional quantitative structure-activity relationship study of heparin-binding epidermal growth factor shedding inhibitors using comparative molecular field analysis. *J Med Chem* 2002;45(4):781–788.

[52]. Fernández M, Caballero J, Tundidor-Camba A. Linear and nonlinear QSAR study of N-hydroxy-2-[(phenylsulfonyl)amino]acetamide derivatives as matrix metalloproteinase inhibitors. *Bioorg Med Chem* 2006;14(12):4137–4150.

[53]. Campestre C, Agamennone M, Tortorella P, et al. N-hydroxyurea as zinc binding group in matrix metalloproteinase inhibition: Mode of binding in a complex with MMP-8. *Bioorg Med Chem Lett* 2006;16(1):20–24.

[54]. Amin EA, Welsh WJ. Highly predictive CoMFA and CoMSIA models for two series of stromelysin-1 (MMP-3) inhibitors elucidate S1' and S1-S2' binding modes. *J Chem Inf Model* 2006;46(4):1775–1783.

[55]. Amin EA, Welsh WJ. A preliminary in silico lead series of 2-phthalimidinoglutaric acid analogues designed as MMP-3 inhibitors. *J Chem Inf Model* 2006;46(5):2104–2109.

[56]. Ambrose Amin E, Welsh WJ. Three-dimensional quantitative structure-activity relationship (3D-QSAR) models for a novel class of piperazine-based stromelysin-1 (MMP-3) inhibitors: Applying a "divide and conquer" strategy. *J Med Chem* 2001;44(23):3849–3855.

[57]. Amadasi A, Cozzini P, Incerti M, et al. Molecular modeling of binding between amidi-nobenzisothiazoles, with antidegenerative activity on cartilage, and matrix metalloproteinase-3. *Bioorg Med Chem* 2007;15(3):1420–1429.

[58]. Tuccinardi T, Ortore G, Santos MA, et al. Multitemplate alignment method for the development of a reliable 3D-QSAR model for the analysis of MMP-3 inhibitors. *J Chem Inf Model* 2009;49(7):1715–1724.

[59]. Durrant JD, de Oliveira CA, McCammon JA. Pyrone-based inhibitors of metalloproteinase types 2 and 3 may work as conformation-selective inhibitors. *Chem Biol Drug Des* 2011;78(2):191–198.

[60]. Senn N, Ott M, Lanz J, et al. Targeted polypharmacology: Discovery of a highly potent non-hydroxamate dual matrix metalloproteinase (MMP)-10/-13 inhibitor. *J Med Chem* 2017;60(23):9585–9598.

[61]. Crascì L, Basile L, Panico A, et al. Correlating in vitro target-oriented screening and docking: Inhibition of matrix metalloproteinases activities by flavonoids. *Planta Med* 2017;83(11):901–911.

[62]. He YL, Xiao Z, Yang S, et al. A phlorotanin, 6,6'-bieckol from Ecklonia cava, against photoaging by inhibiting MMP-1, -3 and -9 expression on UVB-induced HaCaT keratinocytes. *Photochem Photobiol* 2022;98(5):1131–1139.

[63]. Jerah A, Hobani Y, Kumar BV, et al. Curcumin binds in silico to anti-cancer drug target enzyme MMP-3 (human stromelysin-1) with affinity comparable to two known inhibitors of the enzyme. *Bioinformation* 2015;11(8):387–392.

[64]. Chin LT, Liu KW, Chen YH, et al. Cell-based assays and molecular simulation reveal that the anti-cancer harmine is a specific matrix metalloproteinase-3 (MMP-3) inhibitor. *Comput Biol Chem* 2021;94:107556.

13 Modeling Inhibitors of Matrilysin

Suvankar Banerjee, Sandip Kumar Baidya,
Nilanjan Adhikari, and Tarun Jha

CONTENTS

ABSTRACT

Matrilysins, which include MMP-7 and MMP-26, are a subset of the MMP family, and overexpression was observed in several cancer conditions, including lung, breast, colorectal, stomach, head, and neck, as well as squamous cell carcinomas. X-ray crystal structure and NMR solution structures of various matrilysins have been reported in this context. Additionally, this chapter discusses in detail a variety of LBDD and SBDD tactics that have already been undertaken on matrilysin inhibitors and explains a concept related to the design and development of novel matrilysin inhibitors in the future.

Keywords: Matrilysin; Hydroxamates; Aminoproline; Rhodanine

13.1 INTRODUCTION

Two different MMP isoforms—MMP-7 (matrilysin-1) and MMP-26 (matrilysin-2)—are enzymes that fall under the matrilysin sub-category of matrix metalloproteinases. Despite being members of the MMP family, very little work has been conducted on these two isoforms (MMP-7 and MMP-26) [1]. Among these two matrilysin isoforms, MMP-7 is also known as punctuated metalloproteinase/putative metalloproteinase/PUMP1, and its overexpression was observed in several cancer conditions, including lung, breast, colorectal, stomach, head, and neck, as well as squamous cell carcinomas [2]. Again, overexpression of MMP-7 is noticed in carcinoma cells compared with stromal cells, and an MMP-7 overexpression was seen in the ovarian

DOI: 10.1201/9781003303282-16

cancer cell line [2]. In addition, MMP-7 is also associated with several other disease conditions, such as reduced renal function in children, ureteropelvic junction obstruction [3], biliary atresia [4], depressive disorder, schizophrenia [5], nephropathies [6], atrial fibrosis [7], and so on. Studies have been performed on the MMP-7 isoform and its related inhibitors. Apart from MMP-7, MMP-26 is also found to be associated with pathophysiological conditions such as pancreatic adenocarcinoma [8] and skin carcinogenesis [9], where overexpression of MMP-26 is observed. In this context, matrilysin isoforms, especially MMP-7, can be a biomolecule of interest for the design and development of selective MMP inhibitors for effective anticancer therapy related to its enzymatic activity.

13.2 STRUCTURAL ASPECTS OF MMP-7 AND MMP-26

The first discovery of MMP-7 was made from a rat uterus in 1980, which was purified for further characterization in 1988 [10, 11]. The representative structures of these matrilysins are shown in Figure 13.1.

13.3 X-RAY CRYSTAL STRUCTURE AND NMR SOLUTION STRUCTURES OF MATRILYSINS

Several X-ray crystal structures and NMR solution structures of different matrilysins have been reported and incorporated in the protein data bank (PDB) [12]. Among these structures, several matrilysins are ligand-bound and, therefore, may unveil the binding pattern of the ligand and how it binds to the amino acid residues of the catalytic site. Details of these structures are listed in Table 13.1.

13.4 LIGAND- AND STRUCTURE-BASED DRUG DESIGN STRATEGIES ON MATRILYSIN INHIBITORS

Considering the significance of the matrilysin isoforms, a few molecular modeling studies were conducted on reported MMP-7 inhibitors to understand the structural requirements of small molecules of MMP-7 inhibitors that can assist the future development of effective MMP-7 inhibitors.

To understand the binding pattern of MMPIs at the MMP-7 active site, Scozzafava and co-workers [13] used the crystallographic data of the inhibitor-bound active site of MMP-7. The X-ray crystal structure disclosed that the zinc-binding hydroxamates function of the succinate hydroxamate inhibitors formed strong bi-dentate chelation with the MMP-7 catalytic Zn^{2+} ion using its carbonyl and hydroxyl functions (Figure 13.2). Apart from zinc chelation, the hydroxamate zinc binding group (ZBG) compounds also contributed to hydrogen bonding interactions at the active site. The carbonyl oxygen atom and the amide nitrogen atom of the ZBG, compounds formed hydrogen bond interaction with Glu219 and Ala182 residues at the active site. In addition, two of the succinyl carbonyl oxygen atoms showed hydrogen bond contacts with Leu181 and Tyr240 residues, while the backbone amide function between the two carbonyl groups contacted with Pro238 Ω-loop residue, depicting a strong and effective binding at the active site.

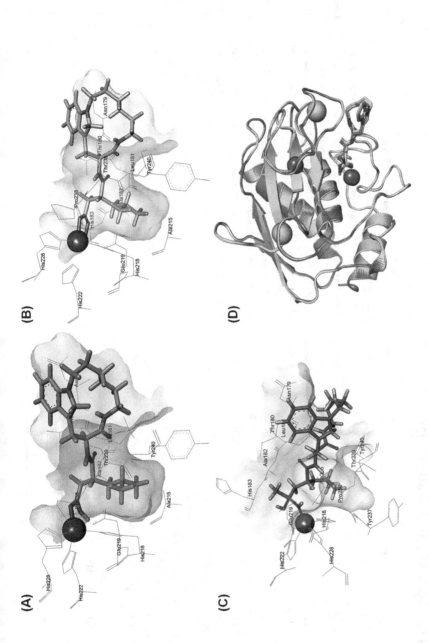

FIGURE 13.1 (A) Active site of MMP-7 with a carboxylate ZBG containing inhibitor (PDB: 1MMP); (B) active site of MMP-7 with a hydroxamate ZBG containing inhibitor (PDB: 1MMQ); (C) active site of MMP-7 with sulfodiimine ZBG containing inhibitor (PDB: 1MMR); (D) alignment of all the matrilysins catalytic domains with inbound ligands.

TABLE 13.1
Details of the Crystal Structures of MMP-7 [12]

PDB ID	Type	Structure	Resolution	Sequence length	Substrate/inhibitor	Year of release
1MMP	X-ray	—	2.39	170	5-methyl-3-(9-oxo-1,8-diaza-tricyclo[10.6.1.013,18]nona deca-12(19),13,15,17-tetraen-10-ylcarbamoyl)-hexanoic acid	1996
1MMQ	X-ray	—	1.90	170	N4-hydroxy-2-isobutyl-N1-(9-oxo-1,8-diaza-tricyclo[10.6.1.01 3,18]nonadeca-12(19),13,15,17-tetraen-10-yl)-succinamide	1996
1MMR	X-ray	—	2.40	170	4-methyl-3-(9-oxo-1,8-diaza-tricyclo[10.6.1.0(13,18)]nonadec a-12(19),13(18),15,17-tetraene-10-carbamoyl)penta-methylsulf onediimine	1996
2DDY	NMR	—	—	173	(1R)-N,6-dihydroxy-7-methoxy-2-[(4-methoxyphenyl)sulfon yl]-1,2,3,4-tetrahydroisoquinoline-1-carboxamide	2007
2Y6C	X-ray	—	1.70	165	N-[[4-chloro-3-(trifluoromethyl)phenyl]sulfonyl]-L-tryptophan	2011
2Y6D	X-ray	—	1.60	174	N-[[4-chloro-3-(trifluoromethyl)phenyl]sulfonyl]-L-tryptophan	2011
2MZE	NMR	pro-MMP-7 with zwitterionic membrane	—	250	—	2015
2MZH	NMR	pro-MMP-7 with anionic membrane	—	248	—	2015
2MZI	NMR	—	—	250	—	2016
5UE2	NMR	pro-MMP-7 with heparin octa saccharide bridging between domains	—	247	—	2017
5UE5	NMR	pro-MMP-7 with heparin octa saccharide bound to the catalytic domain	—	247	—	2017
7WXX	X-ray	—	1.50	175	—	2022

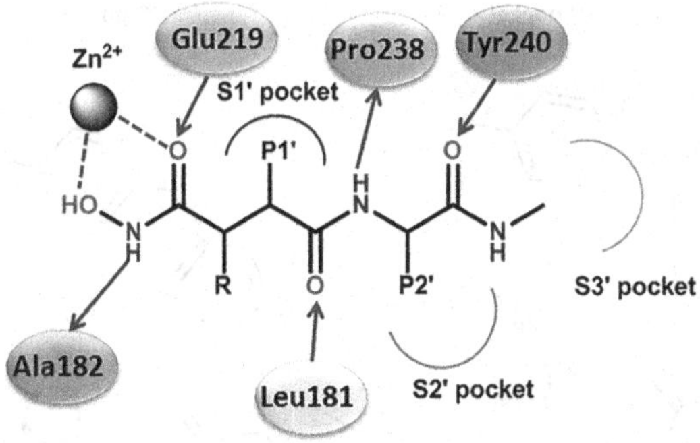

FIGURE 13.2 Binding mode of interaction of hydroxamate derivative at the catalytic site of MMP-7.

In the study of hydantoin-containing MMP-7 inhibitors [14, 15], the regression-based 2D-QSAR model performed on 13 (n = 13) MMP-7 inhibitors displayed an R^2 of 0.937, LOO-cross-validated R^2 (Q^2) of 0.908, and an F value of 74.365. The 2D-QSAR model revealed a positive contribution of the Crippen hydrophobic parameter (ClogP) and a negative correlation of McGowan's volume (MgVol) that suggested the positive influence of lipophilicity and the negative impact of the steric effect of these molecules for MMP-7 inhibition.

Intending to optimize the Zn^{2+} parameters and increase the binding affinity, Hu et al. [16] performed a molecular docking mediated structure-based drug designing approach of MMP inhibitors toward MMPs. Among the molecular docking studies and binding mode analyses of the MMPIs at the active site of MMPs, there is a binding of hydroxamate-containing aryl sulfonamide derivatives at the catalytic site of MMP-1, MMP-2, MMP-7, and MMP-13 (Figure 13.3). It is observed that after the Zn^{2+} chelation by the hydrogen functions, the hydrophobic P1' moiety of the RS-113456 (compound **13.1**) occupied the large and tunnel-like S1' pocket of MMP-2 and MMP-13 (Figure 13.3A and 13.3B, respectively), whereas, in the case of MMP-7, due to a smaller S1' pocket, the outer halfway through the MMP-1 S1' pocket, due to a shorter pocket, the S1' group bounded to the cleft due to distorted geometry (Figure 13.3C and 13.3D, respectively).

A 2D-QSAR study was performed on several hydroxamate-based aryl sulfonyl derivatives as antibacterial agents [17]. In this study, physicochemical properties, such as steric, electrostatic, and hydrophobic features, were correlated with the MMP-inhibitory potency of these compounds. From this regression-based 2D-QSAR study, the authors suggested the negative contribution of electrostatic property at the aryl (P1') substituents of these molecules for their MMP-7 inhibition. The 2D-regression model of these MMP-7 inhibitors (n = 3) showed a correlation coefficient (R) value of 0.940, a standard error of 0.180, and an F value of 8.030. From this regression model, the negative contribution of the R_1 (P1') group F value (f^{R1}; electronic effect on R_1) suggested that the presence of lesser electronic functions in the R_1 group is beneficial for the MMP-7 inhibition of these molecules (Figure 13.4).

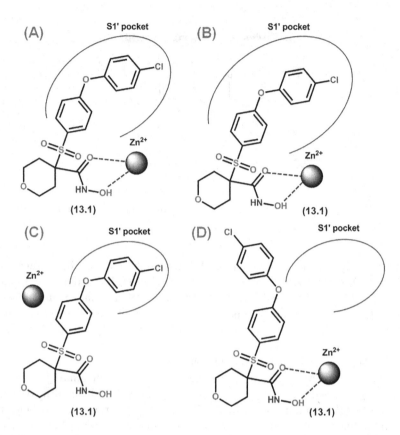

FIGURE 13.3 Binding mode of interaction of hydroxamate-containing aryl sulfonamide derivative (compound **13.1**) at the active site of (A) MMP-2; (B) MMP-13; (C) MMP-1; and (D) MMP-7.

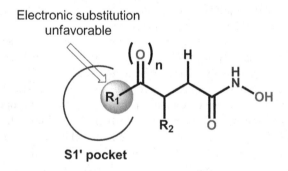

FIGURE 13.4 Crucial structural features of hydroxamate-based aryl sulfonyl derivatives for MMP-7 inhibition.

In 2003, a series of 4-amino proline-based hydroxamate derivatives as MMP inhibitors were considered for the 2D-QSAR study. In this study, Gupta and co-workers correlated the MMP-7 inhibitory activity of these MMP-7 inhibitors with their physicochemical properties [18, 19]. The 2D-regression-based QSAR models performed on 12 (n = 12) and 27 MMP-7 inhibitors displayed an R of 0.866 and 0.903 and adjusted squared correlation coefficients (R^2_A) of 0.660 and 0.760, a cross-validated R^2 (R^2cv) of 0.470 and 0.680 along with a standard error (SE) of 0.100 and 0.250, with an F value of 8.010 and 14.710, respectively. The study disclosed the importance of the electrotopological state-atom index of the sulfur atom (S_S) of these MMP-7 inhibitors, suggesting the significance of π and lone pair electrons on the sulfur atom for MMP-7 inhibition. It was suggested that the presence of the sulfonyl group of these molecules may provide higher chances of hydrogen bond contacts at the MMP-7 active site through partial negative charge of the sulfonyl oxygen atoms (Figure 13.5). The intrinsic state descriptor for the W substituent (I_W) showed a significant effect on MMP-7 inhibitory potency, suggesting the importance of the W substituent and the cyclic amide ring of these compounds. It was suggested that due to the possible steric effects, the cyclic amide group ($^1X^V_N$) contributed negatively to MMP-7 inhibition. On the other hand, the significance of the R substituent ($^1X^V_R$) was described in the study, indicating the negative contribution toward MMP-7 inhibition of these hydroxamate derivatives. It was interesting to note that the previous study performed by Hu and co-workers [16] described the improper fitting of the inhibitors at the small MMP-7 S1′ pocket due to large P1′ substituents that were also validated by the negative contribution of the R substituent for potent MMP-7 inhibition.

To identify the ligand-selectivity landscape of MMP inhibitors, Pirard and Matter [20] performed a GRID-force field-based PCA analysis of 56 MMP structures and one tumor necrosis factor-α converting enzyme (TACE) structure. In their study, it was suggested that the S3′ pocket of the MMP-7 was characterized by Asn162 residue, whereas the size of the pocket was determined by Ile193, which was also found to contribute to the pocket polarity. Therefore, it was also suggested

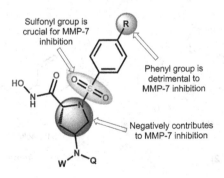

FIGURE 13.5 Important structural requirements of 4-amino proline-based hydroxamates for MMP-7 inhibition.

that the size of the S3′ pocket of MMPs is decided by the various conformations and length of the 193rd amino acid residue. A larger P3′ substituent can greatly improve the MMP-7 selectivity up to 40-fold compared to the methyl P3′ substituent. On the other hand, it was also postulated that such a larger P3′ substituent can be detrimental to the collagenase-binding of these molecules. It was also suggested that the S3′ pocket, due to its solvent-exposed nature, showed favorable polar probe discrimination due to the presence of polar Ile193 amino acid residue and the Asn162 side chain of MMP-7. Regarding the shallow S2′ subsite, the nature of MMP-7-ligand interaction was suggested to be influenced by the Thr159 residue of MMP-7, whereas it was indicated that a favorable interaction region was near the sulfonyl oxygen atom for MMP-7. It was also supported by the 2D-QSAR study performed previously by Gupta et al. [18], where the molecular modeling study revealed the importance of the sulfonyl group for higher hydrogen bonding interaction at the MMP-7 active site.

In the study of designing rhodanine ZBG-containing MMP inhibitors, Hu et al. [21] explored the binding mode of triazole-containing rhodanine derivatives (compound **13.2**) at the active site of MMP-7. From this study, it was noticed that the sulfur atom of the rhodanine ZBG chelated with the catalytic Zn^{2+} ion of MMP-7, whereas the N-2-ethoxyphenyl triazolyl moiety of the molecule comfortably fitted the S1′ pocket (Figure 13.6A), unlike the fitting of the molecule at the large active site S1′ pocket of MMP-13 (Figure 13.6B).

In the study of MMP-7 inhibitors [22], the 2D regression-based QSAR study of seven MMP-7 inhibitors (n = 7), the regression model produced an R value of 0.879 and an R^2_{CV} value of 0.730 along with a SE value of 0.210 and an F value of 54.63. The regression model identified the contribution of the electronic property of the substitution of the P1′ phenyl ring and suggested the negative effect of the electronic group substitution at that position. This indicates that the presence of a low electronic feature at the P1′ phenyl ring is more suitable for interacting inside the MMP-7 S1′ pocket for better MMP-7 inhibition of the pyranyl-based sulfonamide hydroxamate derivatives.

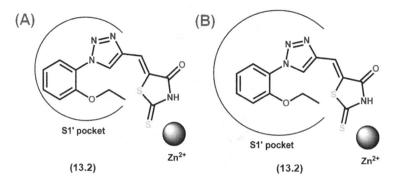

FIGURE 13.6 Binding mode of interaction of rhodanine-derivative (**13.2**) at the active site of (A) MMP-7 and (B) MMP-13.

In a recent *in silico* study to design potent MMP-7 inhibitors, Katari et al. [23] performed an E-pharmacophore modeling study of the available five MMP-7 co-crystal-bound inhibitors. They were able to screen a library of more than two million compounds. Also, the performed rigid-receptor, quantum-polarized, and induced-fit docking study of the 5,000 screened molecules yielded four potential lead molecules as promising MMP-7 inhibitors. In the post-docking evaluation, the lead molecules showed a receiver-operating curve (ROC) matrix of 0.930 when evaluated using the co-crystal-bound ligands and 1,000 decoy molecules at the E-pharmacophore analysis. Interestingly, one of these lead molecules (lead 1) in complex with MMP-7 exhibited the root mean square error (RMSE) of 2.35Å and the root mean square fluctuation (RMSF) of 0.66Å in the molecular dynamics (MD) simulation study performed for 1,000 ns (1 μs) while displaying strong metallic contact with Glu220 residue at the MMP-7 active site.

13.5 SUMMARY

In the sub-category of matrilysin isoforms, the importance of MMP-7 has been disclosed in a variety of cancer conditions as well as in other pathophysiological conditions such as neuronal and kidney-related disorders where the overexpression of MMP-7 has been noted in most of these cases. These pieces of evidence suggest the possibility of MMP-7 becoming a potential target for therapeutic development for different disease conditions. Compared with such a possibility, studies of the structure of MMP-7 and its potential inhibitors have not been performed in large quantities over the years. A few structures of MMP-7 and pro-MMP-7 are available as solution NMR and X-ray crystallographic data (Table 13.1) that can assist MMP-7-related selective inhibitor development. Among the molecular modeling studies conducted on MMP-7 and its inhibitors, it was interesting to note that the observations of several of these studies have agreed with each other. Despite having fewer MMP-7 and its inhibitor-related molecular modeling studies, there have been a few crucial observations and factors such as the smaller size of the S1' pocket of MMP-7 compared with other MMP isoforms (i.e., MMP-2 and MMP-13), the size and polarity of the S3' pocket, and the nature (steric, hydrophobic, electronic properties) of the P1' substituent of MMP-7 inhibitors that are important for designing selective MMP-7 inhibitors. However, it is acknowledged that fewer MMP-7-related molecular modeling studies offer less information. It is important to conduct more research on the structure of MMP-7 and its inhibitors. This can assist in the development of selective MMP-7 inhibitors for treating various pathophysiological conditions in the future.

REFERENCES

[1]. Nagase H, Visse R, Murphy G. Structure and function of matrix metalloproteinases and TIMPs. *Cardiovasc Res* 2006;69(3):562–573.

[2]. Wang FQ, So J, Reierstad S, Fishman DA. Matrilysin (MMP-7) promotes invasion of ovarian cancer cells by activation of progelatinase. *Int J Cancer* 2005;114(1):19–31.

[3]. Wang HS, Cho PS, Zhi H, et al. Association between urinary biomarkers MMP-7/ TIMP-2 and reduced renal function in children with ureteropelvic junction obstruction. *PLOS ONE* 2022;17(7):e0270018.

[4]. Nomden M, Beljaars L, Verkade HJ, et al. Current concepts of biliary atresia and matrix metalloproteinase-7: A review of literature. *Front Med (Lausanne)* 2020;7:617261.

[5]. Omori W, Hattori K, Kajitani N, et al. Increased matrix metalloproteinases in cerebrospinal fluids of patients with major depressive disorder and schizophrenia. *Int J Neuropsychopharmacol* 2020;23(11):713–720.

[6]. Zhang J, Ren P, Wang Y, et al. Serum matrix metalloproteinase-7 level is associated with fibrosis and renal survival in patients with IgA nephropathy. *Kidney Blood Press Res* 2017;42(3):541–552.

[7]. Jia M, Li ZB, Li L, et al. Role of matrix metalloproteinase-7 and apoptosisassociated gene expression levels in the pathogenesis of atrial fibrosis in a Beagle dog model. *Mol Med Rep* 2017;16(5):6967–6973.

[8]. Bister V, Skoog T, Virolainen S, et al. Increased expression of matrix metalloproteinases-21 and -26 and TIMP-4 in pancreatic adenocarcinoma. *Mod Pathol* 2007;20(11):1128–1140.

[9]. Ahokas K, Skoog T, Suomela S, et al. Matrilysin-2 (matrix metalloproteinase-26) is upregulated in keratinocytes during wound repair and early skin carcinogenesis. *J Invest Dermatol* 2005;124(4):849–856.

[10]. Woessner JF Jr, Taplin CJ. Purification and properties of a small latent matrix metalloproteinase of the rat uterus. *J Biol Chem* 1988;263(32):16918–16925.

[11]. Woessner JF Jr. Matrix metalloproteinases and their inhibitors in connective tissue remodeling. *FASEB J* 1991;5(8):2145–2154.

[12]. https://www.rcsb.org/ as accessed in October 2022.

[13]. Scozzafava A, Supuran CT. Carbonic anhydrase and matrix metalloproteinase inhibitors: Sulfonylated amino acid hydroxamates with MMP inhibitory properties act as efficient inhibitors of CA isozymes I, II, and IV, and N-hydroxysulfonamides inhibit both these zinc enzymes. *J Med Chem* 2000;43(20):3677–3687.

[14]. Natchus MG, Bookland RG, De B, et al. Development of new hydroxamate matrix metalloproteinase inhibitors derived from functionalized 4-aminoprolines. *J Med Chem* 2000;43(26):4948–4963.

[15]. Patil VM, Gupta SP. Quantitative structure-activity relationship studies on sulfonamide-based MMP inhibitors. *Exp Suppl* 2012;103:177–208.

[16]. Hu X, Shelver WH. Docking studies of matrix metalloproteinase inhibitors: Zinc parameter optimization to improve the binding free energy prediction. *J Mol Graph Modell* 2003;22(2):115–126.

[17]. Gupta MK, Mishra P, Prathipati P, et al. 2D-QSAR in hydroxamic acid derivatives as peptide deformylase inhibitors and antibacterial agents. *Bioorg Med Chem* 2002;10(12):3713–3716.

[18]. Gupta SP, Kumar D, Kumaran S. A quantitative structure-activity relationship study of hydroxamate matrix metalloproteinase inhibitors derived from functionalized 4-aminoprolines. *Bioorg Med Chem* 2003;11(9):1975–1981.

[19]. Gupta SP. Quantitative structure-activity relationship studies on zinc-containing metalloproteinase inhibitors. *Chem Rev* 2007;107(7):3042–3087.

[20]. Pirard B, Matter H. Matrix metalloproteinase target family landscape: A chemometrical approach to ligand selectivity based on protein binding site analysis. *J Med Chem* 2006;49(1):51–69.

[21]. Hu M, Li J, Yao SQ. In situ "click" assembly of small molecule matrix metalloprotease inhibitors containing zinc-chelating groups. *Org Lett* 2008;10(24):5529–5531.

[22]. Verma RP, Hansch C. Matrix metalloproteinases (MMPs): Chemical-biological functions and (Q)SARs. *Bioorg Med Chem* 2007;15(6):2223–2268.

[23]. Katari SK, Pasala C, Nalamolu RM, et al. In silico trials to design potent inhibitors against matrilysin (MMP-7). *J Biomol Struct Dyn* 2021:1–12.

14 Modeling Inhibitors of Membrane-Type MMPs

*Suvankar Banerjee, Sandip Kumar Baidya,
Nilanjan Adhikari, and Tarun Jha*

CONTENTS

ABSTRACT

Membrane-type matrix metalloproteinases (MT-MMPs) play crucial roles in the pathophysiology of several disease conditions, including various cancers and neurodegenerative diseases. Although a large amount of crystallographic data has been available to date, a sufficient amount of work still needs to be done to design and discover promising MT-MMP inhibitors. In this context, ligand- and structure-based drug design approaches (LBDD and SBDD) may play vital roles. Since other membrane-type MMP inhibitors are not available here, in this chapter, drug-designing methods conducted on some MMP-14 inhibitors will be discussed in detail. Application of these LBDD and SBDD processes may broaden the development of novel and potential MMP-14 and other membrane-type MMP inhibitors.

Keywords: MT-MMP; MMP-14; Molecular docking; QSAR studies; X-ray crystal data

14.1 INTRODUCTION

Among zinc-dependent matrix metalloproteinases (MMPs), membrane type-matrix metalloproteinases (MT-MMPs) are associated with the cell membrane through a transmembrane (TM) domain or glycosylphosphatidylinositol (GPI) anchor [1, 2]. To date, six MT-MMPs (namely MT1-MMP/MMP-14, MT2-MMP/MMP-15, MT3-MMP/MMP-16, MT4-MMP/MMP-17, MT5-MMP/MMP-24, and MT6-MMP/MMP-26) have been identified, playing crucial roles in cellular invasion and migration in tumors [1, 3, 4]. Among these MT-MMPs, the versatile roles of MT1-MMP

DOI: 10.1201/9781003303282-17

or MMP-14 are well-studied compared with other MT-MMPs. MMP-14 is found to activate pro-MMP-2. Subsequently, the activated MMP-2 helps to break the basement membrane type IV collagen [1, 5–8]. MMP-14 is found to be directly involved in the progression of various cancers such as breast cancer [9, 10], ovarian cancer [11, 12], pancreatic cancer [13], non-small cell lung cancer (NSCLC) [14], colorectal cancer [15], prostate cancer [16], urinary bladder carcinoma [17], esophageal cancer [18], gastric cancer [19], glioma [20], and melanoma [21]. MMP-14 is accumulated in invadopodia, a specialized ECM-degrading membrane protrusion of invasive cells [22]. In addition, the crucial roles of MMP-14 in neurodegenerative diseases (namely Alzheimer's disease, multiple sclerosis, human amyotrophic lateral sclerosis (ALS), and acute brain trauma), as well as in neuroinflammation and cerebral ischemia, have been shown [23, 24]. Nevertheless, MMP-14 is also involved in developing postmenopausal hypertension [25], atherosclerotic plaque formation [26], deep venous thrombosis (DVT) [27], and diabetic retinopathy [28], as well as periodontal inflammation related to type 2 diabetes mellitus [29]. Furthermore, MMP-14 has a strong correlation with Fuchs endothelial corneal dystrophy [30], glaucoma [31], homeostasis in adult skin [32], and Dupuytren's disease fibroblast-mediated contraction [33]. Also, MMP-14 is found to be involved in modulating genotype VII Newcastle disease virus [34] and sepsis [35].

14.2 STRUCTURAL ASPECTS OF MT-MMPs

Due to the localization of MMP-14 in cancer cells with invasive features, it can be considered a promising target for anticancer therapeutics [36]. MT-MMPs exhibit a high degree of structural resemblance to other MMPs comprising an N-terminal signal peptide, a pro-peptide domain, and a conserved catalytic domain along with a structure of one catalytic Zn^{2+} with two Ca^{2+} ions. Moreover, a hemopexin domain is also followed by the conserved catalytic domain, whereas the presence of a fibronectin domain followed by a cytoplasmic tail at the C-terminal end of these MT-MMPs makes them unique compared with other MMPs [37]. In addition, these MT-MMPs also comprise a hydrophobic phenylalanine residue in the Ω-loop [38, 39]. Again, MMP-14 is bound to the cell membrane through the type 1 transmembrane region and is expressed in an active form on the cell surface by the activity of furin-like serine proteinases [40, 41]. The hemopexin domain may be activated by the protein substrate, which is important for the breakdown of type I collagen [40, 42–44]. The hemopexin domain also participates in the modulation of enzyme and cellular localization [40, 45, 46]. The representative structures of MT-MMPs are depicted in Figure 14.1.

14.3 X-RAY CRYSTAL STRUCTURE AND NMR SOLUTION STRUCTURES OF MT-MMPs

Numerous X-ray crystal structures and NMR solution structures of some MT-MMPs have been identified. Among these MT-MMPs, a few MT-MMPs are ligand bound and, therefore, can be useful in exploring the binding mode of interactions of the ligand at the catalytic site of MT-MMPs. Based on the binding pattern of interactions,

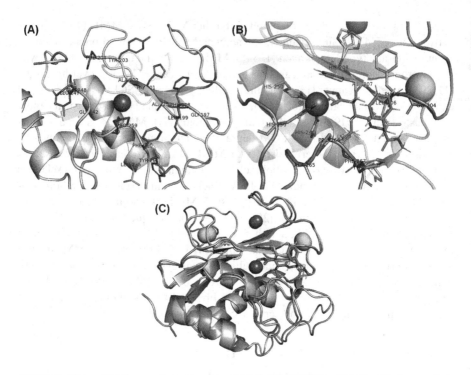

FIGURE 14.1   (A) The catalytic domain of MT1-MMP (PDB: 1BQQ); (B) the catalytic domain of MT3-MMP (PDB: 1RM8); (C) alignment of all the membrane type MMP catalytic domains with ligand bound to MT3-MMP.

newer effective and selective MT-MMP inhibitors can be designed. A detail of X-ray crystal structures and NMR solution structures of MT-MMPs are listed in Table 14.1.

14.4 LIGAND- AND STRUCTURE-BASED DRUG DESIGN STRATEGIES OF MT-MMP INHIBITORS

It is important to note that very little ligand- and structure-based drug design work has been performed to date on MT-MMP inhibitors. Work has mostly been conducted on MMP-14 inhibitors because of the lack of inhibitors of other MT-MMPs. However, considering the role of MMP-14 inhibitors in multiple diseases, including cancer, these ligand- and structure-based drug-design strategies may be considered promising for developing potential MMP-14 inhibitors.

Verma and Hansch [49] performed some QSAR models on various MMP-14 inhibitors. The QSAR model performed on seven benzofuran derivatives produced an R^2 of 0.920 and Q^2 of 0.872. This model reflected that the higher hydrophobicity may reduce the MMP-14 inhibitory activity (Figure 14.2). Again, another QSAR model performed on five phosphinic pseudo-tripeptides showed that molar refractivity may contribute positively to MMP-14 inhibition. Another QSAR model derived

TABLE 14.1

Details of the Crystal Structures of Membrane-Type MMPs [47, 48]

PDB ID	Type	Structure	Resolution	Sequence length	Substrate/Inhibitor	Year of Release
1BQQ#	X-ray	–	2.75	174	TIMP-2	1999
2MQS#	X-ray	–	–	181	TIMP-1	2010
3MA2#	X-ray	Hemopexin-like domain	2.05	196	–	2009
3C7X#	X-ray		1.07			
3X23#	X-ray	–				
4P3D#	X-ray	MT1-MMP:Fab complex	1.95	218	4-(2-hydroxyethyl)-1-piperazine ethanesulfonic acid	2014
4P3C#	X-ray	MT1-MMP:Fab complex	1.94	218	4-(2-hydroxyethyl)-1-piperazine ethanesulfonic acid	2014
5H0U#	X-ray	Catalytic domain	2.24	170	4-(2-hydroxyethyl)-1-piperazine ethanesulfonic acid	2017
6CM1#	Solution NMR	MT1-MMP HPX domain with Blade 2 Loop Bound to Nanodiscs	–	196	1,2-dimyristoyl-sn-glycero-3-phosphocholine	2018
6CLZ#	Solution NMR	MT1-MMP HPX domain with Blade 4 Loop Bound to Nanodiscs	–	196	1,2-dimyristoyl-sn-glycero-3-phosphocholine	2018
1RM8$	X-ray	Catalytic domain	1.80	169	4-(N-hydroxyamino)-2R-isobutyl-2S-(2-thienylthiomethyl)succinyl-L-phenylalanine-N-methylamide	2004

#Structures of MMP-14 (MT1-MMP); $structure of MMP-16 (MT3-MMP).

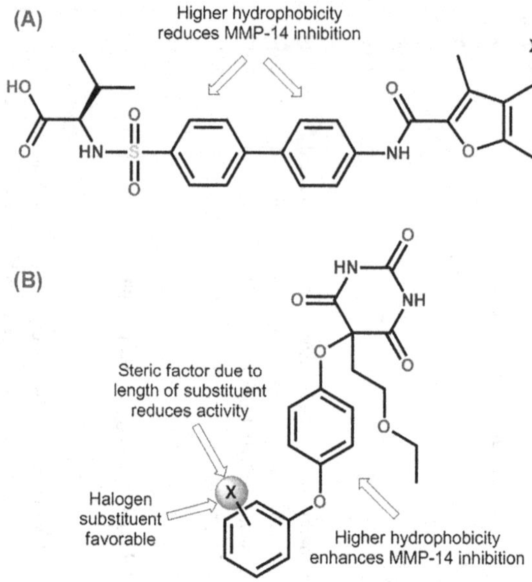

FIGURE 14.2 Structural requirements of potential MMP-14 inhibitors (A) benzofuran derivatives and (B) pyrimidinetrione derivatives.

from 17 pyrimidinetrione derivatives produced an R^2 of 0.877 and a Q^2 of 0.752. This QSAR model disclosed that the higher hydrophobicity and halogen substitution at the X position were crucial for higher MMP-14 inhibition. However, the length of the X substituent may provide some steric effects detrimental to MMP-14 inhibition (Figure 14.2).

Hurst et al. [1] proposed the binding mode of interactions of potential mercapto-sulfide-based MMP-14 inhibitors at the active site of MMP-14. The higher potency may be achieved due to zinc-binding ability, several hydrogen bonding interactions, and favorable van der Waals interactions. Importantly, the type of P1′ substituent may be the key reason for exerting variation in MMP-14 inhibitory activity. Compound **14.1** (MMP-14 K_i = 24 nM) showed that the leucine side chain oriented properly at the S1′ site (Figure 14.3). Four hydrogen bonding interactions were observed between the peptide backbone and the mercaptosulfide inhibitor **14.1**. The carbonyl group of the P1′ substituent formed hydrogen bonding with the amide group of Leu199. Moreover, the amide group at the P2′ substituent formed hydrogen bonding with the carbonyl group of Pro259. Nevertheless, the carbonyl group of the P2′ substituent formed hydrogen bonding with Tyr261. Again, the terminal amide group formed hydrogen bonding with Gly197. Moreover, the Phe198 residue between the Gly197 and Leu199 was found to orient in such a manner that it may form coordination with the Ca^{2+} ion, resulting in a reduction in the flexibility of these residues.

Rahman et al. [50] exhibited molecular docking interactions of phosphonate-containing compounds and MMP-14 (PDB: 1BQQ). The phosphate groups of compound **14.2** were found to form Zn^{2+} chelation as well as interactions with Glu240, backbone amide, and carbonyl groups of Ala200 as well as the amide group of Leu199 and Tyr261 (Figure 14.4).

Chowdhury and co-workers [51] performed molecular docking analysis of green tea catechins with MMP-14. Compound **14.3** showed interactions with Phe198, Leu199, Ala200, His201, Ala202, Val236, Glu240, His249, Pro259, and Phe260 (Figure 14.5A).

Among these residues, Glu240, Ala202, His239, Leu199, Ala200, and Tyr261 formed hydrogen bonding, whereas only His239 formed π-π stacking interaction. Similarly, compound **14.4** formed interactions with Gly197, Phe198, Leu199, Ala200, His201, Ala202, Glu240, His249, Pro259, Phe260, and Tyr261 (Figure 14.5B). Among these residues, Glu240, Ala200, Leu199, and Ala202 formed hydrogen bonding interactions, whereas His243 formed a π-cationic interaction. On the other

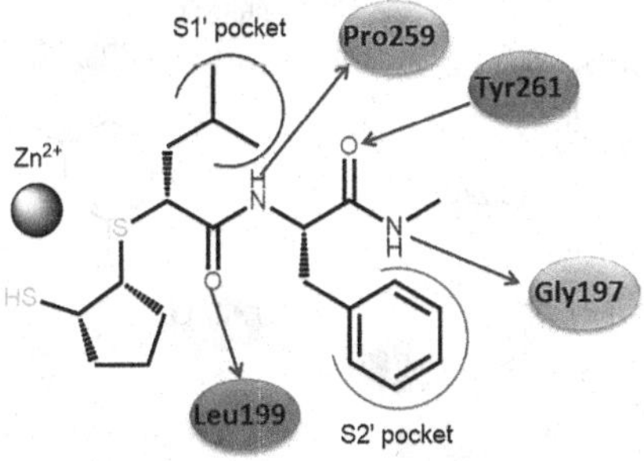

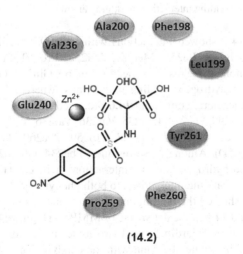

(14.1)

FIGURE 14.3 Binding mode of interaction of compound **14.1** at the active site of MMP-14 (hydrogen bonding interaction: dark gray arrow).

(14.2)

FIGURE 14.4 Binding mode of interaction of compound **14.2** at the active site of MMP-14.

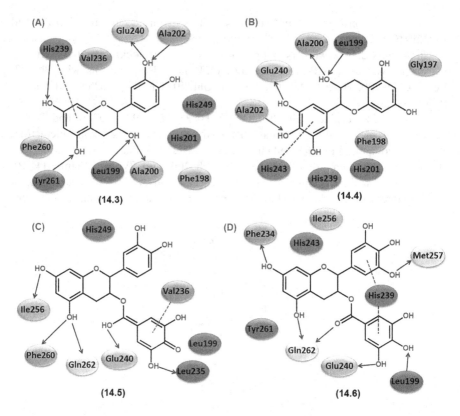

FIGURE 14.5 Binding mode of interaction of (A) compound **14.3**, (B) compound **14.4**, (C) compound **14.5**, and (D) compound **14.6** at the active site of MMP-14 (π-π stacking interaction: gray dotted line; π-cationic interaction: light gray dotted line; π-σ interaction: dark gray dotted line; hydrogen bonding interaction: dark gray arrow)

hand, compound **14.5** showed interactions with Leu199, His201, Leu235, Val236, His239, Glu240, His243, Ile256, Met257, Ala258, Pro259, Phe260, and Gln262 (Figure 14.5C). Among these residues, Ile256, Phe260, Gln262, Glu240, and Leu265 were found to form hydrogen bonding interactions, whereas Val236 formed a π-σ interaction. Furthermore, compound **14.6** produced interactions with amino acid residues Gly197, Leu199, Phe234, Leu235, Val236, Val236, Val238, His239, Glu240, His243, Ser250, Ile256, Met257, Ala258, Pro259, Phe260, Tyr261, Gln262, and Met264 (Figure 14.5D). Among these residues, Phe234, Gln262, Glu240, Met257, and Leu199 formed hydrogen bonding interactions, whereas His239 was found to form both π-π and π-cationic interactions to both phenyl rings.

Sylte et al. [52] showed the binding mode of interactions of galardin (compound **14.7**) and compound **14.8** at the active site of MMP-14 (Figure 14.6).

The hydroxamate of galardin formed two ionic interactions with the catalytic Zn^{2+} ion. It formed bidentate chelation with the catalytic Zn^{2+}. Again, the hydroxy

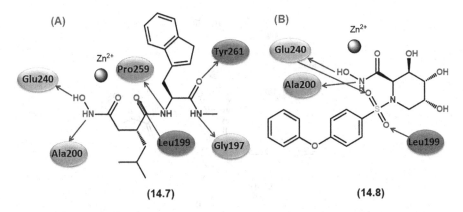

FIGURE 14.6 Binding mode of interaction of (A) galardin (compound **14.7**) and (B) compound **14.8** at the active site of MMP-14 (hydrogen bonding interaction: dark gray arrow).

group of hydroxamate moiety formed hydrogen bonding with Glu240. Moreover, the amide group of hydroxamate moiety formed hydrogen bonding with the carbonyl oxygen of Ala200. The 4-methylpentanoyl group was found at the entrance of the S1' pocket, interacting with side chain amino acid residues His239, Tyr261, Leu199, and Val236. The carboxamido group adjacent to the 4-methylpentanoyl moiety formed two hydrogen bonding interactions. The carbonyl oxygen formed hydrogen bonding with the amide group of Leu199, whereas the amido group formed hydrogen bonding with the carbonyl group of Pro259. The methylamido moiety also formed two hydrogen bonding interactions with Tyr261 and Gly197. On the other hand, the hydroxamate group of compound **14.8** formed strong chelation with the catalytic Zn²⁺ ion. Again, the hydroxy and amide groups formed hydrogen bonding with Glu240 and Ala200, respectively. The sulfonyl oxygen atoms formed hydrogen bonding with main chain amide groups of Ala200 and Leu199. The diphenyl ether moiety entered the S1' pocket, interacting with side chain amino acid residues Leu199, Leu235, Val236, His239, Ile256, Pro259, and Tyr261.

The molecular dynamics (MD) simulation study of compound **14.9** at the MMP-14 active site [53] disclosed that the hydroxamate group was lying close to the catalytic Zn²⁺ ion coordinating three histidine residues (His401, His405, and His411), whereas the amide group of hydroxamate moiety formed hydrogen bonding interaction with Ala189 and one of the sulfonyl oxygen atoms formed hydrogen bonding with Leu188 (Figure 14.7).

Adekoya et al. [54], through molecular docking interactions, showed that amino acid residues Glu240, Ala203, Ala200, Ala202, Ala258, Phe260, and Gln262 are crucial for forming hydrogen bonding interactions at the active site of MMP-14. Similarly, Huang and co-workers, through docking analysis [55], disclosed that amino acid residues, namely Met13, Met18, Arg30, Tyr161, Tyr168, Lys170, Tyr182, and Trp190, at the hemopexin domain of MMP-14 are crucial for binding interactions.

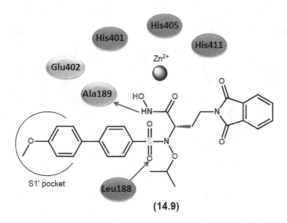

(14.9)

FIGURE 14.7 Binding mode of interaction of compound **14.9** at the active site of MMP-14 (hydrogen bonding interaction: dark gray arrow).

14.5 SUMMARY

MT1-MMP or MMP-14 is one of the prime MMPs that take part in crucial roles in several major diseases, including several cancers, and neurodegenerative diseases. To date, research has been carried out exploring the potential roles of MMP-14 in these diseases. However, there is a large gap in this field regarding the design and discovery of potential MMP-14 inhibitors in particular and other membrane-type MMP inhibitors in general. Interestingly, the structure of MMP-14 is well-explored and the catalytic site is well-defined. Therefore, designing effective and highly selective MMP-14 inhibitors targeting these disease conditions is highly probable. Already, a large number of X-ray crystallographic data and NMR solution structures of MMP-14 have been identified. These can be advantageous because they provide a detailed idea about the 3D arrangement of the inbound ligand at the MMP-14 active site. Nevertheless, crucial amino acid residues and vital structural features may also be identified. In addition, based on these binding modes of interactions, SBDD strategies can be adopted for the development of potent and selective MMP-14 inhibitors. LBDD strategies can also be applied to existing MMP-14 inhibitors to acquire knowledge regarding the crucial structural features of these inhibitors responsible for the higher inhibitory potential. Therefore, with some knowledge regarding LBDD and SBDD, such ideas can unveil a huge scope in the future design and discovery of novel MT-MMP inhibitors.

REFERENCES

[1]. Hurst DR, Schwartz MA, Jin Y, et al. Inhibition of enzyme activity of and cell-mediated substrate cleavage by membrane type 1 matrix metalloproteinase by newly developed mercaptosulphide inhibitors. *Biochem J* 2005;392(3):527–536.
[2]. Hernandez-Barrantes S, Bernardo M, Toth M, et al. Regulation of membrane type-matrix metalloproteinases. *Semin Cancer Biol* 2002;12(2):131–138.

[3]. Hotary KB, Allen ED, Brooks PC, et al. Membrane type I matrix metalloproteinase usurps tumor growth control imposed by the three-dimensional extracellular matrix. *Cell* 2003;114(1):33–45.

[4]. Ueda J, Kajita M, Suenaga N, et al. Sequence-specific silencing of MT1-MMP expression suppresses tumor cell migration and invasion: Importance of MT1-MMP as a therapeutic target for invasive tumors. *Oncogene* 2003;22(54):8716–8722.

[5]. Pei D, Weiss SJ. Transmembrane-deletion mutants of the membrane-type matrix metalloproteinase-1 process progelatinase A and express intrinsic matrix-degrading activity. *J Biol Chem* 1996;271(15):9135–9140.

[6]. Ohuchi E, Imai K, Fujii Y, et al. Membrane type 1 matrix metalloproteinase digests interstitial collagens and other extracellular matrix macromolecules. *J Biol Chem* 1997;272(4):2446–2451.

[7]. Zucker S, Drews M, Conner C, et al. Tissue inhibitor of metalloproteinase-2 (TIMP-2) binds to the catalytic domain of the cell surface receptor, membrane type 1-matrix metalloproteinase 1 (MT1-MMP). *J Biol Chem* 1998;273(2):1216–1222.

[8]. Butler GS, Butler MJ, Atkinson SJ, et al. The TIMP2 membrane type 1 metalloproteinase "receptor" regulates the concentration and efficient activation of progelatinase A. A kinetic study. *J Biol Chem* 1998;273(2):871–880.

[9]. Di D, Chen L, Guo Y, et al. Association of BCSC-1 and MMP-14 with human breast cancer. *Oncol Lett* 2018;15(4):5020–5026.

[10]. Karamanou K, Franchi M, Vynios D, et al. Epithelial-to-mesenchymal transition and invadopodia markers in breast cancer: Lumican a key regulator. *Semin Cancer Biol* 2020;62:125–133.

[11]. Vos MC, van der Wurff AAM, van Kuppevelt TH, et al. The role of MMP-14 in ovarian cancer: A systematic review. *J Ovarian Res* 2021;14(1):101.

[12]. Vos MC, Hollemans E, Ezendam N, et al. MMP-14 and CD44 in epithelial-to-mesenchymal transition (EMT) in ovarian cancer. *J Ovarian Res* 2016;9(1):53.

[13]. Morcillo MÁ, García de Lucas Á, Oteo M, et al. MT1-MMP as a PET imaging biomarker for pancreas cancer management. *Contrast Media Mol Imaging* 2018;2018:8382148.

[14]. Wang YZ, Wu KP, Wu AB, et al. MMP-14 overexpression correlates with poor prognosis in non-small cell lung cancer. *Tumour Biol* 2014;35(10):9815–9821.

[15]. Kanazawa A, Oshima T, Yoshihara K, et al. Relation of MT1-MMP gene expression to outcomes in colorectal cancer. *J Surg Oncol* 2010;102(6):571–575.

[16]. Harrison GM, Davies G, Martin TA, et al. The influence of CD44v3-v10 on adhesion, invasion and MMP-14 expression in prostate cancer cells. *Oncol Rep* 2006;15(1):199–206.

[17]. Kudelski J, Młynarczyk G, Darewicz B, et al. Dominative role of MMP-14 over MMP-15 in human urinary bladder carcinoma on the basis of its enhanced specific activity. *Med (Baltim)* 2020;99(7):e19224.

[18]. Chen N, Zhang G, Fu J, et al. Matrix metalloproteinase-14 (MMP-14) downregulation inhibits esophageal squamous cell carcinoma cell migration, invasion, and proliferation. *Thorac Cancer* 2020;11(11):3168–3174.

[19]. Kasurinen A, Tervahartiala T, Laitinen A, et al. High serum MMP-14 predicts worse survival in gastric cancer. *PLOS ONE* 2018;13(12):e0208800.

[20]. Wang L, Yuan J, Tu Y, et al. Co-expression of MMP-14 and MMP-19 predicts poor survival in human glioma. *Clin Transl Oncol* 2013;15(2):139–145.

[21]. Stasiak M, Boncela J, Perreau C, et al. Lumican inhibits SNAIL-induced melanoma cell migration specifically by blocking MMP-14 activity. *PLOS ONE* 2016;11(3):e0150226.

[22]. Poincloux R, Lizárraga F, Chavrier P. Matrix invasion by tumour cells: A focus on MT1-MMP trafficking to invadopodia. *J Cell Sci* 2009;122(17):3015–3024.

[23]. Langenfurth A, Rinnenthal JL, Vinnakota K, et al. Membrane-type 1 metalloproteinase is upregulated in microglia/brain macrophages in neurodegenerative and neuroinflammatory diseases. *J Neurosci Res* 2014;92(3):275–286.

[24]. Candelario-Jalil E, Yang Y, Rosenberg GA. Diverse roles of matrix metalloproteinases and tissue inhibitors of metalloproteinases in neuroinflammation and cerebral ischemia. *Neuroscience* 2009;158(3):983–994.

[25]. Dai Q, Lin J, Craig T, et al. Estrogen effects on MMP-13 and MMP-14 regulation of left ventricular mass in dahl salt-induced hypertension. *Gend Med* 2008;5(1):74–85.

[26]. Li C, Jin XP, Zhu M, et al. Positive association of MMP 14 gene polymorphism with vulnerable carotid plaque formation in a Han Chinese population. *Scand J Clin Lab Investig* 2014;74(3):248–253.

[27]. Dahi S, Lee JG, Lovett DH, et al. Differential transcriptional activation of matrix metalloproteinase-2 and membrane type-1 matrix metalloproteinase by experimental deep venous thrombosis and thrombin. *J Vasc Surg* 2005;42(3):539–545.

[28]. Ünal A, Baykal O, Öztürk N. Comparison of matrix metalloproteinase 9 and 14 levels in vitreous samples in diabetic and non-diabetic patients: A case control study. *Int J Retina Vitreous* 2022;8(1):44.

[29]. Kim JB, Jung MH, Cho JY, et al. The influence of type 2 diabetes mellitus on the expression of inflammatory mediators and tissue inhibitor of metalloproteinases-2 in human chronic periodontitis. *J Periodont Implant Sci* 2011;41(3):109–116.

[30]. Xu I, Thériault M, Brunette I, et al. Matrix metalloproteinases and their inhibitors in Fuchs endothelial corneal dystrophy. *Exp Eye Res* 2021;205:108500.

[31]. Golubnitschaja O, Yeghiazaryan K, Liu R, et al. Increased expression of matrix metalloproteinases in mononuclear blood cells of normal-tension glaucoma patients. *J Glaucoma* 2004;13(1):66–72.

[32]. Zigrino P, Brinckmann J, Niehoff A, et al. Fibroblast-derived MMP-14 regulates collagen homeostasis in adult skin. *J Investig Dermatol* 2016;136(8):1575–1583.

[33]. Wilkinson JM, Davidson RK, Swingler TE, et al. MMP-14 and MMP-2 are key metalloproteases in Dupuytren's disease fibroblast-mediated contraction. *Biochim Biophys Acta* 2012;1822(6):897–905.

[34]. Hu Z, Gu H, Ni J, et al. Matrix metalloproteinase-14 regulates collagen degradation and migration of mononuclear cells during infection with genotype VII Newcastle disease virus. *J Gen Virol* 2021;102(1). https://doi.org/10.1099/jgv.0.001505.

[35]. Idowu TO, Etzrodt V, Seeliger B, et al. Identification of specific Tie2 cleavage sites and therapeutic modulation in experimental sepsis. *Elife* 2020;9:e59520.

[36]. Nakahara H, Howard L, Thompson EW, et al. Transmembrane/cytoplasmic domain-mediated membrane type 1-matrix metalloprotease docking to invadopodia is required for cell invasion. *Proc Natl Acad Sci U S A* 1997;94(15):7959–7964.

[37]. Mondal S, Adhikari N, Banerjee S, et al. Matrix metalloproteinase-9 (MMP-9) and its inhibitors in cancer: A minireview. *Eur J Med Chem* 2020;194:112260.

[38]. Fernandez-Catalan C, Bode W, Huber R, et al. Crystal structure of the complex formed by the membrane type 1-matrix metalloproteinase with the tissue inhibitor of metalloproteinases-2, the soluble progelatinase A receptor. *EMBO J* 1998;17(17):5238–5248.

[39]. Lang R, Braun M, Sounni NE, et al. Crystal structure of the catalytic domain of MMP-16/MT3-MMP: Characterization of MT-MMP specific features. *J Mol Biol* 2004;336(1):213–225.

[40]. Hurst DR, Schwartz MA, Ghaffari MA, et al. Catalytic- and ecto-domains of membrane type 1-matrix metalloproteinase have similar inhibition profiles but distinct endopeptidase activities. *Biochem J* 2004;377(3):775–779.

[41]. Yana I, Weiss SJ. Regulation of membrane type-1 matrix metalloproteinase activation by proprotein convertases. *Mol Biol Cell* 2000;11(7):2387–2401.

[42]. Murphy G, Knäuper V. Relating matrix metalloproteinase structure to function: Why the "hemopexin" domain? *Matrix Biol* 1997;15(8–9):511–518.

[43]. Lauer-Fields JL, Juska D, Fields GB. Matrix metalloproteinases and collagen catabolism. *Biopolymers* 2002;66(1):19–32.

[44]. Overall CM. Molecular determinants of metalloproteinase substrate specificity: Matrix metalloproteinase substrate binding domains, modules, and exosites. *Mol Biotechnol* 2002;22(1):51–86.

[45]. Lehti K, Lohi J, Juntunen MM, et al. Oligomerization through hemopexin and cytoplasmic domains regulates the activity and turnover of membrane-type 1 matrix metalloproteinase. *J Biol Chem* 2002;277(10):8440–8448.

[46]. Mori H, Tomari T, Koshikawa N, et al. CD44 directs membrane-type 1 matrix metalloproteinase to lamellipodia by associating with its hemopexin-like domain. *EMBO J* 2002;21(15):3949–3959.

[47]. https://www.rcsb.org as accessed in November 2022.

[48]. Baidya SK, Banerjee S, Adhikari N, et al. Selective inhibitors of medium-size s1' pocket matrix metalloproteinases: A stepping stone of future drug discovery. *J Med Chem* 2022;65(16):10709–10754.

[49]. Verma RP, Hansch C. Matrix metalloproteinases (MMPs): Chemical-biological functions and (Q)SARs. *Bioorg Med Chem* 2007;15(6):2223–2268.

[50]. Rahman F, Nguyen TM, Adekoya OA, et al. Inhibition of bacterial and human zinc-metalloproteases by bisphosphonate- and catechol-containing compounds. *J Enzyme Inhib Med Chem* 2021;36(1):819–830.

[51]. Chowdhury A, Nandy SK, Sarkar J, et al. Inhibition of pro-/active MMP-2 by green tea catechins and prediction of their interaction by molecular docking studies. *Mol Cell Biochem* 2017;427(1–2):111–122.

[52]. Sylte I, Dawadi R, Malla N, et al. The selectivity of galardin and an azasugar-based hydroxamate compound for human matrix metalloproteases and bacterial metalloproteases. *PLOS ONE* 2018;13(8):e0200237.

[53]. Nuti E, Cantelmo AR, Gallo C, et al. N-O-isopropyl sulfonamido-based hydroxamates as matrix metalloproteinase inhibitors: Hit selection and in vivo antiangiogenic activity. *J Med Chem* 2015;58(18):7224–7240.

[54]. Adekoya OA, Sjøli S, Wuxiuer Y, et al. Inhibition of pseudolysin and thermolysin by hydroxamate-based MMP inhibitors. *Eur J Med Chem* 2015;89:340–348.

[55]. Huang Y, Cui J, Liang Z, et al. Virtual screening of lead chemicals based on HPX domain of MT1-MMP. In *2011 5th International Conference on Bioinformatics and Biomedical Engineering*, 2011, 1–4.

15 Modeling Inhibitors of Other MMPs

Suvankar Banerjee, Sandip Kumar Baidya,
Nilanjan Adhikari, and Tarun Jha

CONTENTS

ABSTRACT

MMPs divided into other types of MMPs are MMP-12, MMP-19, MMP-20, MMP-21, MMP-27, and MMP-28. There has not been a lot of research done on these MMPs. Although there are different forms of MMPs, MMP-12 has been the focus of most research. MMP-12 has been recognized as a promising biomolecular target in numerous disease states, particularly in chronic obstructive pulmonary disease, asthma, and respiratory distress. In this context, X-ray crystal data and NMR solution data of MMP-12 are provided, which is useful for understanding the essential structural characteristics of the ligands at the MMP-12 active site. The different MMP-12 inhibitors studied using ligand-based drug design (LBDD) and structure-based drug design (SBDD) methods are depicted in this chapter. These findings can be used to design, produce, and biologically test a new chemical substance targeting MMP-12. However, other MMPs like MMP-19, MMP-20, MMP-21, MMP-28, and MMP-29 lack both knowledge and biological experimental data. Thus, there may be a huge scope for designing such inhibitors if proper experiments are done; hence, these inhibitors will be discovered in the future.

Keywords: MMP-12; MMP-19; MMP-20; MMP-21; MMP-27; MMP-28

15.1 INTRODUCTION

Among the other category of MMPs, there are several MMPs, namely MMP-12, MMP-19, MMP-20, MMP-21, MMP-27, and MMP-28 [1]. However, except for MMP-12, most of these MMPs have not been studied in detail. Therefore, there is a

DOI: 10.1201/9781003303282-18

huge scope to explore the relationship among these other types of MMPs with several disease conditions, including designing their respective inhibitors to combat various disease states. Among the other classes of MMPs, MMP-12 is the most widely studied MMP. A number of studies have been carried out on MMP-12, showing that it plays a pivotal role in the modulation of various disease conditions. Among these diseases, MMP-12 has a direct association with chronic obstructive pulmonary disease (COPD) [2–7], emphysema [8], inflammatory respiratory diseases like asthma [9–11], allergic rhinitis [12], allergic airway inflammation [13], chronic rhinosinusitis with nasal polyposis [14], neuroinflammation and neurological diseases [15, 16], heart-related diseases like chronic heart disease [17], ischemic stroke [18], coronary artery disease [19, 20], abdominal aortic aneurysms [21], experimental autoimmune encephalomyelitis [22], osteoarthritis [23], rheumatoid arthritis [24, 25], and several cancers such as endometrial adenocarcinoma [26], oral squamous cell carcinoma [27], non-small cell lung cancer [28], gastric cancer [29], and colorectal cancer [30], as well as other diseases like Crohn's disease [31], dermatitis [32], and viral infection [33]. In this context, it may be postulated that MMP-12 is a potential biomolecular target for designing useful drug candidates to effectively manage such disease conditions. On the other hand, due to a lack of biological activity or unavailability of data related to other MMPs (namely MMP-19, MMP-20, MMP-21, MMP-27, and MMP-28), molecular modeling studies on these MMPs have not been conducted.

15.2 STRUCTURAL ASPECTS OF MMP-12

MMP-12 possesses three domains, having a common structural resemblance with other MMPs. Among these, MMP-12 displays 49% structural similarity with MMP-1 and MMP-3. Domain I of MMP-12 is the N-terminal domain, which is a short signal peptide. It comprises a highly conserved cysteine residue that is found to coordinate the catalytic Zn^{2+} ion [34–36]. Moreover, domain II is a catalytic domain that comprises the zinc-binding sequence motif (i.e., HExxHxxGxxH) [34, 37, 38]. Again, domain III of MMP-12 is the C-terminal domain. The hemopexin-like C-terminal domain exerts a sequence similarity with vitronectin and hemopexin [34]. The active site of MMP-12 comprises three unprimed (called S1, S2, and S3) and three primed pockets (called S1′, S2′, and S3′). Based on the S1′ pocket size, MMP-12 has been categorized as the intermediate or medium-sized S1′ pocket MMP [39]. Considering the size, shape, and variability among the amino acid residues at the S1′ pocket and the binding mode of interactions, novel, promising, and selective MMP-12 inhibitors can be designed.

15.3 X-RAY CRYSTAL STRUCTURES AND NMR SOLUTION STRUCTURES OF MMP-12

Many X-ray crystal structures and NMR solution structures have been explored. Many of these MMP-12 enzyme structures are ligand-bound, thus showing how they bind to the catalytic domain amino acid residues. Based on the interaction pattern, newer effective and selective MMP-12 inhibitors can be designed. The detail of these structures is in Table 15.1.

TABLE 15.1
Details of the Crystal Structures of MMP-12 [34, 40]

PDB ID	Type	Structure	Resolution	Sequence length	Substrate/inhibitor	Year of release
1JK3	X-ray	–	1.09	158	4-(N-hydroxyamino)-2r-isobutyl-2s-(2-thienylthiomethyl)succinyl-L-phenylalanine-N-methylamide	2001
1JIZ	X-ray	–	2.60	166	N-hydroxy-2(R)-[[(4-methoxyphenyl)sulfonyl](3-Picolyl)amino]-3-methylbutanamide hydrochloride	2002
1RMZ	X-ray	Catalytic domain	1.34	159	N-isobutyl-N-[4-methoxyphenylsulfonyl]glycyl hydroxamic Acid	2004
1UTT	X-ray	–	2.20	159	2-(1,3-dioxo-1,3-dihydro-2H-isoindol-2-yl)ethyl-4-(4-ethoxy[1,1-biphenyl]-4-yl)-4-oxobutanoic acid	2004
1UTZ	X-ray	–	2.50	159	(2R)-3-({[4-[(pyridin-4-yl)phenyl]-thien-2-yl}carboxamido)(phenyl)propanoic acid	2004
1ROS	X-ray	–	2.00	163	2-(1,3-dioxo-1,3-dihydro-2H-isoindol-2-yl)ethyl-4-(4-ethoxy[1,1-biphenyl]-4-yl)-4-oxobutanoic acid	2004
1Y93	X-ray	Catalytic domain	1.03	159	Acetohydroxamic acid	2005
2HU6	X-ray	–	1.32	159	Acetohydroxamic acid and bicyclic inhibitor	2006
2OXU	X-ray	–	1.24	159	–	2007
2Z2D	Solution NMR	–	–	164	Gamma-keto butanoic acid inhibitor	2007
2K2G	Solution NMR	Wild-type catalytic domain	–	165	N-(dibenzo[b,d]thiophen-3-ylsulfonyl)-L-valine	2008
2JXY	Solution NMR	hemopexin-like domain	–	194	–	2008
3BA0	X-ray	Full-length MMP-12	3.00	365	–	2008
3F1A	X-ray	Catalytic domain	1.25	158	N-(2-nitroso-2-oxoethyl)benzene sulfonamide	2008
3F15	X-ray	Catalytic domain	1.70	158	(S)-N-(2,3-dihydroxypropyl)-4-methoxy-N-(2-nitroso-2-oxoethyl)benzene sulfonamide	2008
2WO9	X-ray	–	1.70	164	Beta hydroxy carboxylic acid	2009

(Continued)

TABLE 15.1 (CONTINUED)
Details of the Crystal Structures of MMP-12 [34, 40]

PDB ID	Type	Structure	Resolution	Sequence length	Substrate/inhibitor	Year of release
2WOA	X-ray	—	2.30	164	Beta hydroxy carboxylic acid	2009
3EHX	X-ray	—	1.90	158	(R)-2-(biphenyl-4-ylsulfonamido)-4-methylpentanoic acid	2009
3EHY	X-ray	—	1.90	158	(R)-2-(4-Methoxyphenylsulfonamido)propanoic acid	2009
3LIR	X-ray	—	1.90	159	Non-zinc chelating inhibitor	2010
3LJG	X-ray	—	1.31	159	Non-zinc chelating inhibitor	2010
3LIL	X-ray	—	1.80	159	Non-zinc chelating inhibitor	2010
3N2U	X-ray	Catalytic domain	1.81	158	N-hydroxy-2-(4-methoxy-N(2-(3,4,5-trihydroxy-6-(hydroxymethyl)tetrahydro-2H-pyran-2-yloxy)ethyl)phenylsulfonamido)acetamide	2010
3N2V	X-ray	Catalytic domain	1.55	158	N-hydroxy-2-(N-hydroxyethyl)biphenyl-4-ylsulfonamido)acetamide	2010
3LK8	X-ray	Catalytic domain	1.80	158	Para-methoxy-sulfonyl-glycine hydroxamate	2010
3NX7	X-ray	Catalytic domain	1.80	159	N-hydroxy-2-(N-(2-hydroxyethyl)4-methoxyphenylsulfonamido)acetamide	2010
3RTS	X-ray	Catalytic domain	1.81	158	N-hydroxy-2-(2-phenylethylsulfonamido)acetamide	2012
3RTT	X-ray	Catalytic domain	1.82	158	(R)-N-hydroxy-1-(phenethylsulfonyl)pyrrolidine-2-carboxamide	2012
3TSK	X-ray	—	2.00	159	L-glutamate motif inhibitor	2012
4GQL	X-ray	Catalytic domain	1.15	159	RXP470.1	2013
4GR0	X-ray	Catalytic domain	1.50	159	RXP470B	2013
4GR3	X-ray	Catalytic domain	1.49	159	RXP470A	2013
4GR8	X-ray	Catalytic domain	1.30	152	RXP470C	2013

(Continued)

TABLE 15.1 (CONTINUED)
Details of the Crystal Structures of MMP-12 [34, 40]

PDB ID	Type	Structure	Resolution	Sequence length	Substrate/inhibitor	Year of release
2MLR	Solution NMR	Membrane bilayer complex with matrix metalloproteinase-12 (at alpha face)	–	164	1,2-dimyristoyl-Sn-Glycero-3-Phosphocholine	2014
2MLS	Solution NMR	Membrane bilayer complex with matrix metalloproteinase-12 (at beta face)	–	164	1,2-dimyristoyl-Sn-glycero-3-phosphocholine	2014
2N8R	Solution NMR	–	–	164	–	2016
5L7F	X-ray	MMP-12 mutant K421A	1.80	159	RXP470.1 conjugated with fluorophore Cy5.5 in space group P21	2016
5L79	X-ray	–	2.07	159	RXP470.1 conjugated with fluorophore Cy5.5 in space group P21212	2016
5I0L	X-ray	Catalytic domain	2.45	159	DC27	2016
5I4O	X-ray	Catalytic domain	2.05	159	DC28	2016
5I3M	X-ray	Catalytic domain	2.17	159	DC31	2016
5I43	X-ray	Catalytic domain	1.95	159	DC32	2016
5I2Z	X-ray	Catalytic domain	2.30	159	DC24	2016
5N5J	X-ray	–	1.80	158	3-(5-(1,2-dithiolan-3-yl)pentanamido)propane-1-sulfonate	2017
5N5K	X-ray	Catalytic domain	1.80	156	5-(1,2-dithiolan-3-yl)-N-(3-hydroxypropyl) pentanamide	2017
6EOX	X-ray	–	1.30	159	LP165	2018
6ENM	X-ray	–	1.59	159	LP168	2018
6ELA	X-ray	–	1.49	159	BE4	2018
6EKN	X-ray	–	1.20	159	BE7	2018

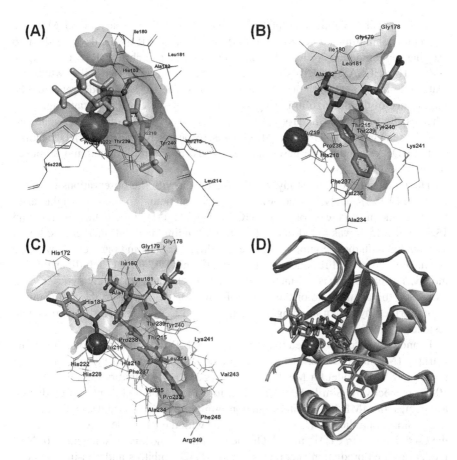

FIGURE 15.1 Ligand binding mode of (A) hydroxamic acid ZBG containing MMP-12 inhibitor (PDB ID: 1RMZ); (B) non-ZBG-containing MMP-12 inhibitor (PDB ID: 3LIR); (C) phosphonic acid ZBG containing MMP-12 inhibitors (PDB ID: 4GQL) at the active site of MMP-12 as observed in X-ray co-crystal structures; (D) superimposed structure of the inhibitor-bound catalytic domain of MMP-12 (light gray: 1RMZ; dark gray: 3LIR; gray: 4GQL).

Structurally, MMP-12 is well-explored, and a vast amount of X-ray crystal data has been disclosed to date. The structure of MMP-12 bound with ligands is depicted in Figure 15.1.

15.4 LIGAND- AND STRUCTURE-BASED DRUG DESIGN STRATEGIES ON MMP-12 INHIBITORS

Considering the importance of MMP-12 inhibitors in various disease conditions, several ligand- and structure-based molecular modeling studies have been performed for a better understanding of the crucial structural features and the binding mode of interactions modulating MMP-12 inhibitory potential.

Shamsara and Shahir-Sadr [41] performed an HQSAR study of 35 MMP-12 inhibitors containing a dibenzofuran scaffold. The HQSAR model developed on 26 training set compounds provided good internal predictive ability ($R^2 = 0.986$, $Q^2 = 0.697$). This HQSAR model also provided good external predictive ability while validated on nine test set compounds ($R^2_{Pred} = 0.873$). The HQSAR model reflected the importance of the dibenzofuran ring as suggested by the gray/dark gray fragments, whereas the substituted heterocyclic scaffold showed good to moderate contributions, as seen in gray and light gray fragments, respectively (Figure 15.2). Depending on the HQSAR model, five new compounds (**n1–n5**) were designed and proposed (Figure 15.3).

The molecular docking study was in agreement with the observations obtained from the HQSAR analysis. The newly designed compound (**n3**) with a slight variation from the most potent compound ($IC_{50} = 114.288$ μM) of the dataset (compound **15.1**, Figure 15.4) was found to exert a similar binding mode of interactions. It was noticed that both these compounds produced three π-π stacking interactions with the active site amino acid residues, namely His218 and Tyr240, through dibenzofuran moiety. The carboxylic acid function was found to chelate with the catalytic Zn^{2+} ion and fused the phenyl ring of the dibenzofuran moiety. Moreover, the sulfonamido group formed hydrogen bonding interactions with Leu181 and Ala182 amino acid residues at the enzyme active site.

Li and co-workers [42] tried to predict some MMP-12 inhibitors through machine learning (ML) approaches. The average prediction accuracies of the support vector machine (SVM) model for MMP-12 inhibitors and non-inhibitors were 96.15% and 100%, respectively. Similarly, the random forest (RF) method displayed prediction accuracies for MMP-12 inhibitors and non-inhibitors of 98.08% and 93.62%, respectively. Similar prediction accuracies compared with the RF model were observed for the C4.5 decision tree (DT) model. On the other hand, the k-nearest neighbor (*k*-NN) model revealed prediction accuracies for MMP-12 inhibitors and non-inhibitors as

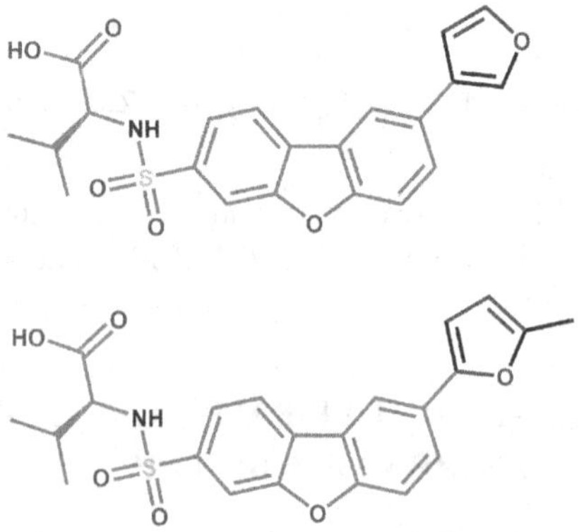

FIGURE 15.2 The extremely good (dark gray), very good (gray), good (light gray), and moderate (medium gray) fragments modulating MMP-12 inhibitory activity of dibenzofuran analogs.

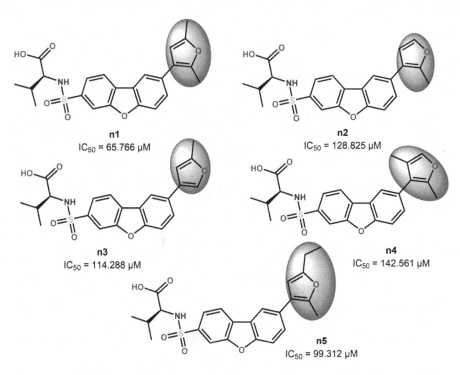

FIGURE 15.3 Newly designed compounds based on the observations of HQSAR modeling (light gray encircled positions are modified).

98.08% and 89.36%, respectively. Based on these machine learning (ML) models, it was assumed that the dibenzofuran sulphonamido-based carboxylic acid derivatives were the most promising selective MMP-12 inhibitors (Figure 15.5).

Hitaoka and co-workers [43] performed a QSAR analysis on 80 arylsulfone-based hydroxamates and carboxylic acid derivatives as MMP-12 inhibitors using a linear expression of representative energy terms (LERE). The LERE-QSAR analysis reproduced the variation in the overall free-energy change by determining the contributions of representative free-energy changes associated with the complex formation of MMP-12 and these respective MMP-12 inhibitors. In addition, the fragment molecular orbital (FMO) method-dependent inter-fragment interaction energy difference (FMO-IFIED) analysis explored quantitatively that there may be significant energy differences between the carboxylic acid and hydroxamate moieties while binding to the Zn^{2+} ion. Such types of binding interaction energy may play a crucial role in the MMP-12 inhibitory efficacy of such compounds. Nevertheless, the variations in the dispersion interaction energies of the aryl substituents and the surrounding amino acid residues may play a vital role in the free energy changes among various aryl substituents. Based on these observations, newer effective MMP-12 inhibitors as drug candidates may be designed for the treatment of COPD.

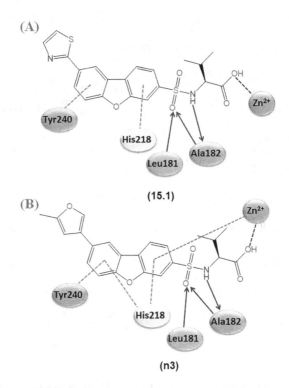

FIGURE 15.4 Binding mode of interactions of (A) the best active molecule (compound **15.1**) of the dataset and (B) the newly designed compound **n3** at the MMP-12 active site (π-π stacking interaction: light gray dotted line; hydrogen bonding interaction: arrow; π-cationic interaction: gray dotted line; Zinc binding interaction: dark gray dotted line).

Verma and Hansch [44] performed a QSAR study on some phosphinic acid-based MMP-12 inhibitors. It was noticed that the lipophilicity (cLogP) of these compounds contributes positively to MMP-12 inhibitors (Figure 15.6A). Again, another QSAR model was developed on 6H-1,3,4-thiadiazine-based MMP-12 inhibitors, and it was found that the length of the Y substituent, as well as the presence of the halogen moiety as the Y substituent, may have a detrimental effect on MMP-12 inhibition (Figure 15.6B).

Santamaria et al. [45] performed a kinetic characterization analysis of some N-O-isopropyl sulphonamide-based hydroxamates as dual MMP-12/MMP-13 inhibitors. Among these molecules, compound **15.2** exhibits potent but dual inhibitory efficacy of MMP-12/MMP-13. It (compound **15.2**) was further subjected to molecular docking analysis at the MMP-12 active site (PDB ID: 3F17) to identify the binding mode of interactions (Figure 15.7).

The molecular docking interactions revealed that the hydroxamate moiety coordinated with the Zn^{2+} ion through a bidentate fashion at the enzyme active site. Nevertheless, the hydroxamate moiety also formed a hydrogen bonding interaction with the carbonyl group of Ala182. The sulphonamido group was found to be crucial

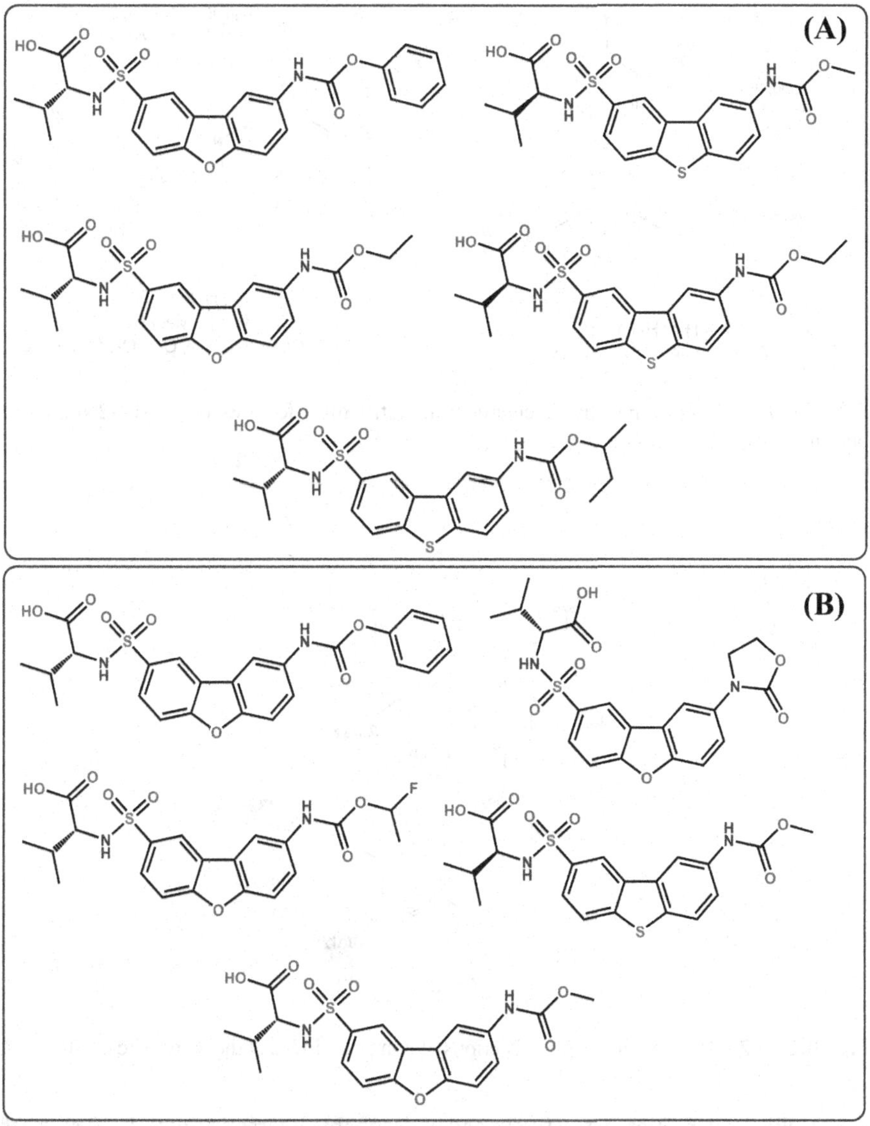

FIGURE 15.5 (A) Molecules best predicted by the SVM model; (B) molecules better predicted by the RF model.

because it produced hydrogen bonding interactions with Leu181 and Ala182 and subsequently helped to plunge the P1′ substituent, i.e., *p*-chloro benzyloxy biphenyl moiety deep inside the S1′ pocket. Moreover, the chloro atom formed a T-shaped interaction with the aromatic ring of Phe248. Again, the *p*-chlorobenzyl moiety formed hydrophobic interactions with Leu214, Val243, and Val235 side chain amino acid residues. Nevertheless, the phenyl ring adjacent to the sulphonamide moiety formed

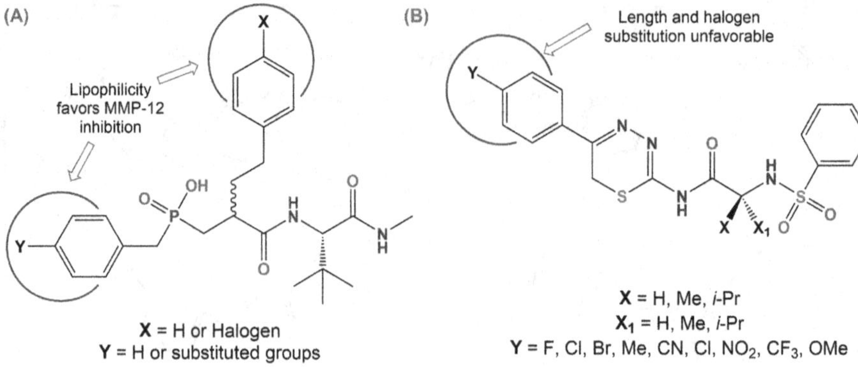

FIGURE 15.6 Important physicochemical and structural features of MMP-12 inhibitors obtained by QSAR analysis.

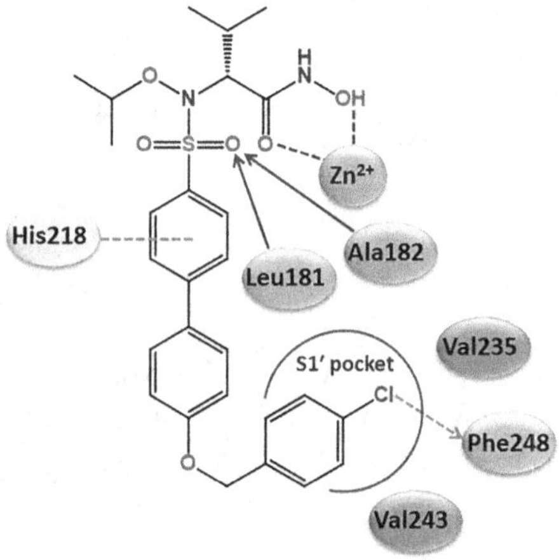

(15.2)

FIGURE 15.7 Binding mode of interactions of compound **15.2** at the active site of MMP-12.

π-π stacking interaction with His218 and hydrophobic interaction with Leu181. Such types of interactions at the MMP-12 active site suggested the higher inhibitory activity of compound **15.2** against MMP-12.

Nuti et al. [46] disclosed the design, synthesis, biological evaluation, and binding mode of interaction analysis of some arylsulfone derivatives as potent and selective MMP-12 inhibitors. The molecular docking study of several molecules displayed that these compounds were perfectly placed into the active site of MMP-12 (PDB ID: 1RMZ). The molecular docking interaction of compound **15.3** displayed that the p-methoxyphenoxyphenyl group was inserted deep inside the S1' pocket of MMP-12. The sulfonyl group formed interactions with Leu181 and Ala182. Nevertheless, the hydroxy group of the hydroxamate ZBG formed a hydrogen bonding interaction with Ala182 without any interaction with Glu219 (Figure 15.8).

Similarly, compound **15.4** resulted in a properly coordinated ZBG group and Zn^{2+} due to an introduction of the methylene group between ZBG and the aromatic ring. However, in this case, the hydroxy and the amide functions of the hydroxamate moiety formed hydrogen bonding interactions with Ala182 and Glu219. Again, the sulfonyl group formed hydrogen bonding interactions with Leu181 and Ala182 (Figure 15.8). The *p*-methoxyphenoxyphenyl moiety was also found inserted deep inside the S1' pocket. Also, similar interactions like compound **15.4** were noticed for compound **15.5** (Figure 15.8).

Mori et al. [47] performed a structure-based optimization process of some arylsulfonamide-based molecules (Figure 15.9). The hydroxamate ZBG of compound

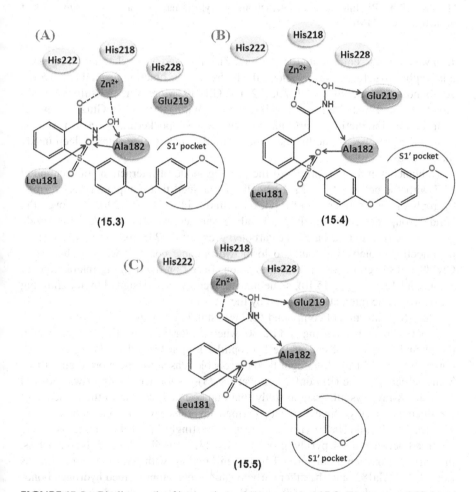

FIGURE 15.8 Binding mode of interactions of (A) compound **15.3**, (B) compound **15.4**, and (C) compound **15.5** at the active site of MMP-12.

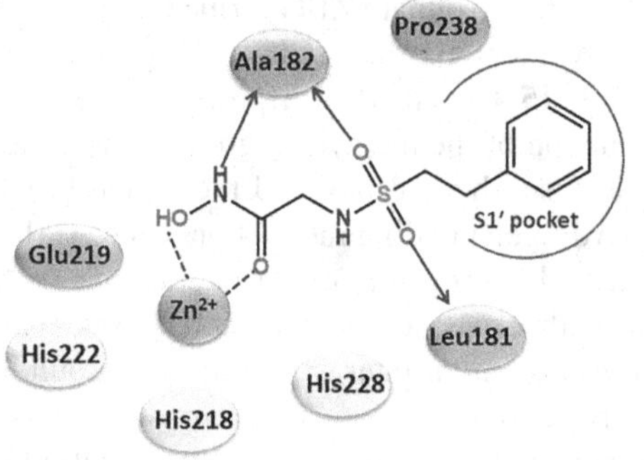

(15.6)

FIGURE 15.9 Binding mode of interactions of arylsulfonamido-based compound **15.6** at the active site of MMP-12.

15.6 was found to coordinate the catalytic Zn^{2+} ion, and it correlated with co-crystalographic structures. Nevertheless, the hydroxamate function formed two hydrogen bonding interactions with Ala182 and Glu219. Moreover, the sulphonamido moiety formed hydrogen bonding interactions with Ala182 and Glu219. Several hydrophobic interactions were noticed with the S1′ pocket amino acid residues. Due to the presence of methylene moiety, the P1′ substituents entered deep inside the S1′ pocket.

Dublanchet et al. [48] proposed the binding mode of interactions of compound **15.7** with the active site of MMP-12. It was noticed that compound **15.7** formed hydrophobic interactions with S1′ pocket amino acid residue Tyr240. Moreover, the amide group formed two hydrogen bonding interactions with the backbone amide group of Leu181 and the backbone carbonyl group of Pro238, respectively. The morpholinoethyl moiety was found to form hydrophobic contacts with the backbone Gly179-Ile180 peptide bond for stabilization. Based on the docking interactions of compound **15.7** (Figure 15.10), some new molecules were designed by maximizing the hydrophobic interactions exerted by the P1′ substituents.

The (R)- conformer of compound **15.8** was stabilized by the hydrophobic interactions between the phenyl ring and Ile180, whereas, for the respective (S)-conformer, the phenyl ring was placed at the hydrophilic region instead of the hydrophobic region (Figure 15.10). This might be the probable reason for the more than 50-fold higher efficacy of the (R)-conformer over the (S)-conformer. Again, it was noticed from the X-ray crystallographic study that compound **15.9,** due to the presence of the thienyl 4-pyridyl phenyl moiety, formed favorable hydrophobic contacts with Thr215, Tyr240, and His218 (Figure 15.10). Interestingly, lipophilic interactions were observed between the 4-pyridyl group and Lys241, as well as Val235. Nevertheless, the carbonyl oxygen atom formed hydrogen bonding with backbone amino acids Leu181 and Ala182, and the other carboxylate oxygen atom formed hydrogen bonding with the backbone amide of Tyr240. However, the other carboxylate oxygen atom formed water-mediated hydrogen bonding with Gly179.

Devel and co-workers [49] designed some selective MMP-12 inhibitors. The molecular modeling study at the MMP-12 active site revealed one of the glutamic acid residues in close proximity to the Thr239 at the S2' pocket. Moreover, the other glutamic acid residue is close to Lys177 at the S3' pocket. Nevertheless, the P1' substituent side chain is near several amino acids of the S1' pocket.

Nuti and co-workers [50] further reported some sugar-based arylsulfonamido carboxylates as selective MMP-12 inhibitors. As per their observation, there exists a complete difference in the binding pattern between the thioureido derivatives and the triazole derivatives, where it was noticed that the sugar moieties attached to both these moieties did not overlap completely at the active site of MMP-12. Moreover, the length and shape of the P1' substituent are key features for the higher potency and selectivity toward MMP-12 over MMP-9. Therefore, 4-(4'-chlorobenzyl-oxy) biphenyl thioureido moiety was a suitable P1' substituent for designing potent and highly selective MMP-12 inhibitors.

Recently, Baidya and co-workers [39] analyzed the binding mode of interactions of some selective MMP-12 inhibitors. It was noticed that for almost all such compounds, the bulky aryl group firmly entered into the S1' cavity and made proper interactions. Moreover, the ZBG group (either hydroxamate or carboxylate) showed proper Zn^{2+} chelating ability. Comparatively, the MMP-12 selectivity of these molecules over other MMPs mainly depends on several features. These are the interactions with the Ω-loop amino acids, interactions with flexible parts of molecules and the backbone amino acid residues, some favorable hydrophobic and van der Waals interactions at the MMP-12 active site, or a closer binding pattern to the catalytic

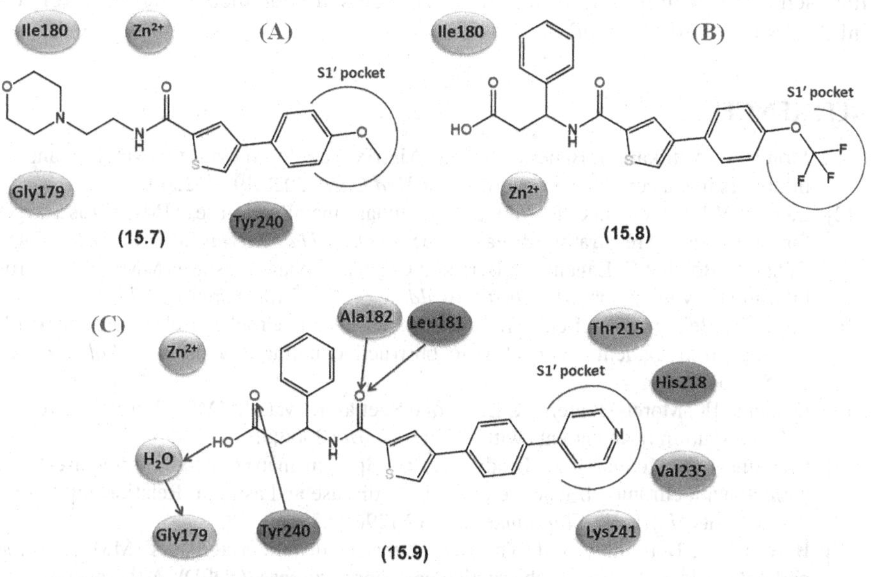

FIGURE 15.10 Binding mode of interactions at the active site of MMP-12: (A) compound 15.7, (B) compound 15.8, and (C) compound 15.9.

Zn^{2+} ion, as well as with the S2' pocket amino acid residues. Therefore, proper orientation at the catalytic site due to the flexible features of molecules may be a prime factor for MMP-12 selectivity.

15.5 SUMMARY

Among other categories of MMPs, MMP-12 is the prime target for drug design due to its involvement in major diseases, including asthma, COPD, inflammatory diseases, arthritis, and several cancers. Only MMP-12, among other classes of MMPs, has been studied extensively, as other MMPs (namely MMP-19, MMP-20, MMP-21, MMP-28, and MMP-29) have not yet been explored like MMP-12. In this context, there may be scope for designing disease-specific selective MMP-12 inhibitors. A huge amount of X-ray crystal data and NMR solution data of MMP-12 have already been made available. Such an amount of data may be effective not only in determining crucial structural features of these ligands at the MMP-12 active site but also in acquiring knowledge of the binding patterns and crucial amino acid residues at the MMP-12 active site. Furthermore, ligand- and structure-based drug design strategies conducted on various MMP-12 inhibitors may be beneficial in designing potent and selective MMP-12 inhibitors. Depending on such observations, a new chemical entity targeting MMP-12 can be designed, synthesized, and biologically evaluated. In contrast, there is a lack of information and biological experimental data available in the case of other MMPs such as MMP-19, MMP-20, MMP-21, MMP-28, and MMP-29. Thus, molecular modeling studies are quite impossible for such MMPs to date. However, there may be scope for designing such types of inhibitors if proper experiments are conducted, and thus, related inhibitors can be discovered.

REFERENCES

[1]. Mondal S, Adhikari N, Banerjee S, et al. Matrix metalloproteinase-9 (MMP-9) and its inhibitors in cancer: A minireview. *Eur J Med Chem* 2020;194:112260.

[2]. Lagente V, Le Quement C, Boichot E. Macrophage metalloelastase (MMP-12) as a target for inflammatory respiratory diseases. *Expert Opin Ther Targets* 2009;13(3):287–295.

[3]. Nénan S, Boichot E, Lagente V, Bertrand CP. Macrophage elastase (MMP-12): A proinflammatory mediator? *Mem Inst Oswaldo Cruz* 2005;100(Suppl 1):167–172.

[4]. Molet S, Belleguic C, Lena H, et al. Increase in macrophage elastase (MMP-12) in lungs from patients with chronic obstructive pulmonary disease. *Inflamm Res* 2005;54(1):31–36.

[5]. Demedts IK, Morel-Montero A, Lebecque S, et al. Elevated MMP-12 protein levels in induced sputum from patients with COPD. *Thorax* 2006;61(3):196–201.

[6]. Chaudhuri R, McSharry C, Brady J, et al. Sputum matrix metalloproteinase-12 in patients with chronic obstructive pulmonary disease and asthma: Relationship to disease severity. *J Allergy Clin Immunol* 2012;129(3):655–663.e8.

[7]. Belvisi MG, Bottomley KM. The role of matrix metalloproteinases (MMPs) in the pathophysiology of chronic obstructive pulmonary disease (COPD): A therapeutic role for inhibitors of MMPs? *Inflamm Res* 2003;52(3):95–100.

[8]. Gharib SA, Manicone AM, Parks WC. Matrix metalloproteinases in emphysema. *Matrix Biol* 2018;73:34–51.

[9]. Abd-Elaziz K, Jesenak M, Vasakova M, Diamant Z. Revisiting matrix metalloproteinase 12: Its role in pathophysiology of asthma and related pulmonary diseases. *Curr Opin Pulm Med* 2021;27(1):54–60.

[10]. Chiba Y, Yu Y, Sakai H, Misawa M. Increase in the expression of matrix metalloproteinase-12 in the airways of rats with allergic bronchial asthma. *Biol Pharm Bull* 2007;30(2):318–323.

[11]. Mukhopadhyay S, Sypek J, Tavendale R, et al. Matrix metalloproteinase-12 is a therapeutic target for asthma in children and young adults. *J Allergy Clin Immunol* 2010;126(1):70–6.e16.

[12]. Zhou Y, Xu M, Gong W, et al. Circulating MMP-12 as potential biomarker in evaluating disease severity and efficacy of sublingual immunotherapy in allergic rhinitis. *Mediators Inflammm* 2022;2022:3378035.

[13]. Makino A, Shibata T, Nagayasu M, et al. RSV infection-elicited high MMP-12-producing macrophages exacerbate allergic airway inflammation with neutrophil infiltration. *iScience* 2021;24(10):103201.

[14]. Lygeros S, Danielides G, Kyriakopoulos GC, et al. Evaluation of MMP-12 expression in chronic rhinosinusitis with nasal polyposis. *Rhinology* 2022;60(1):39–46.

[15]. Chelluboina B, Nalamolu KR, Klopfenstein JD, et al. MMP-12, a promising therapeutic target for neurological diseases. *Mol Neurobiol* 2018;55(2):1405–1409.

[16]. Liu Y, Zhang M, Hao W, et al. Matrix metalloproteinase-12 contributes to neuroinflammation in the aged brain. *Neurobiol Aging* 2013;34(4):1231–1239.

[17]. Polonskaya YV, Kashtanova EV, Murashov IS, et al. Association of matrix metalloproteinases with coronary artery calcification in patients with CHD. *J Pers Med* 2021;11(6):506.

[18]. Wang CY, Zhang CP, Li BJ, et al. MMP-12 as a potential biomarker to forecast ischemic stroke in obese patients. *Med Hypotheses* 2020;136:109524.

[19]. Jguirim-Souissi I, Jelassi A, Slimani A, et al. Matrix metalloproteinase-1 and matrix metalloproteinase-12 gene polymorphisms and the outcome of coronary artery disease. *Coron Artery Dis* 2011;22(6):388–393.

[20]. Jguirim-Souissi I, Jelassi A, Addad F, et al. Plasma metalloproteinase-12 and tissue inhibitor of metalloproteinase-1 levels and presence, severity, and outcome of coronary artery disease. *Am J Cardiol* 2007;100(1):23–27.

[21]. Longo GM, Buda SJ, Fiotta N, et al. MMP-12 has a role in abdominal aortic aneurysms in mice. *Surgery* 2005;137(4):457–462.

[22]. Goncalves DaSilva A, Liaw L, Yong VW. Cleavage of osteopontin by matrix metalloproteinase-12 modulates experimental autoimmune encephalomyelitis disease in C57BL/6 mice. *Am J Pathol* 2010;177(3):1448–1458.

[23]. Kaspiris A, Khaldi L, Chronopoulos E, et al. Macrophage-specific metalloelastase (MMP-12) immunoexpression in the osteochondral unit in osteoarthritis correlates with BMI and disease severity. *Pathophysiology* 2015;22(3):143–151.

[24]. Chen YE. MMP-12, an old enzyme plays a new role in the pathogenesis of rheumatoid arthritis? *Am J Pathol* 2004;165(4):1069–1070.

[25]. Liu M, Sun H, Wang X, et al. Association of increased expression of macrophage elastase (matrix metalloproteinase 12) with rheumatoid arthritis. *Arthritis Rheum* 2004;50(10):3112–3117.

[26]. Yang X, Dong Y, Zhao J, et al. Increased expression of human macrophage metalloelastase (MMP-12) is associated with the invasion of endometrial adenocarcinoma. *Pathol Res Pract* 2007;203(7):499–505.

[27]. Saleem Z, Shaikh AH, Zaman U, et al. Estimation of salivary matrix metalloproteinases-12 (MMP-12) levels among patients presenting with oral submucous fibrosis and oral squamous cell carcinoma. *BMC Oral Health* 2021;21(1):205.

[28]. Hofmann HS, Hansen G, Richter G, et al. Matrix metalloproteinase-12 expression correlates with local recurrence and metastatic disease in non-small cell lung cancer patients. *Clin Cancer Res* 2005;11(3):1086–1092.

[29]. Zheng J, Chu D, Wang D, et al. Matrix metalloproteinase-12 is associated with overall survival in Chinese patients with gastric cancer. *J Surg Oncol* 2013;107(7):746–751.

[30]. Zucker S, Vacirca J. Role of matrix metalloproteinases (MMPs) in colorectal cancer. *Cancer Metastasis Rev* 2004;23(1–2):101–117.

[31]. Di Sabatino A, Saarialho-Kere U, Buckley MG, et al. Stromelysin-1 and macrophage metalloelastase expression in the intestinal mucosa of Crohn's disease patients treated with infliximab. *Eur J Gastroenterol Hepatol* 2009;21(9):1049–1055.

[32]. Salmela MT, Pender SL, Reunala T, et al. Parallel expression of macrophage metalloelastase (MMP-12) in duodenal and skin lesions of patients with dermatitis herpetiformis. *Gut* 2001;48(4):496–502.

[33]. Bassiouni W, Ali MAM, Schulz R. Multifunctional intracellular matrix metalloproteinases: Implications in disease. *FEBS Journal* 2021;288(24):7162–7182.

[34]. Nar H, Werle K, Bauer MM, et al. Crystal structure of human macrophage elastase (MMP-12) in complex with a hydroxamic acid inhibitor. *J Mol Biol* 2001;312(4):743–751.

[35]. Becker JW, Marcy AI, Rokosz LL, et al. Stromelysin-1: Three-dimensional structure of the inhibited catalytic domain and of the C-truncated proenzyme. *Protein Sci* 1995;4(10):1966–1976.

[36]. Morgunova E, Tuuttila A, Bergmann U, et al. Structure of human pro-matrix metalloproteinase-2: Activation mechanism revealed. *Science* 1999;284(5420):1667–1670.

[37]. Bode W, Grams F, Reinemer P, et al. The metzincin-superfamily of zinc-peptidases. *Adv Exp Med Biol* 1996;389:1–11.

[38]. Bode W, Fernandez-Catalan C, Tschesche H, et al. Structural properties of matrix metalloproteinases. *Cell Mol Life Sci* 1999;55(4):639–652.

[39]. Baidya SK, Banerjee S, Adhikari N, et al. Selective inhibitors of medium-size S1' pocket matrix metalloproteinases: A stepping stone of future drug discovery. *J Med Chem* 2022;65(16):10709–10754.

[40]. https://www.rcsb.org/ as accessed in September 2022.

[41]. Shamsara J, Shahir-Sadr A. A predictive HQSAR model for a series of tricycle core containing MMP-12 inhibitors with dibenzofuran ring. *Int J Med Chem* 2014;2014:630807.

[42]. Li B, Hu L, Xue Y, et al. Prediction of matrix metal proteinases-12 inhibitors by machine learning approaches. *J Biomol Struct Dyn* 2019;37(10):2627–2640.

[43]. Hitaoka S, Chuman H, Yoshizawa K. A QSAR study on the inhibition mechanism of matrix metalloproteinase-12 by arylsulfone analogs based on molecular orbital calculations. *Org Biomol Chem* 2015;13(3):793–806.

[44]. Verma RP, Hansch C. Matrix metalloproteinases (MMPs): Chemical-biological functions and (Q)SARs. *Bioorg Med Chem* 2007;15(6):2223–2268.

[45]. Santamaria S, Nuti E, Cercignani G, et al. N-O-Isopropyl sulfonamido-based hydroxamates: Kinetic characterisation of a series of MMP-12/MMP-13 dual target inhibitors. *Biochem Pharmacol* 2012;84(6):813–820.

[46]. Nuti E, Panelli L, Casalini F, et al. Design, synthesis, biological evaluation, and NMR studies of a new series of arylsulfones as selective and potent matrix metalloproteinase-12 inhibitors. *J Med Chem* 2009;52(20):6347–6361.

[47]. Mori M, Massaro A, Calderone V, et al. Discovery of a new class of potent MMP inhibitors by structure-based optimization of the arylsulfonamide scaffold. *ACS Med Chem Lett* 2013;4(6):565–569.

[48]. Dublanchet AC, Ducrot P, Andrianjara C, et al. Structure-based design and synthesis of novel non-zinc chelating MMP-12 inhibitors. *Bioorg Med Chem Lett* 2005;15(16):3787–3790.

[49]. Devel L, Rogakos V, David A, et al. Development of selective inhibitors and substrate of matrix metalloproteinase-12. *J Biol Chem* 2006;281(16):11152–11160.

[50]. Nuti E, Cuffaro D, D'Andrea F, et al. Sugar-based arylsulfonamide carboxylates as selective and water-soluble matrix metalloproteinase-12 inhibitors. *ChemMedChem* 2016;11(15):1626–1637.

Part D

Conclusion and Future Perspective

16 Conclusion and Future Perspectives

Nilanjan Adhikari, Sandip Kumar Baidya,
Suvankar Banerjee, and Tarun Jha

Matrix metalloproteinases (MMPs) belonging to Zn^{2+}-dependent endopeptidases are highly interlinked with the breakdown of the extracellular matrix (ECM). MMPs are secreted in the body from various proinflammatory cells and connective tissues, namely osteoblasts, fibroblasts, endothelial cells, neutrophils, lymphocytes, and macrophages [1, 2]. MMPs are strongly overexpressed in various pathophysiological conditions and major diseases including several cancers [1, 3–4], rheumatoid arthritis and osteoarthritis [5, 6], cardiovascular disorders [7, 8], atherosclerosis [9], COPD [10], asthma [11], diabetes [12], periodontal disease [13], various neurological disorders [14, 15], and several other diseases such as allergic airway inflammation [16], dermatitis [17], sepsis [18], Crohn's disease [19], ulcerative colitis [20], inflammatory bowel disease [21], coronary artery disease [22], liver fibrosis [23], and many more. Therefore, MMPs can be targeted as tremendously valuable biomolecular targets for drug discovery and development against these abovementioned disease conditions. Considering the crucial roles of various MMPs, the earlier chapters focused on the in-depth knowledge of several potential matrix metalloproteinase inhibitors (MMPIs) and their efficacy in various disease conditions. However, there is still a gap in identifying promising MMPIs as efficacious drug molecules in the market despite the long journey of the last 50 years in the research area of MMPs and related inhibitors [24, 25]. To date, various hydroxamate-based MMPIs (namely batimastat, marimastat, prinomastat, ilomastat, BB-1101, CGS-27023A, CP-471358, solimastat, RO-32-3555, and RS-130830) and several non-hydroxamate MMPIs (such as doxycycline, minocycline, metastat, tanomastat, and PG-530742) have been evaluated in various phases of preclinical and clinical trials [25]. However, these molecules failed to proceed further in the market for several reasons: poor oral bioavailability and dose-dependent toxicities, variability in results among human and animal models, or complex mechanisms during broad-spectrum metalloenzyme inhibition [25]. Despite this, MMPs remain promising drug targets, but no drug candidates have reached the market yet. Therefore, developing specific and selective MMPIs is urgently needed, but the structural similarity among different MMPs makes the design process challenging and time-consuming. It is also important to note that MMPIs are mainly taken into consideration for the treatment of various types of solid tumors. However, their utility in various hematological cancers has not yet been evaluated in detail. Therefore, considering the crucial intercorrelations of MMPs

DOI: 10.1201/9781003303282-20

in various leukemic conditions, potent and selective MMPIs can be considered for developing promising antileukemic therapeutics [25].

In this context, several ligand-based drug design (LBDD) approaches have been applied by several groups of researchers [26–37] to acquire knowledge about preferable fragments or features required for designing selective MMPIs. Such types of features can also be considered for designing novel selective MMPIs. In addition, ligand-bound X-ray crystallographic structures, along with various NMR solution structures, have unveiled the binding pattern of MMPI interactions, which can be utilized further in discovering novel MMPIs [25, 38].

It is important to have a thorough knowledge regarding the prime amino acid residues at the respective active sites of MMPs and their binding patterns of interactions and orientations with respective MMPIs to improve activity and selectivity. Considering the spatial orchestrations of MMPIs at the active site of specific MMPs, further structure-based drug design (SBDD) strategies such as molecular docking followed by molecular dynamic simulations can be adapted to extract highly selective MMPIs before multi-step synthesis and rigorous biological screening. Importantly, higher selectivity toward a specific MMP can be crucial to reduce the dose-related and off-target adverse effects. Considering this fact, it may be assumed that several ligand-bound structures of MMPIs and their binding orientations toward specific MMPs have unveiled a huge scope for designing highly selective MMPIs. Also, the knowledge of crucial amino acids at the MMP active site and the respective binding patterns may unveil a new horizon in the development of drug-like MMPIs [25].

Regarding the design of selective MMPIs, various crucial aspects should be considered. The size and shape of the S1′ pocket are important features. Despite the resemblance in shape among MMPs, the size and volume of S1′ pockets differ a lot. Furthermore, the distance between the S1′ pocket and the respective MMP differs. This may be one of the prime reasons behind the variability among the binding modes of a specific MMP inhibitor in various MMPs. Thus, considering this aspect, the variable distance between the S1′ pocket and the Zn^{2+} ion of respective MMPs should be considered while designing specific MMPIs [25].

The S1′ pockets of most of these MMPs are hydrophobic in nature and have a narrow tunnel-like shape. Therefore, P1′ substituents should be optimized during the design of selective MMPIs. In a number of cases, the P1′ substituents of such MMPIs comprise more than two aryl or heteroaryl groups. Again, the overall distance of the tunnel-like S1′ pocket is a prime factor for interactions with amino acid residues with these P1′ substituents of MMPIs. This factor should be kept in mind when designing potent and selective MMPIs. Nevertheless, the size and hydrophobicity of the P1′ group should be optimized as extreme hydrophobic groups may produce a negative impact on the druggable characteristics and pharmacokinetic profile of these MMPIs. However, higher hydrophobicity of the P1′ substituent may offer potency and selectivity toward a particular MMP but may drastically affect the drug-likeliness, subsequently affecting pharmacokinetic and metabolic features [25].

Despite the crucial feature of P1′ substituent regulating the inhibitory potential and specific MMP inhibition, other pockets (i.e., S1, S2, and S2′) can also be targeted to design specific MMPIs. Many of these isoform-selective MMPIs were designed by considering such smaller pockets. Thus, the shape, size, and distance of such pockets with the Zn^{2+} ion should also be optimized for designing selective MMPIs. The conformational changes (for example, S and R conformations) of MMPIs should also be kept in mind [25].

While binding, both MMPI and the active site amino acids need stability. Amino acids forming various hydrophobic pockets offer various dynamic characteristics due to the variations of amino acids present in the Ω-loop and S1' pocket. Such variations may be responsible for the alterations of both the volume and dynamic features of the S1' pocket and P1' substituents and, therefore, influence the binding stability of MMPIs toward specific MMP isoforms. Similarly, the dynamic behavior of other hydrophobic pockets should also be taken into consideration. Therefore, both the dynamic features and the distances among these pockets, including the Zn^{2+} ion along with their shapes and volumes, should be optimized during the selective design of MMPIs [25].

Regarding MMPIs, most of these MMPIs are designed to comprise a ZBG group that coordinates to the catalytic Zn^{2+} ion with good affinity. Among these ZBGs, hydroxamate is the strongest ZBG that can produce potent MMPIs due to the formation of bidentate chelation. Noticeably, the hydroxamate group not only has the binding ability to interact with MMP family members but also with other Zn^{2+}-dependent metalloenzymes, which may be one of the prime factors for dose-related and off-target side effects. On the other hand, other ZBGs, such as carboxylates or phosphonates, were also considered for designing potential and selective MMPIs. However, due to their weaker affinity to the catalytic Zn^{2+} ion, there may be alterations of binding affinity and mode of interactions compared with hydroxamates, and thus, MMPIs comprising such ZBGs bind in a different fashion to the Zn^{2+} ion, subsequently influencing the MMP isoform selectivity [25]. Binding with the catalytic Zn^{2+} ion of MMPs and respective MMPIs is one of the major issues responsible for the modulation of higher potency. However, to eliminate the associated off-target adverse effects of these MMPIs, the discovery of non-zinc chelating selective MMPIs, along with pocket-selective and mechanism-based MMPIs, can be taken into consideration. Therefore, the design of such types of selective MMPIs that may interact with the amino acid residues of the Ω-loop and the S1' pocket can be carried out [25]. Considering these crucial aspects, potential and isoform-selective MMPIs can be designed before experimental validation to manage diseases associated with MMPs.

REFERENCES

[1]. Mondal S, Adhikari N, Banerjee S, et al. Matrix metalloproteinase-9 (MMP-9) and its inhibitors in cancer: A minireview. *Eur J Med Chem* 2020;194:112260.

[2]. Adhikari N, Amin SA, Jha T. Collagenases and gelatinases and their inhibitors as anticancer agents. In Gupta SP, Ed. *Cancer-Leading Proteases*, Academic Press, 2020, pp. 265–294.

[3]. Majumder A, Ray S, Banerji A. Epidermal growth factor receptor-mediated regulation of matrix metalloproteinase-2 and matrix metalloproteinase-9 in MCF-7 breast cancer cells. *Mol Cell Biochem* 2019;452(1–2):111–121.

[4]. Gong Y, Chippada-Venkata UD, Oh WK. Roles of matrix metalloproteinases and their natural inhibitors in prostate cancer progression. *Cancers (Basel)* 2014;6(3):1298–1327.

[5]. Hu Q, Ecker M. Overview of MMP-13 as a promising target for the treatment of osteoarthritis. *Int J Mol Sci* 2021;22(4):1742.

[6]. Wan Y, Li W, Liao Z, et al. Selective MMP-13 inhibitors: Promising agents for the therapy of osteoarthritis. *Curr Med Chem* 2020;27(22):3753–3769.

[7]. Yabluchanskiy A, Ma Y, Iyer RP, et al. Matrix metalloproteinase-9: Many shades of function in cardiovascular disease. *Physiol (Bethesda)* 2013;28(6):391–403.

[8]. Wang GY, Bergman MR, Nguyen AP, et al. Cardiac transgenic matrix metalloproteinase-2 expression directly induces impaired contractility. *Cardiovasc Res* 2006;69(3):688–696.

[9]. Lenglet S, Mach F, Montecucco F. Role of matrix metalloproteinase-8 in atherosclerosis. *Mediators Inflammm* 2013;2013:659282.

[10]. Molet S, Belleguic C, Lena H, et al. Increase in macrophage elastase (MMP-12) in lungs from patients with chronic obstructive pulmonary disease. *Inflamm Res* 2005;54(1):31–36.

[11]. Abd-Elaziz K, Jesenak M, Vasakova M, et al. Revisiting matrix metalloproteinase 12: Its role in pathophysiology of asthma and related pulmonary diseases. *Curr Opin Pulm Med* 2021;27(1):54–60.

[12]. Opdenakker G, Abu El-Asrar A. Metalloproteinases mediate diabetes-induced retinal neuropathy and vasculopathy. *Cell Mol Life Sci* 2019;76(16):3157–3166.

[13]. Romero-Castro NS, Vázquez-Villamar M, Muñoz-Valle JF, et al. Relationship between TNF-α, MMP-8, and MMP-9 levels in gingival crevicular fluid and the subgingival microbiota in periodontal disease. *Odontology* 2020;108(1):25–33.

[14]. Stomrud E, Bjorkqvist M, Janciauskiene S, et al. Alterations of matrix metalloproteinases in the healthy elderly with increased risk of prodromal Alzheimer's disease. *Alzheimers Res Ther* 2010;2(3):20.

[15]. Gu Z, Cui J, Brown S, et al. A highly specific inhibitor of matrixmetalloproteinase-9 rescues laminin from proteolysis and neurons from apoptosis in transient focal cerebral ischemia. *J Neurosci* 2005;25(27):6401–6408.

[16]. Makino A, Shibata T, Nagayasu M, et al. RSV infection-elicited high MMP-12-producing macrophages exacerbate allergic airway inflammation with neutrophil infiltration. *iScience* 2021;24(10):103201.

[17]. Salmela MT, Pender SL, Reunala T, et al. Parallel expression of macrophage metalloelastase (MMP-12) in duodenal and skin lesions of patients with dermatitis herpetiformis. *Gut* 2001;48(4):496–502.

[18]. Sivula M, Hästbacka J, Kuitunen A, et al. Systemic matrix metalloproteinase-8 and tissue inhibitor of metalloproteinases-1 levels in severe sepsis-associated coagulopathy. *Acta Anaesthesiol Scand* 2015;59(2):176–184.

[19]. Di Sabatino A, Saarialho-Kere U, Buckley MG, et al. Stromelysin-1 and macrophage metalloelastase expression in the intestinal mucosa of Crohn's disease patients treated with infliximab. *Eur J Gastroenterol Hepatol* 2009;21(9):1049–1055.

[20]. Rath T, Roderfeld M, Halwe JM, et al. Cellular sources of MMP-7, MMP-13 and MMP-28 in ulcerative colitis. *Scand J Gastroenterol* 2010;45(10):1186–1196.

[21]. Vizoso FJ, González LO, Corte MD, et al. Collagenase-3 (MMP-13) expression by inflamed mucosa in inflammatory bowel disease. *Scand J Gastroenterol* 2006;41(9):1050–1055.

[22]. Jguirim-Souissi I, Jelassi A, Slimani A, et al. Matrix metalloproteinase-1 and matrix metalloproteinase-12 gene polymorphisms and the outcome of coronary artery disease. *Coron Artery Dis* 2011;22(6):388–393.

[23]. Uchinami H, Seki E, Brenner DA, et al. Loss of MMP 13 attenuates murine hepatic injury and fibrosis during cholestasis. *Hepatology* 2006;44(2):420–429.

[24]. Gross J, Lapiere CM. Collagenolytic activity in amphibian tissues: A tissue culture assay. *Proc Natl Acad Sci U S A* 1962;48(6):1014–1022.

[25]. Baidya SK, Banerjee S, Adhikari N, et al. Selective inhibitors of medium-size S1' pocket matrix metalloproteinases: A stepping stone of future drug discovery. *J Med Chem* 2022;65(16):10709–10754.

[26]. Sanapalli BKR, Yele V, Jupudi S, et al. Ligand-based pharmacophore modeling and molecular dynamic simulation approaches to identify putative MMP-9 inhibitors. *RSC Adv* 2021;11(43):26820–26831.

[27]. Sanyal S, Amin SA, Adhikari N, et al. Ligand-based design of anticancer MMP-2 inhibitors: A review. *Future Med Chem* 2021;13(22):1987–2013.

[28]. Guti S, Baidya SK, Banerjee S, et al. A robust classification-dependent multi-molecular modelling study on some biphenyl sulphonamide based MMP-8 inhibitors. *SAR QSAR Environ Res* 2021;32(10):835–861.

[29]. Verma RP, Hansch C. Matrix metalloproteinases (MMPs): Chemical-biological functions and (Q)SARs. *Bioorg Med Chem* 2007;15(6):2223–2268.

[30]. Hitaoka S, Chuman H, Yoshizawa K. A QSAR study on the inhibition mechanism of matrix metalloproteinase-12 by arylsulfone analogs based on molecular orbital calculations. *Org Biomol Chem* 2015;13(3):793–806.

[31]. Asawa Y, Yoshimori A, Bajorath J, et al. Prediction of an MMP-1 inhibitor activity cliff using the SAR matrix approach and its experimental validation. *Sci Rep* 2020;10(1):14710.

[32]. Tabti K, Ahmad I, Zafar I, et al. Profiling the structural determinants of pyrrolidine derivative as gelatinases (MMP-2 and MMP-9) inhibitors using in silico approaches. *Comput Biol Chem* 2023;104:107855.

[33]. Prathipati P, Saxena AK. Evaluation of binary QSAR models derived from LUDI and MOE scoring functions for structure based virtual screening. *J Chem Inf Model* 2006;46(1):39–51.

[34]. Jana S, Singh SK. Identification of selective MMP-9 inhibitors through multiple e-pharmacophore, ligand-based pharmacophore, molecular docking, and density functional theory approaches. *J Biomol Struct Dyn* 2019;37(4):944–965.

[35]. Jha T, Adhikari N, Saha A, et al. Multiple molecular modelling studies on some derivatives and analogues of glutamic acid as matrix metalloproteinase-2 inhibitors. *SAR QSAR Environ Res* 2018;29(1):43–68.

[36]. Adhikari N, Amin SA, Saha A, et al. Understanding chemico-biological interactions of glutamate MMP-2 inhibitors through rigorous alignment-dependent 3D-QSAR analyses. *ChemistrySelect* 2017;2(26):7888–7898.

[37]. Adhikari N, Amin SA, Saha A, et al. Exploring in house glutamate inhibitors of matrix metalloproteinase-2 through validated robust chemico-biological quantitative approaches. *Struct Chem* 2018;29(1):285–297.

[38]. https://www.rcsb.org/.

Index

Printed in the United States
by Baker & Taylor Publisher Services